IMMUNOLOGY
A Short Course

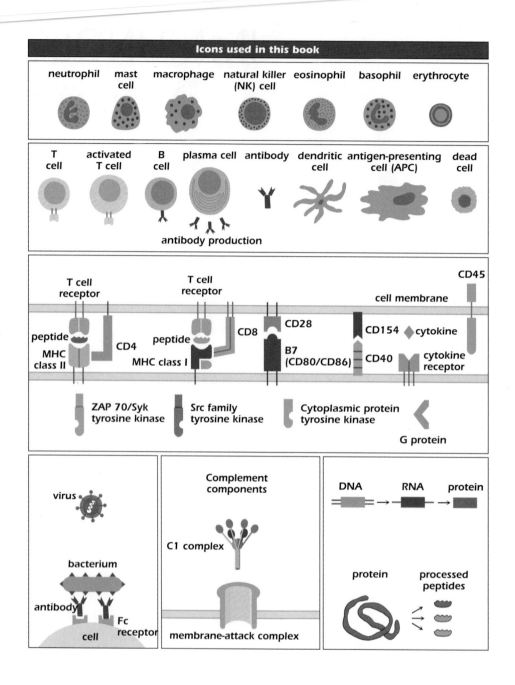

Icons used in this book

neutrophil   mast cell   macrophage   natural killer (NK) cell   eosinophil   basophil   erythrocyte

T cell   activated T cell   B cell   plasma cell   antibody   dendritic cell   antigen-presenting cell (APC)   dead cell

antibody production

T cell receptor   T cell receptor   CD45   cell membrane

peptide   MHC class II   CD4   peptide   MHC class I   CD8   CD28   B7 (CD80/CD86)   CD154   cytokine   CD40   cytokine receptor

ZAP 70/Syk tyrosine kinase   Src family tyrosine kinase   Cytoplasmic protein tyrosine kinase   G protein

virus

bacterium

antibody   Fc receptor   cell

Complement components

C1 complex

membrane-attack complex

DNA → RNA → protein

protein   processed peptides

IMMUNOLOGY
A Short Course

SIXTH EDITION

Richard Coico
Professor of Microbiology and Immunology
Temple University School of Medicine

Geoffrey Sunshine
Senior Scientist, Heath Effects Institute,
and Lecturer, Tufts University School of Medicine

⟨W⟩WILEY-BLACKWELL

A JOHN WILEY & SONS, INC., PUBLICATION

Library of Congress Cataloging-in-Publication Data:

Coico, Richard.
   Immunology : a short course / Richard Coico, Geoffery Sunshine. –6th ed.
      p. ; cm.
   Includes bibliographical references and index.
   ISBN: 978-0-470-08158-7 (pbk.)
  1. Immunology. I. Sunshine, Geoffrey. II. Title.
   [DNLM: 1. Allergy and Immunology. 2. Immunity. QW 504 C6785i 2008]
   QR181.B395 2008
   616.07'9–dc22

                         2008038576

Printed in the United States of America

10 9 8 7 6 5 4 3 2 1

To
Lisa, Jonathan, and Jennifer
R.C.

To
Ilene, Caroline, Alex, and Pearl
G.C.

CONTENTS IN BRIEF

CONTENTS

ABOUT THE AUTHORS

Richard Coico is Professor of Microbiology and Immunology and Senior Associate Dean for Research at Temple University School of Medicine, Philadelphia, Pennsylvania. His major research interest concerns the study of the physiologic role of IgD—a B-cell membrane immunoglobulin coexpressed with IgM. Another area of research concerns computational approaches to the identification of candidate vaccines for several hemorrhagic viruses, including Lassa fever virus. He serves on several editorial boards, including *Current Protocols in Immunology* and *Current Protocols in Microbiology*, both of which are published by John Wiley and Sons, Inc.

Geoffrey Sunshine is a Senior Scientist at the Health Effects Institute in Boston, Massachusetts, which funds research worldwide on the health effects of air pollution. He is also a lecturer in the Tufts School of Medicine immunology course. For several years, he has directed a course in immunology for graduate dental students at Tufts University School of Dental Medicine and previously directed a course for veterinary students at Tufts University School of Veterinary Medicine. He was also a member of the Sackler School of Graduate Biomedical Sciences at Tufts University, doing research on antigen presentation and teaching immunology to medical graduate and undergraduate students.

CONTRIBUTORS

Susan R.S. Gottesman
Department of Pathology
State University of New York
Health Science Center at Brooklyn
Brooklyn, New York

Linda Spatz
Department of Microbiology and Immunology
City University of New York Medical School
New York, New York

PREFACE AND ACKNOWLEDGMENTS

The sixth edition of *Immunology: A Short Course* preserves our commitment to the motto *less is more,* the watchword of the Short Course title since its first edition over 20 years ago. Since the publication of the fifth edition, our knowledge of how the immune system develops and functions and ways in which these physiological phenomena can fail or be compromised and thereby cause disease has significantly expanded. To reflect this new knowledge, every chapter in the sixth edition has been updated, rewritten to incorporate new findings, or streamlined to delete information that no longer reflects current thinking.

Recent advances in immunology have led to a better understanding of the human immune system and the mechanisms of infectious and immune-mediated diseases. These include infectious diseases such as malaria and tuberculosis—major causes of mortality around the world which account for more than three million deaths each year—as well as parasitic diseases, respiratory infections, and diseases caused by vector-borne pathogens. Although the immune system is essential for survival in the face of these pathogens, it can also cause disease in some circumstances. These include immunodeficiency diseases, such as severe combined immune deficiency (SCID); asthma; allergic diseases; contact dermatitis; autoimmune diseases such as systemic lupus erythematosus, multiple sclerosis, insulin-dependent diabetes mellitus, and type 1 diabetes; acute and chronic inflammatory disorders such as Crohn's disease; and rejection of transplanted organs, tissues, and cells. Success against these diseases depends on fundamental scientific research, including how the immune system and pathogens interact, how the immune system develops and is regulated, and the pathologic mechanisms by which the immune system causes damage when it fails to carry out its physiologic functions.

The sixth edition of *Immunology: A Short Course* is intended to provide the reader with a clear and concise overview of our current understanding of the physiology of the immune system as well as the pathophysiology associated with various immune-mediated diseases. Concurrent with the sixth edition we are pleased to announce the publication of *Immunology: Clinical Case Studies and Disease Pathophysiology* (Wiley, 2009), a companion book by Warren Strober (NIAID/NIH) and

Susan Gottesman (SUNY-Downstate) that builds on the information presented in our text and provides a deeper clinical context. Throughout the 6th edition of *Immunology: A Short Course*, we have cross-referenced clinical cases presented in this companion book. We are confident that the synergy created by the pairing of these two books will be a true asset to students of medicine as well as those in other health professions.

We are very grateful to Dr. Linda Spatz (CUNY Medical School), who contributed Chapter 12 (Tolerance and Autoimmunity). We would also like to thank Dr. Susan Gottesman (SUNY-Downstate) who updated Chapter 17 (Immunodeficiency Disorders and Neoplasias of Lymphoid System). Finally, we wish to acknowledge Dennis Kunkel, who prepared the immune cell images used to create the cover of the sixth edition (http://www.denniskunkel.com).

This is the first edition of *Immunology: A Short Course* to be written without Eli Benjamini. Dr. Benjamini wrote the first two editions with Dr. Sidney Leskowitz and he has contributed to all the other editions up to the fifth. We gratefully acknowledge the contributions of Dr. Benjamini and Dr. Leskowitz in establishing *Immunology: A Short Course* and hope that the new edition lives up to their high standards.

Richard Coico would like acknowledge the loving, enduring support of his wife, Lisa, during the writing of this book. Her encouragement and inspiration is second to none with two possible exceptions, namely, their children, Jonathan and Jennifer. Jonathan, a talented budding writer himself, and Jennifer, an emerging global health advocate, are each blessed with patience and bright inquisitive minds—the ideal mix of attributes for children and students alike. He also wishes to acknowledge his cousin, Frank Coico, who selflessly cheered him on with encouragement during his training years. "That made all the difference." Special thanks is extended to the following list of colleagues who generously provided their insightful scientific expertise and many helpful suggestions for the sixth edition: Dr. Ethan Shevach (NIH), Dr. Warren Strober (NIH), and Dr. Joanne Manns (Temple University School of Medicine). Special thanks are also extended to his coworkers, including secretaries, office assistants, and other staff members, who helped with the preparation of the manuscript. Finally, he would like to thank his late mentor, Dr. G. Jeanette Thorbecke, who greatly influenced his commitment and passion to the field of immunology.

Geoffrey Sunshine would like to thank his colleagues Peter Brodeur and Arthur Rabson, with whom he teaches immunology at Tufts University Medical School, for many stimulating discussions about how best to present information to medical students and other health professionals. Grateful thanks also goes to Peter Brodeur for his many

helpful suggestions during the preparation of the current edition. In addition, Geoffrey would like to thank his wife, Ilene, for her continued support and understanding during the writing.

Finally, the authors wish to express their appreciation to the staff members of John Wiley and Sons, Inc., who helped to publish the sixth edition, especially Developmental Editor Karen Trost, Senior Editor Thomas Moore, Illustration Manager Dean Gonzalez, and Senior Production Editor II Danielle Lacourciere.

IMMUNOLOGY: A SHORT COURSE 6TH EDITION ON THE INTERNET

The new edition of Immunology: A Short Course offers an online resource for students and instructors. This can be accessed at the following url: (http://www.wiley.com/college/coico). The following features are included at this Web site:

- Description
- Table of Contents
- Detailed Contents

- Information about the Authors
- New to this edition
- Sample Chapter

Reviews (as they become available)

In addition, Instructors may access complete electronic versions of all of the figures from the book by registering at the "Instructor Companion Site" and setting up a username and password.

OVERVIEW OF THE IMMUNE SYSTEM

● INTRODUCTION

Anyone who has had the good fortune to hear a brilliant orchestra performance of a symphony composed by one of the great masters knows that each of the carefully tuned musical instruments contributes to the collective, harmonious sound produced by the musicians. In many ways, the normally tuned immune system continuously plays an orchestrated symphony to maintain homeostasis in the context of host defenses. However, as William Shakespeare noted, "untune that string, and, hark, what discord follows!" (Troilus and Cressida). Similarly, an untuned immune system can cause discord, which manifests as autoimmunity, cancer, or chronic inflammation. Fortunately, for most of us, our immune systems are steadfastly vigilant in monitoring themselves to ensure that each cellular component behaves and interacts symbiotically to generate protective immune responses that ensure good health.

In his penetrating essays discussing symbiosis and parasitism, scientist–author Lewis Thomas described the forces that would drive all living matter into one huge ball of protoplasm if regulatory and recognition mechanisms did not allow us to distinguish *self* from *nonself*. The origins of these mechanisms go far back in evolutionary history; many originated as markers allowing cells to recognize and interact with one another to set up symbiotic households. For example, genetically related sponge colonies that are placed close together tend to grow toward one another and fuse into one large colony. However, unrelated colonies react differently, destroying cells that come in contact and leaving a zone of rejection between the colonies.

In the plant kingdom, similar types of recognition occur. In self-pollinating species, a pollen grain landing on the stigma of a genetically related flower will send a pollen tube down the style to the ovary for fertilization. A pollen grain from a genetically distinct plant reacts in one of two ways: (1) it will fail to germinate or (2) the pollen tube will disintegrate in the style. The opposite occurs in cross-pollinating species: self-marked pollen grains disintegrate, but nonself grains germinate and fertilize.

The nature of these primitive recognition mechanisms has not been completely worked out, but it almost certainly involves cell surface molecules that are able to specifically bind and adhere to other molecules on opposing cell surfaces. This simple method of molecular recognition has evolved over time into the very complex immune system that retains, as its essential feature, the ability of a protein molecule to recognize and bind specifically to a particular structure on another molecule. Such molecular recognition is the underlying principle involved in the discrimination between self and nonself during an immune response. It is the purpose of this book to describe how the fully mature immune system—which has evolved from this simple beginning—makes use of this principle of recognition in increasingly complex and sophisticated ways.

The study of immunology as a science has gone through several periods of quiescence and active development; the latter usually occurs following the introduction of a new technique or a changed paradigm for

Immunology: A Short Course, Sixth Edition, By Richard Coico and Geoffrey Sunshine
Copyright © 2009 John Wiley & Sons, Inc.

thinking about the subject. Perhaps the biggest catalyst for progress in this and many other biomedical areas has been the advent of molecular biologic techniques. It is important to acknowledge, however, that the reverse is also true: Certain technological advances in the field of molecular biology were made possible by earlier progress in the field of immunology. For example, the importance of immunologic methods (Chapter 5) used to purify proteins as well as identify specific complementary deoxyribonucleic acid (cDNA) clones cannot be understated. These advances were greatly facilitated by the pioneering studies of Kohler and Milstein (1975), who developed a method for producing monoclonal antibodies. Their achievement, which was rewarded with the Nobel Prize in Medicine, revolutionized research efforts in virtually all areas of biomedical science. Some monoclonal antibodies produced against so-called tumor-specific antigens have now been approved by the U.S. Food and Drug Administration for use to treat certain human malignancies. Monoclonal antibody technology is an excellent example of how the science of immunology has transformed not only medicine but also fields ranging from agriculture to the food science industry. Given the rapid advances occurring in immunology and many other biomedical sciences, including the sequencing of the human genome, every contemporary biomedical science textbook runs a considerable risk of being outdated before it appears in print. Nevertheless, we take solace from the observation that new formulations generally build on and expand existing information rather than replacing or negating it completely. We begin, therefore, with an overview of innate and acquired immunity, which continues to serve as a conceptual compass, orienting our fundamental understanding of host defense mechanisms.

● INNATE AND ACQUIRED IMMUNITY

The English word *immunity*, which refers to all the mechanisms used by the body as protection against environmental agents that are foreign to the body, arose from the Latin term *immunis*, meaning "exempt." The environmental agents may be microorganisms or their products, foods, chemicals, drugs, pollen, or animal hair, and dander. Immunity may be innate or acquired.

Innate Immunity

Innate immunity is conferred by a diverse array of cellular and subcellular components with which an individual is born. They are always present and available at very short notice to protect the individual from challenges by foreign invaders. Most of these elements are discussed in detail in Chapter 2. Table 1.1 summarizes and compares some of the major properties of the innate and adaptive immune systems. Elements of the innate immune system include body surfaces and internal components, such as the skin, the mucous membranes, and the cough reflex, all of which present effective barriers to environmental agents.

Chemical influences, such as pH and secreted fatty acids, also constitute effective barriers against invasion by many microorganisms. Another noncellular element of the innate immune system is the complement system. As in the previous editions of this book, we cover the subject of complement in a separate chapter (Chapter 13).

Numerous other features of innate immunity include fever; interferons (Chapter 11); other substances released by leukocytes; pattern recognition molecules (*innate receptors*), which can bind to various microorganisms (e.g., Toll-like receptors; Chapter 2); and serum proteins such as β-lysin, the enzyme lysozyme, polyamines, and the kinins. All of these elements either affect pathogenic invaders directly or enhance the effectiveness of host reactions to them. Phagocytic cells such as granulocytes, macrophages, and microglial cells of the central nervous system, which participate in the destruction and elimination of foreign material that has penetrated the body's physical and chemical barriers, are also considered part of the innate immune system.

Acquired Immunity

Acquired immunity came into play relatively late in evolutionary terms and is present only in vertebrates.

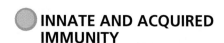 TABLE 1.1. Major Properties of the Innate and Adaptive Immune Systems

Property	Innate	Adaptive
Characteristics	Antigen nonspecific	Antigen specific
	Rapid response (minutes-hours)	Slow response (days)
	No memory	Memory
Immune components	Natural barriers (e.g., skin, mucous membranes)	Lymphocytes
	Phagocytes and Natural Killer cells	Antigen recognition molecules (B- and T-cell recptors)
	Soluble mediators (e.g., complement)	Secreted molecules (e.g., antibody)
	Pattern recognition molecules	

Although an individual is born with the capacity to mount immune responses to a foreign substance, the number of B and T cells available for initiating such responses must be expanded before you are said to be immune to that substance. This is achieved following contact with an antigen by activation of lymphocytes bearing antigen-specific receptors. Antigenic stimulation of B cells, T cells, and antigen-presenting cells initiates a chain of events that leads to proliferation of activated cells, along with a genetic program of differentiation events that generate the B cells or T cells responsible for the humoral or cell-mediated responses, respectively. These events take days to weeks to unfold. Fortunately, the cellular and noncellular components of the innate immune system are mobilized more rapidly (within minutes to hours) to eliminate or neutralize the foreign substance. One way to think about this host defense strategy is to consider this as a one–two punch: (1) innate cells and noncellular elements of the immune system are always available to quickly remove or cordon off the invader; (2) cells of the acquired immune system (B and T cells) are programmed by virtue of their antigen-specific receptors to react with specific foreign substances. The clonal expansion of the cells of the acquired immune system gives rise to an arsenal of antigen-specific cells available for rapid responses to the same antigen in the future, a phenomenon referred to as *memory responses*. By this process, the individual acquires the immunity to withstand and resist a subsequent attack by or exposure to the same offending agent.

The discovery of acquired immunity predates many of the concepts of modern medicine. It has been recognized for centuries that people who did not die from such life-threatening diseases as bubonic plague and smallpox were subsequently more resistant to the disease than were people who had never been exposed to it. The rediscovery of acquired immunity is credited to the English physician Edward Jenner, who, in the late-eighteenth century, experimentally induced immunity to smallpox. If Jenner performed his experiment today, his medical license would be revoked, and he would be the defendant in a sensational malpractice lawsuit: He inoculated a young boy with pus from a lesion of a dairy maid who had cowpox, a relatively benign disease that is related to smallpox. He then deliberately exposed the boy to smallpox. This exposure failed to cause disease! Because of the protective effect of inoculation with cowpox, the process of inducing acquired immunity has been termed *vaccination* (*vaccinia*, from the Latin word *vacca*, meaning "cow").

The concept of vaccination or immunization was expanded by Louis Pasteur and Paul Ehrlich almost 100 years after Jenner's experiment. By 1900, it had become apparent that immunity could be induced against not only microorganisms but also their products. We now know that immunity can be induced against innumerable natural and synthetic compounds, including metals, chemicals of relatively low molecular weight, carbohydrates, proteins, and nucleotides.

The compound that induces the acquired immune response is termed an *antigen*, a term initially coined because these compounds were known to cause *anti*body responses to be *gen*erated. Of course, we now know that antigens can generate both antibody-mediated and T-cell-mediated responses.

Active, Passive, and Adoptive Immunization

Acquired immunity is induced by immunization, which can be achieved in several ways:

- *Active immunization* refers to immunization of an individual by administration of an antigen.
- *Passive immunization* refers to immunization through the transfer of specific antibody from an immunized individual to a nonimmunized individual.
- *Adoptive immunization* refers to the transfer of immunity by the transfer of immune cells.

Major Characteristics of the Acquired Immune Response. The acquired immune response has several general features that distinguish it from other physiologic systems, such as circulation, respiration, and reproduction:

- *Specificity* is the ability to discriminate among different molecular entities and to respond only to those uniquely required, rather than making a random, undifferentiated response.
- *Adaptiveness* is the ability to respond to previously unseen molecules that may in fact never have naturally existed before on earth.
- *Discrimination between self and nonself* is a cardinal feature of the specificity of the immune response; it is the ability to recognize and respond to molecules that are foreign (nonself) and to avoid making this response to those molecules that are self. This distinction, and the recognition of antigen, is conferred by specialized cells (lymphocytes) that bear antigen-specific receptors on their surface.
- *Memory* a property shared with the nervous system, is the ability to recall previous contact with a foreign molecule and respond to it in a learned manner—that is, with a more rapid and larger response. Another term often used to describe immunologic memory is *anamnestic response*.

By the time you reach the end of this book, you should understand the cellular and molecular bases of these features of the immune response.

Cells Involved in the Acquired Immune Response. For many years, immunology remained an empirical subject involving the study of the effects of injecting various substances into hosts. Most progress came in the form of more quantitative methods for detecting the products of the immune response. However, a major shift in focus occurred in the 1950s. The revelation that lymphocytes were the major cellular players in immune responses caused the birth of an entirely new field of study, cellular immunology.

A convenient way to define the cell types involved in acquired immunity is to divide the host defense mechanisms into two categories: B-cell responses and T-cell responses. While this is an oversimplified definition, it is, by and large, the functional outcome of acquired immune responses. B and T cells are derived from a common lymphoid precursor cell but differentiate along different developmental lines, as discussed in detail in Chapters 7 and 8, respectively. In short, B cells develop and mature in the bone marrow, and T cells develop in the bone marrow but undergo critical maturation steps in the thymus.

Antigen-presenting cells (APC), such as macrophages and dendritic cells, constitute the third cell type participating in the acquired immune response. Although these cells do not have antigen-specific receptors themselves, they process and present antigen to the antigen-specific receptors expressed by T cells. The APC express a variety of cell-surface molecules that facilitate their interaction with T cells. Among these are the ***major histocompatibility complex*** (***MHC***) molecules discussed in Chapter 8. MHC molecules are encoded by a set of polymorphic genes expressed within a population. In clinical settings, MHC molecules determine the success or failure of organ and tissue transplantation. In fact, this observation facilitated their discovery and the current terminology (major *histocompatibility* complex) used to define these molecules. (We now understand that their physiologic role is concerned with T cell–APC interactions.) Physiologically, APC process protein antigens intracellularly, resulting in the constellation of peptides that noncovalently bind to MHC molecules and ultimately get displayed on the cell surface.

Other cell types, such as neutrophils and mast cells, also participate in acquired immune responses. In fact, they participate in both innate and acquired immunity. While these cells have no specific antigen recognition properties and can be activated by a variety of substances, they are an integral part of the network of cells that participate in host defenses and often display potent immunoregulatory properties.

CLONAL SELECTION THEORY

A turning point in immunology came in the 1950s with the introduction of a Darwinian view of the cellular basis of specificity in the immune response. The now universally accepted ***clonal selection theory*** was proposed and developed by Jerne and Burnet (both Nobel Prize winners) and by Talmage. The clonal selection theory had a truly revolutionary effect on the field of immunology. It dramatically changed our approach to studying the immune system and affected all research carried out during the last half of the twentieth century. This work ultimately provided us with knowledge regarding the molecular machinery behind the activation and regulation of cellular elements of the immune system. The essential postulates of this theory are summarized below.

As discussed earlier, the specificity of immune responses is based on the ability of B and T lymphocytes to recognize particular foreign molecules (antigens) and respond to them in order to eliminate them. The process of clonal expansion of these cells is highly efficient, but there is always the rare chance that errors or mutations will occur. Such errors can result in the generation of B and T lymphocytes with receptors that bind to self-antigens and therefore display ***autoreactivity***. Under normal conditions, nonfunctioning cells may survive or be aborted with no deleterious consequences to the individual. In contrast, the rare self-reactive cells are clonally deleted or suppressed by other regulatory cells of the immune system charged with this role. If such a mechanism were absent, autoimmune responses might occur routinely. It is noteworthy that during the early stages of development, lymphocytes with receptors that bind to self-antigens are produced, but fortunately they are eliminated or functionally inactivated. This process gives rise to the initial repertoire of mature lymphocytes that are programmed to generate antigen-specific responses. As noted above, some errors can occur during this process, leading to the development of autoreactive cells (Fig. 1.1). The circumstances and predisposing genetic conditions that may lead to the latter phenomenon are discussed in Chapter 12.

As we have already stated, the immune system is capable of recognizing innumerable foreign antigens. How is a response to any one antigen accomplished? In addition to the now-proven postulate that self-reactive clones of lymphocytes are functionally inactivated or aborted, the clonal selection theory proposed the following:

- T and B lymphocytes of myriad specificities exist before there is any contact with the foreign antigen.
- Lymphocytes participating in an immune response express antigen-specific receptors on their surface membranes. As a consequence of antigen binding to the lymphocyte, the cell is activated and releases various products. In the case of B lymphocytes, these receptors, so-called ***B-cell receptors (BCRs)*** are the very molecules that subsequently get secreted as antibodies following B-cell activation.

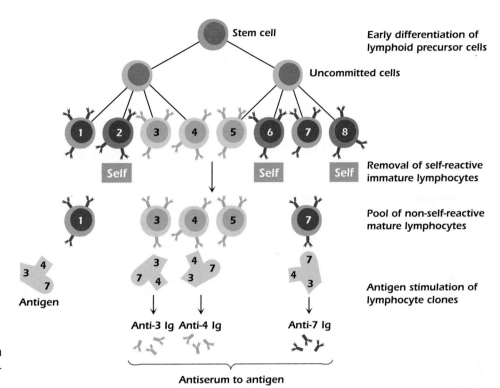

Figure 1.1. Clonal selection theory of B cells leading to antibody production.

- T cells have receptors denoted as **T-cell receptors** (**TCRs**). Unlike the B cell, the T-cell products are not the same as their surface receptors. Instead, other protein molecules, called cytokines, participate in elimination of the antigen by regulating the many cells needed to mount an effective immune response.

- Each lymphocyte carries on its surface receptor molecules of only a single specificity, as demonstrated in Figure 1.1. This is true for both B and T cells.

These three postulates describe the existence of a large repertoire of possible specificities formed by cellular multiplication and differentiation *before* there is any contact with the foreign substance requiring a response. Upon introduction of the foreign antigen, those cells with specificity for the antigen bind to it.

The remaining postulates of the clonal selection theory account for this process of selection by the antigen from among all the available cells in the repertoire:

- Surface receptors of the immunocompetent lymphocytes combine with the foreign antigen, or a portion of it, termed the **epitope** or **antigenic determinant**. The cells expressing these epitope-specific receptors are then activated under appropriate conditions to proliferate and differentiate into clones of cells with the corresponding epitope-specific receptors.

- With B-cell clones, this process will lead to the synthesis of antibodies having specificity for the same antigen. In most cases, the antigen stimulating the response is complex and contains many different epitopes, each capable of activating a clone of epitope-specific B cells. Hence, the clonally secreted antibodies collectively constitute what is often referred to as polyclonal antiserum capable of interacting with the multiple epitopes expressed by the antigen. Several distinct regions (epitopes) of an antigen can be recognized; thus, several different clones of B cells will be stimulated to produce antibody. The collective response produces an antiserum that is made up of antigen-specific antibodies (Fig. 1.1);

- T cells are similarly selected by appropriate epitopes. Each selected T cell will be activated to divide and produce clones with specificity for the same antigen. Thus the clonal response to the antigen will be amplified, and subsequent exposure to the same antigen will now result in the activation of many cells or clones of that specificity. Instead of synthesizing and releasing antibodies like the B cells, the T cells synthesize and release cytokines. These cytokines, which are soluble mediators, exert their effect on other cells to grow or become activated, facilitating elimination of the antigen. All of the T-cell clones that recognize various epitopes on the same antigen will be activated to perform their function.

A final postulate was added to account for the ability to recognize self-antigens without making a response:

• Circulating self-antigens that reach the developing lymphoid system before some undesignated maturational step will serve to shut off those cells that recognize it specifically, and no subsequent immune response will be induced.

HUMORAL AND CELLULAR IMMUNITY

Acquired immune responses have historically been divided into two separate arms of defense, namely, B-cell-mediated or *humoral immunity* and T-cell-mediated or *cellular immunity*. Today, while we recognize that B and T cells have very distinct yet complementary molecular and functional roles within our immune system, we understand that the two arms are fundamentally interconnected at many levels. "Experiments of nature" was a term coined by Robert A. Good in the 1950s when describing the immune status of mice with a congenital mutation associated with an athymic phenotype (a similar phenomenon in humans is called DiGeorge syndrome). Good's experiments have provided significant insights into the interdependence of these two arms of the immune system. Athymic mice, those that fail to develop thymic tissue, develop a profound T-cell deficiency with accompanying abnormalities in B-cell function. Without T-cell help, B cells are unable to generate normal antibody responses and, in particular, to undergo immunoglobulin class switching (see Chapters 7 and 17). The help normally provided by T cells is delivered in several ways, including the synthesis and secretion of a variety of cytokines that regulate many events required for proliferation and differentiation of B cells (see Chapter 11).

B cells are initially activated to secrete antibodies after binding of antigens to antigen-specific *immunoglobulin* (*Ig*) molecules expressed by B cells. All serum globulins with antibody activity are referred to as immunoglobulins (see Chapter 4). It has been estimated that each B cell expresses 10^5 BCRs of identical specificity. Once ligated, the B cell receives signals to begin making the secreted form of this immunoglobulin, a process that initiates the full-blown antibody response with the purpose of eliminating the antigen from the host. Antibodies are a heterogeneous mixture of serum globulins, all of which share the ability to bind individually to specific antigens.

Immunoglobulins have common structural features which enable them to do two things: (1) recognize and bind specifically to a unique structural entity on an antigen (the epitope) and (2) perform a common biologic function after combining with the antigen. Immunoglobulin molecules consist of two identical light (L) chains and two identical heavy (H) chains linked by disulfide bridges. The resultant structure is shown in Figure 1.2. The portion of the molecule that binds antigen consists of an area composed of the amino-terminal regions of both H and L chains. Thus, each immunoglobulin molecule composed of 2H and 2L chains is symmetric and is capable of binding two identical epitopes, either on the same antigen molecule or on two different molecules. There are other differences among immunoglobulin molecules in addition to variations in the antigen-binding portion, the most important of which occur in the H chains. There are five major classes of H chains (termed γ, μ, α, ε, and δ). On the basis of differences in their H chains, immunoglobulin molecules are divided into five major classes: IgG, IgM, IgA, IgE, and IgD. Each class has several unique biologic properties. For example, IgG is the only class of immunoglobulin that crosses the placenta, conferring the mother's immunity on the fetus, and IgA is the major antibody found in secretions such as tears and saliva. It is important to remember that antibodies in all five classes may possess precisely the same specificity against an antigen (antigen-combining regions), while at the same time having different functional (biologic effector) properties. The binding between antigen and antibody is not covalent but depends on many relatively weak forces, such as hydrogen bonds, van der Waals forces, and hydrophobic interactions. Since these forces are weak, successful binding between antigen and antibody depends on a very close fit over a sizable area, much like the contacts between a lock and a key.

Besides the help provided by T cells in the generation of antibody responses, noncellular components of the innate immune system, collectively termed the *complement system*, play a key role in the functional activity of antibodies when they interact with antigen (Chapter 13). The reaction between antigen and antibody serves to activate this system, which consists of a series of serum enzymes. The end result is lysis of the target in the case of microbes such as bacteria or enhanced *phagocytosis* (ingestion of the antigen) by phagocytic cells. The activation of complement also results in the recruitment of highly *phagocytic polymorphonuclear* (**PMN**) cells or neutrophils, which are active in innate immunity.

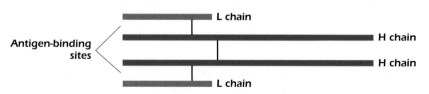

Figure 1.2. Typical antibody molecule composed of two heavy (H) and two light (L) chains. Antigen-binding sites are noted.

Cell-Mediated Immunity

In contrast to humoral immune responses that are mediated by antibodies, cell-mediated responses are T-cell mediated. However, this is an oversimplified definition. The effector cell responsible for the elimination of a foreign antigen such as a pathogenic microbe can be an activated T cell expressing a pathogen-specific TCR or a phagocytic cell that gets activated by innate receptors which they express and the cytokines produced by activated T cells (Fig. 1.3). Unlike B cells, which produce soluble antibody that circulates to bind specific antigens, each T cell, bearing approximately 10^5 identical antigen receptors (TCRs), circulates directly to the site of antigen expressed on APC and interacts with these cells in a *cognate* (cell-to-cell) fashion (Chapter 10).

There are several phenotypically distinct subpopulations of T cells, each of which may have the same specificity for an antigenic determinant (epitope). However, each subpopulation may perform different functions. This is somewhat analogous to the different classes of immunoglobulin molecules, which may have identical specificity but different biologic functions. Several major subsets of T cells exist, including helper T cells (T_H cells), which express molecules called CD4, and cytotoxic T cells (T_C cells), which express CD8 molecules on their surface. Another population of T cells possessing suppressor activity is the T-regulatory cell (T_{reg} cells).

The functions ascribed to the various subsets of T cells include the following:

- **B-cell help**. T_H cells cooperate with B cells to enhance the production of antibodies. T_H cells function by releasing cytokines, which provide various activation signals for the B cells. As mentioned earlier, cytokines are soluble substances, or mediators that can regulate proliferation and differentiation of B cells. Additional information about cytokines is presented in Chapter 11.

- **Inflammatory effects**. On activation, certain T_H cells releases cytokines that induce the migration and activation of monocytes and macrophages, leading to inflammatory reactions (Chapter 16).

- **Cytotoxic effects**. Certain T cells, called T-cytotoxic (T_C) cells, are able to deliver a lethal hit on contact with their target cells, leading to their death. In contrast to T_H cells, T_C cells express molecules called CD8 on their membranes and are, therefore, CD8$^+$ cells.

- **Regulatory effects**. Helper T cells can be further subdivided into different functional subsets that are commonly defined by the cytokines they release. As you will learn in subsequent chapters, these subsets (T_H1, T_H2) have distinct regulatory properties that are mediated by the cytokines they release (Chapter 11). T_H1 cells can negatively cross-regulate T_H2 cells and vice versa. Another population of regulatory or suppressor T cells coexpresses CD4 and a molecule called CD25 (CD25 is part of a cytokine receptor known as the interleukin 2 receptor α chain; Chapter 11). The regulatory activity of these CD4$^+$/CD25$^+$cells and their role in actively suppressing autoimmunity are discussed in Chapter 12.

- **Cytokine effects**. Cytokines produced by each of the T-cell subsets (principally T_H cells) exert numerous effects on many cells, lymphoid and nonlymphoid. Thus, directly or indirectly, T cells communicate and collaborate with many cell types.

For many years, immunologists have recognized that cells activated by antigen manifest a variety of effector phenomena. It is only in the last few decades that researchers began to appreciate the complexity of events that take place in activation by antigen and communication with other cells. We know today that just mere contact of the TCR with antigen is not sufficient to activate T cells. At least two signals must be delivered to the antigen-specific T cell for activation to occur: Signal 1 involves the binding of the TCR to antigen, which must be presented in the appropriate manner by APC. Signal 2 involves costimulators, including cytokines such as interleukin 1 (IL-1), IL-4, and IL-6 (Chapter 11) and cell surface molecules expressed on APC, such as CD40 and CD86 (Chapter 10). Recently, the term **costimulator** has been broadened to include stimuli such as microbial products (infectious nonself) and damaged tissue (Matzinger's "danger hypothesis") that will enhance signal 1 when that signal is relatively weak.

Once T cells are optimally signaled for activation, a series of events takes place and the activated cell undergoes proliferation and synthesizes and releases cytokines. In turn, these cytokines come in contact with appropriate cell surface receptors on different cells and exert their effect on these cells.

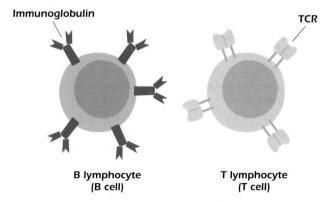

Figure 1.3. Antigen receptors expressed as transmembrane molecules on B and T lymphocytes.

Although the humoral and cellular arms of acquired immune responses have been considered as separate and distinct components, it is important to understand that the response to any particular pathogen may involve a complex interaction between them along with components of innate immunity. All this ensures a maximal survival advantage for the host by eliminating the antigen and, as we shall see, by protecting the host from mounting an immune response against self.

GENERATION OF DIVERSITY IN THE IMMUNE RESPONSE

The most recent tidal surge in immunologic research represents a triumph of the marriage of molecular biology and immunology. Although cellular immunology had outlined the cellular basis and exquisite specificity of a large and diverse repertoire of responses, arguments abounded regarding the exact genetic mechanisms that enabled all these specificities to become part of the immune response in every individual of the species.

Briefly, the arguments were as follows:

- By various calculations, the number of antigenic specificities against which an immune response could possibly be mounted could range upward of 10^6–10^7.
- If every specific response, in the form of either antibodies or T-cell receptors, were encoded by a single gene, did this mean that $>10^7$ genes (one for each specific antibody or TCR) were required in every individual? How was this massive amount of DNA carried intact from individual to individual?

The pioneering studies of Tonegawa (a Nobel laureate) and Leder, using molecular biologic techniques, finally addressed these issues by describing a unique genetic mechanism by which immunologic receptors expressed on B cells (BCRs) of enormous diversity could be produced with a modest amount of DNA.

The technique evolved by nature was one of genetic recombination, in which a protein could be encoded by a DNA molecule composed of a set of recombined minigenes that made up a complete gene. Given small sets of these minigenes, which could be randomly combined to make the complete gene, it was possible to produce an enormous repertoire of specificities from a limited number of gene fragments. This idea is discussed in detail in Chapter 6.

Although this mechanism was first elucidated to explain the enormous diversity of antibodies that not only are released by B cells but also, in fact, constitute the antigen- or epitope-specific BCRs, it was subsequently established that the same mechanisms operate in generating diversity of the antigen-specific TCR. The mechanisms involved in generating diversity of TCRs are discussed in

Chapter 8. For now, all you need to know is that various techniques of molecular biology, which permit genes to be both analyzed and moved from one cell to another, have continued the onrushing tide of progress in the field of immunology.

BENEFITS OF IMMUNOLOGY

So far we have discussed the theoretical aspects of immunology. However, its practical applications are of paramount importance for survival.

The field of immunology has been in the limelight since the successful use of polio vaccines in the mid-twentieth century. More recently, the transplantation of the human heart and other major organs, such as the liver, has been the focus of a great deal of publicity. Public interest in immunology has intensified in light of the potential application of immune responses to the detection and management of cancer. In the 1980s, awareness of immunology among the general public was also heightened because of the alarming spread of acquired immunodeficiency syndrome (AIDS).

The innate and acquired immune systems play an integral role in the prevention of and recovery from infectious diseases and are, without question, essential to the survival of the individual. In the 1800s, Metchnikoff was the first to propose that phagocytic cells formed the first line of defense against infection and that the inflammatory response could actually serve a protective function for the host. Indeed, innate immune responses are responsible for the detection and rapid destruction of most infectious agents that we encounter in daily life. We now know that innate immune responses operate in concert with adaptive immune responses to generate antigen-specific effector mechanisms that lead to the death and elimination of the invading pathogen. Chapter 20 presents information about the response of our immune systems to microorganisms and exploitation of these mechanisms through immunoprophylaxis. Vaccination against infectious diseases has been and continues to be an effective form of prophylaxis. Immunoprophylaxis against the virus that causes poliomyelitis has significantly reduced the incidence of this devastating disease. Indeed, one of the most widespread diseases, smallpox, has been virtually eliminated from the face of the earth. The last documented case of natural transmission of smallpox virus was in 1972. Unfortunately, the threat of biologic weapons has prompted new concerns regarding the reemergence of smallpox and certain other infectious diseases. Fortunately, public health vaccination initiatives can prevent or significantly curtail the threat of weaponized microbiological agents.

Recent developments in immunology also hold the promise of immunoprophylaxis against malaria and several other parasitic diseases that plague many parts of the world and affect billions of people. Vaccination against diseases of livestock promises to increase the production of meat in developing countries, while inoculations targeting various substances that play roles in the reproductive processes in mammals offer the possibility of long-term contraception in humans and companion animals such as cats and dogs.

DAMAGING EFFECTS OF THE IMMUNE RESPONSE

The enormous survival value of immune responses is self-evident. Acquired immunity directed against a foreign material has as its ultimate goal the elimination of the invading substance. In the process, some tissue damage may occur as the result of the accumulation of components with nonspecific effects. This damage is generally temporary. As soon as the invader is eliminated, the situation at the site of the immune response reverts to normal.

There are instances in which the power of the immune response, although directed against innocuous foreign substances—such as some medications, inhaled pollen particles, or substances deposited by insect bites—produces a response that may result in severe pathologic consequences and even death. These responses are known collectively as hypersensitivity reactions or allergic reactions. An understanding of the basic mechanisms underlying these disease processes has been fundamental in their treatment and control. In addition, studying these processes has contributed much to our knowledge of normal immune responses. Normal and hyperreactive immune responses both utilize essentially identical mechanisms; however, in hypersensitivity, these mechanisms are misdirected or out of control (see Chapters 14–16).

Given the complexity of immune responses and their potential for inducing damage, they must operate under carefully regulated conditions, like any other physiologic system. These multiple controls include feedback inhibition by soluble products and cell–cell interactions of many types, which may either heighten or reduce the response. The net result is to maintain a state of homeostasis so that, when the system is disrupted by a foreign invader, just enough response is generated to control the invader, and then the system returns to equilibrium—in other words, the immune response is shut down. However, memory of that particular invader is retained so that a more rapid and heightened response will occur should the invader return. A disturbance in these regulatory mechanisms may be caused by a condition such as a congenital defect, hormonal imbalance, or certain infections, any of which can have disastrous consequences. AIDS is a timely example; AIDS is associated with an infection of T lymphocytes that participate in regulating immune responses. As a result of infection with the human immunodeficiency virus (HIV), which causes AIDS, there is a decrease in occurrence and function of a vital subpopulation of T cells, which leads to immunologic deficiency and renders the patient powerless to resist infections by microorganisms that are normally benign.

Another important form of regulation is the prevention of immune responses against self-antigens. During the developmental stages leading to the generation of mature B and T lymphocytes, there are checkpoints that eliminate or functionally silence these self-reactive cells (discussed in Chapter 12). Sometimes, however, rare autoreactive cells may develop, causing the body to mount an immune response against its own tissues. This type of immune response is termed autoimmunity and is the cause of diseases such as some forms of arthritis, thyroiditis, and type I diabetes, which are very difficult to treat.

THE FUTURE OF IMMUNOLOGY

A peek into the world of the future of immunology suggests many exciting areas of research. The application of molecular and computational techniques promises significant dividends. To cite just a few examples, we focus on vaccine development and control of immune responses. Rather than the laborious, empirical search for an attenuated virus or bacterium for use in immunization, it is now possible to use pathogen-specific protein sequence data and sophisticated computational methods (*bioinformatics*) to identify candidates to be tested. Alternatively, DNA vaccines involving the injection of DNA vectors that encode immunizing proteins may revolutionize vaccination protocols in the not-too-distant future. The identification of various genes and the proteins or peptides that they are encoding makes it possible to design vaccines against a wide spectrum of biologically important compounds.

Another area of great promise is control of immune responses. Techniques of gene isolation, clonal reproduction, the polymerase chain reaction, and biosynthesis have contributed to rapid progress in the characterization and synthesis of various cytokines that enhance and control the activation of various cells associated with immune responses. Powerful and important modulators have been synthesized using recombinant DNA technology and are being tested for their therapeutic efficacy in a variety of diseases, including many different cancers. In some cases, cytokine research efforts have already moved from the bench to the bedside with the development of therapeutic agents used to treat patients.

Finally, probably one of the most exciting areas of research is the genetic engineering of cells and even whole animals, such as mice, that lack one or more specific traits (gene knockout) or that carry a specific trait (transgenic). These and other immune-based experimental systems are the subject of Chapter 5. They allow the immunologist to study the effects of such traits on the immune system and on the body as a whole with the goals of understanding the intricate regulation, expression, and function of immune responses and controlling the trait to benefit the individual. Our growing understanding of the functioning of the immune system, combined with the recently acquired ability to alter and manipulate its components, carries enormous implications for the future of humankind.

 ## THE SHORT COURSE BEGINS HERE

This brief overview of the immune system is intended to introduce you to the complex yet fascinating subject of immunology. In the remaining chapters we provide a more detailed account of the workings of the immune system. We begin with its cellular components (Chapter 2), followed by a description of the structure of the reactants (Chapters 3 and 4) and the general methodology for measuring their reactions (Chapter 5). This is followed by chapters describing the formation and activation of the cellular and molecular components of the immune apparatus required to generate a response (Chapters 6–9). A discussion of the control mechanisms that regulate the scope and intensity of immune responses completes the description of the basic nature of immunity (Chapter 10). Next is a chapter on cytokines (Chapter 11), the soluble mediators that regulate immune responses and play a significant role in hematopoiesis, followed by chapters that deal with the great variety of immune-mediated diseases. These vary from responses to self-antigens (autoimmunity; Chapter 12) to those produced by aberrant immune responses (hypersensitivity; Chapters 14–16) to ineffective or absent immune responses (immunodeficiency; Chapter 17). Also included in this group is a chapter on the complement system (Chapter 13). Following the chapters that describe the role of the immune response in transplantation (Chapter 18) and antitumor reactions (Chapter 19), a final

chapter focuses on the spectrum of microorganisms that challenge the immune system and how immune responses are mounted in a vigilant, orchestrated fashion to protect the host from infectious diseases. Included in Chapter 20 is a discussion of immunoprophylaxis using vaccines that protect us from a variety of pathogenic organisms. Without question, the successful use of vaccines helped revolutionize the field of medicine in the twentieth century. What lies ahead in the twenty-first century are research efforts related to the development of crucial new vaccines to protect humankind from naturally occurring pathogenic viruses and microorganisms that have just begun to plague us (such as bird flu), have been engineered as potential biologic weapons, or have yet to be identified.

As you read the chapters that follow, we urge you to take note of cross-references to clinical correlations associated with basic immunologic concepts that appear as clinical cases in the companion book by W. Strober and S.R.S. Gottesman (*Immunology: Clinical Case Studies and Pathophysiology*). These will appear in the form of icons and clinical case titles such as the example below:

**X-linked
Agammaglobulinemia**

With the enormous scope of the subject and the extraordinary richness of detail available, we have made every effort to adhere to fundamental elements and basic concepts required to achieve an integrated, if not extensive, understanding of the immune response. If your interest has been piqued, many current books, articles, and reviews and growing numbers of educational Internet sites, including the one that supports this textbook (see the Preface), are available to help you further explore the exciting field of immunology.

REFERENCES

Baxter AG, Hodgkin PD (2002): Activation rules: The two-signal theories of immune activation. *Nature Rev Immunol.* 2:439.

Blom B, Spits H (2006): Development of human lymphoid cells. *Annu Rev Immunol* 24:287.

Boehm T, Bleul CC (2007): The evolutionary history of lymphoid organs. *Nature Immunol* 8:131.

Matzinger P (1994): Tolerance, danger and the extended family. *Annu Rev Immunol* 12:991.

Shevach EM (2002): CD4$^+$, CD25$^+$ suppressor T cells: More questions than answers. *Nature Rev Immunol* 2:389.

ELEMENTS OF INNATE AND ACQUIRED IMMUNITY

 INTRODUCTION

Every living organism is confronted by continual intrusions from its environment. Our immune systems are equipped with a network of mechanisms to safeguard us from infectious microorganisms that would otherwise take advantage of our bodies for their own survival. In short, the immune system has evolved as a surveillance system poised to initiate and maintain protective responses against virtually any harmful foreign element we might encounter. These defenses range from physical barriers, such as our skin, to highly sophisticated systems, such as acquired immune responses. This chapter describes the defense systems: the elements that constitute the defense, the participating cells and organs, and the action of the participants in the immune response to foreign substances that invade the body.

In vertebrates, immunity against microorganisms and their products or against other foreign substances that may invade the body is divided into two major categories: *innate immunity* and *acquired immunity*. The cellular components and interrelationships of these two types of immunity are discussed in this chapter. Here and in the chapters that follow, it will become apparent that innate immune responses are important not only because they are an independent arm of the immune system but also because they profoundly influence the nature of acquired immune responses.

 INNATE IMMUNITY

Innate immunity is present from birth and its principal role is to provide a first line of defense against pathogens. Most microorganisms encountered daily in the life of a healthy individual are detected and destroyed within minutes to hours by innate defense mechanisms. Innate immunity is carried out by nonspecific physical and chemical barriers (e.g. the skin), cellular barriers (e.g., phagocytes), and molecular pattern-based reactions (e.g., the Toll-like receptors, or TLRs). This section, which describes the major components of innate immunity, serves as an important backdrop for subsequent discussions of the links between innate and adaptive immunity.

Physical and Chemical Barriers of Innate Immunity

Most organisms and foreign substances cannot penetrate intact skin but can enter the body if the skin is damaged. Some microorganisms can enter through sebaceous glands and hair follicles. However, the acid pH of sweat and sebaceous secretions and the presence of various *fatty acids* and *hydrolytic enzymes* (e.g., *lysozymes*) all have some antimicrobial effects, which minimizes the importance of this route of infection. In addition, soluble proteins, including the interferons and certain members of the complement system found in the serum (see Chapter 13), contribute to nonspecific immunity. *Interferons* are a group of proteins made by cells in response to virus infection which essentially induce a generalized antiviral state in surrounding cells (see Chapter 11). Activation of the *complement system* in response to certain microorganisms results in a controlled enzymatic cascade which targets the membrane of pathogenic organisms and leads to their destruction. An important innate immune mechanism involved in the protection of many areas of the body, including the respiratory and gastrointestinal tracts, is the coverage of surfaces in these areas with mucus. In these areas, the mucous membrane barrier traps microorganisms, which are then swept toward the external openings by ciliated epithelial cells. The hairs in the nostrils and the cough reflex are also helpful in preventing organisms from infecting the respiratory tract. Alcohol consumption, cigarette smoking, and narcotics suppress this entire defense system.

The elimination of microorganisms from the respiratory tract is aided by pulmonary or alveolar macrophages, which, as we shall see later, are phagocytic cells able to engulf and destroy some microorganisms. Other microorganisms that have penetrated the mucous membrane barrier can be picked up by macrophages or otherwise transported to lymph nodes, where many are destroyed. The environment of the gastrointestinal tract is made hostile to many microorganisms by other innate mechanisms, including the hydrolytic enzymes in saliva, the low pH of the stomach, and the proteolytic enzymes and bile in the small intestine. The low pH of the vagina serves a similar function.

Intracellular and Extracellular Killing of Microorganisms

Once an invading microorganism has penetrated the various physical and chemical barriers that constitute the first line

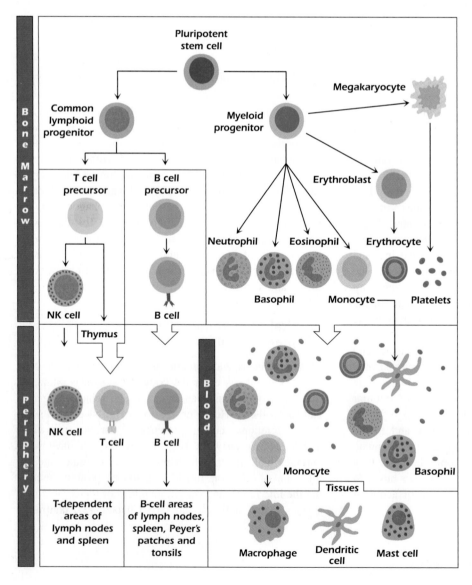

Figure 2.1. Developmental pathways of various cell types from pluripotential bone marrow stem cells.

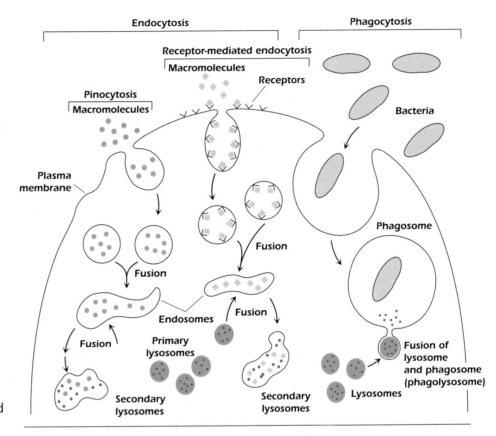

Figure 2.2. Endocytosis and phagocytosis by macrophages.

of defense, it encounters the next line of defense, which consists of various specialized cells whose purpose is to destroy the invader. These include the polymorphonuclear leukocytes, monocytes, and macrophages each of which is derived from hematopoietic precursor cells. The developmental pathways of the various hematopoietic cells are shown in Figure 2.1. Before we discuss the innate host defense mechanisms carried out by these cells, it is important to understand two fundamental cellular activities associated with many members of this group of cells: endocytosis and phagocytosis.

Endocytosis. *Endocytosis* is the ingestion by cells of macromolecules present in extracellular fluid. This can occur either by *pinocytosis*, which involves nonspecific membrane invagination, or by *receptor-mediated endocytosis*, a process involving the selective binding of macromolecules to specific membrane receptors. In both cases, ingestion of the foreign macromolecules generates endocytic vesicles filled with the foreign material, which then fuse with acidic compartments called *endosomes*. Endosomes then fuse with *lysosomes* containing degradative enzymes (e.g., nucleases, lipases, proteases) to reduce the ingested macromolecules to small breakdown

products, including nucleotides, sugars, and peptides (Fig. 2.2).

Phagocytosis. *Phagocytosis*, the ingestion by individual cells of invading foreign particles such as bacteria, is a critical protective mechanism of the immune system. Many microorganisms release substances that attract phagocytic cells. Phagocytosis may be enhanced by a variety of factors that make the foreign particle an easier target. These factors, collectively referred to as *opsonins* (Greek word meaning "prepare food for"), consist of antibodies and various serum components of complement (see Chapter 13). After ingestion, the foreign particle is entrapped in a phagocytic vacuole (*phagosome*), which fuses with lysosomes to form the *phagolysosome* (Fig. 2.2). The phagolysosome releases its powerful enzymes, which digest the particle.

Phagocytes can also damage invading pathogens through the generation of toxic products in a process known as the *respiratory burst*. Production of these toxic metabolites is induced during phagocytosis of pathogens such as bacteria and is catalyzed by a set of interrelated enzyme pathways. The most important toxic products produced by the respiratory burst are nitric oxide [catalyzed by inducible nitric oxidase synthase), hydrogen peroxide and superoxide anion (catalyzed by phagocyte nicotinamide adenine dinucleotide phosphate (NADPH) oxidase], and hypochlorous acid (catalyzed by myeloperoxidase). In addition to being toxic to bacteria, each of these microbicidal products can also damage host cells. Fortunately, a series of protective enzymes produced by phagocytes primarily limits their microbicidal activity to the phagolysosome (see Fig. 2.2), thereby focusing their toxicity on ingested pathogens. These protective enzymes include catalase, which degrades hydrogen peroxide, and superoxide dismutase, which converts the superoxide anion into hydrogen peroxide and oxygen. The absence of or an abnormality in any one of the respiratory burst components results in a form of immunodeficiency that predisposes individuals to repeated infections (Chapter 17).

Cells Involved in the Innate Immune System

As noted above, several cell types participate in innate host defense mechanisms. These cell types are defined in more detail in this section. Upon activation (e.g., contact with microorganisms) these cells produce and often release biologically active soluble substances, including potent antimicrobial products (e.g., peroxide) and cytokines, which have different effects on the various host cells (see Chapter 11). They are also involved in key steps in the induction of acquired immune responses mediated by B and T cells. One example of this interrelationship is *antigen presentation* by so-called APC carried out by particular cell types within the innate immune system. As will be discussed in great detail in subsequent chapters, T cells must interact with APC displaying particular antigens in order to generate antigen-specific responses. Thus, while the descriptions of the cells below primarily describe their involvement in innate immune responses, it is important to recognize their important role in acquired immune responses at this early stage of your study of the immune system.

Polymorphonuclear (PMN) Leukocytes. **PMN leukocytes** are a population of cells also referred to as **granulocytes**. These include the **basophils**, **mast cells**, **eosinophils**, and **neutrophils**. Granulocytes are short-lived phagocytic cells that contain enzyme-rich lysosomes, which can facilitate destruction of infectious microorganisms (Fig. 2.3). They also produce peroxide and superoxide radicals, which are toxic to many microorganisms. Some lysosomes also contain bactericidal proteins such as lactoferrin. PMN leukocytes play a major role in protection against infection. Defects in PMN cell function are accompanied by chronic or recurrent infection.

Macrophages. **Macrophages** are phagocytes derived from blood monocytes (Fig. 2.4). The **monocyte** is a small, spherical cell with few projections, abundant

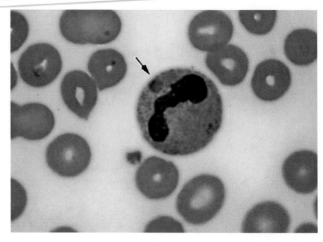

Figure 2.3. A PMN leukocyte (surrounded by erythrocytes in blood smear) with trilobed nucleus and cytoplasmic granules (×950). [Reproduced with permission from Olana and Walker, *Infect Med* 19:318 (2002).]

cytoplasm, little endoplasmic reticulum, and many granules. Following migration of monocytes from the blood to various tissues, they undergo further differentiation into a variety of histologic forms, all of which play a role in phagocytosis, including the following:

- *Kupffer cells*, in the liver; large cells with many cytoplasmic projections.
- *Alveolar macrophages*, in the lung.
- *Splenic macrophages*, in the white pulp of the spleen.

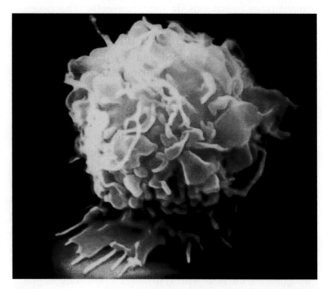

Figure 2.4. Scanning electron micrograph of macrophage with ruffled membranes and surface covered with microvilli (×5200). [Reproduced with permission from *J Clin. Invest* 117 (2007).]

- *Peritoneal macrophages*, free floating in peritoneal fluid.
- *Microglial cells*, in the central nervous tissue.

Each of these macrophage populations constitutes part of the cellular members of the *reticuloendothelial system (RES)*, which is widely distributed throughout the body. The major function of the RES is to phagocytize microorganisms and foreign substances that invade the bloodstream and various tissues. The RES also functions in the destruction of aged and imperfect cells, such as effete erythrocytes.

Although associated with diverse names and locations, many macrophages share common features, such as the ability to bind and engulf particulate materials and antigens. Because of their location along capillaries, these cells are most likely to make first contact with invading pathogens and antigens and, as we shall see later, play a large part in the success of innate as well as acquired immunity.

In general, macrophages have two major functions. One, as their name ("large eater") implies, is to engulf and break down trapped materials into simple amino acids, sugars, and other substances for excretion or reuse, with the aid of the degradative enzymes in their lysosomal granules. Thus these cells play a key role in the removal of bacteria and parasites from the body. As noted above and discussed in detail in later chapters, the second major function of macrophages is to take up antigens, process them by denaturation or partial digestion, and present the fragments to antigen-specific T cells (i.e., the process of antigen presentation).

Dendritic Cells. *Dendritic cells* are long-lived and reside in an immature state in most tissues where they recognize and phagocytize pathogens and other antigens. They are found as *interdigitating cells of the thymus*. Dendritic cells found in the skin are called *Langerhans cells*. These cells are derived from the same hematopoietic precursor cells as monocytes. Direct contact of all dendritic cells with pathogens leads to their maturation and allows them to significantly increase in their antigen presentation capacity. Moreover, mature dendritic cells have the ability to activate naïve antigen-specific T cells. This is discussed in detail in subsequent chapters describing the cellular and molecular features of T-cell activation. Given these general properties of dendritic cells, it should be clear that these cells are important players in both innate immunity and the initiation of acquired immune responses.

Natural Killer Cells. Altered features of the membranes of abnormal cells, such as those found on virus-infected or cancer cells, are recognized by *natural killer (NK) cells*, which are cytotoxic. NK cells probably play a role in the early stages of viral infection or tumorogenesis, before the large numbers of activated cytotoxic T lymphocytes are generated. Histologically, NK cells

are large granular lymphocytes. The intracellular granules contain preformed biologically potent molecules that are released when NK cells make contact with target cells. Some of these molecules cause the formation of pores in the membrane of the target cell, leading to its lysis. Other molecules enter the target cell and cause *apoptosis* (programmed cell death) of the target cell by enhanced fragmentation of its nuclear DNA. Hence, they are able to lyse certain virus-infected cells and tumor cells without prior stimulation.

Unlike cytotoxic T lymphocytes, which recognize target cells in an antigen-specific fashion due to their expression of TCRs, NK cells lack antigen-specific receptors. How, then, do they seek and destroy their targets? They use a mechanism involving cell–cell contact, which allows them to determine whether a potential target cell has lost a particular self-antigen, namely, *MHC class I* molecules. MHC class I is expressed on virtually all nucleated cells. NK cells express receptors called *killer-cell inhibitory receptors (KIRs)*, which bind to MHC class I molecules expressed on normal cells. When KIRs bind to MHC class I molecules, intracellular signals are generated which cause inhibition of specific transcription factors. This results in inhibition of NK cell activation and subsequent degranulation and destruction of the target cells. Virus-infected or transformed (tumor) cells have significantly reduced numbers of MHC class I molecules on their surfaces. Thus, when such cells encounter NK cells, they fail to effectively engage KIRs and become susceptible to NK-cell-mediated cytotoxicity (Fig. 2.5)

Natural Killer T Cells. Recognized more than a decade ago, *natural killer T (NKT) cells* differentiate from thymic precursors through signals emanating from cortical thymocytes during TCR engagement. Like other T cells, these cells express TCRs, although with restricted

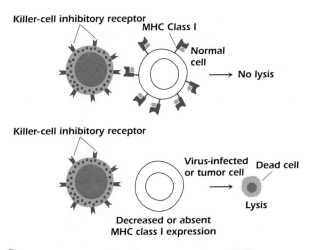

Figure 2.5. NK-cell inhibitory receptors and killing.

variability. Their semi-invariant TCRs recognize a mammalian glycosphingolipid (isoglobotrihexosylceramide) as well as microbial α-glycuronylceramides found in the cell walls of Gram-negative bacteria. NKT cells are unique in terms of their functional status because they fall somewhere between the innate and the adaptive immune systems. Following activation, they secrete several regulatory cytokines, including IL-4 and interferon-γ, and kill target cells via Fas–Fas ligand interactions, which cause apoptosis (see Chapter 10). NKT cells also regulate a range of immunopathologic conditions, but the mechanisms and the ligands involved remain unknown.

From these brief descriptions, you can see that each of the cellular components of the innate immune system has diverse roles in the achievement of two common goals: (1) eliminating foreign substances and pathogens from the host and (2) generating antigen-specific acquired immune responses that ultimately give rise to long-term immunity. Finally, as producers of an array of cytokines, these cells influence the functional properties of many other cell types within the immune system. For example, they can enhance the phagocytic activity of macrophages to enhance their killing of pathogens as well as the cytotoxic effects of NK cells. Thus, innate immune cells are pivotal players in strategies employed by the immune system to ensure protection of the host against infectious microorganisms. They are also called into play whenever physical barriers of defense are compromised (e.g., skin wounds). In either case, mobilization of innate immune cells following injury or infection generates a physiologic response known as inflammation, the topic of the next section.

Inflammation

An important function of phagocytic cells is their participation in inflammatory reactions. The word *inflammation* comes from the Latin *inflammare* ("to set on fire"). In some disorders the inflammatory process, which under normal conditions is self-limiting, becomes continuous, causing the development of chronic inflammatory diseases.

Inflammation, a major component of the body's defense mechanisms, is a physiologic process typically initiated by tissue damage from endogenous factors such as tissue necrosis or bone fracture as well as exogenous factors. Exogenous factors include mechanical injury (e.g., cuts), physical injury (e.g., burns), chemical injury (e.g., exposure to corrosive chemicals), immunologic injury (e.g., hypersensitivity reactions; see Chapters 14–16), and biologic injury (e.g., infections caused by pathogenic microorganisms; see Chapter 20). While perhaps paradoxical in light of the discomfort associated with certain types of inflammatory responses (e.g., hypersensitivity to poison ivy), inflammation is a normal immunologic process designed to restore immune homeostasis by bringing the injured tissue back to its normal state.

Hallmark Signs of Inflammation. The triad of clinical signs of inflammation are ***pain, redness***, and ***heat***. These can be explained by increased blood flow, elevated cellular metabolism, vasodilatation, release of soluble mediators, extravasation of fluids that move from the blood vessels to surrounding tissue, and cellular influx. Pain is caused by increased vascular diameter, which leads to increased blood flow, thereby causing heat and redness in the area. A subsequent reduction in blood velocity and concomitant cytokine- and kinin-induced increased expression of adhesion molecules on the endothelial cells lining the blood vessel promote the binding of circulating leukocytes to the vessel. These events facilitate the attachment and entry of leukocytes into tissues and the recruitment of neutrophils and monocytes to the site of inflammation. Another major change in the local blood vessels is increased vascular permeability. This results from the separation of the tightly joined endothelial cells lining the blood vessels, which leads to the exit of fluid and proteins from the blood and their accumulation in the tissue. These events account for the swelling (*edema*) associated with inflammation, which contributes significantly to the pain and attendant redness and heat associated with the accumulation of cells at the site.

Within minutes after injury, the inflammatory process begins with the activation and increased concentration of pharmacologically powerful substances, including proteins known as ***acute-phase proteins***. The emerging ***acute-phase response*** induces additional responses, both localized and systemic. Localized inflammatory responses are generated, in part, as a result of the activation of the kinins and the coagulation system (clotting).

Localized Inflammatory Responses. Once activated, the ***kinins*** have several important localized effects on cells and organ systems:

- They act directly on local smooth muscle and cause muscle contraction.
- They act on axons to block nervous impulses, leading to a distal muscle relaxation.
- Most important, kinins such as the vasoactive peptide bradykinin act on vascular endothelial cells, causing them to contract (leading to an increase in vascular permeability) and to express ***endothelial cell adhesion molecules*** (ECAMs), leading to leukocyte adhesion and extravasation.
- Kinins are very potent nerve stimulators and are the molecules most responsible for pain (and itching) associated with inflammation.

Kinins are rapidly inactivated by proteases generated during these localized responses.

The **coagulation pathway** consists of plasma enzymes that are activated in a cascading manner following damage to blood vessels. Its role in the inflammatory response is to form a physical barrier (**clot**) that prevents microorganisms from entering the bloodstream. The simultaneous activation of kinins and the coagulation system during inflammatory responses thus produce inhospitable conditions for invading pathogens as well as new physical barriers to limit their ability to use the circulatory system to gain entry to distal tissues and organs.

Systemic Inflammatory Responses. Systemic inflammatory responses include the induction of fever (discussed below), increased white blood cell production, increased synthesis of hydrocortisone and adrenocorticotropic hormone (ACTH), and production of the acute-phase proteins (see Chapter 11). An important acute-phase protein is *C-reactive protein*, which is capable of binding to certain microorganisms and activating the complement system (Chapter 13). This results in the lysis of the microorganism, enhanced phagocytosis by phagocytic cells, and several other important host defense functions, as you shall see later.

Cytokines play a key role in the inflammatory response. IL-1, IL-6, and tumor necrosis factor-α (TNF-α) are among the most important *proinflammatory cytokines* involved (Chapter 11). As noted above, these cytokines, are released principally by activated macrophages and induce the expression of adhesion molecules on the membranes of vascular endothelial cells to which neutrophils, monocytes, and lymphocytes adhere before moving out of the vessel—a process called *extravasation*—to the affected tissue. These cytokines also promote coagulation and increased vascular permeability. Other cytokines, including IL-8 and interferon-γ, exert additional effects, such as increased leukocyte chemotaxis and activation of phagocytes. All these effects result in edema and the accumulation of leukocytes in the injured areas. The response becomes amplified as additional biologically active compounds are transported to the site and released from the accumulated cells, attracting and activating still more cells.

Most of the cells involved in inflammatory responses are phagocytic cells, primarily PMN leukocytes. The PMN leukocytes accumulate within 30–60 min, phagocytize the intruder, and release their lysosomal enzymes in an attempt to destroy the intruder. If the cause of the inflammatory response persists, within 4–6 h the area harboring the invading microorganism or foreign substance will be infiltrated by macrophages and lymphocytes. The macrophages supplement the phagocytic activity of the PMN leukocytes. They also process and present antigens to T cells, which then generate antigen-specific responses.

Activated T cells synthesize and release a variety of cytokines, which proactively stimulate antigen-specific B cells, facilitating antibody production. Within five to seven days, antibodies produced by these B cells are detectable as serum antibodies and thus become part of the humoral immune defense arsenal.

Chronic Inflammation. Many substances activated during the inflammatory process participate in repairing the injury. During this remarkable process, many cells, including leukocytes, are being destroyed. The macrophages present in the area phagocytize the debris, the inflammation subsides, and a state of homeostasis at the site of injury is restored. Under these conditions, the tissue returns to its normal state or scar tissue may be formed.

Sometimes it is difficult or impossible to remove the causes of inflammation. *Chronic inflammation* occurs in situations of chronic infection (e.g., tuberculosis) or chronic activation of the immune response (e.g., rheumatoid arthritis and glomerulonephritis). In such cases, the inflammatory response continues and can be modified only temporarily by the administration of anti-inflammatory agents such as aspirin, ibuprofen, and cortisone. These agents, other drugs, and biologic therapies act on several of the metabolic pathways involved in the elaboration and activation of the pharmacologic mediators of inflammation. However, they do not affect the root cause of the inflammation; when they are withdrawn, the symptoms may return.

Fever

Although *fever*, an elevation in body temperature, is one of the most common manifestations of infection and inflammation, there is still limited information about the significance of fever in the course of infection in mammals. Fever is caused by many bacterial products, most notably the *endotoxins* of Gram-negative bacteria. Fever results when cytokines called *endogenous pyrogens* are produced by innate immune cells (monocytes and macrophages) in response to the presence of endotoxins. Examples of cytokines with endogenous pyrogenic properties include IL-1 and certain interferons (see Chapter 11). Cells in other tissues can also produce these cytokines. For example, the keratinocytes present in skin contain IL-1. Interestingly, when the skin is overexposed to the ultraviolet rays of the sun (sunburn), keratinocytes are physically damaged, causing the release of their contents, including IL-1. Within a few hours, the increased IL-1 levels can cause fever, with accompanying chills and malaise—a phenomenon you may have experienced after a summer day at the beach. Fortunately, a variety of topical sunscreens can block ultraviolet rays, preventing both sunburn and fever.

Biologically Active Substances

Many tissues also synthesize substances that are harmful to microorganisms. Examples are *degradative enzymes, toxic free radicals, and acute-phase proteins*. Certain interferons also have the ability to interfere with viral replication, making them components of our innate defense arsenal. In short, depending on their ability to synthesize substances that act directly or indirectly to kill microorganisms, many tissues may have a heightened resistance to infection by some infectious pathogens.

Receptors Involved in the Innate Immune System

The innate immune system lacks the specificity of the B and T cells of the acquired immune system, which use clonally expressed, antigen-specific receptors to recognize and respond to antigens (BCRs TCRs, respectively). Instead, innate immune cells utilize a diverse set of membrane receptors that are not clonally expressed to recognize antigen. Unlike BCRs and TCRs, these innate receptors are encoded in the germline of these cells. Therefore, all members of cells of the same lineage (e.g., monocytes/macrophages) express identical receptors.

In the section that follows, we focus our discussion of innate immunity receptors on their utility in host cell recognition of microorganisms. As you might expect, the

microbial molecules to which these receptors bind are not present on host cells, so they are recognized as foreign.

Pattern Recognition Receptors

Microbes display highly conserved molecules on their surface that are often referred to as *molecular patterns*. The recognition of these signatures of certain classes of pathogens by *pattern recognition receptors* leads to a range of responses by the host. These innate receptors, like pieces of a puzzle, "fit" with a distinct pattern of a corresponding "piece" of a pathogen. Host defense outcomes depend on the effector cell engaged and the receptor type involved. The innate immune system has evolved to take advantage of these patterns which, in effect, serve as flags alerting responding cells to the presence of an invading microorganism.

One class of pattern recognition receptor is the *Toll-like receptor* (*TLR*). The Toll gene family was originally studied for its contribution to dorsoventral patterning in *Drosophila melanogaster* embryos. Later studies showed that Toll genes encode proteins that play a critical role in the fly's innate immune response to microbial infection. Further investigation confirmed the existence of homologous proteins in mammals (TLRs) that can activate phagocytes and tissue dendritic cells in response to pathogens. TLRs are a large family of receptors, each of which recognizes specific microbial

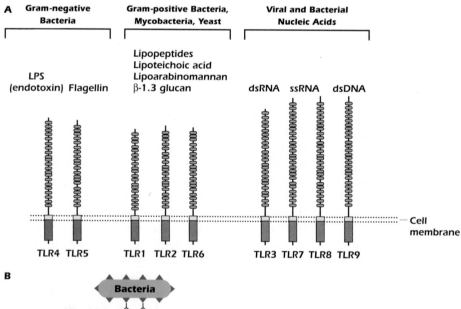
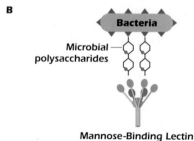

Figure 2.6. (A) Pattern recognition receptors called TLRs binding to molecules with specific pattern motifs expressed by various pathogens. (B) Soluble MB lectin binding to bacterial polysacchrides (terminal mannose residues in this case).

molecular patterns. Activation of cells expressing TLRs following receptor ligation also facilitates initiation of acquired immune responses due to the production of proinflammatory cytokines by these activated cells (Fig. 2.6). This phenomenon illustrates, yet again, the important relationship between the innate and acquired immune systems.

As you have learned, TLRs play a crucial role in innate cell recognition of extracellular pathogens. Another group of pattern recognition receptors, called nucleotide-binding oligomerization domain (NOD)–like receptors (NLRs), are cytosolic receptors that recognize and alert cells to invasion by intracellular pathogens. NLRs are activated by characteristic bacterially derived molecules, such as peptidoglycan, ribonucleic acid (RNA), toxins, and flagellin, in the cytosol. NLRs contain a central nucleotide-binding oligomerization domain (NACHT), an N-terminal effector-binding domain, and C-terminal leucine-rich repeats (LRRs). Following the binding of these microbial molecules, NLRs initiate a program of cellular activities that facilitate inflammatory responses and other host defense mechanisms. Recent studies have described the genetic association of mutations in NLR genes with several chronic inflammatory barrier diseases, such as Crohn's disease and asthma, and with rare autoinflammatory syndromes, including familial cold urticaria, Muckle–Wells syndrome, and Blau syndrome.

Phagocytes utilize pattern recognition receptors to facilitate their physical attachment to microbes and other substances—a process that initiates phagocytosis. A second class of pattern recognition receptor involved in this phenomenon is the *mannan-binding (MB) lectin*. MB lectin allows phagocytes to recognize microbial polysaccharides with a sugar composition and residue spacing not found on host cells. Ligation (binding) of the phagocyte MB lectin with these sugars initiates and activates the MB lectin pathway of complement (Fig. 2.6B; discussed further in Chapter 13). This results in the generation of specific complement components that innately coat the microorganism triggering the response—a process known as *opsonization*—by virtue of their affinity for other molecular patterns. Coating microbes with complement makes them more susceptible to phagocytosis. How does this happen? Phagocytes express receptors for certain complement components; when these components are bound to microorganisms, they serve as a bridge to facilitate close contact between the phagocyte and the microbe and, ultimately, cause phagocytosis (see Chapter 13).

A third type of pattern recognition receptor is the *scavenger receptor*. These receptors recognize specific anionic polymers and acetylated low-density lipoproteins expressed by certain pathogens. They also recognize dying (*effete*) red blood cells, leading to the removal of these cells. The removal of red blood cells is carried out mainly within the spleen, which contains large numbers of macrophages expressing scavenger receptors.

Finally, certain cells within the innate immune system play a role in mobilizing other host defense cells to the site of infection. How do these cells sound the alarm? One way is through their recognition of N-formylated peptides expressed by certain bacteria. Neutrophils express the *f-Met–Leu–Phe receptor* which specifically binds to N-formylated peptides. Ligation of N-formylated peptides expressed by microbes to the f-Met–Leu–Phe receptor on neutrophils causes the neutrophils to increase the expression of adherence molecules. The adherence molecules facilitate the binding of neutrophils to vascular endothelial cells. This is advantageous to the host for several reasons. First, the site of infection becomes infiltrated with large numbers of neutrophils which can rapidly participate in the innate immune response that is already underway. Second, cytokines released by neutrophils serve as chemotactic factors that attract other immune cells of both the innate and acquired immune systems to the site of infection. This process will be discussed in more detail in Chapter 11.

ACQUIRED IMMUNITY

When an infectious organism is not eliminated by innate immune mechanisms, acquired immune responses ensue with the generation of *antigen-specific lymphocytes* (effector cells) and *memory cells* that can prevent reinfection with the same organism. These responses (sometimes called adaptive immune responses) take more time to develop (>96 h) because the rare B and T cells specific for the invading microorganism must undergo clonal expansion before they can differentiate into effector cells to help eliminate the infection. In contrast to innate immunity, which is an attribute of virtually every living organism in one form or another, *acquired immunity* is a more specialized form of immunity. It developed late in evolution and is found only in vertebrates. As discussed earlier in this chapter, the various elements that participate in innate immunity exhibit broad specificity against foreign agents by recognizing molecules not found in the host (e.g., N-formylated peptides). By contrast, acquired immunity always exhibits antigenic specificity. As its name implies, acquired immunity is a consequence of an encounter with a foreign substance. The first encounter with a particular foreign substance triggers a chain of events that stimulates an acquired immune response with specificity against that foreign substance, often referred to as *primary immune responses*. Details of how this happens within the B- and T-cell lineages will be presented in the chapters that follow.

CELLS AND ORGANS INVOLVED IN ACQUIRED IMMUNITY

In contrast with innate immunity, acquired immune responses are antigen-specific. As we have already discussed, the effector cells responsible for acquired immune responses are the B and T cells. B cells expressing antigen-specific BCRs synthesize and secrete antibody into the bloodstream. This is often termed *humoral immunity*. T cells, which also exhibit antigen specificity by virtue of their expression of antigen-specific, TCRs, do not make antibodies. Their participation in acquired immune responses is as varied as the T-cell subsets and cytokines they produce. Historically, T-cell-mediated responses are often referred to as *cell-mediated responses* or *cellular immunity*.

Unlike B cells, which express BCRs that bind directly to antigens for which they are specific, T cells are incapable of binding to antigens by themselves. They recognize and bind to antigenic peptides when they come in contact with *APC* such as macrophages and dendritic cells which display processed, MHC-bound peptides derived from the antigen. However, even this APC-dependent recognition of peptides is insufficient to activate the responding T cell. Two signals are required to activate T cells: (1) T-cell expression of peptide (epitope)–specific TCRs and (2) ligation of costimulatory molecules expressed by T cells with complementary membrane molecules expressed by APC. The costimulatory signaling step initiates a cascade of intracellular and nuclear events that measurably change the behavior of responding T cells. Thus, T cells begin to express and release new gene products (e.g., cytokines), they undergo clonal expansion to increase the number of TCR-expressing cells within the T-cell repertoire, and they differentiate to create a pool of memory cells. These events occur in the secondary lymphoid organs (lymph nodes and spleen), which you will learn more about in the next section of this chapter.

T-cell activation greatly facilitates the activation and differentiation of B cells responding to antigen. This is achieved primarily by the binding of T-cell-derived cytokines to specific cytokine receptors expressed by B cells. Functional consequences of this assistance from T cells include B-cell proliferation, generation of memory B cells, and diversification of the kinds of immunoglobulins produced (class switching). The recurring theme of cytokine involvement in normal immune responses is underscored by the fact that B cells are dependent on T cells for optimal antibody responses to most antigens; thus, these antigens are often referred to as *T-cell-dependent antigens*.

The Lymphatic Organs

The lymphatic system includes organs in which lymphocyte maturation, differentiation, and proliferation take place. They are generally divided into two categories, primary and secondary organs. The *primary or central lymphoid organs* are those in which the maturation of B and T lymphocytes into antigen-recognizing lymphocytes occurs. In other words, functional antigen-specific BCRs and TCRs are expressed by B and T cells, respectively, in these organs. Mature B cells differentiate to fully mature cells within the *bone marrow*. Historically, the term "B cell" derived from developmental studies in birds which demonstrated that antibody-forming lymphocytes differentiate within an organ unique to birds called the *bursa of Fabricius* (hence, "B" for bursa). In contrast, T cells differentiate only partially within the bone marrow. Precursor cells destined to become mature T cells undergo final maturation within the *thymus gland* (hence, "T" for thymus). Histologic characteristics of the thymus are discussed in the next section.

Mature B and T cells migrate through the bloodstream and lymphatic system to the peripheral lymphoid tissues, including the lymph nodes and spleen, collectively referred to as the *secondary lymphoid organs*. It is here that antigen-driven activation (proliferation and differentiation) of B and T cells takes place (Fig. 2.7). Histologic properties of the secondary lymphoid organs are also presented below.

The Thymus Gland: A Primary Lymphoid Organ.
The thymus gland is a bilobed structure derived from the endoderm of the third and fourth pharyngeal pouches (Fig. 2.8). During fetal development, the size of the thymus increases. At puberty growth of the thymus stops, and the organ atrophies slowly throughout adulthood.

The thymus is a *lymphoepithelial* organ. It consists of epithelial cells organized into *cortical* (outer) and *medullary* (central) areas that are infiltrated with lymphoid cells (*thymocytes*). The cortex is densely populated with lymphocytes of various sizes, most of which are immature, and scattered macrophages involved in clearing apoptotic thymocytes.

Secondary Lymphoid Organs.
The secondary lymphoid organs have two major functions: (1) They are highly efficient in trapping and concentrating foreign substances and (2) they are the main sites of production of antibodies and the induction of antigen-specific T lymphocytes. The major secondary lymphoid organs are the *spleen* and the *lymph nodes*. In addition, the tonsils, the appendix, clusters of lymphocytes distributed in the lining of the small intestine (*Peyer's patches*), and lymphoid aggregates spread throughout mucosal tissue are considered secondary lymphoid organs. Lymphoid aggregates are

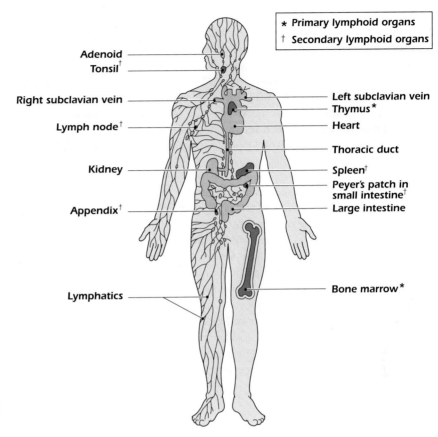

* Primary lymphoid organs
† Secondary lymphoid organs

Adenoid
Tonsil†
Right subclavian vein
Lymph node†
Kidney
Appendix†
Lymphatics

Left subclavian vein
Thymus*
Heart
Thoracic duct
Spleen†
Peyer's patch in small intestine†
Large intestine
Bone marrow*

Figure 2.7: Distribution of lymphoid tissues in the body.

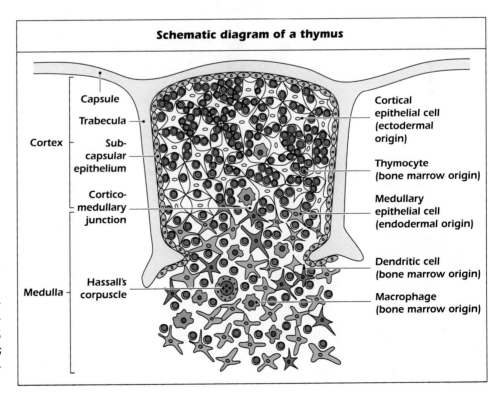

Schematic diagram of a thymus

Cortex
Capsule
Trabecula
Sub-capsular epithelium
Cortico-medullary junction

Medulla
Hassall's corpuscle

Cortical epithelial cell (ectodermal origin)
Thymocyte (bone marrow origin)
Medullary epithelial cell (endodermal origin)
Dendritic cell (bone marrow origin)
Macrophage (bone marrow origin)

Figure 2.8. Cellular organization of the thymus. (Reproduced with permission from FS Rosen and RS Geha, *Case Studies in Immunology*, Garland Publishing.)

found in various areas of the body, such as the linings of the digestive tract, the respiratory and genitourinary tracts, the conjunctiva, and the salivary glands, where mature lymphocytes interact with antigen and undergo activation. These mucosal lymphoid organs have been given the name *mucosa-associated lymphoid tissue* (MALT). Those lymphoid tissues associated with the gut are termed *gut-associated lymphoid tissue* (GALT); those associated with the bronchial tree are often referred to as *bronchus-associated lymphoid tissue* (BALT).

The Spleen.   The spleen is the largest of the secondary lymphoid organs (Fig. 2.9) and is highly efficient in trapping and concentrating foreign substances carried in the blood. It is the major organ in the body in which antibodies are synthesized and from which they are released into the circulation. The spleen is composed of *white pulp*, rich in lymphoid cells, and *red pulp*, which contains many sinuses as well as large quantities of erythrocytes and macrophages, some lymphocytes, and a few other cell types.

The areas of white pulp are located mainly around small arterioles with peripheral regions rich in T cells; B cells are present mainly in germinal centers. Approximately 50% of spleen cells are B lymphocytes; 30–40% are T lymphocytes. After antigenic stimulation, the germinal centers contain large numbers of B cells and plasma cells. These cells synthesize and release antibodies.

Lymph Nodes.   Lymph nodes are small ovoid structures (normally <1 cm in diameter) found in various regions throughout the body (Fig. 2.10). They are close to major junctions of the lymphatic channels, which are connected to the thoracic duct. The thoracic duct transports lymph and lymphocytes to the vena cava, the vessel that carries blood to the right side of the heart (Fig. 2.11). From there they are redistributed throughout the body.

Lymph nodes are composed of a medulla with many sinuses and a cortex, which is surrounded by a capsule of connective tissue (Fig. 2.10A). The cortical region contains primary *lymphoid follicles*. After antigenic stimulation, these structures enlarge to form secondary lymphoid follicles with germinal centers containing dense populations of lymphocytes (mostly B cells) that are undergoing mitosis. In response to antigen stimulation, antigen-specific B cells proliferating within these germinal centers also undergo a process known as *affinity maturation* to generate clones of cells that produce high-affinity antigen-specific antibodies

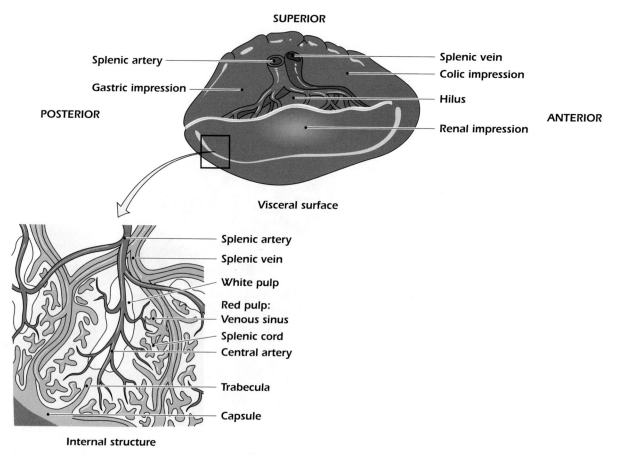

Figure 2.9. Overall and section views of the spleen.

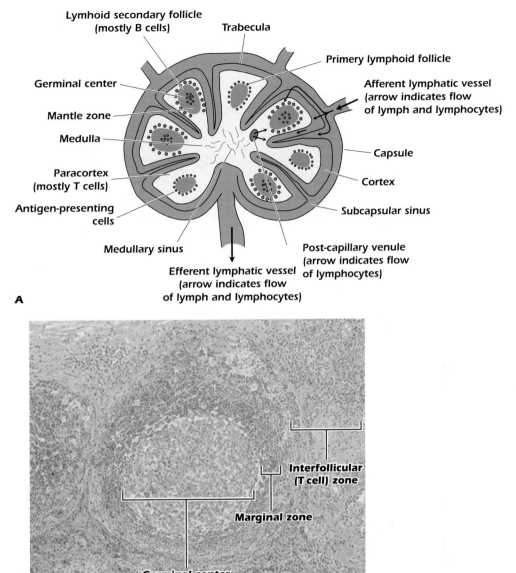

Figure 2.10. (A) Section of a lymph node. Arrows represent the flow of lymph and lymphocytes. (B) Section through a lymph node showing T-cell zone, marginal zone, and germinal center.

(see Chapter 7). The remaining antigen-nonspecific B cells are pushed to the outside to form the mantle zone. The deep cortical area, or *paracortical region*, contains T cells and dendritic cells. Antigens are brought into these areas by dendritic cells, which present antigenic peptides to T cells, resulting in T-cell activation. The medullary area of the lymph node contains antibody-secreting plasma cells that have traveled from the cortex to the medulla via lymphatic vessels.

Lymphocyte Migration and Recirculation

Lymph nodes are highly efficient in trapping antigen that enters through the *afferent lymphatic vessels*. Within the lymph node, antigens interact with macrophages, T cells, and B cells, and that interaction brings about an immune response, manifested by the generation of antibodies and antigen-specific T cells. Lymph, antibodies, and cells leave the lymph node through the efferent lymphatic vessel, which is just below the medullary region.

Blood lymphocytes enter the lymph nodes through *postcapillary venules* and leave the lymph nodes through *efferent lymphatic vessels*, which eventually converge in the *thoracic duct*. This duct empties into the *vena cava*, the vessel that returns the blood to the *heart*, thus providing for the continual recirculation of lymphocytes (Fig. 2.11).

The spleen functions in a similar manner. Arterial blood lymphocytes enter the spleen through the hilus and pass into the trabecular artery, which along its course becomes narrow and branched. At the farthest branches of the trabecular artery, capillaries lead to lymphoid

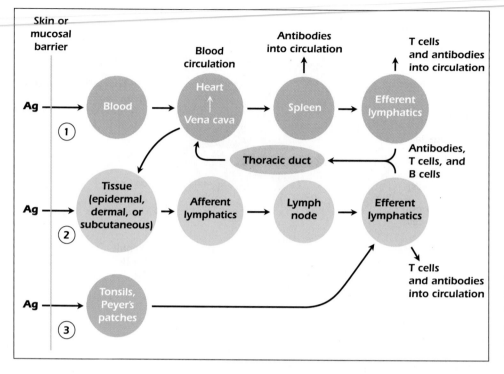

Figure 2.11. Circulation of lymph and fate of antigen following penetration through (1) bloodstream, (2) skin, and (3) gastrointestinal or respiratory tract.

nodules. Ultimately, the lymphocytes return to the venous circulation through the trabecular vein. Like lymph nodes, the spleen contains efferent lymphatic vessels. Through the efferent lymphatic vessels the lymph empties into the lymphatics, is recirculated throughout the body, and returns to the afferent vessels.

The migration of lymphocytes between various lymphoid and nonlymphoid tissues and their *homing* to a particular site is highly regulated by means of various *cell surface adhesion molecules* (CAMs) and their receptors. With the exception of the spleen, where small arterioles end in the parenchyma, blood lymphocytes must generally cross the endothelial vascular lining of postcapillary vascular sites, termed **high endothelial venules** (HEVs), in a process called *extravasation*. Recirculating lymphocytes selectively bind to specific receptors on the HEV of lymphoid tissue or inflammatory tissue spaces and appear to completely ignore other vascular endothelium. In addition, it appears that there is more selective binding between the HEV and various distinct subsets of lymphocytes, further regulating the migration of lymphocytes into the various lymphoid and nonlymphoid tissues. Recirculating monocytes and granulocytes express adhesion molecule receptors and migrate to tissue sites using a similar mechanism.

The migration of lymphocytes between lymphoid and nonlymphoid tissues ensures that, upon exposure to an antigen, the antigen and the lymphocytes specific to that antigen are sequestered in the lymphoid tissue, where the lymphocytes undergo proliferation and differentiation. This results in expansion of antigen-specific B and

T lymphocytes as well as long-lived, antigen-specific memory cells. The latter are disseminated throughout the secondary lymphoid tissues to ensure long-lasting immunity to the antigen.

FATE OF ANTIGEN AFTER PENETRATION

The RES is designed to trap foreign antigens that have penetrated the body and to subject them to ingestion and degradation by the phagocytic cells of the system. Also, there is constant movement of lymphocytes throughout the body, and this movement permits deposition of lymphocytes in strategic places along the lymphatic vessels. The system not only traps antigens but also provides locations (the secondary lymphoid organs) where antigen, macrophages, T cells, and B cells can interact within a very small area to initiate an immune response.

The fate of an antigen that has penetrated the body's physical barriers and confronted the cellular and antibody components of the ensuing immune response is shown in Figure 2.11. Three major routes may be followed by an antigen after it has entered the body:

- Antigen entering the body through the bloodstream is carried through circulatory system to the spleen where it interacts with APC, such as dendritic cells and macrophages. As we have discussed earlier, a major function of these APC is to take up, process, and then present components of the antigen to the T cells that express the appropriate antigen-specific TCR. This interaction, together with the other costimulatory signals derived from cell–cell interaction, activates the T cells. Splenic B cells expressing antigen-specific BCRs are also activated following exposure to antigen—a process facilitated by the cytokines produced by antigen-activated T cells.

- Antigens may lodge in the epidermal, dermal, or subcutaneous tissues to stimulate inflammatory responses. From these tissues, the antigen, either free or trapped by APC, is transported through the afferent lymphatic channels into the regional draining lymph node. In the lymph node, the antigen, macrophages, dendritic cells, T cells, and B cells interact to generate an immune response. After synthesis in the lymph node, antigen-specific T cells and antibodies enter the circulation and are transported to the various tissues. Antigen-specific T and B cells and antibodies also enter the circulation via the thoracic duct.

- The antigen may enter the gastrointestinal or respiratory tract, where it lodges in the MALT and interacts with macrophages and lymphocytes. Antibodies synthesized in these organs are deposited in the local tissue. In addition, lymphocytes entering the efferent lymphatics are carried through the thoracic duct to the circulation and redistributed to various tissues.

Frequency of Antigen-Specific Naïve Lymphocytes

It has been estimated that in a *naïve* (nonimmunized) animal, only one in every 10^3–10^5 lymphocytes is capable of recognizing a typical antigen. Therefore, the probability that an antigen will encounter these cells is very low.

The problem is compounded by the fact that two different kinds of lymphocytes, the T and B lymphocytes, each with specificity against this particular antigen, must interact for synthesis of antibody to ensue.

Statistically, the chances for the interaction of specific T lymphocytes with their particular antigen and then with B lymphocytes specific for the same antigen are very low. However, nature has devised an ingenious mechanism for bringing these cells into contact with antigen: The antigen is carried via the draining lymphatics to the secondary lymphoid organs. In these organs, the antigen is exposed on the surface of fixed specialized cells. Because both T and B lymphocytes circulate at a rather rapid rate, making the rounds every several days, some circulating lymphocytes with specificity for the particular antigen should pass by the antigen within a relatively short time. When these lymphocytes encounter the antigen for which they are specific, the lymphocytes become activated, and the acquired immune response, with specificity against this antigen, is triggered.

● INTERRELATIONSHIP BETWEEN INNATE AND ACQUIRED IMMUNITY

The innate and acquired branches of the immune system have developed a beautiful interrelationship. The intricate and ingenious communication among the various cytokines and cell adhesion molecules allows components of innate and acquired immunity to interact, send signals, activate one another, and work together toward the final goal of destroying and eliminating the invading microorganism and its products. The interrelationship between innate and acquired immunity is summarized in Figure 2.12.

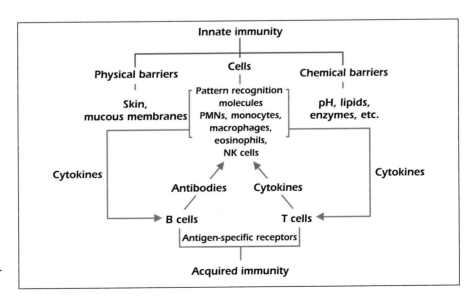

Figure 2.12. Interrelationship between innate and acquired immunity.

SUMMARY

1. There are two forms of immunity: innate and acquired.

2. Innate immune responses are rapid (minutes to hours); acquired immune responses require more time (days).

3. Unlike acquired immunity, innate immunity does not exhibit memory to antigenic exposure.

4. Many non-cellular and cellular elements participate in innate immunity, including various physical barriers (e.g., skin), chemical barriers (e.g., low pH in stomach), pattern recognition receptors (e.g., TLRs), phagocytes, NK cells, etc.

5. Two major types of cells participate as effector cells in acquired immunity: B and T cells.

6. Macrophages constitute an essential part of the RES and function to trap, process, and present antigen to T cells, thus assuming an important function in both innate and acquired immunity.

7. B and T cells express antigen-specific receptors, namely BCRs and TCRs, respectively.

8. Precursor cells of the B and T lineages are found in the bone marrow—a primary lymphoid organ.

B lymphocytes fully differentiate within the bone marrow to become mature B cells.

9. T cells are derived from the same lymphoid progenitor cells as B cells and differentiate in the thymus to become functional cells before migrating to the peripheral lymphoid organs.

10. Mature B and T lymphocytes differentiate and proliferate in response to antigenic stimulation. These events generally take place in secondary lymphoid organs.

11. B lymphocytes synthesize and secrete antibodies. T lymphocytes participate in cell-mediated immunity; they help B cells make antibodies by providing them with soluble growth and differentiation factors (cytokines) needed for B-cell activation. They also participate in various other regulatory aspects of the immune response by releasing cytokines.

12. Lymphocytes continuously recirculate among the blood, lymph, lymphoid organs, and tissues. Receptors on lymphocytes interact with CAMs located on specialized HEVs, facilitating extravasation to tissue sites where immune-cell activation occurs.

REFERENCES

Aderem A, Underhill DM (1999): Mechanisms of phagocytosis in macrophages. *Annu Rev Immunol* 17: 593.

Akira S, Takeda K, Kaiso T (2001): Toll-like receptors: Critical proteins linking innate and acquired immunity. *Nature Immunol* 2: 675.

Beutler B, Jiang Z, Georgel P, Crozat P, Croker B, Rutschmann S, Du X, Hoebe K (2007): Genetic analysis of host resistance:

Toll-like receptor signaling and immunity at large. *Annu Rev Immunol* 24: 353.

Lanier, LL (1998): NK cell receptors. *Annu Rev Immunol* 16: 359.

Pancer Z, Cooper MD (2007): The evolution of adaptive immunity. *Annu Rev Immunol* 24: 497.

Stekel DJ, Parker CE, Nowak MA (1997): A model for lymphocyte recirculation. *Immunol Today* 18: 216.

 REVIEW QUESTIONS

For each question, choose the ONE BEST answer.

1. Which of the following generally does *not* apply to bone marrow (a primary lymphoid organ)?
   A) cellular proliferation
   B) differentiation of lymphocytes
   C) cellular interaction
   D) antigen-dependent responses

2. Which of the following applies uniquely to secondary lymphoid organs?

   A) presence of precursor B and T cells
   B) circulation of lymphocytes
   C) terminal differentiation
   D) cellular proliferation

3. Recognition of intracellular pathogens in innate immune cells involves
   A) Toll-like receptors (TLRs)
   B) antibody
   C) NOD-like receptors (NLRs)
   D) NKT cells

4. The major function of the lymphoid system is:
   A) innate immunity
   B) inflammation
   C) phagocytosis
   D) acquired immunity

5. Removal of the bursa of Fabricius from a chicken results in:
   A) a markedly decreased number of circulating T lymphocytes
   B) anemia.
   C) a delayed rejection of skin grafts
   D) low serum levels of antibodies
   E) a deficient innate immunity

6. The germinal centers found in the cortical region of lymph nodes and the peripheral region of splenic periarteriolar lymphatic tissue:
   A) support the development of immature B and T cells
   B) remove damaged erythrocytes from the circulation
   C) act as the major source of stem cells and thus help maintain hematopoiesis
   D) provide an infrastructure that on antigenic stimulation contains large populations of B lymphocytes and plasma cells
   E) are the sites of NKT-cell differentiation

7. Which of these statements about NK cells is true?
   A) They proliferate in response to antigen.
   B) They kill target cells by phagocytosis and intracellular digestion.
   C) They are a subset of polymorphonuclear cells.
   D) They kill target cells in an extracellular fashion.
   E) They are particularly effective against certain bacteria.

8. Mature dendritic cells are capable of which of the following?
   A) activation of naïve antigen-specific T cells
   B) removal of red blood cells
   C) production of bradykinin
   D) extracellular killing of target cells

ANSWERS TO REVIEW QUESTIONS

1. *D* Cellular proliferation, differentiation of lymphocytes, and cellular interactions can take place in the bone marrow (or the bursa of Fabricius in birds). However, antigen-dependent responses occur only in the secondary lymphoid organs, such as the spleen and lymph nodes.

2. *C* Terminal differentiation of B cells into plasma cells occurs only in secondary lymphoid organs, such as the spleen and lymph nodes. Circulation of lymphocytes and cellular proliferation take place in both the primary and secondary lymphoid organs. The bone marrow, a primary lymphoid organ, is the site where pluripotent stem cells differentiate into precursor B and T cells.

3. *C* The NLRs are a group of cytosolic innate receptors that recognize microbes that infect cells. Once ligated, they initiate a set of cellular activities that facilitate inflammatory responses and other host defense mechanisms.

4. *D* The major function of the lymphoid system is the recognition of foreign antigen by lymphocytes, which leads to the acquired immune response. Functions such as phagocytosis and inflammation do not necessarily require the lymphoid system, and they constitute part of innate immunity.

5. *D* Removal of the bursa of Fabricius from a chicken results in low levels of antibodies in serum, since this organ serves as a primary lymphoid organ in which B lymphocytes (which eventually synthesize and secrete antibodies) undergo maturation. The removal of the organ will not result in a marked decrease in the number of circulating T lymphocytes or in anemia, characterized by a marked decrease in erythrocyte count, since erythrocytes undergo maturation outside the bursa. Bursectomy has no effect on rejection of skin grafts.

6. *D* On antigenic stimulation, the germinal centers contain large populations of B lymphocytes undergoing mitosis and plasma cells secreting antibodies. Virgin immunocompetent lymphocytes are developed in the primary lymphoid organs, not in the secondary lymphoid organs, such as the spleen and lymph nodes. Germinal centers do not participate in the removal of damaged erythrocytes, and are not a source of stem cells; stem cells are found in the bone marrow.

7. *D* NK cells are large granular lymphocytes. Their number does not increase in response to antigen. Their killing is extracellular, and their target cells are virus-infected cells or tumor cells. They are not particularly effective against bacterial cells.

8. *A* When immature dendritic cells are activated following phagocytosis of pathogens, they mature and become more efficient at antigen presentation and, in fact, can activate antigen-specific naïve T cells.

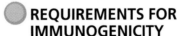

IMMUNOGENS AND ANTIGENS

 INTRODUCTION

Immune responses arise as a result of exposure to foreign stimuli. The compound that evokes the response is referred to as either antigen or immunogen. The distinction between these terms is functional. An ***antigen*** is any agent capable of binding specifically to components of the immune system, such as the BCR on B lymphocytes and soluble antibodies. By contrast, an ***immunogen*** is any agent capable of inducing an immune response and is therefore ***immunogenic***. The distinction between the terms is necessary because there are many compounds that are incapable of inducing an immune response, yet they are capable of binding with components of the immune system that have been induced specifically against them. Thus all immunogens are antigens, but not all antigens are immunogens. This difference becomes obvious in the case of low-molecular-weight compounds, a group of substances that includes many antibiotics and drugs. By themselves, each of these compounds is incapable of inducing an immune response, but when coupled with a much larger entity, such as a protein, the resultant conjugate induces an immune response that is directed against various parts of the conjugate, including the low-molecular-weight compound. When manipulated in this manner, the low-molecular-weight compound is referred to as a ***hapten*** (from the Greek *hapten*, which means "to grasp"); the high-molecular-weight compound

to which the hapten is conjugated is referred to as a ***carrier***. Thus a hapten is a compound that, by itself, is incapable of inducing an immune response; however, an immune response can be induced against the hapten when it is conjugated to a carrier.

Immune responses have been demonstrated against all the known biochemical families of compounds, including carbohydrates, lipids, proteins, and nucleic acids. Similarly, immune responses to drugs, antibiotics, food additives, cosmetics, and small synthetic peptides can also be induced, but only when these are coupled to a carrier. In this chapter, we discuss the major attributes of compounds that render them antigenic and immunogenic.

 REQUIREMENTS FOR IMMUNOGENICITY

A substance must possess the following characteristics to be immunogenic: (1) foreignness, (2) high molecular weight, (3) chemical complexity, and in most cases (4) degradability and interaction with the host's MHC.

Foreignness

Animals normally do not respond immunologically to self. Thus, for example, if a rabbit is injected with its own serum albumin, it will not mount an immune response;

Immunology: A Short Course, Sixth Edition, By Richard Coico and Geoffrey Sunshine
Copyright © 2009 John Wiley & Sons, Inc.

it recognizes the albumin as self. By contrast, if rabbit serum albumin is injected into a guinea pig, the guinea pig recognizes the rabbit serum albumin as foreign and mounts an immune response because it recognizes the substance as foreign. Thus, the first requirement for a compound to be immunogenic is foreignness. The more foreign the substance, the more immunogenic it is.

In general, compounds that are part of self are not immunogenic to the individual. However, there are exceptional cases in which an individual mounts an immune response against his or her own tissues. This condition is termed autoimmunity (see Chapter 12).

High Molecular Weight

The second requirement for immunogenicity is a certain minimum molecular weight. In general, small compounds that have a molecular weight less than 1000 Da (e.g., penicillin, progesterone, aspirin) are not immunogenic; those of molecular weight between 1000 and 6000 Da (e.g., insulin, ACTH) may or may not be immunogenic; and those of molecular weight greater than 6000 Da (e.g., albumin, tetanus toxin) are generally immunogenic. In short, relatively small substances have decreased immunogenicity, and large substances have increased immunogenicity.

Chemical Complexity

The third characteristic of immunogenicity is a certain degree of physicochemical complexity. For example, simple molecules such as homopolymers of amino acids (e.g., a polymer of lysine with a molecular weight of 30,000 Da) are seldom good immunogens. Similarly, even though it has a molecular weight of 50,000 Da, the homopolymer of poly-γ-D-glutamic acid (the capsular material of *Bacillus anthracis*) is not immunogenic. These compounds, although of high molecular weight, are not sufficiently chemically complex to be immunogenic. However, if complexity is increased by attaching various moieties—such as dinitrophenol or other low-molecular-weight compounds—that, by themselves, are not immunogenic, the entire macromolecule becomes immunogenic. The resulting immune response is directed against not only the coupled low-molecular-weight compounds but also the high-molecular-weight homopolymer. In general, an increase in the chemical complexity of a compound is accompanied by an increase in its immunogenicity. Thus, copolymers of several amino acids, such as polyglutamine and lysine (poly-GAT), tend to be highly immunogenic.

The acquired immune response recognizes many structural features and chemical properties of compounds. Because many immunogens are proteins, it is important to understand the structural features of these molecules.

Each of the four levels of protein structure contributes to the molecule's immunogenicity. For example, antibodies can recognize a protein's *primary structure* (the amino acid sequence), *secondary structures* (the organization of the backbone of the polypeptide chain, such as an α helix or β-pleated sheet), and *tertiary structures* (formed by the three-dimensional configuration of the protein, which is conferred by the folding of the polypeptide chain and held by disulfide bridges, hydrogen bonds, hydrophobic interactions, etc.) (Fig. 3.1). The immune system can also respond to *quaternary structures* (formed by the juxtaposition of separate parts if the molecule is composed of more than one protein subunit) (Fig. 3.2).

Degradability

For antigens that activate T cells to stimulate immune responses, interactions with MHC molecules expressed on APC must occur (see Chapter 9). Before they can express antigenic *epitopes* (small fragments of the immunogen) on their surface, APC must first degrade the antigen through a process known as *antigen processing* (enzymatic degradation of antigen). Once degraded and noncovalently bound to MHC, epitopes stimulate the activation and clonal expansion of antigen-specific effector T cells. A protein antigen's susceptibility to enzymatic degradation largely depends on two properties: (1) It has to be sufficiently stable so that it can reach the site of interaction with B or T cells necessary for the immune response and (2) it must be susceptible to the partial enzymatic degradation that takes place during antigen processing by APC. Peptides composed of D-amino acids are resistant to enzymatic degradation so they are not immunogenic, but their L-isomers are susceptible to enzymes and do demonstrate immunogenicity. Carbohydrates are not processed or presented and are thus unable to activate T cells, although they can activate B cells.

In general, a substance must have all four of the characteristics described in order to be immunogenic: it must be foreign to the individual in whom it is administered, have a relatively high molecular weight, possess a certain degree of chemical complexity, and be degradable.

Haptens

As noted earlier, substances called haptens fail to induce immune responses in their native form because of their low molecular weight and their chemical simplicity. These compounds are not immunogenic unless they are conjugated to high-molecular-weight, physiochemically complex carriers. Thus an immune response can be evoked to thousands of chemical compounds, those of high molecular weight and those of low molecular weight, provided the latter is conjugated to high-molecular-weight complex carriers.

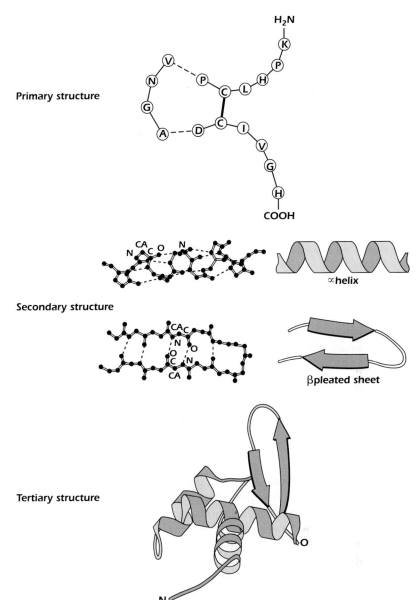

Figure 3.1. Levels of protein organizational structure. The primary structure is indicated by the linear arrangement of amino acids (using single-letter code) and includes any intrachain disulfide bonds, as shown. The secondary structure derives from the folding of the polypeptide chain into α helices and β-pleated sheets. The tertiary structure, shown as a ribbon diagram, is formed by the folding of regions between secondary features. (Adapted with permission from P Sun and JC Boyington, *Current Protocols in Protein Science*, John Wiley and Sons, Inc., Hoboken, NJ.)

Further Requirements for Immunogenicity

Several other factors play roles in determining whether a substance is immunogenic. The genetic makeup (genotype) of the individual plays an important role in determining whether a given substance will stimulate an immune response. Genetic control of immune responsiveness is largely controlled by genes mapping within the MHC. Another factor that plays a crucial role in immunogenicity relates to the individual's B- and T-cell repertoires. Acquired immune responses are triggered following the binding of antigenic epitopes to antigen-specific receptors on B and T lymphocytes. If an individual lacks a particular clone of lymphocytes bearing the identical antigen-specific receptor needed to respond to the stimulus, an immune response to that antigenic epitope will not take place. Finally, practical issues such as the *dosage* and *route of administration* of antigens play a role in determining whether the substance is immunogenic.

Insufficient doses of antigen may not stimulate an immune response for one of two reasons: (1) The amount administered fails to activate enough lymphocytes or (2) such a dose renders the responding cells unresponsive. The latter phenomenon induces a state of tolerance to that antigen (discussed further in Chapter 12). The number of doses administered also affects the outcome of the immune response generated. As discussed below, repeated administration of antigen is required to stimulate a strong immune response.

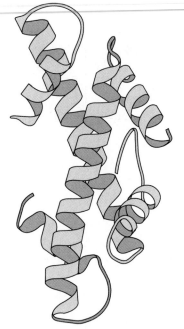

Quarternary structure

Figure 3.2. The quaternary structure of proteins results from the association of two or more polypeptide chains, which form a polymeric protein. (Adapted with permission from P Sun and JC Boyington, *Current Protocols in Protein Science*, John Wiley and Sons, Inc., Hoboken, NJ.)

Finally, the route of administration can affect the outcome of the immunization strategy because it determines which organs and cell populations will be involved in the response. Antigens administered via the most common route, **subcutaneously**, generally elicit the strongest immune responses because Langerhans cells in the skin, which are responsible for antigen uptake, processing, and presentation to T cells, are among the most potent APC. Responses to subcutaneously administered antigens take place in the lymph nodes draining the injection site. **Intravenously** administered antigens are carried first to the spleen, where they can induce immune unresponsiveness or tolerance or, if presented by APC, generate an immune response. Orally administered antigens (**gastrointestinal route**) elicit local antibody responses within the intestinal lamina propria but often produce a systemic state of tolerance (antigen unresponsiveness) (see Chapter 12 for a detailed discussion about tolerance). Finally, administration of antigens via the respiratory tract (**intranasal route**) often elicits allergic responses (see Chapter 14).

Since immune responses depend on multiple cellular interactions, the type and extent of the immune response is affected by the cells populating the organ in which the antigen is ultimately delivered. The stringent requirements outlined above constitute only a portion of the control mechanisms in charge of the delicate balance between activation of the acquired immune response and protection of the individual from detrimental responses.

PRIMARY AND SECONDARY IMMUNE RESPONSES

The first exposure of an individual to an immunogen is referred to as the **primary immunization**, which generates a **primary response**. As we shall see in subsequent chapters, many events take place during this primary immunization. Cells process antigen, triggering antigen-specific lymphocytes to proliferate and differentiate. T-lymphocyte subsets interact with other subsets and induce the latter to differentiate into T lymphocytes with specialized functions. T lymphocytes also interact with B lymphocytes, inducing them to synthesize and secrete antibodies.

A second exposure to the same immunogen results in a **secondary response**. This may occur after the response to the first immune event has leveled off or has totally subsided (within weeks or even years). The secondary response differs from the primary response in many respects. Most notably and biologically relevant is the much quicker onset and the much higher magnitude of the response. In a sense, this secondary (and subsequent) exposure occurs as if the body remembered that it had been previously exposed to that same immunogen. In fact, secondary and subsequent responses exploit the expanded number of antigen-specific lymphocytes generated in response to the primary immune response. Thus, the increased arsenal of responding lymphocytes accounts, in part, for the magnitude of the observed response. The secondary response is also called the **memory** or **anamnestic response**, and the B and T lymphocytes that participate in the memory response are termed **memory cells**. The kinetics of antibody production after immunization are described in detail in Chapter 4 and Figure 4.12.

ANTIGENICITY AND ANTIGEN-BINDING SITE

An immune response induced by an antigen generates antibodies or lymphocytes that react specifically with the antigen. The antigen-binding site of an antibody or a receptor on a lymphocyte has a unique structure that allows a complementary fit to some structural aspect of the specific antigen. The portion of the immunoglobulin that specifically binds to the antigenic determinant or epitope is concentrated in several hypervariable regions of the molecule, which form the **complementarity-determining region** (**CDR**). Additional structural features of the immunoglobulin molecule are described in Chapter 4.

Various studies indicate that the size of an epitope that combines with the CDR on a given antibody is approximately equivalent to five to seven amino acids. These dimensions were calculated from experiments that involved the binding of antibodies to polysaccharides and to peptide epitopes. Such dimensions would also be expected to correspond roughly to the size of the complementary antibody-combining site, termed the *paratope*, and this expectation has been confirmed by X-ray crystallography. The small size of an epitope (peptide) that binds to a specific TCR (peptides with 8–12 amino acids) is made functionally larger, since it is noncovalently associated with MHC proteins of the APC. This bimolecular epitope–MHC complex then binds to the TCR, forming a *trimolecular complex* (TCR–epitope–MHC).

EPITOPES RECOGNIZED BY B AND T CELLS

According to a large body of evidence, the properties of many epitopes recognized by B cells differ from those recognized by T cells (Table 3.1). In general, membrane-bound antibody present on B cells recognizes and binds free antigen in solution. Thus, these epitopes are typically on the outside of the molecule, accessible for interaction with the B-cell receptor. Terminal side chains of polysaccharides and hydrophilic portions of protein molecules generally constitute B-cell epitopes. An example of an antigen with five *linear* B-cell epitopes located on the exposed surface of myoglobulin is shown in Figure 3.3. B-cell epitopes may also form as a result of the folded conformation of molecules, as shown in Figure 3.4. In such epitopes, called *conformational* or *discontinuous epitopes*, noncontiguous residues along a polypeptide chain are brought together by the folded conformation of the protein shown in Figure 3.3.

In contrast to B cells, T cells are unable to bind soluble antigen. The interaction of an epitope with the TCR requires APC to process the antigen; after enzymatic degradation takes place, the resulting small peptides associate with MHC. Thus, T-cell epitopes can only be *continuous* or linear since they are composed of a single segment of a polypeptide chain. Figure 3.5 illustrates the structural organization of a class I MHC bound to an antigenic peptide. Generally such processed epitopes are internal denatured linear hydrophobic areas of proteins. Polysaccharides, on the other hand, are not processed by APC and are not known to bind or activate T cells. Thus polysaccharides contain epitopes recognized solely by B cells, but protein epitopes can be recognized by both B and T cells (Table 3.1). Antigenic epitopes may have the characteristics shown schematically in Figure 3.6.

TABLE 3.1. Antigen Recognition by B and T Cells

Characteristic	B Cells	T Cells
Antigen interaction	BCR binds Ag	TCR binds antigenic peptides bound to MHC
Nature of antigens	Protein, polysaccharide, lipid	Peptide
Binding soluble antigens	Yes	No
Epitopes recognized	Accessible, sequential, or nonsequential	Internal linear peptides produced by antigen processing (proteolytic degradation)

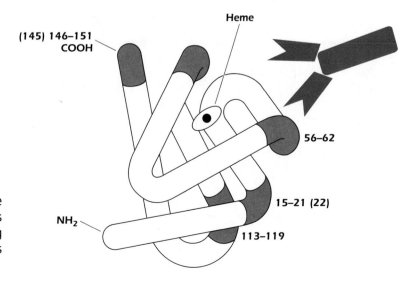

Figure 3.3. Example of antigen (sperm whale myoglobin) containing five linear B-cell epitopes (*red*), one of which is bound to antibody-binding site of antibody specific for amino acid residues 56–62.

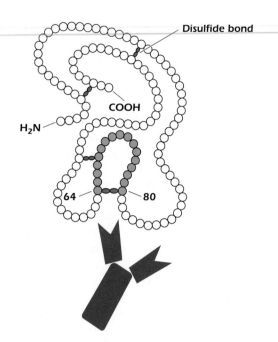

Figure 3.4. Antigen showing amino acid residuces (*circles*), which form nonsequential epitope "loop" (*blue*) resulting from disulfide bond between residues 64 and 80. Note the binding of an epitope-specific antibody to the nonsequential amino acids that constitute the epitope.

Thus, they may consist of a single epitope (hapten) or have varying numbers of the same epitope on the same molecule (e.g., polysaccharides). The most common antigens (proteins) have varying numbers of different epitopes on the same molecule.

MAJOR CLASSES OF ANTIGENS

The following major chemical families may be antigenic:

1. *Carbohydrates* (**polysaccharides**). Polysaccharides can induce antibody responses in the absence of T cell help. Polysaccharides that form part of more complex molecules (glycoproteins) will elicit T-cell-dependent immune responses, part of which is directed specifically against the polysaccharide moiety of the molecule. An immune response, consisting primarily of antibodies, can be induced against many kinds of polysaccharide molecules, such as components of microorganisms (e.g., teichoic acid of Gram-negative bacteria). In addition, polysaccharides associated with the ABO blood groups on the surface of red blood cells are also good examples of carbohydrates that are immunogenic.

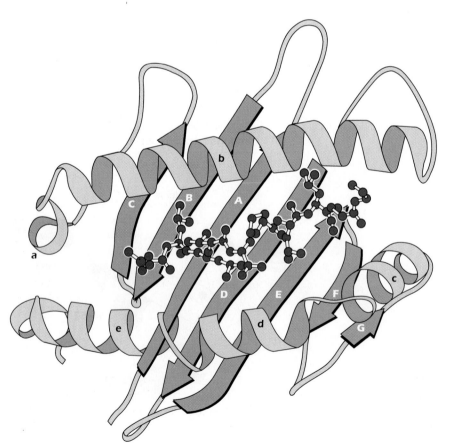

Figure 3.5. Structure of MHC class I molecule (*ribbon diagram*) with antigenic peptide (*ball-and-stick model*).

	Description	Example
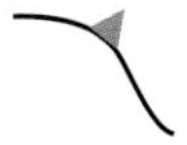	One epitope	Haptens
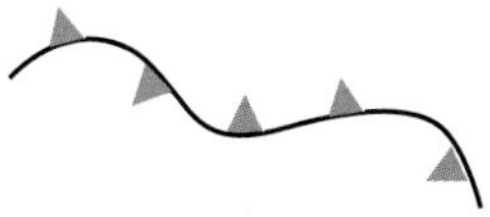	Many epitopes of the same specificity	Many polysaccharides, homopolymers
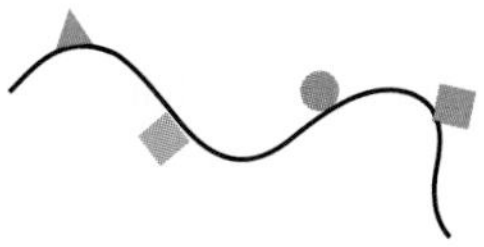	Many epitopes of different specificities	Proteins

Figure 3.6. Some possible antigenic structures containing single and multiple epitopes.

2. **Lipids.** Lipids are rarely immunogenic, but an immune response to lipids may be induced if the lipids are conjugated to protein carriers. Thus, in a sense, lipids may be regarded as haptens. Immune responses to glycolipids and to sphingolipids have also been demonstrated.
3. **Nucleic acids.** Nucleic acids are poor immunogens by themselves, but they become immunogenic when they are conjugated to protein carriers. DNA, in its native helical state, is usually nonimmunogenic in normal animals. However, immune responses to nucleic acids have been reported in many instances. One important clinical example is the appearance of anti-DNA antibodies in patients with systemic lupus erythematosus (discussed in detail in Chapter 12).

Systemic Lupus Erythematosus

4. **Proteins.** Because virtually all proteins are immunogenic, the most common immune responses are those to proteins. The greater the degree of complexity of the protein, the more vigorous the immune response to that protein will be. Because of their size and complexity, proteins contain multiple epitopes.

 BINDING OF ANTIGEN TO ANTIGEN-SPECIFIC ANTIBODIES OR T CELL RECEPTORS

The binding between antigen and antibodies is discussed in detail in Chapters 4 and 5. The interactions of antigen with both B and T cells and subsequent activation events are discussed in Chapter 10. At this point, it is important to emphasize only that the binding of antigen with antibodies or TCRs does not involve covalent bonds. The **noncovalent binding** may involve **electrostatic** **interactions, hydrophobic interactions, hydrogen bonds**, and **van der Waals forces**. Since these interactive forces are relatively weak, the fit between the antigen and its antigen receptor must occur over an area large enough to allow the summation of all possible interactions. This requirement is the basis for the exquisite specificity observed in immunologic interactions.

CROSS-REACTIVITY

Since macromolecular antigens contain several distinct epitopes, some of these antigens can be altered without totally changing the immunogenic or antigenic structure of the entire molecule. This concept is important in relation to immunization against highly pathogenic microorganisms or highly toxic compounds. Obviously, immunization with pathogenic toxins is unwise. However, it is possible to destroy the biologic activity of such toxins and a broad variety of other toxins (e.g., snake venoms) without appreciably affecting their immunogenicity. A toxin that has been modified to the extent that it is no longer toxic but still maintains some of its immunochemical characteristics is called a **toxoid**. Thus we can say that a toxoid *cross-reacts* immunologically with the toxin. Accordingly, it is possible to immunize individuals with the toxoid and induce immune responses to some of the epitopes that the toxoid still shares with the native toxin. Although the molecules of toxin and toxoid differ in many physicochemical and biologic respects, they nevertheless cross-react immunologically: They share enough epitopes to allow the immune response to the toxoid to mount an effective defense against the toxin itself. An immunologic reaction in which the immune components, either cells or antibodies, react with two molecules that share epitopes but are otherwise dissimilar is called a **cross-reaction**. Another form of cross-reactivity is seen when antibodies or cells with specificity to one epitope bind, usually more weakly, to another epitope that has a structural resemblance but is not identical to the first epitope. To denote that the antigen used for immunization is different from the one with which the induced immune components are then allowed to react, the terms homologous and heterologous are used. ***Homologous*** denotes that the antigen and the immunogen are the same; ***heterologous*** indicates that the substance used to induce the immune response is different from the substance that is then used to react with the products of the induced response.

Although the hallmark of immunology is specificity, immunologic cross-reactivity has been observed on many levels. This means not that the immunologic specificity has been diminished but rather that the substances that cross-react share antigenic determinants. In the example described above, a toxin and its corresponding toxoid represent two molecules, the toxin being the native molecule and the toxoid being a modified molecule that cross-reacts with the native molecule.

In other examples of immunologic cross-reactivity, the two cross-reacting substances are unrelated to each other except that they share one or more areas that have similar three-dimensional characteristics. Such substances are referred to as ***heterophile antigens***. For example, human blood group A antigen reacts with antiserum raised against pneumococcal capsular polysaccharide (type XIV). Similarly, human blood group B antigen reacts with antibodies to certain strains of *Escherichia coli*. In these examples of cross-reactivity, the antigens of the microorganisms are referred to as the heterophile antigens (with respect to the blood group antigen).

ADJUVANTS

To enhance the immune response to a given immunogen, various additives or vehicles are often used. An ***adjuvant*** (from the Latin *adjuvare*, "to help") is a substance that,

when mixed with an immunogen, enhances the immune response against the immunogen. It is important to distinguish between a carrier for a hapten and an adjuvant. A hapten will become immunogenic when conjugated covalently to a carrier; it will not become immunogenic if mixed with an adjuvant. Thus, an adjuvant enhances the immune response to immunogens but does not confer immunogenicity on haptens.

Adjuvants have been used to augment immune responses to antigens for almost a century. Interest in the identification of adjuvants for use with vaccines is growing because many new vaccine candidates lack sufficient immunogenicity. This is particularly true of peptide-based vaccines. Adjuvant mechanisms include (1) increasing the biologic or immunologic half-life of vaccine antigens, (2) increasing the production of local inflammatory cytokines, and (3) improving antigen delivery and antigen processing and presentation by APC, especially the dendritic cells. Empirically, it has been found that adjuvants containing microbial components (e.g., mycobacterial extracts) are the best adjuvants. Pathogen components induce macrophages and dendritic cells to express costimulatory molecules and to secrete cytokines. More recently, it has been shown that such induction by microbial components involves pattern recognition molecules (e.g., TLR) expressed by these cells. Binding of microbial components to TLRs signals the cells to express costimulatory molecules and to release cytokines.

While many adjuvants have been developed in animal models (Table 3.2) and tested experimentally in humans, only one has been accepted for routine vaccination. Currently, aluminum hydroxide and aluminum phosphate (alum) are the only adjuvants approved for human vaccines administered to normal individuals in the United States. As an inorganic salt, alum binds to proteins, causing them

TABLE 3.2. Common Adjuvants and Their Mechanism of Action

Adjuvant	Composition	Mechanism of Action
Aluminum hydroxide or aluminum phosphate (alum)	Aluminum hydroxide gel	Enhanced uptake of antigen by APC; delayed release of antigen
Alum with a mycobacterial-derived dipeptide	Aluminum hydroxide gel with muramyl dipeptide	Enhanced uptake of antigen by APC; delayed release of antigen; induction of costimulatory molecules on APC
Alum with *Bordetella pertussis*	Aluminum hydroxide gel with killed *B. pertussis*	Enhanced uptake of antigen by APC; delayed release of antigen; induction of costimulatory molecules on APC
Freund's complete adjuvant	Oil in water with killed mycobacteria	Enhanced uptake of antigen by APC; delayed release of antigen; induction of costimulatory molecules on APC
Freund's incomplete adjuvant	Oil in water	Enhanced uptake of antigen by APC; delayed release of antigen
Immune stimulatory complexes	Open cagelike structures containing cholesterol and a mixture of saponins	Delivery of antigen to cytosol, allowing induction of cytotoxic T-cell responses

to precipitate, and elicits an inflammatory response that nonspecifically increases the immunogenicity of antigen. When injected, the precipitated antigen is released more slowly than antigen alone at the injection site. Moreover, the increased size of the antigen, which occurs as a consequence of precipitation, increases the probability that the macromolecule will be phagocytized.

Many adjuvants have been used in experimental animals. One commonly used adjuvant, **Freund's complete adjuvant**, consists of killed *Mycobacterium tuberculosis* or *Mycobacterium butyricum* suspended in oil, which is then emulsified with an aqueous antigen solution. The oil-emulsified state of the adjuvant–antigen mixture allows the antigen to be released slowly and continuously, helping sustain the recipient's exposure to the immunogen.

Other microorganisms used as adjuvants are bacille Calmette-Guerin (BCG) (an attenuated mycobacterium), *Corynebacterium parvum*, and *Bordetella pertussis*. In reality, many of these adjuvants exploit the immune cell activation properties of microbe-expressed molecules, including lipopolysaccharide (LPS), bacterial DNA containing unmethylated CpG dinucleotide motifs, and bacterial heat-shock proteins. Many of these microbial cell adjuvants bind to TLRs to facilitate adaptive B- and T-cell responses. Dendritic cells are important APC involved in the activity of microbial adjuvants. They respond by secreting cytokines and expressing costimulatory molecules; the costimulatory molecules in turn stimulate the activation and differentiation of antigen-specific T cells.

SUMMARY

1. Immunogenicity is the capacity of a compound to induce an immune response. Immunogenicity requires that a compound (a) be foreign to the immunized individual, (b) possess a certain minimal molecular weight, (c) possess a certain degree of chemical complexity, and (d) be degradable or susceptible to antigen processing and presentation through its interaction with MHC.

2. Antigenicity refers to the ability of a compound to bind with antibodies or with cells of the immune system. This binding is highly specific; the immune components are capable of recognizing various physicochemical aspects of the compound. The binding between antigen and immune components involves several weak forces operating over short distances (van der Waals forces, electrostatic interactions, hydrophobic interactions, and hydrogen bonds); it does not involve covalent bonds.

3. The smallest unit of antigen that is capable of binding with antibodies is called an antigenic determinant or epitope. Compounds may have one or more epitopes capable of reacting with immune components. The immune response against these compounds involves the production of antibodies or the generation of cells with specificities directed against most or all of the epitopes.

4. B-cell membrane immunoglobulin or secreted antibody tends to recognize amino acid sequences that are accessible, usually hydrophilic and mobile. These can be contiguous or noncontiguous amino acids (conformational determinants), which are brought into proximity by the three-dimensional folding of the protein. B-cell membrane immunoglobulins and antibody are capable of recognizing polysaccharides and lipids.

5. T cells recognize internal amino acid sequences of proteins in the context of MHC class I or class II molecules. Peptide fragments of protein antigens generated by antigen processing may associate with MHC molecules and be presented to T cells.

6. Immunologic cross-reactivity denotes a situation in which two or more substances with various degrees of dissimilarity share epitopes and would, therefore, react with the immune components induced against any one of these substances. Thus a toxoid, a modified form of toxin, may have one or more epitopes in common with the native toxin. Immunization with the toxoid leads to an immune response capable of reacting not only with the toxoid but also with the toxin.

7. Adjuvants are substances that can accelerate, prolong, and enhance the quality of specific immune responses. When administered with antigens, adjuvants facilitate immune responses that are specific for the antigen (not for adjuvant itself) since the adjuvant nonspecifically amplifies the response. The principal mechanisms of adjuvant activity include increased antigen presentation by APC (especially dendritic cells), induction of costimulatory molecules, and induction of local inflammatory cytokine responses.

REFERENCES

Atassi MZ (1977): *Immunochemistry of Proteins*, Vols 1 and 2. New York: Plenum.

Benjamin DC, Berzofsky JA, East IJ, Gurd FRN, Hannum C, Leach SJ, Margoliash E, Michael JG, Miller A, Prager EM, Reichlin M, Sercarz EE, Smith-Gill SJ, Todd PE, Wilson AC (1984): The antigenic structure of proteins: A reappraisal. *Annu Rev Immunol* 2:67.

Davis DR, Cohen GH (1996): Interactions of protein antigens with antibodies. *Proc Natl Acad Sci USA* 93:7.

Davis MM, Boniface JJ, Reich Z, Lyons D, Hampl J, Arden B, Chien Y (1998): Ligand recognition by αβ T cell receptors. *Annu Rev Immunol* 16:523.

Freund J, Calals J, Hosmer EP (1937): Sensitization and antibody formation after injection of tubercle bacilli and paraffin oil. *Proc Soc Exp Biol Med* 37:509.

Ishii KJ, Akira S (2007): Toll or toll-free adjuvant path toward the optimal vaccine development. *J Clin Immunol* 27:363.

Krishnan J, Selvarajoo K, Tsuchiya M, Lee G, Choi S (2007): Toll-like receptor signal transduction. *Exp Mol Med* 39:421.

Kwissa M, Kasturi SP, Pulendran B (2007): The science of adjuvants. *Expert Rev Vaccines* 6:673.

Paul, WE (2003): *Fundamental Immunology*. Philadelphia, PA: Lippincott, Williams, and Wilkins.

 ## REVIEW QUESTIONS

For each question, choose the ONE BEST answer.

1. A large protein has been enzymatically digested in the laboratory to yield a mixture of peptides ranging in size from four to six amino acids in length. Which of the following would be expected if the peptide mixture were administered to an experimental animal together with an adjuvant such as Freund's complete adjuvant?
   A) Peptide-specific antibodies would be generated using the peptide mixture alone.
   B) Peptide-specific antibodies would be generated only if an adjuvant were administered with the peptide mixture.
   C) Peptide-specific antibodies would be generated if they were first coupled to a protein carrier.
   D) Peptide-specific antibody and T-cell responses would be generated using the peptide mixture alone.
   E) There would be neither a humoral immune response nor a cell-mediated immune response to the peptides in the mixture.

2. The protection against smallpox virus infection afforded by prior infection with cowpox virus represents:
   A) antigenic specificity
   B) antigenic cross-reactivity
   C) enhanced viral uptake by macrophages
   D) innate immunity
   E) passive protection

3. Converting a toxin to a toxoid:
   A) makes the toxin more immunogenic
   B) renders the toxin safe for use as an immunogen
   C) enhances binding with antitoxin
   D) induces only innate immunity
   E) increases phagocytosis

4. Haptens:
   A) require carrier molecules to be immunogenic
   B) react with specific antibodies when homologous carriers are not employed
   C) interact with specific antibody even if the hapten is monovalent
   D) cannot stimulate secondary antibody responses without carriers
   E) all of the above

5. An adjuvant is a substance that:
   A) increases the size of the immunogen
   B) enhances the immunogenicity of haptens.
   C) increases the chemical complexity of the immunogen
   D) enhances the immune response to the immunogen
   E) enhances immunologic cross-reactivity

6. An antibody made against a large protein antigen reacts with it even when the protein is denatured by disrupting all disulfide bonds. Another antibody against the antigen fails to react when it is similarly denatured. The most likely explanation can be stated as follows:
   A) The first antibody is specific for several epitopes expressed by the antigen.
   B) The first antibody is specific for the primary amino acid sequence of the antigen, and the second is specific for conformational determinants.
   C) The second antibody is specific for disulfide bonds.
   D) The first antibody has a higher affinity for the antigen.

ANSWERS TO REVIEW QUESTIONS

1. *E* Peptides ranging from four to six amino acids in length are low-molecular-weight molecules that are unable to generate antibody responses or T-cell responses due to their small size. If these peptides were coupled or bound to a protein carrier, they could be immunogenic.

2. *B* The protection against smallpox provided by prior infection with cowpox is an example of antigenic cross-reactivity. Immunization with cowpox leads to the production of antibodies capable of reacting with smallpox because the two viruses share several identical, or structurally similar, determinants.

3. *B* Conversion of a toxin to a toxoid is performed in order to allow it to be used as a safe, immunogen. Immune responses to toxoids cross-react with toxins.

4. *E* Haptens are substances, usually of low molecular weight and univalent, that, by themselves, cannot induce immune responses (primary or secondary) but can do so if conjugated to high-molecular-weight carriers. The haptens can and do interact with the induced antibodies, with or without being conjugated to the carrier.

5. *D* An immunologic adjuvant is a substance that, when mixed with an immunogen, enhances the immune response against that immunogen by mechanisms that depend upon the specific adjuvant used (e.g., enhanced antigen presentation, delayed release of antigen). It does not increase its size or chemical complexity. In addition, it does not enhance the immune response against a hapten, which requires conjugation to an immunogenic carrier to induce a response. The adjuvant has no relevance to possible toxicity of an immunogen.

6. *B* Antibodies can recognize single epitopes formed by primary sequence structures or secondary, tertiary, and quaternary conformational structures. Denaturing a protein by disrupting disulfide bonds generally destroys conformational determinants. Therefore it is likely that the first antibody reacts with a primary amino acid sequence determinant that is present on both native and denatured antigen, while the second antibody sees a conformational determinant only on the native antigen.

4

ANTIBODY STRUCTURE AND FUNCTION

 INTRODUCTION

One of the major functions of the immune system is the production of soluble proteins that circulate freely and exhibit properties that contribute specifically to immunity and protection against foreign material. These soluble proteins are the ***antibodies***, which belong to the class of proteins called globulins because of their globular structure. Initially, owing to their migratory properties in an electrophoretic field, they were called γ-globulins (in relation to the more rapidly migrating albumin, α-globulin, and β-globulin); today they are known collectively as ***immunoglobulins***.

Immunoglobulins can be membrane bound or secreted. Membrane-bound antibody is present on the surface of B cells, where it serves as the antigen-specific receptor. The membrane-bound form of antibody is associated with a heterodimer called Igα/Igβ to form the BCR. As will be discussed in Chapter 7, the Igα/Igβ heterodimer mediates the intracellular signaling mechanisms associated with B-cell activation. Secreted antibodies are produced by ***plasma cells***—the terminally differentiated B cells that serve as antibody factories and are housed largely within the bone marrow.

The structure of immunoglobulins incorporates several features essential for their participation in the immune response. The two most important features are specificity and biologic activity. ***Specificity*** is attributed to a defined region of the antibody molecule containing the hypervariable region or complimentarity-determining region (CDR). This restricts the antibody to combine only with those substances that contain a particular antigenic structure. The existence of a vast array of potential antigenic determinants which, as we discussed in Chapter 3, are also known as epitopes, prompted the evolution of a system for producing an enormous repertoire of antibody molecules, each of which is capable of combining with a particular antigenic structure. Thus, antibodies collectively exhibit great diversity, in terms of the types of molecular structures with which they are capable of reacting, but individually they exhibit a high degree of specificity, since each is able to react with only one particular antigenic structure.

Despite the large numbers of antigen-specific antibodies, the biologic effects of antigen–antibody reactions are rather few in number. Depending on the nature of the antigen, these include neutralization of toxins, immobilization of microorganisms, neutralization of viral activity, agglutination (clumping together) of microorganisms or antigenic particles (see Chapter 5), or binding with soluble antigen leading to the formation of precipitates. The latter is an example of how the acquired immune system collaborates with the innate immune system, since precipitated antigens are readily phagocytized and destroyed by phagocytic cells (see Chapter 2). Other examples of the collaboration of antigen–antibody complexes with the innate immune system include activation of complement

Immunology: A Short Course, Sixth Edition, By Richard Coico and Geoffrey Sunshine
Copyright © 2009 John Wiley & Sons, Inc.

to facilitate the lysis of microorganisms (see Chapter 13) and complement-mediated opsonization, which also results in phagocytosis and destruction of microbes. Yet another important biologic function of antibodies, the ability of certain classes of immunoglobulins to cross the placenta from the mother to the fetus, is discussed in more detail later in this chapter.

The differences in the various biologic activities of antibodies are attributed to structural properties conferred by the germline-encoded portions of the Ig molecule. Thus, not all antibody molecules are equal in the performance of all of the biologic tasks described above. In the simplest terms, antibody molecules contain structural components that are shared with other antibodies within their *class*, and an antigen-binding component that is unique to a given antibody. This chapter deals with these structural and biologic properties of immunoglobulins.

ISOLATION AND CHARACTERIZATION OF IMMUNOGLOBULINS

Serum, the liquid portion left when blood has been withdrawn and allowed to clot, is the antibody-containing component of blood. Unless measures are taken to prevent clotting of blood in the vacutainer in which blood is collected (e.g., addition of heparin), clotting factors will be activated and a cellular clot will form. When the serum component is subjected to *electrophoresis* (separation in an electrical field) at slightly alkaline pH (8.2), five major components can normally be visualized (see Fig. 4.1). The slowest in terms of migration toward the anode, called γ-globulin, contains the immunoglobulins. This was demonstrated by a simple comparison of the electrophoretic pattern of antiserum from a *hyperimmune* rabbit (one that had received multiple immunizations with a test antigen) both before and

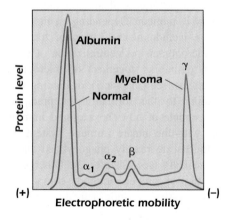

Figure 4.1. Electrophoretic mobility of serum proteins obtained from normal individual (lower tracing in blue) and from patient with IgG myeloma (upper tracing in red).

after removal of the test antigen-specific antibody by precipitation with the antigen. Only the size of the γ-globulin fraction was diminished by this procedure. Analysis showed that when this fraction was collected separately, all measurable antibodies were contained within it. Later it was shown that antibody activity is present not only in the γ-globulin fraction but also in a slightly more anodic area. Consequently, all globular proteins with antibody activity are generically referred to as immunoglobulins, as exemplified by the γ peak (see Fig. 4.1).

From the broad electrophoretic peaks, it is clear that a heterogeneous collection of Ig molecules with slightly different charges is present. This heterogeneity was one of the early obstacles in attempts to determine the structure of antibodies, since analytical chemistry requires homogeneous, crystallizable compounds as starting material. This problem was solved, in part, by the discovery of *myeloma proteins*, homogeneous immunoglobulins produced by the progeny of a single plasma cell that has become neoplastic in the malignant disease called *multiple myeloma*. The presence of myeloma proteins in the serum of a patient with this disease is demonstrated by the γ-globulin spike in the electrophoretic pattern of serum proteins (see Fig. 4.1). When it became clear that some myeloma proteins bound antigen, it also became apparent that they could be dealt with as typical Ig molecules.

Another aid to structural studies of antibodies was the discovery of *Bence Jones proteins* in the urine. These were named after Henry Bence Jones (1813–1873), a British physician who discovered them. Bence Jones proteins are homogeneous proteins, produced in large quantities by some patients with multiple myeloma, consisting of dimers of immunoglobulin κ or λ light chains. Historically, they have proved to be very useful in the determination of the structure of the light-chain portion of the Ig molecule. Today, the powerful technique of cell–cell hybridization, which allows for the *in vitro* immortalization of antibody-producing B cells, permits the production of hybridoma cell lines that make large quantities of monoclonal antibody of virtually any specificity (see Chapter 5).

STRUCTURE OF LIGHT AND HEAVY CHAINS

Analysis of the structural characteristics of antibody molecules really began in 1959 with two discoveries that revealed for the first time that the molecule could be separated into analyzable parts suitable for further study. In 1948, a British immunologist named Rodney Porter found that proteolytic treatment with the enzyme *papain* split the Ig molecule (molecular weight 150,000 Da) into three fragments of about equal size (Fab, Fab, and Fc; see Fig. 4.2). Two of the fragments, referred to as

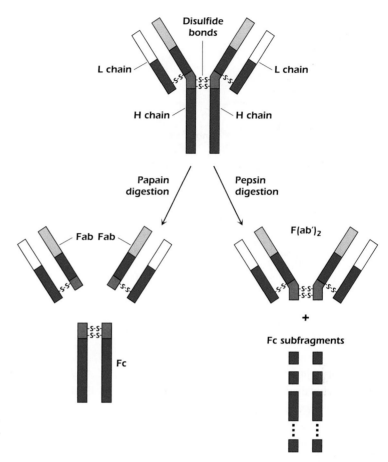

Figure 4.2. Proteolytic digestion of immunoglobulin using papain and pepsin.

Fab (fragment antigen-binding), were found to retain the antibody's ability to bind antigen specifically. However, unlike the intact molecule, they could no longer precipitate the antigen from solution. Fab fragments are considered to be univalent; each one possesses a single binding site and is identical to the other in every way. The third fragment could be crystallized out of solution, a property indicative of its apparent homogeneity. This fragment, called the *Fc fragment* (fragment crystallizable), cannot bind antigen, but, as was subsequently shown, it is responsible for the biologic functions of the antibody molecule after antigen has been bound to the Fab part of the intact molecule.

Several years after Porter's discovery of the proteolytic effects of papain on immunoglobulins, Gerald M. Edelman in the United States discovered that when γ-globulin was extensively reduced by treatment with mercaptoethanol (a reagent that breaks disulfide bonds), the molecule fell apart into four chains: two identical light chains with a molecular weight of about 53,000 Da each and two others of about 22,000 Da each. The larger molecules were designated *heavy chains* (often abbreviated as *H chains*) and the smaller ones, *light chains* (often abbreviated as *L chains*). On the basis of these results, the structure of Ig molecules, as depicted in Figure 4.2, was proposed. This model was subsequently shown to be essentially correct, and Porter

and Edelman shared the Nobel Prize for the elucidation of antibody structure. All Ig molecules consist of a basic unit of four polypeptide chains, two identical heavy chains and two identical light chains, held together by several disulfide bonds. It should be noted that papain digestion of the Ig molecule results in cleavage N-terminally to the disulfide bridge between the heavy chains at the hinge region, yielding two monovalent Fab fragments and an Fc fragment. On the other hand, studies carried out in Edelman's laboratory showed that pepsin digestion cleaved immunoglobulins C terminally to the disulfide bridge. This results in a divalent fragment referred to as **F(ab)'$_2$**, consisting of two Fab fragments joined by the disulfide bond, along with several Fc subfragments. A more detailed diagram of a generic Ig molecule, consisting of two glycosylated heavy chains and two light chains, is shown in Figure 4.3.

As you might expect, immunoglobulins of one species are immunogenic in another species. In other words, the use of immunoglobulins of a given species as immunogens in another species produces antisera that can then be used to investigate the various features of different Ig chains. This serologic approach to studying immunoglobulins, together with several biochemical strategies, has revealed important insights into the structural properties of these molecules. For example, almost all species studied have two major

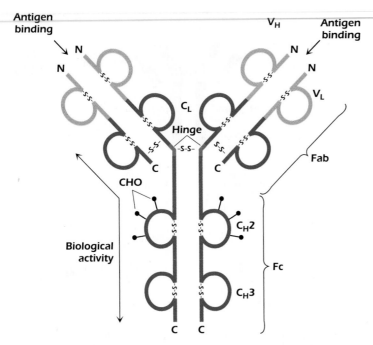

Figure 4.3. Schematic representation of the Ig molecule showing Ig-fold domains formed by intrachain disulfide bonds.

classes of light chains, called **κ chains** and **λ chains**. Any one individual of a species produces both types of light chain, but the ratio of κ chains to λ chains varies with the species (mouse 95% κ; human 60% κ). However, in any one Ig molecule, the light chains are always identical—both κ or both λ.

Another important characteristic of immunoglobulins revealed in this early work was that the heavy chains of immunoglobulins of virtually all species studied can be divided into five different **classes** or **isotypes**: IgM, IgD, IgG, IgA, and IgE. These are distinguished from one another based upon so-called **constant regions** of the heavy chains, which differ from one another with regard to their protein sequences, carbohydrate content, and size. As noted earlier, these portions of the various Ig classes also confer different biologic functions associated with each isotype. The constant regions of the Ig heavy chains are derived from Ig heavy-chain genes (discussed in detail in Chapter 6) and designated with Greek letters as shown below:

Immunoglobulin	Heavy-Chain Gene
IgM	μ
IgD	δ
IgG	γ
IgA	α
IgE	ε

The genes encoding these constant (C) regions responsible for the μ, δ, γ, α, and ε heavy chains are called Cμ, Cδ, Cγ, Cα, and Cε respectively.

Any individual of a species makes all five Ig isotypes, in proportions characteristic of the species, but, just as the case with light chains described above, in any one antibody molecule both heavy chains are always identical (e.g., 2γ or 2ε). Thus, an antibody molecule of the IgG class could have the structure $\kappa_2\gamma_2$ with two identical kappa light chains and two identical gamma heavy chains. Alternatively, it could have the structure $\lambda_2\gamma_2$ with two identical lambda light chains and two identical gamma heavy chains. In contrast, an antibody of the IgE class could have the structure $\kappa_2 \varepsilon_2$ or $\lambda_2 \varepsilon_2$. In each case, it is the nature of the heavy chains that confers on the molecule its unique biologic properties, such as its half-life in the circulation, its ability to bind to certain receptors, and its ability to activate enzymes (see Chapter 13) when combined with antigen.

Further characterization of these isotypes by specific antisera has led to the designation of several subclasses with more subtle differences. The major class of human IgG can be subdivided into the **subclasses** IgG_1, IgG_2, IgG_3, and IgG_4. IgA has been divided similarly into two subclasses, IgA_1 and IgA_2. The subclasses differ from one another in numbers and arrangement of interchain disulfide bonds as well as by alterations in other structural features. These alterations, in turn, produce some changes in functional properties that will be discussed later.

IMMUNOGLOBULIN DOMAINS

In addition to interchain disulfide bonds between the light and heavy chains and between the two heavy chains, intrachain disulfide bonds form loops *within* the chains. These intrachain bonds result in regions called ***immunoglobulin*** *fold domains*, which create the antiparallel β-pleated sheet structure characteristic of antibody molecules The **globular structure** of immunoglobulins and the ability of enzymes to cleave these molecules into large entities instead of degrading them to oligopeptides and amino acids are indicative of a very compact structure. Furthermore, the presence of intrachain disulfide bonds at regular, approximately equal intervals of about 100–110 amino acids leads to the prediction that each loop in the peptide chains should form a compactly folded **globular domain**. In fact, each light chain has two domains, and each heavy chain has four or five domains, separated by a short unfolded stretch (see Fig. 4.3). These configurations have been confirmed by direct observation and by genetic analysis (see Chapter 6).

Immunoglobulin molecules are assemblies of separate domains, each centered on a disulfide bond. The extensive homology of the domains suggests that they evolved from a single ancestral gene which duplicated several times and then mutated, resulting in a change in amino acid sequence that enabled the resultant different domains to fulfill different functions. Each domain is designated by a letter that indicates whether it is on a light chain or a heavy chain and a number that indicates its position. As we shall soon discuss in more detail, the amino acid sequence of the first domain on light and heavy chains is highly variable from one antibody to the next, so the first domain is designated V_L or V_H (see Fig. 4.3). The amino acid sequences of the second and subsequent domains on both heavy chains are much more constant, so the domains are designated C_L or C_H1, C_H2, and C_H3 (Fig. 4.3). In addition to their interchain disulfide bonding, the globular domains bind to each other in homologous pairs, largely by hydrophobic interactions, as follows: $V_H V_L$, $C_H1 C_L$, $C_H2 C_H2$, and $C_H3 C_H3$.

IMMUNOGLOBULIN HINGE REGION

The hinge region of immunoglobulins is typically composed of a short segment of amino acids and is found between the C_H1 and C_H2 regions of the heavy chains (see Fig. 4.3). Exceptions are IgD and IgE, which have relatively long hinge regions compared to those of other Ig isotypes. This hinge segment is made up predominantly of cysteine and proline residues. The cysteines are involved in formation of interchain disulfide bonds, and the proline residues prevent folding in a globular structure. This region of the heavy chain is important structurally because it permits flexibility between the two Fab arms of the Y-shaped antibody molecule. It allows the arms to open and close to accommodate binding to two epitopes, separated by a fixed distance, as might be found on the surface of a bacterium. Additionally, since this stretch of amino acids is open and as accessible as any other nonfolded peptide, it can be cleaved by proteases, such as papain, to generate the Fab and Fc fragments described above (see Fig. 4.2).

IMMUNOGLOBULIN VARIABLE REGION

As discussed earlier, it is the variable region of an immunoglobulin that binds to a specific antigen. A major problem for immunologists was to determine how so many individual specificities, which are required to meet the enormous variety of antigenic challenges, are generated from the variable region. As we shall see in Chapter 6, this issue has been largely resolved and is explained by the phenomenon of gene rearrangement associated with B cells (and T cells for the TCR, as you will learn in Chapter 8). We will briefly introduce the concept of hypervariability regions of immunoglobulins in this section as it relates to the concept of antibody specificity, since it is important to an understanding of topics covered later in this chapter.

Significant insights into the antigen-binding region of antibodies have been obtained from examination of the amino acid sequences of Ig molecules derived from sera or urine of individuals suffering from multiple myeloma. Why were these sera and urine samples chosen for examination? As discussed earlier in this chapter, the sera of multiple myeloma patients contains copious amounts of Ig molecules, all identical in structure and specificity by virtue of their production by the neoplastic plasma cells causing the disease. In addition, urine from such patients contains large amounts of light-chain molecules associated with these myeloma proteins (i.e., Bence Jones proteins). Using these sera and urine samples, it was found that the greatest variability existed in the 110 N-terminal amino acids of both the light and heavy chains. Kabat and Wu compared the amino acid sequences of many different V_L and V_H regions. They plotted the variability in the amino acids at each position in the chain and showed that the greatest amount of variability (defined as the ratio of the number of different amino acids at a given position to the frequency of the most common amino acid at that position) occurred in three regions of the light and heavy chains. These regions are called **hypervariable regions**. The less variable stretches, which occur between these hypervariable regions, are called framework regions. It is now clear that the hypervariable regions participate in the binding with antigen and form the region complementary in structure to the antigen. Consequently, hypervariable regions are termed **complementarity-determining regions** (CDR) of the light and heavy chains: CDR1, CDR2, and CDR3 (see Fig. 4.4).

Although they are separated in the linear, two-dimensional model of the peptide chains, the hypervariable regions of the light chain and the heavy chain are actually brought together in the folded form of the intact antibody molecule. Together they constitute the combining site, which is complementary to the epitope (Fig. 4.5). The variability in these CDRs provides the diversity required for the function of antibodies of different specificities. All the known forces involved in antigen–antibody interactions

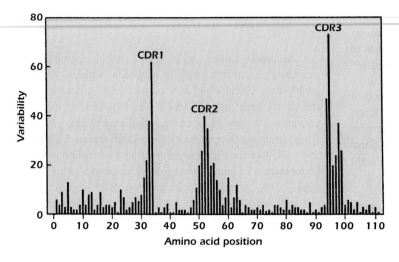

Figure 4.4. Variability of amino acids representing N-terminal residues of V_H in representative Ig molecule.

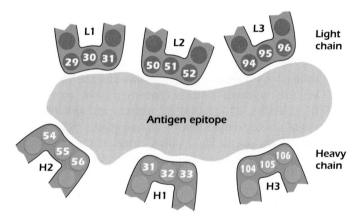

Figure 4.5. Schematic representation of complementarity between an epitope and antibody-combining site consisting of hypervariable areas of the L and H chains. Numbered letters denote CDR of heavy (H1, H2, H3) and light (L1, L2, L3) chains; circled numbers denote the number of the amino acid residue in the CDRs.

are weak, noncovalent interactions (e.g., ionic bonds, hydrogen bonds, van der Waals forces, and hydrophobic interactions). It is therefore necessary that there be a close fit between antigen and antibody over a sufficiently large region to allow a total binding force that is adequate for stable interaction. Both the heavy and the light chains contribute to the binding between epitope and antibody.

It should now be apparent that two antibody molecules with different antigenic specificities must have different amino acid sequences in their hypervariable regions and that those with similar sequences will generally have similar specificities. However, it is possible for two antibodies with different amino acid sequences to have specificity for the same epitope. In this case, the *binding affinities* (a measure of the strength of binding) of the antibodies with the epitope will probably be different because there will be differences in the number and types of binding forces available to bind identical antigens to the different binding sites of the two antibodies.

An additional source of variability involves the size of the combining site on the antibody, which is usually (but not always) considered to take the form of a depression or

cleft. In some instances, especially when small, hydrophobic haptens are involved, the epitopes do not occupy the entire combining site, yet they achieve sufficient affinity of binding. It has been shown that antibodies specific for such a hapten may, in fact, react with other antigens that

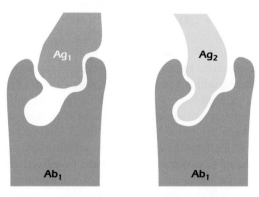

Figure 4.6. Representation of how an antibody of a given specificity (Ab) can exhibit binding with two different epitopes (Ag₁ and Ag₂).

have no obvious similarity to the hapten (e.g., dinitrophenol and sheep red cells). These dissimilar antigens bind either to a larger area or to a different area of the combining site on the antibody (see Fig. 4.6). Thus, a particular antibody-combining site may have the ability to combine with two (or more) apparently diverse epitopes, a property called **redundancy**. The ability of a single antibody molecule to cross-react with an unknown number of epitopes may reduce the number of different antibodies needed to defend an individual against a broad range of antigenic challenges.

 ## IMMUNOGLOBULIN VARIANTS

The three types of Ig variants are discussed below and summarized in Figure 4.7.

Isotypes

As you learned earlier in the chapter, the five isotypes or classes of immunoglobulins are IgA, IgG, IgM, IgD, and IgE. Why has the immune system evolved to provide this level of Ig diversity? To optimize humoral immune defenses against infectious pathogens and other foreign substances, a variety of mechanisms have developed. Each mechanism is dependent on a somewhat different property or function of an Ig molecule. Thus, when a specific antibody molecule combines with a specific antigen or a pathogen, several different effector mechanisms come into play. These different mechanisms derive from the isotypes, each of which may combine with the same epitope but trigger a different biologic response. These differences result from structural variations in heavy chains, which have generated domains that mediate a variety of functions. A summary of the properties of the Ig classes is given in Tables 4.1 and 4.2.

Allotypes

Another form of variation in the structure of immunoglobulins, based on genetic differences between individuals, is **allotypy**. In other words, different allelic forms (**allotypes**) of the heavy- or light-chain constant-region genes give rise to different forms of the same gene at a given locus. As a result of allotypy, a heavy- or light-chain constituent of any immunoglobulin can be present in some members of a species and absent in others. Bear in mind, however, that despite these allotypic differences among Ig classes within a species, the vast majority of the protein sequences of the constant regions (H or L) for a given class are highly conserved. Allotypic differences at known H- and L-chain gene loci usually result in changes in only one or two amino acids in the constant region of a chain. With a few exceptions, the presence of allotypic differences in two identical Ig molecules does not generally affect binding with antigen, but it serves as an important marker for analysis of Mendelian inheritance.

Some known allotype markers constitute a group on the γ chain of human IgG (called **Gm** for IgG markers), a group on the κ chain (called **Km**), and a group on the α chain (called **Am**).

Allotypic markers have been found in the immunoglobulins of several species, usually by the use of antisera generated by immunization of one member of a species with antibody from another member of the same species. As with other allelic systems, allotypes are inherited as dominant Mendelian traits. The genes encoding these markers are expressed codominantly, so that an individual may be homozygous or heterozygous for a given marker.

Idiotypes

As you have seen, the combining site of a specific antibody molecule is made up of a unique combination of amino acids in the variable regions of the light and heavy chains. Since this combination is not present in other antibody molecules, it should be immunogenic and capable of stimulating an immunologic response against itself in an animal of the same species. This prediction was actually found to be accurate. If mice are immunized to generate an antibody response and the antigen-specific antibodies from the immune sera are isolated, the antibodies are capable

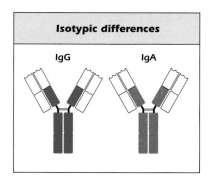 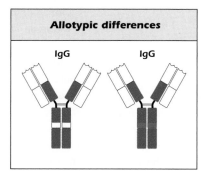 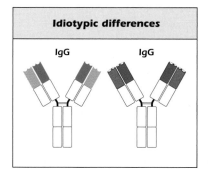

Figure 4.7. Different types of Ig variation.

TABLE 4.1. Most Important Features of Immunoglobulin Isotopes

Feature	Isotype				
	IgG	IgA	IgM	IgD	IgE
Molecular weight	150,000	160,000 for monomer	900,000	180,000	200,000
Additional protein subunits	—	J and S	J	—	—
Approximate concentration in serum (mg/mL)	12	1.8	1	0–0.04	0.00002
Percent of total Ig	80	13	6	0.2	0.002
Distribution	~Equal: intravascular and extravascular	Intravascular and secretions	Mostly intravascular	Present on lymphocyte surface	On basophils and mast cells present in saliva and nasal secretions
Half-life (days)	23	5.5	5	2.8	2.0
Placental passage	++	—	—		
Presence in secretion	—	++	—		
Presence in milk	+	+	0 to trace		
Activation of complement	+	—	+++		
Binding to Fc receptors on macrophages, PMN cells, and NK cells	++	—	—		
Relative agglutinating capacity	+	++	+++		
Antiviral activity	+++	+++	+		
Antibacterial activity (Gram negative)	+++	++ (with lysozyme)	+++ (with complement)		
Antitoxin activity	+++	—	—		
Allergic activity	—	—	—	—	++

TABLE 4.2. Important Differences Among Human IgG Subclasses

Characteristic	IgG$_1$	IgG$_2$	IgG$_3$	IgG$_4$
Occurrence (% of total IgG)	70	20	7	3
Half-life	23	23	7	23
Complement binding	+	+	+++	—
Placental passage	++	±	++	++
Binding of monocytes	+++	+	+++	±

of stimulating anti-antibody responses in mice of the same strain. In fact, these anti-antibody responses are *polyclonal* in nature; they have been shown to be specific for several epitopes present on the antibodies used in the inoculation. Given the fact that the donors and recipients of the anti-serum used in the immunization protocol were members of the same strain (genetically identical), should not the antibodies fail to stimulate a response (i.e., be considered "self" antigens)?

The anti-antibody responses were, in fact, stimulated by the collective variable regions on the H and L chains of the antibody molecules contained in the inoculum. These portions of antibody molecules are called *idiotypes*. Thus, a more accurate designation of the antibodies produced in the antibody-immunized mice described above is *anti-idiotype antibodies*. Evidence has suggested that anti-idotype responses occur normally within individuals. One proposed explanation for these findings is that anti-idiotypic antibodies play a physiologic role in regulating the antibody response to the antigen that stimulated the initial response. In some cases anti-idiotypic sera prevent binding of the antibody with its antigen, in which event the idiotypic determinant is considered to be in or very near the combining site itself. Anti-idiotypic sera that do not block binding of antibody with antigen are probably directed against variable determinants of the framework area outside the combining site (see Fig. 4.8).

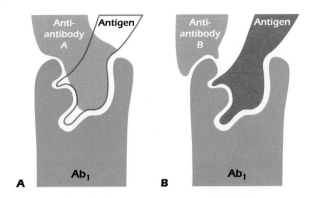

Figure 4.8. Two anti-idiotypic antibodies to Ab_1. (A) The anti-idiotypic antibody is directed to the combining site of Ab_1, preventing binding of Ab_1 with the antigen. (B) The anti-idiotypic antibody binds with framework areas of Ab_1 and does not prevent its binding with antigen.

Although this regulatory role for anti-idiotypic antibodies remains controversial, the concept is consistent with Jerne's network theory for immune regulation, which is discussed further in Chapter 10. In short, this theory postulates that antibodies respond primarily to each other and that foreign antigens merely perturb the normal equilibrium established between idiotypes. In 1984, Jerne shared the Nobel Prize in Medicine with Kohler and Milstein for their contributions to our understanding of development, specificity, and control of immune responses.

Theoretically, it is possible that an anti-idiotypic antibody with a combining site complementary to that of the idiotype bears a resemblance to the epitope, which is also complementary to the idiotype's combining site. Thus, the anti-idiotype may represent a facsimile or an *internal image* of the epitope. Indeed, there are examples of immunization of experimental animals using anti-idiotypic internal images as immunogens. Such immunogens induce antibodies capable of reacting with the antigen that carries the epitope against which the original idiotype is directed. Thus, these antibodies are induced without the immunized animal ever having been introduced to the original antigen.

In some instances, especially with inbred animals, anti-idiotypic antibodies react with several different antibodies that are directed against the same epitope and share idiotypes. These idiotypes are called public or *cross-reacting idiotypes*. This term frequently defines families of antibody molecules. By contrast, sera that react with only one particular antibody molecule define a private idiotype.

In summary, differences between constant regions due to expression of different heavy- and light-chain constant-region genes are called isotypes. Differences due to different alleles of the same constant-region gene are called allotypes. Finally, within a given isotype (e.g., IgG),

differences due to particular rearranged V_H and V_L genes are referred to as idiotypes.

STRUCTURAL FEATURES OF IgG

IgG is the predominant immunoglobulin in blood, lymph fluid, cerebrospinal fluid, and peritoneal fluid. The IgG molecule consists of two γ heavy chains, each with a molecular weight of approximately 50,000 Da, and two light chains (either κ or λ), each with a molecular weight of approximately 25,000 Da. The heavy chains are held together by disulfide bonds and each of the light chains similarly binds to one heavy chain (Fig. 4.9). The entire IgG molecule has a molecular weight of approximately 150,000 Da and a sedimentation coefficient of 7S. Electrophoretically, the IgG molecule is the least anodic of all serum proteins, and it migrates to the γ range of serum globulins, hence its earlier designation as γ-globulin or 7S immunoglobulin.

The IgG class of immunoglobulins in humans contains four subclasses designated IgG_1, IgG_2, IgG_3, and IgG_4, named in order of their abundance in serum, with IgG_1 being the most abundant. Except for their variable regions, all the immunoglobulins within a class (e.g., IgG_1 and IgG_2) have about 90% homology in their amino acid sequences, but there is only 60% homology between classes (e.g., IgG and IgA). This degree of homology means that an antiserum made in mice against human IgG may include antibodies against all members of a given class (e.g., all members of the IgG class) while other antisera may be raised that are specific for determinants found in only one of the subclasses (e.g., in IgG_2). This variation was first detected antigenically by the use of antibodies against various γ chains. The IgG subclasses differ in their chemical properties and, more importantly, in their biologic properties, which are discussed below.

BIOLOGIC PROPERTIES OF IgG

IgG present in the serum of human adults represents about 15% of the body's total protein (other proteins include albumins, globulins, and enzymes). IgG is distributed approximately equally between the intravascular and extravascular spaces.

Except for the IgG_3 subclass, which has a much shorter half-life of 7 days, the half-life of IgG is approximately 23 days, the longest half-life of all Ig isotypes. This persistence in the serum makes IgG the most suitable for passive immunization by transfer of antibodies. Interestingly, as the concentration of IgG in the serum increases (as in cases of multiple myeloma or after the transfer of very high concentrations of IgG), the rate of catabolism of IgG increases, and the half-life of IgG decreases to 15–20 days or even

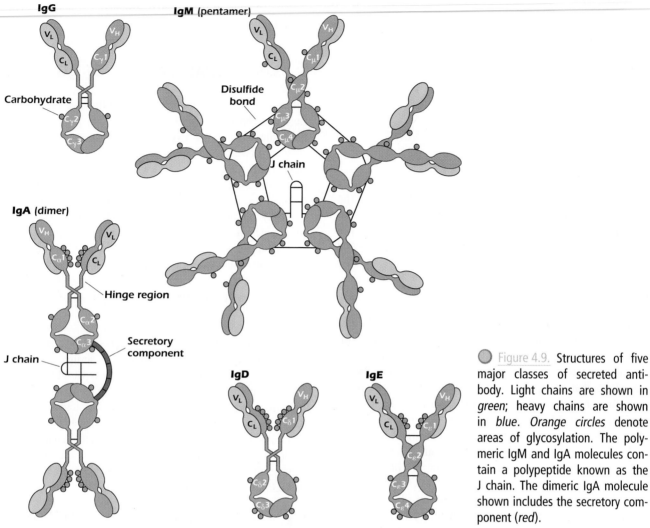

Figure 4.9. Structures of five major classes of secreted antibody. Light chains are shown in *green*; heavy chains are shown in *blue*. *Orange circles* denote areas of glycosylation. The polymeric IgM and IgA molecules contain a polypeptide known as the J chain. The dimeric IgA molecule shown includes the secretory component (*red*).

less. Recent studies have provided a clear explanation for the prolonged survival of IgG relative to other serum proteins and the decrease in its half-life at high concentrations. A saturable IgG receptor that protects the molecule from degradation (protection receptor FcRp, also called the Brambell receptor) has been identified and shown to bind to the Fc region of this isotype. This receptor, found in cellular endosomes, selectively recycles endocytized IgG (e.g., following endocytosis of antigen–antibody immune complexes) back to the circulation. Figure 4.10 illustrates how IgG antibody is cleansed of antigen and harvests antigen for presentation without antibody destruction. Conditions associated with high IgG levels saturate the FcRp receptors, rendering the catabolism of excess IgG indistinguishable from catabolism of albumin or other Ig isotypes.

Agglutination and Formation of Precipitate

IgG molecules can cause the ***agglutination*** or clumping of particulate (insoluble) antigens such as microorganisms.

The reaction of IgG with soluble, multivalent antigens can precipitate antigens out of solution (see Chapter 5). This property of IgG is undoubtedly of considerable survival value since insoluble antigen–antibody complexes are easily phagocytized and destroyed by phagocytic cells. IgG molecules may be made to aggregate by a variety of procedures. For example, precipitation with alcohol, a method employed in the purification of IgG, or heating at 56°C for 10 min, a method used to inactivate complement (see Chapter 13), both cause aggregation. Aggregated IgG can still combine with antigen.

Many of the properties that are attributed to antigen–antibody complexes are exhibited by aggregated IgG (without antigen), such as attachment to phagocytic cells and the activation of complement and other biologically active substances that may be harmful to the body. Such activation is attributable to the juxtaposition of Fc domains by the aggregation process in a way analogous to that produced by antigen-induced immune complex formation. It is therefore imperative that no aggregated IgG be present in passively administered IgG.

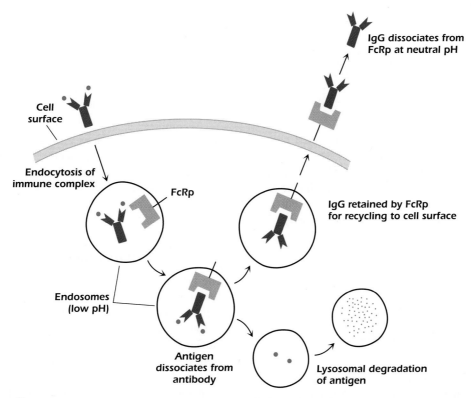

Figure 4.10. Recycling of IgG utilizing protector receptor (FcRp). Circulating monomeric IgG plus antigen (immune complex) enters an antigen-presenting cell through the process of endocytosis. Within the endosome, the complex binds FcRp; IgG and Ag dissociate, allowing the IgG to be directed to the cell surface for recycling. Antigen undergoes lysosomal degredation (antigen processing), and its proteolytic fragments are ultimately expressed on the cell surface in the context of MHC class II molecules.

Passage of Ig Through the Placenta and Absorption in Neonates

The IgG isotype (except for subclass IgG_2) is the only class of immunoglobulin that can pass through the placenta, enabling the mother to transfer her immunity to the fetus. Placental transfer is facilitated by expression of an IgG protection receptor (FcRn) expressed on placental cells. FcRn was recently shown to be identical to the IgG protection receptor (FcRp) found in cellular endosomes. Analysis of fetal immunoglobulins shows that, at the third or fourth month of pregnancy, there is a rapid increase in the concentration of IgG. This IgG must be of maternal origin since the fetus is unable to synthesize immunoglobulins at this age. Then, during the fifth month of pregnancy, the fetus begins to synthesize IgM and trace amounts of IgA. It is not until three or four months after birth, when the level of inherited maternal IgG drops as a result of catabolism, that the infant begins to synthesize its own IgG antibodies. Thus, the resistance of the fetus and the neonate to infection is conferred almost entirely by the mother's IgG, which passes across the placenta. It has been established that passage across the placenta is mediated by the Fc portion of the IgG molecule;

F(ab)'$_2$ or Fab fragments of IgG do not pass through the placenta. Interestingly, the IgG protection receptor (FcRn) expressed on placental cells is transiently superexpressed in the intestinal tissue of neonates. Absorption of maternal IgG contained in the colostrum of nursing mothers is achieved by its binding to these high-density receptors in intestinal tissue. FcRn is down-regulated in intestinal tissue at two weeks of age.

While passage of IgG molecules across the placenta confers immunity to infection on the fetus, it may also be responsible for hemolytic disease of the newborn (erythroblastosis fetalis) (see Chapter 15), which is caused by maternal antibodies to fetal red blood cells. The maternal IgG antibodies to Rh antigen, produced by an Rh$^-$ mother, pass across the placenta and attack the fetal red blood cells that express Rh antigens (Rh$^+$).

Opsonization

When antigens, such as pathogenic microorganisms, bind to antigen-specific IgG, they are more readily phagocytized by phagocytes due to the presence of receptors for the Fc portion of the IgG molecules on these cells. Many

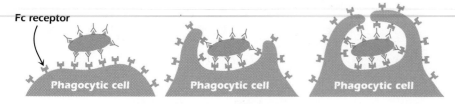

Fc receptor

Phagocytic cell   Phagocytic cell   Phagocytic cell

Figure 4.11. Phagocytosis of particle coated with antibodies.

phagocytic cells, including macrophages and PMN phagocytes, express Fc receptors. This phenomenon is called **opsonization** (from the Greek *opsonin*, which means to prepare for eating). Antibody molecules react with the antigenic epitopes of antigens at their Fab regions, but it is the Fc portion that confers the opsonizing property. The net effect is a zipperlike closure of the surface membrane of the phagocytic cell around the antigen as receptors for Fc and the Fc regions on the antibodies continue to combine, leading to the final engulfing and destruction of the microorganism (see Fig. 4.11).

Antibody-Dependent, Cell-Mediated Cytotoxicity

The IgG molecule plays an important role in antibody-dependent, cell-mediated cytotoxicity (ADCC). In this form of cytotoxicity, the Fab portion binds with the target cell, whether it is a microorganism or a tumor cell, and the Fc portion binds with specific receptors for Fc that are found on certain large granular lymphocytic cells called NK cells (see Chapter 2). By this mechanism, the IgG molecule focuses the killer cells on their target, and the killer cells destroy the target, not by phagocytosis but with the various substances that they release.

Activation of Complement

Chapter 13 will discuss the major properties of complement. In brief, the **complement system** is a set of plasma proteins that can be activated by binding either to certain pathogens or to antibody (e.g., pathogen-specific antibodies). Complement activation is often described as a series of cascading enzymatic events leading to the generation of specific complement components that cause opsonization, phagocytosis of infectious agents, and direct lysis of the invading organism, among other important immunologic phenomena. Structural features of the early complement components involved in the activation cascade dictate the antibody classes to which complement will bind.

IgG molecules are capable of activating the complement system (see Chapter 13). Activation of complement results in the release of several important biologically active molecules and leads to lysis if the antibody is bound to antigen on the surface of a cell. Some of the complement components are also opsonins; they bind to the target antigen and direct phagocytes, which carry receptors specific for these opsonins, to focus their activity on the target antigen. Other components of complement activation are chemotactic; specifically, they attract phagocytic cells. All in all, the activation of complement by IgG has profound biologic effects on the host and on the target antigen, whether it is a live cell, a microorganism, or a tumor cell.

Neutralization of Toxins

The IgG molecule is an excellent antibody for the neutralization of toxins such as tetanus and botulinus or for the inactivation of, for example, snake and scorpion venoms. Because of its ability to neutralize such poisons (mostly by blocking their active sites) and because of its long half-life compared to that of other isotypes, the IgG molecule is the isotype of choice for passive immunization (i.e., the transfer of antibodies) against toxins and venoms.

Immobilization of Bacteria

IgG molecules are efficient in immobilizing various motile bacteria. Reaction of antibodies specific for the flagella and cilia of certain microorganisms causes them to clump, thereby arresting their movement and preventing their ability to spread or invade tissue.

Neutralization of Viruses

IgG antibody is an efficient virus-neutralizing antibody. In one mechanism of neutralization, the antibody binds with antigenic determinants present on various portions of the virus coat, among them the region used by the virus for attachment to the target cell. Inhibition of viral attachment effectively arrests infection. Other antibodies are thought to inhibit viral penetration or the shedding of the viral coat required to induce infection.

The versatility in function of the IgG molecule makes it a very important molecule in the immune response. The effects of immune deficiency disorders in which an individual is unable to synthesize IgG molecules (see Chapter 17) underscore its significance. Affected individuals are prone to infections that may result in toxemias and death.

STRUCTURAL FEATURES OF IgM

As we shall see later in this chapter, IgM is the first immunoglobulin produced following immunization. Its name derives from its initial description as a *macroglobulin (M)*, an immunoglobulin of high molecular weight (900,000 Da). IgM has a sedimentation coefficient of 19S, and it has an extra C_H domain. In comparison to the IgG molecule, which consists of one four-chain structure, IgM is a *pentameric molecule* composed of five such units. Each unit consists of two light and two heavy chains, all joined together by additional disulfide bonds between their Fc portions and by a polypeptide chain called the *J chain* (see Fig. 4.9). The J chain, which, like light and heavy chains, is synthesized in the B cell or plasma cell, has a molecular weight of 15,000 Da. This pentameric ensemble of IgM, which is held together by disulfide bonds, comes apart after mild treatment with reducing agents such as mercaptoethanol.

Surprisingly, each pentameric IgM molecule appears to have a valence of 5 (i.e., five antigen combining sites), instead of the expected valence of 10 predicted by the 10 Fab segments contained in the pentamer. This apparent reduction in valence is probably the result of conformational constraints imposed by polymerization. Pentameric IgM has a planar configuration, so each of its 10 Fab portions cannot open fully with respect to the adjacent Fab when it combines with antigen, as is possible in the case of IgG. Thus, any large antigen bound to one Fab may block a neighboring site from binding with antigen, making the molecule appear pentavalent (or of even lesser valence).

● BIOLOGIC PROPERTIES OF IgM

IgM present in adult human serum is found predominantly in the intravascular spaces. The half-life of the IgM molecule is approximately 5 days. In contrast to IgG, the IgM antibodies are not very versatile; they are poor toxin-neutralizing antibodies, and they are not efficient in the neutralization of viruses. IgM is also found on the surface of mature B cells together with IgD (discussed later in this chapter), where it serves as an antigen-specific BCR. Once the B cell is activated by antigen following ligation of the BCR, it may undergo class switching (see Chapter 6) and begin to secrete and express other membrane Ig isotypes, such as IgG.

Complement Fixation

Because of its pentameric form, IgM is an excellent complement-fixing or complement-activating antibody (see Chapter 13). Unlike other classes of immunoglobulins, a single molecule of IgM can initiate the complement sequence on binding to antigen with at least two of its Fab arms, making it the most efficient immunoglobulin in terms of initiating the lysis of microorganisms and other cells. This ability, taken together with the appearance of IgM as the first class of antibodies generated after immunization or infection, makes IgM antibodies very important as providers of an early line of immunologic defense against bacterial infections.

First Line of Humoral Defense

Unlike IgG, IgM antibodies do not pass through the placenta. However, since this is the only class of immunoglobulins that is synthesized by the fetus, beginning at approximately five months of gestation, elevated levels of IgM in the fetus are indicative of congenital or perinatal infection.

IgM is the isotype synthesized by children and adults in appreciable amounts after immunization or exposure to T-independent antigens, and it is the first isotype that is synthesized after immunization (see Fig. 4.12). Thus, elevated levels of IgM usually indicate either recent infection or recent exposure to antigen.

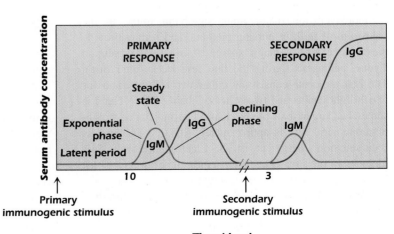

● Figure 4.12. Kinetics of an antibody response.

Agglutination

IgM molecules are efficient agglutinating antibodies. Because of their pentameric form, IgM antibodies can form macromolecular bridges between epitopes on molecules that may be too distant from each other to be bridged by the smaller IgG antibodies. Furthermore, because of their pentameric form and multiple valences, IgM antibodies are particularly well suited to combat antigens that contain repeated patterns of the same antigenic determinant. Examples include polysaccharide antigens or cellular antigens, which are multiply expressed on cell surfaces.

Isohemagglutinins

IgM antibodies include the *isohemagglutinins*, the naturally occurring antibodies against the red blood cell antigens of the ABO blood groups. These antibodies are presumed to arise as a result of immunization by bacteria in the gastrointestinal and respiratory tracts, which bear determinants similar to the oligosaccharides of the ABO blood groups. Thus, without known prior immunization, people with the type O blood group have isohemagglutinins to the A and B antigens; those with the type A blood group have antibodies to the B antigens; and those with type B blood group have antibodies to the A antigen. An individual of the AB group has neither anti-A nor anti-B antibodies. Fortunately, the IgM isohemagglutinins do not pass through the placenta, so incompatibility of the ABO blood groups between mother and fetus poses no danger to the fetus. However, *transfusion reactions*, in which the recipient's isohemagglutinins react with the donor's red blood cells, arise as a result of ABO incompatibility and may have disastrous consequences.

STRUCTURAL AND BIOLOGIC PROPERTIES OF IgA

IgA is the major immunoglobulin in external secretions such as saliva, mucus, sweat, gastric fluid, and tears. It is, moreover, the major immunoglobulin found in the colostrum of milk in nursing mothers, and it may provide the neonate with a major source of intestinal protection against pathogens during the first few weeks after birth. The IgA molecule consists of either two κ light chains or two λ light chains and two α heavy chains. The α chain is somewhat larger than the γ chain. The molecular weight of monomeric IgA is approximately 165,000 Da, and its sedimentation coefficient is 7S. Electrophoretically IgA migrates to the slow β or fast γ region of serum globulins. Dimeric IgA has a molecular weight of 400,000 Da.

The IgA class of immunoglobulins contains two subclasses: IgA_1 (93%) and IgA_2 (7%). Interestingly, if production of all IgA on mucosal surfaces (respiratory, gastrointestinal, and urinary tracts) were taken into account, IgA would be the major immunoglobulin in terms of quantity.

Biologic Properties of IgA

Serum IgA, which has no known biologic function, has a half-life of 5.5 days. The IgA present in serum is predominantly **monomeric** (one four-chain unit) and has presumably been released before dimerization so that it fails to bind to the secretory component. Secretory IgA is very important biologically, but little is known of any function for serum IgA.

Most IgA is present not in the serum but in secretions such as tears, saliva, sweat, and mucus, where it serves an important biologic function as a component of the MALT described in Chapter 2. Within mucous secretions, IgA exists as a **dimer** consisting of two four-chain units linked by the same joining (J) chain found in IgM molecules (see Fig. 4.9). IgA-secreting plasma cells synthesize the IgA molecules and the J chains, which form the dimers. Such plasma cells are located predominantly in the connective tissue called **lamina propria** that lies immediately below the basement membrane of many surface epithelia (e.g., in the parotid gland, along the gastrointestinal tract in the intestinal villi, in tear glands, in the lactating breast, or beneath bronchial mucosa). When these dimeric molecules are released from plasma cells, they bind to the poly-Ig receptor expressed on the basal membranes of adjacent epithelial cells. This receptor transports the molecules through the epithelial cells and releases them into extracellular fluids (e.g., in the gut or bronchi). Release is facilitated by enzymatic cleavage of the poly-Ig receptor, leaving a large 70,000-Da fragment (i.e., the secretory component) of the receptor still attached to the Fc piece of the dimeric IgA molecule (see Fig. 4.13). The secretory component may help to protect the dimeric IgA from proteolytic cleavage. It should be noted that the secretory component also binds and transports pentameric IgM to mucosal surfaces in small amounts.

Role in Mucosal Infections

Because of its presence in secretions such as saliva, urine, and gastric fluid, secretory IgA is of importance in the primary immunologic defense against local respiratory or gastrointestinal infections. Its protective effect is thought to be due to its ability to prevent the invading organism from attaching to and penetrating the epithelial surface. For example, in the case of cholera, the pathogenic *Vibrio* organism attaches to but never penetrates beyond the cells that line the gastrointestinal tract, where it secretes an exotoxin responsible for all symptoms. IgA antibody, which can prevent attachment of the organism to the cells, provides protection from the pathogen. Thus, for protection against local infections, routes of immunization that result

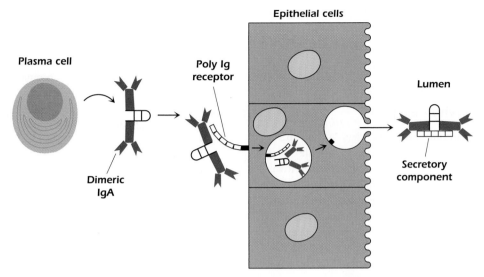

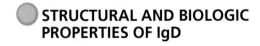 Figure 4.13. Transcytosis of dimeric IgA across epithelia. Plasma cells in close proximity to epithelial basement membranes in the gut, respiratory epithelia, salivary and tear glands, and lactating mammary glands release dimeric IgA. The IgA binds to the poly-Ig receptor and the complex undergoes transcytosis within vesicles across the cell. The poly-Ig receptor is cleaved from the complex at the apical surface to release the IgA from the cell. After exiting the cell, a pentameric fragment of the poly-Ig receptor known as the secretory component remains attached to the dimeric IgA and is believed to protect the antibody within the lumen of several organs that are in contact with the external environment.

in local production of IgA are much more effective than routes that primarily produce antibodies in serum.

Bactericidal Activity

The IgA molecule does not contain receptors for complement and, thus, IgA is not a complement-activating or complement-fixing immunoglobulin. Consequently, it does not induce complement-mediated bacterial lysis. IgA has been shown to possess bactericidal activity against Gram-negative organisms, but only in the presence of lysozyme, which is also present in the same secretions that contain secretory IgA.

Antiviral Activity

Secretory IgA is an efficient antiviral antibody, preventing viruses from entering host cells. In addition, secretory IgA is an efficient agglutinating antibody.

STRUCTURAL AND BIOLOGIC PROPERTIES OF IgD

The IgD molecule consists of two light chains, either both κ or both λ, and two δ heavy chains (see Fig. 4.9). IgD is a monomer with a molecular weight of 180,000 Da and a sedimentation coefficient of 7S. It migrates to the fast γ region of serum globulins. No heavy-chain allotypes or subclasses have been reported for the IgD molecule.

IgD is present in serum in very low and variable amounts, probably because it is not secreted by plasma cells and because, among immunoglobulins, it is highly susceptible to proteolytic degradation due to its long hinge region. In addition, following B-cell activation, transcription of the δ heavy-chain protein is down-regulated rapidly—a phenomenon that also helps explain the low serum IgD levels.

IgD is coexpressed with IgM on the surface of mature B cells and, like IgM, functions as an antigen-specific BCR. Its presence on the surface marks the differentiation of B cells to a more mature form. Thus, during ontogeny of B cells, expression of IgD lags behind that of IgM (see Chapter 7).

While the function of IgD has not been fully elucidated, expression of membrane IgD appears to correlate with the elimination of B cells with the capacity to generate self-reactive antibodies. Thus, during development, the major biologic significance of IgD may be in silencing autoreactive B cells. In mature B cells, IgD serves as an antigen-binding surface immunoglobulin with coexpressed IgM.

STRUCTURAL AND BIOLOGIC PROPERTIES OF IgE

The IgE molecule consists of two light chains (κ or λ) and two heavy ε chains. Like IgM molecules, IgE has an extra

C_H domain (see Fig. 4.9). IgE has a molecular weight of approximately 200,000 Da, its sedimentation coefficient is 8S, and it migrates electrophoretically to the fast γ region of serum globulins.

Importance of IgE in Parasitic Infections and Hypersensitivity Reactions

IgE, also called *reaginic antibody*, has a half-life in serum of 2 days, the shortest half-life of all classes of immunoglobulins. It is present in serum in the lowest concentration of all immunoglobulins. These low levels are due in part to a low rate of synthesis and to the unique ability of the Fc portion containing the extra C_H domain to bind with very high affinity to receptors (Fcε receptors) found on mast cells and basophils. Once bound to these high-affinity receptors, IgE may be retained by these cells for weeks or months. When antigen reappears, it combines with the Fab portion of the IgE attached to these cells, causing cross-linking of IgE molecules and, hence, indirect cross-linking of Fcε receptors. When this occurs, mast cells and basophils become activated and release the contents of their granules: histamine, heparin, leukotrienes, and other pharmacologically active compounds that trigger the immediate hypersensitivity reactions. These reactions may be mild, as in the case of a mosquito bite, or severe, as in the case of bronchial asthma; they may even result in systemic anaphylaxis, which can cause death within minutes (see Chapter 14).

IgE is not an agglutinating or complement-activating antibody; nevertheless, it has a role in protection against certain parasites, such as helminths (worms). This protection is achieved by activation of the same acute inflammatory response seen in a more pathologic form of immediate hypersensitivity responses. Elevated levels of IgE in serum have been shown to occur during infections with ascaris (a roundworm). In fact, immunization with ascaris antigen induces the formation of IgE.

KINETICS OF ANTIBODY RESPONSES FOLLOWING IMMUNIZATION

Primary Response

As mentioned in Chapter 3, the first exposure of an individual to a particular immunogen is referred to as the primary immunization and the measurable response that ensues is called the primary response. As shown in Figure 4.12, the primary antibody response may be divided into several phases as follows:

1. *Latent or lag period*: After initial exposure to an antigen, a period of one to two weeks follows

before antibody is detectable in the serum. The actual length of time depends on the species immunized, the nature of the antigen used to stimulate the response, and other factors that will become apparent in subsequent chapters. The length of the latent period also depends heavily on the sensitivity of the assay used to measure the product of the response. As we shall see in more detail in subsequent chapters, the latent period includes the time taken for T and B cells to make contact with the antigen, to proliferate, and to differentiate. B cells must also secrete antibody in sufficient quantity so that it can be detected in the serum. The less sensitive the assay used for detection of antibody, the more antibody will be required for detection and the longer the apparent latent period will be.

2. *Exponential phase*: During this phase, the concentration of antibody in the serum increases exponentially.

3. *Steady state*: During this period, production and degradation of antibody are balanced.

4. *Declining phase*: Finally, the immune response begins to shut down, and the concentration of antibody in serum declines rapidly.

The first class of antibody detected in primary responses is generally IgM, which, in some instances, may be the only class of immunoglobulin that is produced. If production of IgG antibody ensues, its appearance is generally accompanied by a rapid cessation of production of IgM (see Fig. 4.12).

Secondary Response

Although production of antibody after primary immunization with antigen may cease entirely within a few weeks (see Fig. 4.12), the immunized individual is left with a pool of long-lived *memory cells* capable of mounting a secondary response as well as any other future responses to the antigen. Experimentally, this secondary or memory response (also called the *anamnestic response*) becomes apparent when a response is triggered by a second injection of the same antigen. After the second injection, the lag phase is considerably shorter and antibody may appear in less than half the time required for the primary response. The magnitude of antibody produced in the secondary response is much greater than in the primary response; significantly higher concentrations of antibody are detectable in the serum. The production of antibody may also continue for a longer period, with persistent levels remaining in serum months or even years later.

There is a marked change in the type of antibody produced in the secondary response; different classes of immunoglobulins with the same antigen specificity appear. This shift is known as ***class switching;*** IgG antibodies appear at higher concentrations and with greater persistence than IgM antibodies. IgM levels may be greatly reduced or the immunoglobulin may disappear altogether. IgA and IgE may also appear. In addition, ***affinity maturation*** occurs—a phenomenon in which the average affinity (binding constant) of the antibodies for the antigen increases as the secondary response develops (see Chapter 7). The driving force for this increase in affinity may be a selection process during which B cells compete with free antibody to capture a decreasing amount of antigen. Thus, only those B-cell clones with high-affinity Ig receptors on their surfaces will bind enough antigen to ensure that the B cells are triggered to differentiate into plasma cells. These plasma cells, which arise from preferentially selected B cells, synthesize this antibody with high affinity for antigen.

The capacity to make a secondary response may persist for a long time (years in humans), and it provides an obvious selective advantage for an individual who survives the first contact with an invading pathogen. Establishment of this memory for generating a specific response is, of course, the purpose of public health immunization programs.

THE IMMUNOGLOBULIN SUPERFAMILY

The shared structural features of Ig heavy and light chains, which include the Ig -fold domains (see Figs. 4.3 and 4.4), are also seen in a large number of proteins. Most of these have been found to be membrane-bound glycoproteins. Because of this structural similarity, these proteins are classified as members of the ***immunoglobulin superfamily***. The redundant structural characteristic seen in these proteins suggests that the genes that encode them arose from a common primordial gene. Duplication and subsequent divergence of this primordial gene would explain the existence of the large number of membrane proteins that possess one or more regions homologous to the Ig-fold domain. Genetic and functional analyses of these Ig superfamily proteins have indicated that these genes have evolved independently, since they do not share genetic linkage or function. Figure 4.14 provides examples of proteins that are members of the Ig superfamily. Numerous other examples are discussed in other chapters. As can be seen in the figure, each molecule contains the characteristic Ig-fold structure (loops) formed as a result of intrachain disulfide bonds and consists of approximately 110 amino acids. These Ig-fold domains are believed to facilitate interactions between membrane proteins (e.g., CD4 molecules on helper T cells and class II MHC molecules on APC).

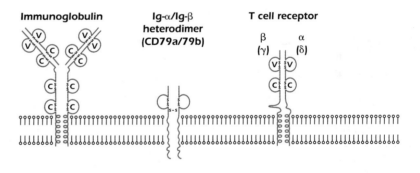

Figure 4.14. Representative members of Ig superfamily. The Ig-fold domains (shown as circular loops in blue) form the common structural features of these molecules. In all cases, the carboxyl-terminal end of the molecules shown are anchored in the membrane.

SUMMARY

1. Immunoglobulins of all classes have a fundamental four-chain structure, consisting of two identical light (L) and two identical heavy (H) chains. Through disulfide bonds each light chain is linked to a heavy chain and the two heavy chains are linked to each other.

2. In the native state, L and H chains fold into domains stabilized by an intrachain disulfide bond. A group of other proteins (e.g., TCR, CD4, class I and class II MHC molecules) also contain these Ig-fold domains, making them all members of the Ig superfamily.

3. Immunoglobulins are expressed in two forms: a membrane-bound antibody present on the surface of B cells and a secreted antibody produced by plasma cells. Membrane-bound antibodies associate with a heterodimer called Igα/Igβ to form the BCR.

4. The variable (V) regions, the N-terminal domains of both heavy and light chains, contain the hypervariable regions, also called complementarity-determining regions. CDRs make up the combining site of the antibody and vary according to the specificity of the antibody.

5. The constant (C) region domains of L and H chains are similar within each of the L- and H-chain isotypes, respectively.

6. The Fc regions of the heavy chains are responsible for the different biologic functions carried out by each class of antibody.

7. Immunoglobulin heavy- and light-chain isotypes are distinguished by the structure of their constant regions. Differences in regions of the H-chain constant regions are due to variations in genetic alleles that cause a change in one or two amino acids. Immunoglobulin molecules with such differences are called allotypes. Allotypes distinguish individuals within a species.

8. By contrast, idiotypic regions of antibody molecules are represented by the unique combinations of amino acids that make up the antigen-combining site of an antibody molecule; they are thus unique for that particular antibody.

9. IgG is a versatile class of antibody capable of carrying out numerous biologic functions that range from neutralization of toxins to activation of complement and opsonization. IgG is the only class of immunoglobulin that passes through the placenta and confers maternal immunity on the fetus. The half-life of IgG (23 days) is the longest of all immunoglobulin classes.

10. IgM is expressed on the surface of mature B cells (as a monomer) and is secreted as a pentameric antibody held together by a J chain; of all classes of immunoglobulin it functions as the best agglutinating and complement-activating antibody.

11. IgA antibody is present in monomeric and dimeric forms. The dimeric IgA is found in secretions and is referred to as secretory IgA. Secretory IgA is an important antiviral immunoglobulin.

12. IgD is present on the surface of mature B cells and is co-expressed and shares antigen specificity with IgM. The functional properties of IgD have not been fully elucidated.

13. IgE, also called reaginic antibody, is of paramount importance in allergic reactions. It also appears to be of importance in protection against parasitic infections. The Fc portion of IgE binds with high affinity to receptors on certain cells, including mast cells. On contact with antigen, IgE triggers the degranulation of such cells, resulting in the release of pharmacologically active substances that mediate the hypersensitivity (allergic) reactions.

14. Following first exposure to an antigen, a primary antibody response occurs. This response consists mainly of the production of IgM antibodies. The second exposure to the same antigen results in a secondary or anamnestic (memory) response, which is more rapid than the primary response and in which the response shifts from IgM production to the synthesis of IgG and other isotypes. The secondary response lasts much longer than the primary response.

REFERENCES

Alzari PM, Lascombe MB, Poljak RJ (1988): Three dimensional structure of antibodies. *Annu Rev Immunol* 6:555.

Capra D, Edmundson AB (1977): The antibody combining site. *Sci Am* 236:50.

Davies DR, Metzger H (1983): Structural basis of antibody function. *Annu Rev Immunol* 1:87.

Eisen HN (2001): Specificity and degeneracy in antigen recognition: Yin and yang in the immune response. *Annu Rev Immunol* 19:1.

Jefferis R (1993): What is an idiotype? *Immunol Today* 14:19.

Junghans RP, Anderson CL (1996): The protection receptor for IgG catabolism is the β2-microglobulin-containing neonatal intestinal transport receptor. *Proc Natl Acad Sci USA* 93:5512.

Kolar GR, Capra JD (1999): Immunoglobulins: Structure and function. In eds Paul WE (ed): *Fundamental Immunology*, 4th ed. New York: Raven.

Koshland ME (1985): The coming of age of the immunoglobulin J chain. *Annu Rev Immunol* 3:425.

Mestecky J, McGhee JR (1987): Immunoglobulin A (IgA): Molecular and cellular interactions involved in IgA biosynthesis and immune response. *Adv Immunol* 40:153.

Stanfield RL, Fisher TM, Lerner R, Wilson IA (1990): Crystal structure of an antibody to a peptide and its complex with peptide antigen at 2.8 D. *Science* 248:712.

Tomasi TB (1992): The discovery of secretory IgA and the mucosal immune system. *Immunol Today* 13:416.

Williams AF, Barclay AN (1988): The immunoglobulin superfamily. *Annu Rev Immunol* 6:381.

 REVIEW QUESTIONS

For each question, choose the ONE BEST answer.

1. Functional properties of immunoglobulins such as binding to Fc receptors are associated with:
   A) light chains
   B) J chains
   C) disulfide bonds
   D) heavy chains
   E) variable regiosn

2. The idiotype of an antibody molecule is determined by the amino acid sequence of the:
   A) constant region of the light chain
   B) variable region of the light chain
   C) constant region of the heavy chain
   D) constant regions of the heavy and light chains
   E) variable regions of the heavy and light chains

3. Which of the following would generate a polyclonal rabbit antiserum specific for human γ heavy chain, κ chain, λ chain, and Fc regions of Ig?
   A) Bence Jones proteins
   B) pooled IgG
   C) pepsin-digested IgG
   D) purified Fab
   E) purified F(ab′)2

4. A polyclonal antiserum raised against pooled human IgA will react with:
   A) human IgM
   B) κ light chains
   C) human IgG
   D) J chain
   E) all of the above

5. An individual was found to be heterozygous for IgG1 allotypes 3 and 12. The different possible IgG1 antibodies produced by this individual will never have:
   A) two heavy chains of allotype 12
   B) two light chains of either κ or λ

   C) two heavy chains of allotype 3
   D) two heavy chains, one of allotype 3 and one of allotype 12

6. Papain digestion of an IgG preparation of antibody specific for the antigen hen egg albumin (HEA) will:
   A) lose its antigen specificity
   B) precipitate with HEA
   C) lose all interchain disulfide bonds
   D) produce two Fab molecules and one Fc fragment
   E) none of the above

7. If an individual who is highly allergic to cat dander is exposed to a pet cat in a friend's house, which class of immunoglobulin would most likely be found to be elevated soon after exposure?
   A) IgA
   B) IgE
   C) IgG
   D) IgM
   E) IgD

8. Which of the following immunoglobulins can activate complement as a single molecule when bound to an antigen?
   A) IgA
   B) IgE
   C) IgG
   D) IgM
   E) IgD

9. The relative level of pathogen-specific IgM antibodies can be of diagnostic significance because:
   A) IgM is easier to detect than the other isotypes.
   B) Viral infection often results in very high IgM responses.
   C) IgM antibodies are more protective against reinfections than the other isotypes.
   D) Relatively high levels of IgM often correlate with a first or recent exposure to the inducing agent.

10. Primary and secondary antibody responses differ in:
   A) the predominant isotype generated
   B) the number of lymphocytes responding to antigen
   C) the speed at which antibodies appear in the serum
   D) the biologic functions manifested by the Ig isotypes produced
   E) all of the above

ANSWERS TO REVIEW QUESTIONS

1. *D* The C-terminal end of the constant region of the heavy chain contains the domains that are associated with biologic activity of immunoglobulins.

2. *E* The idiotype is the antigenic determinant of an Ig molecule, which involves its antigen-combining site. The antigen-combining site consists of contributions from the variable regions of both the light and heavy chains.

3. *B* Only pooled IgG, containing a mixture of IgG molecules each expressing the γ heavy chain (thus the Fc region) and either the κ or λ light chains, would generate an antiserum to each of these Ig components. None of the other answer choices would stimulate antibodies to all of these components. Bence Jones proteins are dimers of light chains found in the urine of patients with multiple myeloma. Pepsin treatment of IgG results in the digestion of the Fc region. Purified Fab and F(ab′)₂ fragments lack the γ heavy chain (thus the Fc region).

4. *E* All are correct statements. Antibody to IgA will have antibody specific for κ and λ light chains, which, of course, will react with IgG and IgM, both of which have κ and λ chains. Antibody will also be present against J chain if the IgA used for immunization was dimeric.

5. *D* In any immunoglobulin produced by a single cell, the two heavy chains and the two light chains are identical. Therefore, any antibody molecule in this individual would have either allotype 3 heavy chains or allotype 12 heavy chains, not a mixture. Similarly, the antibody would have either two κ or two λ chains.

6. *D* Papain digestion cleaves the IgG molecules above the hinge region, generating two Fab molecules and an Fc fragment. The Fab fragments can still bind to HEA, but since they are not held together by disulfide bonds, they cannot precipitate the antigen. This contrasts with the effects of pepsin treatment of IgG, which cleaves below the hinge region, leaving intact one divalent F(ab′)₂ molecule capable of precipitating the antigen. Fragments of pepsin-treated HEA-specific antibody will have the same affinity for the antigen as the original Fab regions of the antibody, since the CDR regions of the molecules are preserved.

7. *B* The major class of immunoglobulin produced in response to allergens is IgE.

8. *D* Only IgM can activate or fix complement when a single molecule is bound to antigen. This is due to the pentameric form of this Ig class.

9. *D* Only the last statement is correct. Relatively high levels of IgM often correlate with first recent exposure to an inducing agent, since IgM is the first isotype synthesized in response to an immunogen.

10. *E* All are correct. The statements are self-explanatory.

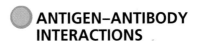

5

ANTIGEN–ANTIBODY INTERACTIONS, IMMUNE ASSAYS, AND EXPERIMENTAL SYSTEMS

● INTRODUCTION

In previous chapters, we have, by necessity, touched upon several techniques and assays that have been used to help us understand some fundamental aspects of innate and adaptive immunity. In this chapter we discuss, in greater detail, *in vitro* techniques, assays, and experimental systems that are used in research and diagnostic laboratories. Some of these are strictly antibody based (e.g., serologic methods). Others employ molecular biological methods, genetic engineering, cell culture techniques, and *in vivo* animal models that have greatly contributed to our understanding of the physiology and pathophysiology of the immune system. Since the sequencing of the human genome in 2000 and with aggressive efforts to sequence microbial genomes, approaches that use bioinformatics and computational biology (so-called *in silica* analyses) have emerged as promising methods for the study of the immune system. Using information derived from genomic and proteomic databases, powerful software tools and algorithms, there is great promise for the field of immunology and, in particular, for the development of future vaccines. Although this topic is beyond the scope of this chapter, it is important to keep in mind that future progress in the field of immunology will come from a combination of in vitro, in vivo, and *in silica* approaches.

We begin this chapter with a discussion of physical dynamics of antigen–antibody interactions.

● ANTIGEN–ANTIBODY INTERACTIONS

The reaction between antigen and serum antibodies (*serology*) serves as the basis for many immune assays. Because of the exquisite specificity of immune responses, the interaction between antigen and antibody *in vitro* is widely used for diagnostic purposes for the detection and identification of either antigen or antibody. An example of the use of serology for the identification and classification of antigens is the *serotyping* of various microorganisms by the use of specific antisera.

The interaction of antigen with antibodies may result in a variety of consequences, including *precipitation* (if the antigen is soluble), *agglutination* (if the antigen is particulate), and *activation of complement*. All of these outcomes are caused by the interactions between multivalent antigens and antibodies that have at least two combining sites per molecule. The consequences of antigen–antibody interaction listed above do not represent the primary interaction between antibodies and a given epitope. Instead, they depend on secondary phenomena which result from the interactions between multivalent antigens and antibodies. Phenomena such as the formation of precipitates, agglutination, and complement activation would not occur if the antibody with two or more combining sites reacted with a hapten (i.e., a unideterminant, univalent antigen) or as a result of the interaction between a univalent fragment of

Immunology: A Short Course, Sixth Edition, By Richard Coico and Geoffrey Sunshine
Copyright © 2009 John Wiley & Sons, Inc.

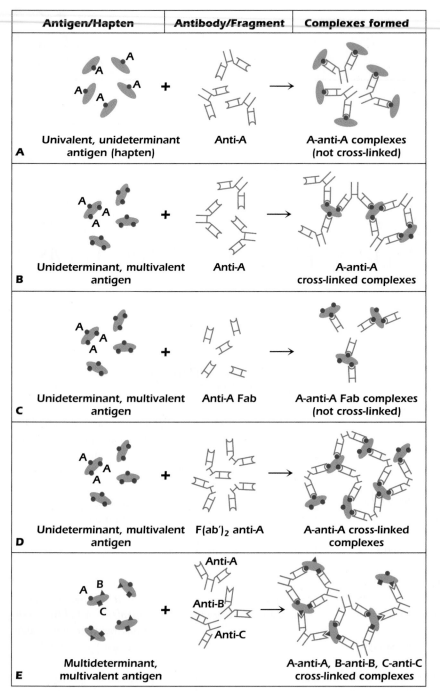

Antigen/Hapten	Antibody/Fragment	Complexes formed

A Univalent, unideterminant antigen (hapten) — Anti-A → A-anti-A complexes (not cross-linked)

B Unideterminant, multivalent antigen — Anti-A → A-anti-A cross-linked complexes

C Unideterminant, multivalent antigen — Anti-A Fab → A-anti-A Fab complexes (not cross-linked)

D Unideterminant, multivalent antigen — F(ab')₂ anti-A → A-anti-A cross-linked complexes

E Multideterminant, multivalent antigen — Anti-A, Anti-B, Anti-C → A-anti-A, B-anti-B, C-anti-C cross-linked complexes

Figure 5.1. Reactions between antibody or antibody fragments and antigens or hapten: (A) between antibody and a hapten; (B) between antibody and an unideterminant, multivalent antigen; (C) between Fab and a unideterminant, multivalent antigen; (D) between F(ab)₂' and a unideterminant, multivalent antigen; (E) between antibodies to determinants A, B, and C and a multivalent, multideterminant antigen with determinants A, B, and C.

antibody, such as Fab, and an antigen, even if the antigen were multivalent. The reasons for these differences are depicted in Figure 5.1. *Cross-linking* of various antigen molecules by antibody is required for precipitation, agglutination, or complement activation, and it is possible only if the antigen is multivalent and the antibody is divalent [either intact, or F(ab)₂'] (see Fig. 5.1). By contrast, no cross-linking is possible if the antigen or the antibody is univalent.

PRIMARY INTERACTIONS BETWEEN ANTIBODY AND ANTIGEN

No covalent bonds are involved in the interaction between antibody and an epitope. Consequently, the binding forces are relatively weak. They consist mainly of *van der Waals forces, electrostatic forces*, and *hydrophobic forces*, all of which require the interacting moieties to be in very close proximity. The very close fit required between an epitope and the antibody is often compared to that between a lock and a key. Because of the low levels of energy involved in the interaction between antigen and antibody, antigen–antibody complexes can be readily dissociated by low or high pH, by high salt concentrations, or by chaotropic ions, such as cyanates, which efficiently interfere with the hydrogen bonding of water molecules.

Association Constant

The reaction between an antibody (Ab) and an epitope of an antigen (Ag) is exemplified by the reaction between antibody and a univalent hapten. Because an antibody molecule is symmetric, with two identical Fab antigen-combining sites, one antibody molecule binds with two identical monovalent hapten molecules, each Fab binding in an independent fashion with one hapten molecule. The binding of a monovalent Ag with each site can be represented by the equation

$$Ag + Ab \underset{k_{-1}}{\overset{k_1}{\rightleftharpoons}} Ab - Ag$$

where k_1 represents the forward (association) rate constant and k_{-1} represents the reverse (dissociation) rate constant. The ratio k_1/k_{-1} is the **association constant, K**, a measure of affinity. It can be calculated by determining the ratio of bound antibody–antigen complex to the concentration of unbound antigen and antibody. Thus,

$$K = \frac{k_1}{k_{-1}} = \frac{[Ab - Ag]}{[Ab][Ag]}$$

The association constant (K) is really a measure of the affinity of the antibody for the epitope (see below). When all the antibody molecules that bind a given hapten or epitope are identical (as in the case of monoclonal antibodies), then K represents the intrinsic association constant. However, because even those serum antibodies binding to a single epitope are heterogeneous, an average association constant of all the antibodies to the epitope is referred to as K_0. The interaction between antibodies and each epitope of a multivalent antigen follows the same kinetics and energetics as those involved in the interaction between antibodies and haptens because each epitope of the antigen reacts with its corresponding antibody in the same manner described above.

The association constant K can be determined using **equilibrium dialysis**. In this procedure, a dialysis chamber is used; two compartments are separated by a semipermeable membrane that allows free passage of appropriately sized molecules from one side to the other. Antibody is placed on one side of the semipermeable membrane and cannot pass through due to its size. A known amount of small, permeable, radiolabeled hapten molecules, oligosaccharides, or oligopeptides composing the epitope of the complex carbohydrate or protein is added on the antigen side of the membrane. At time zero, the hapten or antigenic epitope used (hereafter referred to as the ligand) will then diffuse across the membrane; at equilibrium, the concentration of free ligand will be the same on both sides. However, the total amount of ligand will be greater on the Ab-containing side because some of the ligand will be bound to the antibody molecules. The difference in the ligand concentration in the two compartments represents the concentration of the ligand bound to antibody (i.e., the [AgAb] complex). The higher the affinity of the antibody, the more ligand that is bound.

Since the concentration of antibody added to the equilibrium dialysis chamber can be predetermined and kept constant, varying concentrations of ligand can be used. This approach facilitates the so-called **Scatchard analysis** of the antibody, useful in determining whether a given antibody preparation is homogeneous (e.g., monoclonal antibody) or heterogeneous (e.g., polyclonal antiserum) and in measuring the average affinity constant (K_0).

Affinity and Avidity

As noted above, the intrinsic association constant that characterizes the binding of an antibody with an epitope or a hapten is termed **affinity**. When the antigen consists of many repeating identical epitopes or when antigens are multivalent, the association between the entire antigen molecule and antibodies depends not only on the affinity between each epitope and its corresponding antibody but also on the sum of the affinities of all the epitopes involved. For example, the affinity of binding of anti-A with multivalent A (shown in Fig. 5.1B) may be four or five orders of magnitude higher than binding between anti-A and univalent A (Fig. 5.1A). This is because the pairing of anti-A with multivalent A is influenced by the increased number of sites with which anti-A can react.

While the term affinity denotes the intrinsic association constant between antibody and a univalent ligand such as a hapten, the term **avidity** is used to denote the overall binding energy between antibodies and a multivalent antigen. Thus, in general, IgM antibodies are of higher avidity than IgG antibodies, although the binding with ligand of each Fab in the IgM antibody may be of the same affinity as that of the Fab in IgG.

SECONDARY INTERACTIONS BETWEEN ANTIBODY AND ANTIGEN

Agglutination Reactions

Referring again to Figure 5.1, the reactions of antibody with a multivalent antigen that is **particulate** (i.e., an insoluble particle) results in the cross-linking of the various antigen particles by the antibodies (Figs. 5.1D and E). This cross-linking eventually results in the clumping or agglutination of the antigen particles by the antibodies.

Titer.   The ability of an antibody to cause antigens to agglutinate requires an optimal proportion of antibody relative to antigen. A method sometimes used to measure the level of serum antibody specific for a particulate antigen is the agglutination assay. More sensitive, quantitative assays [e.g., enzyme-linked immunosorbent assay (ELISA), discussed later in this chapter] have largely replaced the agglutination assay for measuring antibody levels in serum. Indeed, the agglutinating titer of a certain serum is only a semiquantitative expression of the antibodies present in the serum; it is not a quantitative measure of the concentration of antibody (weight/volume).

The assay is performed by mixing twofold serial dilutions of serum with a fixed concentration of antigen. High dilutions of serum usually do not cause antigen agglutination because at such dilutions there are not enough antibodies to cause appreciable, visible agglutination. The highest dilution of serum that still causes agglutination but beyond which no agglutination occurs is termed the ***titer***. It is a common observation that agglutination may not occur at high concentrations of antibody, even though it does take place at higher dilutions of serum. The tubes with high concentrations of serum, where agglutination does not occur, represent a ***prozone***. In the prozone, antibodies are present in excess. The reason for the absence of agglutination in the prozone is that every epitope on a single particle of antigen may bind only to a single antibody molecule, preventing cross-linking between different particles.

Because of the prozone phenomenon, in testing for the presence of agglutinating antibodies to a certain antigen, it is imperative that the antiserum be tested at several dilutions. Testing serum at only one concentration may give misleading conclusions if no agglutination occurs because the absence of agglutination might reflect either a prozone or a lack of antibody.

Zeta Potential.   The surfaces of certain particulate antigens may possess an electrical charge, such as the net negative charge on the surface of red blood cells caused by the presence of sialic acid. When such charged particles are suspended in saline solution, an electrical potential termed the ***zeta potential*** is created between particles, preventing them from getting very close to one another. This introduces a difficulty in agglutinating charged particles by antibodies, in particular red blood cells by IgG antibodies. The distance between the Fab arms of the IgG molecule, even in its most extended form, is too short to allow effective bridging between two red blood cells across the zeta potential. Thus, although IgG antibodies may be directed against antigens on the charged erythrocyte, agglutination may not occur because of the repulsion by the zeta potential. On the other hand, some of the Fab areas of IgM pentamers are far enough apart and can bridge red blood cells separated by the zeta potential. This property of IgM antibodies, together with their pentavalence, is a major reason for their effectiveness as agglutinating antibodies.

Through the years attempts have been made to improve agglutination reactions by decreasing the zeta potential in various ways, none of which was universally applicable or effective. However, an ingenious method was devised in the 1950s by Coombs to overcome this problem. This method, described below, facilitates the agglutination of erythrocytes by IgG antibodies specific for erythrocyte antigens. It is also useful for the detection of nonagglutinating antibodies that are present on the surface of erythrocytes.

Coombs Test.   The ***Coombs test*** is a method that uses antibodies made against immunoglobulins from a different species (heterologous antibodies) to detect the presence of autoantibodies on the surface of red blood cells (Fig. 5.2). It is based on two important facts: (1) that immunoglobulins of one species (e.g., human) are immunogenic when injected into another species (e.g., rabbit) and lead to the production of antibodies against the immunoglobulins and (2) that many of the anti-immunoglobulins (e.g., rabbit antihuman Ig) bind with antigenic determinants present on the Fc portion of the antibody and leave the Fab portions free to react with antigen. For example, if human IgG autoantibodies are attached to erythrocytes, the addition of rabbit–antihuman Ig will form bridges (cross-links) between the red cells and thus cause agglutination.

There are two versions of the Coombs test: the ***direct Coombs test*** and the ***indirect Coombs test***. The

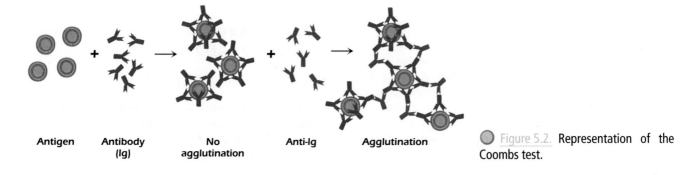

Antigen   Antibody   No   Anti-Ig   Agglutination
           (Ig)   agglutination

Figure 5.2. Representation of the Coombs test.

two versions differ somewhat in mechanics, but both are based on the same principle: using heterologous anti-immunoglobulins to detect a reaction between immuno-globulins and antigen. In the direct Coombs test, anti-immunoglobulins are added to the particles (e.g., red blood cells) that are suspected of having antibodies bound to antigens on their surfaces. For example, if a newborn baby is suspected of having hemolytic disease of the newborn caused by maternal anti-Rh IgG antibodies bound to the baby's erythrocytes, the addition of antihuman immunoglobulin to a suspension of the baby's erythrocytes (the direct Coombs test) would cause red blood cell agglutination to occur. In some cases, the direct Coombs test fails due to the zeta potential. The indirect Coombs test can then be used to determine whether the mother's serum contains anti-Rh antibodies. In this case, the anti-immunoglobulin reagents are added only after the mother's serum is combined with Rh^+ erythrocytes. Thus, the direct Coombs test measures bound antibody, and the indirect test measures serum antibody.

Originally, the Coombs test was used for the detection of human antibodies on the surface of erythrocytes. Today the term is applied to the detection of any immunoglobulin that is bound to antigen through the use of anti-immunoglobulin.

Passive Agglutination.

The agglutination reaction can be used with particulate antigens (e.g., erythrocytes or bacteria) and also with soluble antigens provided that the soluble antigen can be firmly attached to insoluble particles. For example, the soluble antigen thyroglobulin can be attached to latex particles so that the addition of antibodies to the thyroglobulin antigen will cause agglutination of the latex particles coated with thyroglobulin. The addition of soluble antigen to the antibodies before the introduction of the thyroglobulin-coated latex particles will inhibit agglutination because the antibodies will first combine with the soluble antigen. If the soluble antigen is present in excess, the antibodies will not be able to bind with the particulate antigen, a phenomenon referred to as agglutination inhibition. This type of agglutination inhibition should be distinguished from agglutination inhibition between antibodies and viruses. Antibodies to certain viruses inhibit the agglutination of red blood cells by the virus. In such cases, the antibodies are directed to the area or areas on the virus that bind with the appropriate virus receptors on the red blood cells.

When an antigen is a natural constituent of a particle, the agglutination reaction is referred to as *direct agglutination*. When the agglutination reaction takes place between antibodies and soluble antigen attached to an insoluble particle, the reaction is referred to as *passive agglutination*.

Agglutination reactions are widely used in clinical applications. In addition to the examples already given, major applications include erythrocyte typing in blood banks, diagnosis of immunologically mediated hemolytic diseases such as drug-induced autohemolytic anemia, tests for rheumatoid factor (human IgM, anti-human IgG), confirmatory test for syphilis, and the latex test for pregnancy, which involves the detection of human chorionic gonadotropin (HCG) in the urine of pregnant women.

Precipitation Reactions

Reaction in Solutions.

In contrast to the agglutination reaction, which takes place between antibodies and particulate antigen, the *precipitation reaction* takes place when antibodies and soluble antigen are mixed. As in the case of agglutination, precipitation of antigen–antibody complexes occurs because the divalent antibody molecules cross-link multivalent antigen molecules to form a *lattice*. When it reaches a certain size, this antigen–antibody complex loses its solubility and precipitates out of solution. The phenomenon of precipitation is termed the *precipitin reaction*.

Figure 5.3 depicts a qualitative precipitin reaction. Increasing concentrations of antigen are added to a series of tubes that contain a constant concentration of antibodies, causing variable amounts of precipitate to form. The weight of the precipitate in each tube may be determined by a variety of methods. If the amount of the precipitate is plotted against the amount of antigen added, a precipitin curve like the one shown in Figure 5.3 is obtained.

There are three important areas under the curve shown in Figure 5.3: (1) the zone of antibody excess (prozone), (2) the equivalence zone, and (3) the zone of antigen excess. In the equivalence zone, the proportion of antigen to antibody is optimal for maximal precipitation; in the zones of antibody excess and antigen excess, the proportions of the reactants do not lead to efficient cross-linking and formation of precipitate.

It should be emphasized that the zones of the precipitin curve are based on the amount of antigen–antibody complexes precipitated. However, the zones of antigen excess and antibody excess may contain soluble antigen–antibody complexes, particularly the zone of antigen excess, where a minimal amount of precipitate is formed but large amounts of *antigen–antibody complexes* are present in the supernatant. Thus, the amount of precipitate formed is dependent on the proportions of the reactant antigens and antibodies: the correct proportion of the reactions result in maximal formation of precipitate; excess of antigen (or antibody) results in soluble complexes.

Precipitation Reactions in Gels.

Precipitation reactions between soluble antigens and antibodies can take place not only in solution but also in semisolid media such as agar gels. When soluble antigen and antibodies are placed in wells cut in the gel (Fig. 5.4A), the reactants diffuse in the gel and form gradients of concentration, with the highest concentrations closest to the wells.

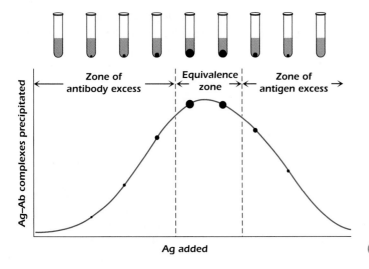

Figure 5.3. Representation of the precipitin reaction.

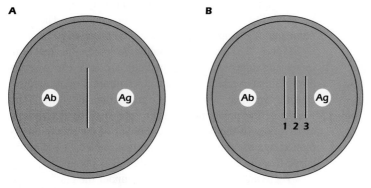

Figure 5.4. Gel diffusion by (A) antibodies and single antigen and (B) antibodies to antigens 1, 2, and 3 and their respective antigens.

Somewhere between the two wells, the reacting antigen and antibodies will be present at proportions that are optimal for formation of a visible precipitate, as shown by the lines between wells in Figure 5.4.

If the antibody well contains antibodies 1, 2, and 3 specific for antigens 1, 2, and 3, respectively, and if antigens 1, 2, and 3 placed in the antigen well diffuse at different rates (with diffusion rates of $1 > 2 > 3$), then three distinct precipitin lines will form. These three precipitin lines form because anti-1, anti-2, and anti-3 antibodies, which diffuse at the same rate, react independently with antigens 1, 2, and 3, respectively, to form three equivalence zones and thus three separate lines of precipitate (Fig. 5.4B). Different rates of diffusion of both antibody and antibody and antigen result from differences in concentration, molecular size, or shape.

Historically this ***double-diffusion method***, developed by Ouchterlony and sometimes referred to as the ***Ouchterlony method***, has been useful for establishing the antigenic relationship between various substances, as shown in Figure 5.5. Three reaction patterns are seen in gel diffusion, each of which is illustrated in Figure 5.5: patterns of identity, patterns of nonidentity, and patterns of partial identity. ***Patterns of identity*** form when the two antigens are identical (Fig. 5.5A). A pattern in which the precipitin lines cross each other is called a ***pattern of nonidentity*** (Fig. 5.5B). Finally, a ***pattern of partial identity*** forms when the test antiserum reacts positively with antigens that contain epitopes that match and some that do not match, causing a precipitin spur to appear in the gel (Fig. 5.5C).

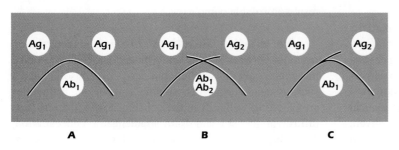

Figure 5.5. Double-gel-diffusion patterns showing (A) pattern of identity, (B) pattern of nonidentity, and (C) pattern of partial identity.

Radial Immunodiffusion. The radial immunodiffusion test, depicted in Figure 5.6, represents a variation of the double-diffusion test. The wells contain antigen at different concentrations, while the antibodies are distributed uniformly in the agar gel. Thus, the precipitin line is replaced by a precipitin ring around the well. The distance the precipitin ring migrates from the center of the antigen well is directly proportional to the concentration of antigen in the well. The relationship between concentration of antigen in a well and the diameter of the precipitin ring can be plotted as shown in the graph in Figure 5.6. If wells such as F and G contain unknown amounts of the same antigen, the concentration of that antigen in these wells can be determined by comparing the diameter of the precipitin ring with the diameter of the ring formed by a known concentration of the antigen.

An important application of radial immunodiffusion is clinical measurement of concentrations of serum proteins. Antiserum to various serum proteins is incorporated in the gel; concentration of a particular protein in a serum sample is determined by comparing the diameter of the resulting precipitin ring with those obtained using known concentrations of the protein.

Immunoelectrophoresis. *Immunoelectrophoresis* involves separation of a mixture of proteins added to a polyacrylamide gel using an electric field (electrophoresis) followed by their detection with antibodies diffusing into the gel. It is very useful for the analysis of a mixture of antigens. For example, in the clinical characterization of human serum proteins, a small drop of human serum is placed in a well cut in the center of a slide that is coated with agar gel. The serum is then subjected to electrophoresis, which separates the various components according to their mobilities in the electric field. After electrophoresis, a trough is cut along the side of the slides, and antibodies to human serum proteins are placed in

the trough. The antibodies diffuse in the agar, as do the separated serum proteins. At an optimal antigen–antibody ratio, each antigen and its corresponding antibodies form precipitin lines. The result is a pattern similar to that depicted in Figure 5.7. Comparison of the pattern and intensity of lines of normal human serum with the results obtained with sera of patients may reveal an absence, overabundance, or other abnormality of one or more serum proteins. In fact, it was through the use of the immunoelectrophoresis assay that the first antibody deficiency syndrome was identified in 1952 (Bruton's agammaglobulinemia) (see Chapter 17).

Western Blots (Immunoblots). In the *Western or immunoblotting* technique, antigen (or a mixture of antigens) is first separated in a gel. The separated material is then transferred onto protein-binding sheets (e.g., nitrocellulose) by using an electroblotting method. Antibody is then applied to the nitrocellulose sheet and binds with its specific antigen. The antibody may be labeled (e.g., with radioactivity) or a labeled anti-immunoglobulin may be used to localize the antibody and the antigen to which it is bound. Western blots are used widely in research and clinical laboratories for the detection and characterization of antigens. A particularly useful example is the confirmatory diagnosis of HIV infection by the application of a patient's serum to the nitrocellulose sheets on which HIV antigens are bound. The finding of specific antibody is strong evidence of infection by the virus (Fig. 5.8).

IMMUNOASSAYS

Direct-Binding Immunoassays

Radioimmunoassay (RIA) employs isotopically labeled molecules and permits measurements of extremely small amounts of antigen, antibody, or antigen–antibody complexes. Concentrations are determined by measuring radioactivity rather than by chemical analysis, increasing the sensitivity of detection by several orders of magnitude. For the development of this highly sensitive analytical method, which has clinical application in hormone assays as well as assays of other substances found at low

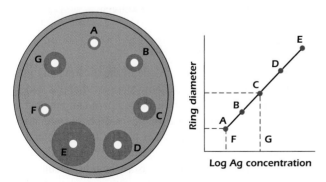

Figure 5.6. Radial diffusion. A, B, C, D, and E represent known concentrations of antigen; F and G represent unknown concentrations that can be determined by comparison of the diameter of their precipitin rings with the diameters of rings formed by known concentrations of the antigen.

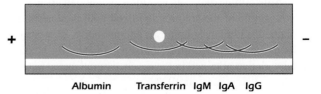

Figure 5.7. Patterns of immunoelectrophoresis of serum proteins.

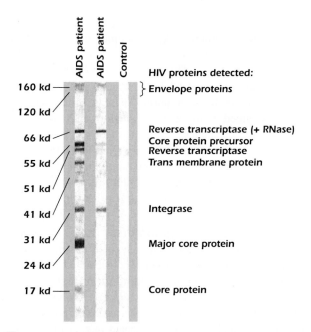

Figure 5.8. Western blots of serum samples from two HIV-infected individuals and one control subject. Note the presence of several bands in the AIDS patient sample lanes indicating serum antibody reactions with HIV proteins.

levels in biological fluids, Rosalyn Yalow received the Nobel Prize.

The principle of RIA is illustrated in Figure 5.9. A known amount of radioactively labeled antigen is reacted with a limited amount of antibody, producing a solution containing antibody-bound labeled antigen as well as some unbound labeled antigen. After separating the antibody-bound antigen from free antigen, the amount of radioactivity bound to antibody is determined. Next, the same amount of labeled antigen is premixed with unlabeled antigen (Fig. 5.10). The mixture is reacted with the same amount of antibody as before, and the antibody-bound antigen is separated from the unbound antigen. Because the unlabeled antigen competes with the labeled antigen for the antibody, less labeled antigen is bound to antibody. The greater the amount of unlabeled antigen present in the reaction mixture, the smaller the ratio of antibody-bound radiolabeled antigen to free radiolabeled antigen. This ratio can be plotted as a function of the concentration of the unlabeled antigen.

To determine the concentration of antigen in a solution, a sample of the solution is mixed with predetermined amounts of radiolabeled antigen and antibody. The ratio of antibody-bound antigen/free antigen radioactivity is compared with that obtained in the absence of unlabeled antigen (the latter value is set at 100%).

An important step in performing a RIA, as described above, is the separation of free antigen from antibody-bound antigen. Depending upon the antigen,

this separation can be achieved in a variety of ways. A principal method is the anti-immunoglobulin procedure.

The anti-immunoglobulin procedure is based on the fact that labeled or unlabeled antigen that is bound to immunoglobulin will be precipitated along with the immunoglobulin following the addition of anti-immunoglobulin antibodies. As a result, only unbound antigen will remain in the supernatant. Radioimmunoassays commonly employ rabbit antibodies to the desired antigens. These rabbit antibody–antigen complexes may be precipitated by the addition of goat antibodies raised against rabbit immunoglobulins.

Since the amounts of antigen and antibody required for RIA are extremely small, the antigen–antibody complexes reacted with anti-immunoglobulin would form only tiny amounts of precipitate. Because it is difficult, if not impossible, to recover these precipitates quantitatively by conventional means in order to determine their radioactivity, it is customary to add immunoglobulins that are not specific for the antigen in the reaction mixture, thereby increasing the total amount of precipitate. Such precipitates consist mainly of the nonspecific immunoglobulins. However, they also contain the extremely small amount of antigen-specific immunoglobulin and any radioactive antigen bound to it.

An alternative method of separating complexes of antibody-bound antigen from free antigen is based on the fact that immunoglobulins become insoluble and precipitate in a solution containing 33% saturated ammonium sulfate. If the antigen does not precipitate in 33% ammonium sulfate, more ammonium sulfate is added until the antibody-bound antigen precipitates, leaving the free antigen in solution. Here, again, the amounts of antibodies reacting with antigen (or free antibodies) are extremely small. As described for the RIA procedure, a sufficient amount of nonspecific immunoglobulins is added to the mixture; an appreciable precipitate will form at 33% saturation ammonium sulfate to allow the separation of free antigen from antibody-bound antigen.

Solid-Phase Immunoassays

Solid-phase immunoassays are one of the most widely used immunologic techniques. It is now automated and is widely used in clinical medicine for the detection of antigen or antibody. A good example is the use of solid-phase immunoassay for the detection of antibodies to HIV (see Chapter 17).

Solid-phase RIAs employ the property of plastics such as polyvinyl or polystyrene to adsorb monomolecular layers of proteins onto their surface. Although the adsorbed molecules may lose some of their antigenic determinants, enough of them can still react with their corresponding antibodies that their presence may be detected by the use of anti-immunoglobulins (Fig. 5.11) labeled with a radioactive tracer or, more commonly, with an enzyme. If it makes

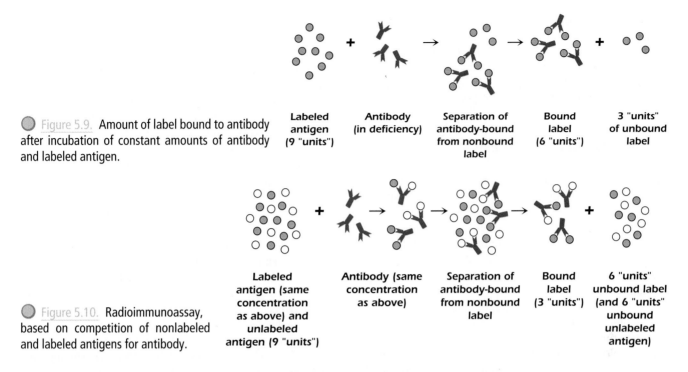

Figure 5.9. Amount of label bound to antibody after incubation of constant amounts of antibody and labeled antigen.

Labeled antigen (9 "units") | Antibody (in deficiency) | Separation of antibody-bound from nonbound label | Bound label (6 "units") | 3 "units" of unbound label

Figure 5.10. Radioimmunoassay, based on competition of nonlabeled and labeled antigens for antibody.

Labeled antigen (same concentration as above) and unlabeled antigen (9 "units") | Antibody (same concentration as above) | Separation of antibody-bound from nonbound label | Bound label (3 "units") | 6 "units" unbound label (and 6 "units" unbound unlabeled antigen)

use of anti-immunoglobulins labeled with an enzyme that can be detected by the appearance of a color on addition of substrate, the test is called an *enzyme-linked immunosorbent assay (ELISA)*.

After coating the plastic surface with antigen, it is imperative to block any uncoated plastic surface to prevent it from absorbing the other reagents, most importantly the labeled reagent. Such blocking is achieved by coating the plastic surface with a high concentration of an unrelated protein, such as gelatin, after the application of the antigen.

Since the plastic wells are usually coated with relatively large amounts of antigen, the higher the concentration of antibodies bound with the antigen, the higher the amount of labeled anti-immunoglobulin that can bind to the

antibodies. Thus, an excess of labeled anti-immunoglobulin is always used to ensure saturation.

Solid-phase immunoassay may be used for qualitative or quantitative evaluations of antigen. Such determinations are performed by mixing the antiserum with varying known amounts of antigen before adding it to the antigen-coated plastic wells. This preliminary procedure results in the binding of the antibodies with the soluble antigen, decreasing the availability of free antibodies. The higher the concentration of the soluble antigen that reacts with antibodies before the addition of the antibody to the wells, the lower the number of antibodies that can bind with the antigen on the plate, and the lower the number of labeled anti-immunoglobulins that can bind to the antigen–antibody complexes. The decrease in the amount

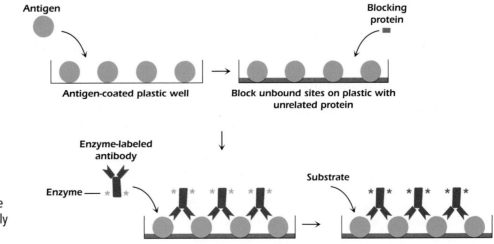

Figure 5.11. Representative ELISA using well coated directly with antigen.

of labeled antibody as a function of the concentration of antigen used can be plotted on a graph; the amount of antigen in an unknown solution can then be determined from the graph by a comparison of the decrease in bound label caused by the unknown solution to the decrease caused by known concentrations of pure antigen.

IMMUNOFLUORESCENCE

A fluorescent compound has the property of emitting light of a certain wavelength when it is excited by exposure to light of a shorter wavelength. Immunofluorescence localizes an antigen through the use of fluorescently labeled antibodies. The procedure, originally described by Coombs, employs antibodies covalently linked to fluorescent groups that do not cause any appreciable change in antibody activity.

One fluorescent compound that is widely used in immunology is fluorescein isothiocyanate (FITC), which fluoresces with a visible greenish color when excited by ultraviolet (UV) light. FITC is easily coupled to free amino groups. Another widely used fluorescent compound is phycoerythrin (PE), which fluoresces red and is also easily coupled to free amino groups. Fluorescence microscopes equipped with a UV light source permit visualization of fluorescent antibody on a microscopic specimen. Immunofluorescence is widely used to localize antigens on various tissues and microorganisms.

There are two important and related procedures that employ fluorescent antibodies: direct immunofluorescence and indirect immunofluorescence.

Direct Immunofluorescence

Direct immunofluorescence, which is used primarily for detection of antigen, involves reacting the target tissue (or microorganism) with fluorescently labeled specific antibodies. It is widely used for clinical purposes such as identifying lymphocytic subsets and confirming the presence of specific protein deposition in certain tissues such as kidney and skin in cases of systemic lupus erythematosus (SLE) (see Chapter 12).

Indirect Immunofluorescence

Indirect immunofluorescence involves reacting the target first with unlabeled specific antibodies and then with fluorescently labeled anti-immunoglobulin.

The indirect immunofluorescence method is more widely used than the direct method, because a single fluorescent anti-immunoglobulin antibody can be used to localize antibody of many different specificities. In addition, since the anti-immunoglobulins contain antibodies to many epitopes on the specific immunoglobulin, the use of

fluorescent anti-immunoglobulins significantly amplifies the fluorescent signal. An excellent example of the use of indirect immunofluorescence is the screening of patients' sera for anti-DNA antibodies in cases of SLE.

FLUORESCENCE-ACTIVATED CELL-SORTING ANALYSIS

A very powerful tool that uses fluorescent antibody specific for cell surface antigens is *fluorescence-activated cell sorting (FACS)*. A cell suspension labeled with specific fluorescent antibody is passed through an apparatus that forms a stream of small droplets, each containing a single cell. These droplets are passed between a laser beam of UV light and a detector that picks up emitted fluorescence from labeled cells. The signal emitted from the detector is passed to an electrode that charges the droplet, leading to its deflection in an electromagnetic field (Fig. 5.12). As the droplets pass through the laser beam, they are counted and can be sorted according to whether they emit a signal (i.e., whether they are labeled or unlabeled). The intensity of fluorescein staining on each cell, which reflects the density of antigen expressed on the cell, may be detected by sophisticated electronics.

With this type of apparatus it is now possible to rapidly develop a flow cytometric profile of a pool of lymphocytes based on their differential expression of cell surface molecules, the relative amount of cell surface molecule expressed on each cell, and the size distribution and numbers of each cell type. It is also possible to use the apparatus to sort a collection of cells stained with five or more different fluorescent labels and obtain a very homogeneous sample of a particular cell type. A variation of this technique uses fluorescent antibodies coupled to magnetic beads to separate cell populations. Cells that bind to the fluorescent antibody can be separated from unstained cells by a magnet. Both FACS and magnetic bead separation methods have resulted in the isolation of very rare cells such as hematopoietic stem cells.

The most common method for phenotyping and sorting cells involves the use of antibodies that react with cell surface proteins identified as *clusters of differentiation (CD) antigens*. The CD nomenclature originates from studies using monoclonal antibodies (discussed later in this chapter) to characterize cells phenotypically. It was found that cell surface markers (CD antigens) are associated with distinct developmental stages. Moreover, these proteins have important biologic functions required for normal cell physiology. The developmental stages of B and T cells and functional subsets of these cells can now be phenotyped based on their expression of CD markers. However, surface expression of a particular molecule may not be specific for just one cell or even for a cell lineage. Nonetheless, cell surface expression can be exploited for purification as well

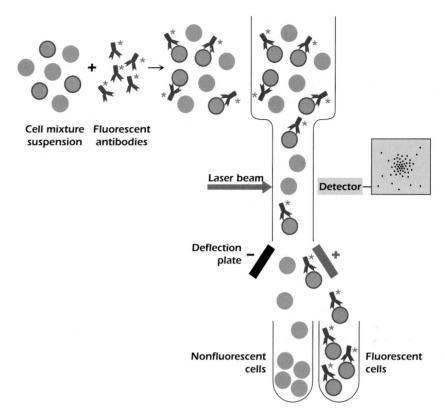

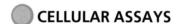
Figure 5.12. Schematic representation of fluorescence-activated cell sorting.

as characterization of cells. For practical purposes, the CD acronym is followed by an arbitrary number that identifies a specific cell surface protein. CD numbers are assigned by the Nomenclature Committee of the International Union of Immunologic Sciences. A list of some of the more important CD antigens expressed by B cells, various T-cell subsets, and other cells can be found in the Appendix.

IMMUNOABSORPTION AND IMMUNOADSORPTION

Because of the specific binding between antigen and antibody, it is possible to trap, or selectively remove, an antigen against which an antibody is directed from a mixture of antigens in solution. Similarly, it is possible to selectively remove antigen-specific antibodies from a mixture of antibodies using the specific antigen.

There are two general, related methods of removal. In one method, the absorption is done with both reagents in solution (*immunoabsorption*). In the other, it is performed with one reagent attached to an insoluble support (*immunoadsorption*). Immunoadsorption is of particular value because the adsorbed material can then be recovered from the complex by careful treatments that dissociate antigen–antibody complexes, such as lowering the pH (HCl–glycine or acetic acid, pH 2–3) or adding chaotropic

ions. This enables the effective purification of antigens or antibodies of interest.

CELLULAR ASSAYS

A number of other immune assays used in the evaluation and study of the cellular components of the immune system are also described in this chapter. Among these are routine methods used to measure lymphocyte function. Assays designed to measure responses of B cells to antigenic or mitogenic stimulation are sometimes used clinically to assess humoral immunocompetence. In experimental settings, these assays help us to understand the regulatory and molecular mechanisms associated with B-cell activation. Similarly, assays for measuring T-cell function are used both clinically and experimentally to measure T-cell proliferative and effector responses and T-cell and cytokine profiles. T-cell assays have contributed significantly to our understanding of T-cell functional diversity and to the identification of the many cytokines produced by cells belonging to a particular subset.

Assays to Assess Lymphocyte Function

Assays used to assess lymphocyte function generally attempt to answer one of the following questions: (1) Do the B or T cells respond normally to mitogenic stimuli that activate cells to undergo a proliferative response? (2) Does mitogenic or antigen-driven stimulation result in antibody production (for B cells) or cytokine production (for T cells)? In addition, given the functional heterogeneity of T cells, T-cell assays can also be used to evaluate the functional integrity of a particular subset. This is particularly useful in the clinical evaluation of patients with suspected immunodeficiency diseases (see Chapter 17). In the case of T-helper-cell assays, the target cell receiving the T-cell help generally determines the functional parameter to be measured. For example, the target population might be B cells in an assay designed to test the ability of T cells to help induce antibody responses. In this example, the assay would quantitate the level of antibody produced. Similarly, if you were interested in learning whether T cells provide the help needed to activate macrophages optimally, the parameters would focus on functional properties associated with these phagocytic cells. Many of the assays used to assess T-cell function also rely on the measurement of specific cytokines, since the cells receiving help may be activated to produce cytokines themselves.

B- and T-Cell Proliferation Assays

Mitogen-stimulated lymphocyte activation triggers biochemical signaling pathways that lead to gene expression, protein synthesis, cell proliferation, and differentiation. The proliferative responses generated in response to mitogens are polyclonal in nature. In addition, mitogens have been identified that selectively stimulate either B- or T-cell populations. Therefore, unlike immunogens that activate only the lymphocyte clones bearing the appropriate antigen receptor, polyclonal activators stimulate many B- or T-cell clones regardless of their antigenic specificity. Mitogens that selectively activate B cells, such as the LPS component of Gram-negative bacterial cell walls, will cause polyclonal stimulation of B cells in mice. The magnitude of cell proliferation in response to mitogenic stimulation can be measured by adding radiolabeled nucleosides (e.g., tritiated thymidine) to the medium during cell culture and then quantitating its incorporation into the DNA of dividing cells using a liquid scintillation counter. Similarly, several sugar-binding proteins called lectins, including *concanavalin A (Con A)* and *phytohemagglutinin (PHA)*, are very effective T-cell mitogens. *Pokeweed mitogen (PWM)* is another example of a lectin with potent mitogenic properties. However, unlike Con A and PHA, PWM stimulates polyclonal activation of both B and T cells.

Assays that Assess Antibody Production by B Cells

Mitogenic stimulation of B and T cells results in the proliferation and differentiation of many clones of cells. In the case of B cells, the polyclonal activators LPS or PWM can be used to assess the ability of a population of B cells to produce antibody. ELISA is the most commonly used quantitative assay for measuring antibody levels. Alternatively, B cells can be stimulated with mitogens or specific antigens *in vitro*, then temporarily cultured in chambers directly on nitrocellulose membranes in a so-called *ELISPOT* assay. The protein-binding property of nitrocellulose facilitates the capture of secreted antibody by individual B cells. This yields discrete foci of antibody bound to the nitrocellulose that can be detected using a secondary, enzyme-labeled antibody specific for the bound antibody, allowing for the enumeration of antibody-secreting cells.

Effector Cell Assays for T and NK Cells

As noted above, the selection of an effector cell assay depends on the questions that need to be answered. T-cell assays are as varied as the functional diverse T-cell subsets known to exist. Thus, various assays measuring T-helper-cell function have been developed that focus on helper activity for B cells and macrophage activation; even other T cells can be used to measure the helper properties of CD4$^+$ T cells. Similarly, several assays that measure cytotoxic activity of CD8$^+$ T cells are available. One such assay (*cytotoxicity assay*) measures the ability of cytotoxic T or NK cells to kill radiolabeled target cells expressing an antigen to which the cytotoxic T cells were sensitized. In a related assay, NK cells are cultured with radiolabeled target cells bound to target cell-specific antibodies. The rationale for this approach is based on the fact that NK cells express membrane Fc receptors that bind to the Fc region of certain Ig isotypes. This method measures an important functional property of NK cells known as antibody-dependent cell-mediated cytotoxicity (see Chapter 4).

 CELL CULTURE

Several experimental systems have revolutionized our ability to investigate a multitude of questions about the development of the immune system, its functional and regulatory properties, and the pathologic mechanisms associated with immunodeficiency and autoimmune diseases. Many of these experimental systems depend on cell culture methods used to maintain cells in vitro. Cell culture systems have facilitated several major scientific breakthroughs, including the development in the 1970s of B-cell hybridoma/monoclonal antibody technology by Kohler and Milstein. Knowledge of the growth factors required to maintain lymphoid cells has made it possible to clone and grow functionally competent cells in vitro. In addition, recombinant DNA techniques have permitted the transfer of genes to cloned cell lines, thereby allowing researchers to answer many questions related to the gene under investigation. Similarly, recombinant DNA techniques have made it possible to develop genetically engineered immune molecules and receptors, which can then be transferred into cells used to elucidate the biologic consequences of receptor expression and receptor triggering (e.g., ligand binding). These *in vitro* systems continue to be used to advance our knowledge of the immune system and, in some cases, to develop new biologic therapies and vaccines for clinical use.

Primary Cell Cultures and Cloned Lymphoid Cell Lines

As with many other fields of biologic science, cell culture systems have served as an essential investigational tool to facilitate our understanding of many developmental/maturational and physiologic properties of cells. The ability to culture primary lymphoid cells consisting of heterogeneous populations of T and/or B cells (albeit for limited periods of time) has allowed immunologists to study the biochemical and molecular mechanisms controlling many important biologic features of B and T cells, including gene rearrangement. Advances in cell culture systems have evolved rapidly during the past few decades, leading to the development of cell-cloning techniques. Transformation of B and T cells derived from a specific parent cell to generate cloned, immortal cell lines has been achieved using a variety of methods. These include exposure of cells to certain carcinogens or viruses such as exposure of B cells to the Epstein-Barr virus and exposure of T cells to human T-cell leukemia virus type 1. Many cell lines are derived from tumors that arise either spontaneously or experimentally (as a result of administration of carcinogens or virus infection). The major advantage of using cloned cell lines is that large numbers of cells can be generated for investigation. A disadvantage in the use of carcinogen- or virus-transformed cells is that they are, by definition, abnormal. Indeed, many transformed cells have abnormal numbers of chromosomes and often display phenotypic and functional properties not seen in normal cells. A major advance in the generation of cloned lymphoid cells came in the late 1970s with the discovery that nontransformed antigen-specific T-cell lines and antigen-specific T-cell clones could be grown indefinitely when a T-cell growth factor (IL-2) was included in the culture along with a source of antigen and antigen-presenting cells. This approach offered several advantages over the use of transformed cells, since the cells derived from such cultures were, for all intents and purposes, normal. Thus, large numbers of nontransformed antigen-specific T cells could be generated for investigation using IL-2. Indeed, many of these cloned T-cell lines have been used in the identification and biochemical characterization of cytokines, leading to the ultimate cloning of genes that encode these proteins.

The combined use of cell-cloning systems, gene transfer methods, and animal models has helped us to understand how lymphoid cells develop self-tolerance and how they can escape tolerance-inducing mechanisms to become disease-causing autoreactive cells. In short, cell culture systems have served as a gateway for research endeavors attempting to shed light on both the physiologic and pathophysiologic properties of lymphoid cells. As will be discussed below, cell culture systems have also been exploited productively in the development of many useful diagnostic and therapeutic reagents, such as monoclonal antibodies.

B-Cell Hybridomas and Monoclonal Antibodies

The specificity of the immune response has served as the basis for serologic reactions in which antibody specificity is used for the qualitative and quantitative determination of antigen. However, the discriminating power of serum antibody is not without limitations; the immunizing antigen, which usually has many epitopes, leads to production of antisera that contain a mixture of antibodies with varying specificity for all the epitopes. Indeed, even antibodies to a single epitope are usually mixtures of immunoglobulins with different fine specificities and therefore different affinities for the determinant. Furthermore, immunization with an antigen expands various populations of antibody-forming lymphocytes. These cells can be maintained in culture for only a short time (on the order of days), so it is impractical, if not impossible, to grow normal cells and obtain clones that produce antibodies of a single specificity. A quantum leap in the resolution and discriminating power of antibodies took place in the 1970s with the development of methods for the generation of monoclonal antibodies by Kohler and Milstein, who shared the Nobel Prize for this development. ***Monoclonal antibodies*** are homogeneous populations of antibody molecules, derived from a single antibody-producing cell, in which all antibodies are identical and of the same precise specificity for a given epitope.

Malignant plasma cells (immortal in cell culture) that do not produce immunoglobulin are used in the production of monoclonal antibodies. The cells are engineered to be deficient in an enzyme hypoxanthine guanine phosphoribosyl transferase (HGPRT) and therefore will not survive in culture unless this enzyme is added to the media in which the cells are grown. These cells are fused (hybridized) with a source of freshly harvested B cells from a mouse recently immunized with antigen (e.g., spleen cells) to form ***B-cell hybridomas*** (Fig. 5.13). The fusion is often accomplished by the use of polyethylene glycol (PEG). Following fusion, the cells are cultured in media lacking HGPRT. Since the antibody-producing B cells produce HGPRT, hybridoma cells will survive in the absence of supplemented HGPRT in the culture medium. Within days, the nonfused HGPRT-negative plasma cells soon die, as do all nonfused B cells. Those hybrid cells synthesizing specific

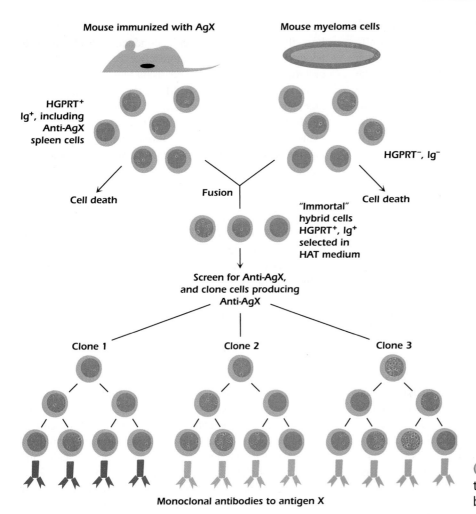

Figure 5.13. Schematic representation of production of monoclonal antibodies.

antibody are selected by some test for antigen reactivity (e.g., ELISA) and then cloned from single cells and propagated in tissue culture, each clone synthesizing antibodies of a single specificity. Those highly specific, monoclonal antibodies are used for numerous procedures, ranging from specific diagnostic tests to biologic agents used in immunotherapy of cancer (see Chapter 19). In immunotherapy, various drugs or toxins are conjugated to monoclonal antibodies, which in turn deliver these substances to the tumor cells against which the antibodies are specifically directed.

T-Cell Hybridomas

In the late 1970s, methods were also developed for the production of hybridomas for T cells. This involves fusing lines of malignant T cells with nonmalignant, antigen-specific T lymphocytes following expansion of the T lymphocyte populations by immunization with antigen. T-cell hybridomas have been very useful in analysis of the relationship between T cells of a single specificity with a corresponding epitope.

Genetically Engineered Molecules and Receptors

To date, most monoclonal antibodies have been created using mouse cells, which are suitable for diagnostic and many other purposes. However, their administration in humans carries with it the potential complication of the formation of antibodies to the mouse immunoglobulins. Attempts to develop *in vitro* human monoclonal antibodies have, by and large, not been very successful.

Human monoclonal antibodies are currently being produced by genetic engineering utilizing several approaches. One method utilizes the technology of recombinant DNA to produce a chimeric mouse–human monoclonal antibody. These so-called **humanized antibodies** consist of the constant region of human immunoglobulin and a variable region of a mouse immunoglobulin. A similar method is used to construct humanized antibodies that consist of a human constant region and a variable region containing a mouse hypervariable region. Another method utilizes the polymerase chain reaction (PCR) to generate gene libraries of heavy and light chains from B-cell hybridomas or plasma cell DNA. With this technology it is now possible to produce millions of clones of different specificities, to screen them rapidly for the desired specificity, and to generate the desired monoclonal Fab constructs without immunization and without the difficulties encountered in the production of monoclonal antibodies.

Genetic engineering of immune proteins is not limited to the production of monoclonal antibodies. Many genes encoding membrane receptors expressed on lymphoid and nonlymphoid cells have been cloned and, in some cases, genetically engineered to allow for gene transfer to cells that do not normally express these receptors. The expression of certain costimulator molecules facilitates cell–cell interactions, such as the physical contact between cytotoxic T cells and target cells, which results in the killing of the latter. The expression of such costimulator molecules (e.g., B7) on tumor cells through gene transfer significantly enhances the ability of T cells to recognize and kill target cells. Experimental vaccination strategies have demonstrated that immunization of tumor-bearing animals with their own tumor cells, which have been removed and transfected with the B7 gene, can potentiate T cells to recognize and destroy the parent tumor cells (a form of immunotherapy). A similar strategy using tumor cells transfected with certain cytokine genes has also been used with some success in animal models. Immunotherapeutic strategies used to treat a variety of diseases are discussed in several chapters of this book (see Chapters 17–19).

 ## EXPERIMENTAL ANIMAL MODELS

Several important *in vivo* animal models have been developed, with experimental value and clinical payoffs similar to those emerging from the use of the *in vitro* systems noted above. These *in vivo* systems rely on the use of inbred mouse strains with a variety of genetic profiles, some of which are genetically engineered. Some inbred strains have an innate predisposition for developing a particular disease (e.g., mammary cancer, leukemia, autoimmune disease, severe combined immunodeficiency disease). Genetically altered animals, on the other hand, have been developed to either express a particular cloned foreign gene (transgenic mice) or interfere with the expression of targeted genes (knockout mice). Such strains are useful in the study of the expression of a particular transgene or in determining the consequences of gene silencing. We begin with a discussion of inbred strains of animals.

Inbred Strains

Many of the classic experiments in the field of immunology have been performed using inbred strains of animals such as mice, rats, and guinea pigs. Selective inbreeding of littermates for more than 20 generations usually leads to the production of an inbred strain. All members of inbred

strains of animals are genetically identical. Therefore, like identical twins, they are said to be **syngeneic**. Immune responses of inbred strains can be studied in the absence of variables associated with genetic differences between animals. As will be discussed in Chapter 18, organ transplants between members of inbred strains are always accepted since their MHC antigens are identical. Indeed, knowledge of the laws of transplantation and the identification of the MHC as the major genetic barrier to transplantation came from research using inbred strains. Experiments using inbred strains led to the identification of class I and class II MHC genes (see Chapter 8). It also explained their main function, the delivery of peptide fragments of antigen to the cell surface, which allows them to be recognized by antigen-specific T cells. Subsequent chapters will elaborate on the important role of the MHC in (1) the generation of normal immune responses, (2) T-cell development, (3) disease susceptibility, and (4) organ transplantation.

Adoptive Transfer

As you learned in Chapter 1, protection against many diseases is conferred through cell-mediated immunity by antigen-specific T cells, rather than through antibody-mediated (humoral) immunity. The distinction between these two arms of the immune response can be demonstrated readily by adoptive transfer of T cells or by passive administration of antiserum or purified antibodies. *Adoptive transfer* of T cells is usually performed using genetically identical donor and recipients (e.g., inbred strains) and results in long-term adoptive immunization following antigen priming. By contrast, passive transfer of serum-containing antibodies, which can be performed across MHC barriers and is effective as long as the transferred antibodies remain active in the recipient, is called passive immunization (see Chapter 1).

SCID Mice

Severe combined immunodeficiency disease (*SCID*) is a disorder in which B and T cells fail to develop, causing the individual to be compromised with respect to lymphoid defense mechanisms. Chapter 17 discusses various causes of SCID in humans. In the 1980s, an inbred strain of mice spontaneously developed an autosomal recessive mutation, resulting in SCID in homozygous *scid/scid* mice. Because of the absence of functional T and B cells, SCID mice are able to accept cells and tissue grafts from other strains of mice or other species. SCID mice can be engrafted with human hematopoietic stem cells to create **SCID-human chimeras**. Such chimeric mice develop mature, functional T and B cells derived from the infused human stem cell precursors. This animal model has become a valuable research tool, since it allows immunologists to manipulate the human immune system *in vivo* and to investigate the development of various lymphoid cells. Moreover, SCID-human mice can be used to test candidate vaccines, including those that might useful in protecting humans from HIV infection.

Thymectomized and Congenically Athymic (Nude) Mice

The importance of the thymus in the development of mature T cells can be demonstrated by using mice that have been neonatally thymectomized, irradiated, and then reconstituted with syngeneic bone marrow. Such mice fail to develop mature T cells. Similarly, mice homozygous for a mutation in a gene called *nu* also fail to develop mature T cells because the mutation results in an athymic (and hairless, hence, the term *nude*) phenotype. In both situations, T-cell development can be restored by grafting these mice with thymic epithelial tissue. Like SCID mice, these animal models have been useful in the study of T-cell development. They have also been useful for the *in vivo* propagation of tumor cell lines and freshly harvested tumor tissue from other strains and other species due to the absence of T cells required for the rejection of foreign cells.

TRANSGENIC MICE AND GENE TARGETING

Transgenic Mice

Another significant animal system used extensively in immunologic research is the ***transgenic mouse***. Transgenic mice are made by injecting a cloned gene (***transgene***) into

fertilized mouse eggs. The eggs are then microinjected into mice rendered pseudopregnant using hormone therapy (Fig. 5.14). The success rate of this technique is rather low, with approximately 10–30% of the offspring expressing the transgene. Since the transgene is integrated into both somatic and germline cells, it is transmitted to the offspring as a Mendelian trait. By constructing a transgene with a particular promoter, it is possible to control the expression of the transgene. For example, some promoters function only in certain tissues (the insulin promoter only functions in the pancreas); others function in response to biochemical signals that can be supplied as a dietary supplement (the metallothionine promoter that functions in response to zinc can be added to drinking water). Transgenic mice have been used to study genes that are not usually expressed *in vivo* (e.g., oncogenes) as well as the effects of transgenes encoding particular Ig molecules, T-cell receptors, MHC class I or class II molecules, and a variety of cytokines. In some transgenic mice, the entire mouse Ig locus has been replaced by human Ig genes. These are useful in generating "human" antibodies in the mouse. There are two disadvantages of the transgenic method. First, the transgene integrates randomly within the genome. Second, it is unphysiologic to express high quantities of transgenes in the wrong tissues, so investigators must use great care in interpreting results obtained in transgenic mice.

Knockout Mice

Sometimes, it is of interest to determine how the removal of a particular gene product affects the immune system.

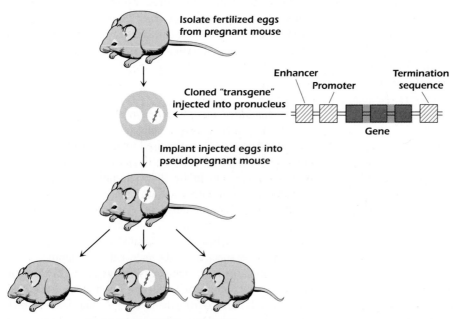

Figure 5.14. General procedure for producing transgenic mice.

Using a *gene-targeting* method, it is possible to replace a normal gene with one that has been mutated or disrupted to generate so-called *knockout mice*. Unlike transgenic mice, knockout mice express transgenes that integrate at specific endogenous genes through a process known as homologous recombination. Virtually any gene for which a mutated or altered transgene exists can be targeted this way. Knockout mice have been generated by using mutated or altered transgenes that target, and therefore silence, the expression of a variety of important genes, including those encoding particular cytokines and MHC molecules. Knockout mice have also been used to identify the parts of genes essential for normal gene function. In order to identify the responsible part of the gene, different mutated copies of the gene are introduced back into the genome by transgenesis to see which one restores normal function.

ANALYSIS OF GENE EXPRESSION: MICROARRAYS

Microarrays, or *gene chips*, are powerful tools for examining the level of expression of thousands of genes simultaneously. The microarray comprises thousands of DNA fragments, each with a unique sequence, attached in an ordered arrangement to a glass slide or other surface. These DNA fragments, in the form of cDNA (generally 500–5000 base pairs long) or oligonucleotides (20–80 base pairs long), can represent genes from all parts of the genome; alternatively, specialized microarrays can be prepared that use DNA from genes thought to be of particular interest. To perform a microarray assay, a sample of total messenger RNA (mRNA; the product obtained from transcription of all active genes) from a cell or tissue is commonly tested with a reference sample to compare gene expression among various samples. For example, different cell types or tissues can be compared, cells can be compared at different stages of differentiation, or tumor cells can be compared with their normal counterparts. The samples added to the microarray are generally not mRNAs; rather, the total mRNA is reverse transcribed into cDNA, which is then labeled with a fluorescent material (a fluorochrome). Different colored fluorochromes are used to distinctly label the different sources of cDNAs. Figure 5.15 illustrates how microarrays are used to compare gene expression in a lymphoid tumor cell population with that of a normal cell population. A red fluorochrome is used to label experimental tumor cell cDNAs, and a green fluorochrome is used for cDNAs prepared from the control normal counterparts. The labeled cDNAs are washed over the microarray and allowed to hybridize by base pairing with matching fragments. cDNA samples derived from both samples are combined so that they compete for binding to the microarray. Unhybridized material is washed away, leaving pockets of fluorescence where matching has occurred. At the end of the hybridization reaction, the microarray is laser scanned to reveal red,

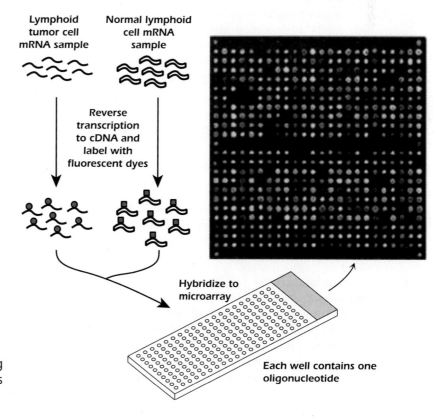

Figure 5.15. Microarray assay comparing samples of mRNA from lymphoid tumor cells and normal lymphoid cells.

green, or yellow spots, indicating higher levels of the experimental tumor cell cDNA (red), higher levels of the control cDNA (green), or equal levels of DNA in the two samples (yellow). To interpret the results, a fluorescence scanner examines each spot on the slide for the precise level of fluorescence. The data are then analyzed by a computer program that typically combines the fluorescence information with a genetic database to determine which

genes are overexpressed or underexpressed in the tested samples. Characterization of the pattern and amount of binding to the microarray has many potential uses in the field of immunology, including clinical diagnosis of lymphoid tumors, drug development, and new gene discovery. For example, candidate immunosuppressive drugs can be tested for their effects on cytokine gene expression.

SUMMARY

1. The reaction between an antibody and an antigen does not involve covalent forces; it involves weak forces of interaction such as electrostatic, hydrophobic, and van der Waals forces. Consequently, for a significant interaction, the antibody-combining site and the antigen require a close fit like a lock and key.

2. Only the reaction between a multivalent antigen and an antibody that is at least bivalent can bring about antigen–antibody reactions that result in the cross-linking of antigen molecules by antibodies. These reactions do not take place with haptens or monovalent Fab.

3. The interaction between a soluble antibody and an insoluble particulate antigen results in agglutination. The extent of agglutination depends on the proportions of the interacting antibody and antigen. At high antibody levels, agglutination may not occur. This is referred to as a prozone. The term *titer* refers to the highest serum dilution at which agglutination still takes place and beyond which (at higher dilution) no agglutination occurs.

4. Precipitation reactions occur on mixing, at the right proportions, soluble multivalent antigen and antibodies that are at least divalent. The precipitation reaction may take place in aqueous media or in gels.

5. The reaction in gels between soluble antigen and antibodies may be used for the qualitative and quantitative analysis of antigen or antibody. Examples include precipitation reactions in gels, radial immunodiffusion, and immunoelectrophoresis.

6. Radioimmunoassay (RIA) is a very sensitive test used to quantitate antibody or antigen. It employs the use of radiolabeled antigen or antibody and is based on competitive inhibition of nonlabeled and labeled antigen. Antibody-bound antigen must be separated from nonbound labeled antigen. Separation is usually achieved by precipitation with anti-immunoglobulins.

7. Solid-phase immunoassay is a test that exploits the ability of many proteins to adhere to plastic and form a monomolecular layer. Antigen is applied to plastic wells, antibodies are added, the well is washed, and any antibodies bound to antigen are measured by the use of radiolabeled or enzyme-linked anti-immunoglobulins.

8. The enzyme-linked immunosorbent assay (ELISA) is a solid-phase immunoassay in which an enzyme is linked to the anti-immunoglobulin. Quantitation is achieved by colorimetric evaluation after the addition of a substrate that changes color in response to enzyme activity.

9. In immunofluorescence, an antigen is detected by the use of fluorescence-labeled immunoglobulins. In direct immunofluorescence, the antibody to the antigen in question carries a fluorescent label. In indirect immunofluorescence, the antigen-specific antibody is not labeled; it is detected by the addition of fluorescently labeled anti-immunoglobulin. Fluorescence-activated cell sorters (FACS) are instruments that can be used to quantitate and sort fluorescently labeled cells.

10. Assays used to assess lymphocyte function typically measure their proliferative responses or effector functions. For example, B cells can be functionally assessed by measuring their ability to proliferate and produce antibodies in response to B-cell mitogens such as LPS. T cells are often assessed by measuring their ability to provide help for other cells (in the case of $CD4^+$ cells) or to kill antigen-bearing targets (in the case of $CD8^+$ cells). In addition, T cells can be assessed by measuring their ability to proliferate and to produce certain cytokines in response to T-cell mitogens such as PHA or Con A.

11. Monoclonal antibodies are highly specific reagents consisting of homogeneous populations of antibodies, all of precisely the same specificity toward an epitope.

REFERENCES

Channing-Rodgers RP (1994): Clinical laboratory methods for detection of antigens and antibodies. In Stites DP, Terr AI, Parslow TG (eds): *Basic and Clinical Immunology*, 8th ed. East Norwalk, CT: Appleton & Lange.

De Groot AS (2006): Immunomics: Discovering new targets for vaccines and therapeutics. *Drug Discov Today* 11: 203.

Harlow E, Lane D (1988): *Antibodies: A Laboratory Manual*. Cold Spring Harbor, NY: Cold Spring Harbor Laboratory.

Hudson L, Hay FC (1989): *Practical Immunology*, 3rd ed. Oxford, UK: Blackwell.

Johnstone A, Thorpe R (1987): *Immunochemistry in Practice*. Oxford, UK: Blackwell.

Köhler G, Milstein C (1975). Continuous cultures of fused cells secreting antibody of predefined specificity. *Nature* 256:495

Koller BH, Smithies O (1992): Altering genes in animals by gene targeting. *Annu Rev Immunol* 10:705.

Louzoun Y (2007): The evolution of mathematical immunology. *Immunol Rev* 216:9.

Mayforth RD (1993): *Designing Antibodies*. San Diego, CA: Academic.

Mishell BB, Shiigi SM (1980): *Selected Methods in Cellular Immunology*. New York: Freeman.

Presta LG (2006): Engineering of therapeutic antibodies to minimize immunogenicity and optimize function. *Adv Drug Deliv Rev* 58:640.

REVIEW QUESTIONS

For each question, choose the ONE BEST answer.

1. Which of the following is required to ensure the integrity and stability of Ig molecules but is not associated with interactions between antigens and antibodies?
    A) covalent bonds
    B) van der Waals forces
    C) hydrophobic forces
    D) electrostatic forces
    E) a very close fit between an epitope and the antibody

2. If an IgG antibody preparation specific for hen egg lysosome (HEL) is treated with papain to generate Fab fragments, which of the following statements concerning the avidity of such fragments is true?
    A) They will have a lower avidity for HEL as compared with the intact IgG.
    B) They will have a higher avidity for HEL as compared with the intact IgG.
    C) They will have the same avidity for HEL as the intact IgG.
    D) They will have lost their avidity to bind to HEL.
    E) They will have the same avidity but will have a lower affinity for HEL.

3. Western blot assays used to test serum samples for the presence of antibodies to infectious agents, such as HIV, are particularly useful as diagnostic assays because:
    A) They are more sensitive than ELISA.
    B) Antibodies specific for multiple antigenic epitopes can be detected.
    C) They provide quantitative data for sample analysis.
    D) They allow multiple samples to be tested simultaneously.
    E) They are less expensive and take less time to perform compared to ELISA.

4. The major difference between transgenic mice and knockout mice is:
    A) Transgenic mice always employ the use of cloned genes derived from other species.
    B) Transgenic mice have foreign genes that integrate at targeted loci through homologous recombination.
    C) Transgenic mice have a functional foreign gene added to their genome.
    D) Knockout mice always have a unique phenotype.

5. SCID mice have a genetic defect that prevents development of functional:
    A) hematopoietic cells
    B) B and T cells
    C) T and NK cells
    D) pluripotential stem cells
    E) myeloid cells

6. Which of the following statements regarding B-cell hybridomas is true?
    A) They are immortal cell lines that produce antibodies with more than one specificity.
    B) They are derived from B cells that are first cloned and grown in cell culture for short periods.
    C) They contain one nucleus.
    D) They are derived by fusing B cells with malignant plasma cells that are unable to secrete immunoglobulin.

7. An ELISA designed to test for the presence of serum antibody for a new strain of pathogenic bacteria is under development. Initially, a monoclonal antibody specific for a single epitope of the organism was used both to sensitize the wells of the ELISA plate and as the enzyme-labeled detecting antibody in a conventional sandwich ELISA. The ELISA failed to detect the antigen despite the use of a wide range of antibody concentrations. What is the most probable cause of this problem?
    A) The antigen used in the assay is too large.
    B) The antibody has a low affinity for the antigen.

C) The monoclonal antibody used to sensitize the wells is blocking access of the epitope, so when the same antibody is enzyme labeled, it cannot bind to the antigen.

D) The enzyme-labeled antibody used should have been a different isotype than the sensitizing antibody.

E) The monoclonal antibody used is probably unstable.

ANSWERS TO REVIEW QUESTIONS

1. A No covalent bonds are involved in the interaction between antibody and antigen. The binding forces are relatively weak and include van der Waals forces, hydrophobic forces, and electrostatic forces. A very close fit between an epitope and the antibody is required.

2. A Avidity denotes the overall binding energy between antigens and multivalent antigens. Since the valency of the Fab fragments is 1 as compared with the HEL-specific IgG molecule, which has a valence of 2 (due to the presence of two Fab regions), the avidity of the fragments will be lower. Choice E is incorrect because the affinity of the Fab fragments will be the same as each of the Fab regions of the intact IgG molecule.

3. B In Western blot assays, electrophoretic separation techniques are used to resolve the molecular mass of a given antigen or mixtures of antigens. Since antibody responses to infectious agents generate polyclonal responses by virtue of the complex antigenic determinants expressed by such agents, Western blot assays can confirm the presence of these antibodies, which react with the electrophoretically separated antigens of known molecular weights.

4. C Cloned foreign genes from either the same or other species are introduced into mice to generate a transgenic strain. Integration is random and occurs in both somatic and germline cells.

Choice D is incorrect because sometimes knockout mice do not have a unique phenotype caused by the replacement of a functional gene with one that is nonfunctional, probably due to the activity of redundant or compensatory mechanisms.

5. B SCID mice possess an autosomal recessive mutation that causes a disorder in which B and T cells fail to develop. Like their human counterparts, SCID mice are compromised with respect to lymphoid defense mechanisms. Pluripotential stem cells present in SCID mice can give rise to other hematopoietic lineages, including cells in the myeloid lineage and NK cells.

6. D The method used to generate B-cell hybridomas employs the fusion of B cells (e.g., from the spleen and lymph nodes) harvested from immunized mice with a selected population of malignant plasma cells unable to secrete immunoglobulin. The process yields a monoclonal antibody secreted by cells that contain nuclei from the B and plasma cells that have fused.

7. C In a sandwich ELISA, an antibody (often monoclonal) used to coat ELISA wells will bind to the epitope for which it is specific. In the example given, the same epitope-specific monoclonal antibody is used as enzyme-labeled detecting antibody. The sensitizing monoclonal antibody is blocking access to the epitope by the enzyme-labeled monoclonal antibody, so it will not bind.

6

THE GENETIC BASIS OF ANTIBODY STRUCTURE

INTRODUCTION

In previous chapters we described the enormous diversity of the immune response, focusing on the diversity of antibodies—immunoglobulin molecules that are the secreted forms of the antigen-specific receptors found on individual B lymphocytes. Estimates of the number of B and T cells with different antigenic specificities that can be generated in a single individual range from 10^{15} to 10^{18}; in other words, every person has the ability to generate 10^{15}–10^{18} different Ig or TCR molecules. The human *genome* (inherited DNA) has now been sequenced and found to contain only 20,000–25,000 genes; the genomes of other mammalian species contain similar numbers of genes. How do so few genes produce so many different antigen receptor molecules?

The work of several investigators over the last 30 years has shown that Ig and TCR genes use a unique strategy involving *combinations* of genes to achieve the required degree of diversity. The first key finding was that the variable and constant regions of an Ig molecule are coded for by different genes. In fact, many different variable- (V) region genes can be linked up to a single constant- (C) region gene. A subsequent crucial finding by Susumu Tonegawa (who was awarded the Nobel Prize in 1987) was that antibody genes can *rearrange* themselves within the genome of a differentiating cell: A V-region gene can move from one position in the DNA of an inherited chromosome (the *germline*) to another during lymphocyte differentiation. This process of rearrangement during differentiation brings together a set of genes that codes for the V and C regions. The set of rearranged genes is then transcribed and translated into a complete heavy (H) or light (L) chain.

Subsequent studies (discussed in more detail in Chapter 8) have shown that TCR genes and the mechanisms used to generate TCR diversity share many common features with Ig genes and the generation of diversity of Ig molecules. To date, the rearrangement strategies used to generate antigen-specific receptors on T and B cells appear unique to lymphocytes. In the remainder of this chapter we describe how Ig genes are organized and rearrange and show how a huge number of Ig polypeptides can be made from a small number of genes.

A BRIEF REVIEW OF NONIMMUNOGLOBULIN GENE STRUCTURE AND GENE EXPRESSION

Before discussing the molecular arrangement and rearrangement of the genes involved in Ig synthesis, we thought it would be helpful to review the organization and expression of nonimmunoglobulin genes. We focus discussion on the components of genes that code for a typical protein expressed at the cell surface, as illustrated in Figure 6.1:

- The genome of an individual consists of linear arrays of genes in the DNA strands of the various chromosomes. A gene is transcribed into RNA, and RNA is translated into protein.

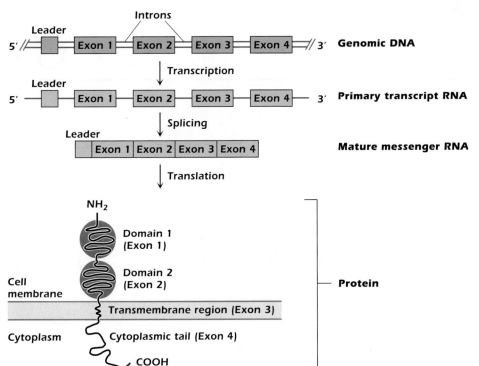

Figure 6.1. Prototypical gene coding for a transmembrane protein: summary of steps involved in expressing protein at the cell surface.

Every diploid cell in the human body contains the same set of genes as every other cell. The only exceptions are lymphocytes, which, as we discuss shortly, differ from other cells and each other in the actual content of genes coding for their antigen-specific receptor. Cells within an individual differ from one another because they transcribe and translate different genes. We say that these cells *express* different patterns of genes.

- The expression of a specific pattern of genes determines the cell's function. For example, every cell contains an insulin gene, but only pancreatic β cells express that gene, enabling them to make insulin. Similarly, all cells contain Ig genes; however, only B lymphocytes (and their differentiated form, plasma cells) express Ig genes and therefore synthesize Ig molecules. Like all other cells except B cells, T cells contain Ig genes but do not express them.
As we discuss further in Chapter 10 regarding the activation of B and T cells, the control of gene expression exists at multiple levels. These include the activity of *transcription factors* (proteins that initiate or modulate transcription, generally by binding to regulatory DNA sequences close to the 5′ end of genes), the rate of transcription, and the half-life of mRNA. Understanding the mechanisms that regulate gene expression and, in particular, how genes are turned on and off in different cell types is an area of intense research interest.
- Most genes coding for a protein have a characteristic structure of exons and introns. *Exons* are sequences

of base pairs that are later transcribed into mature mRNA. Exons are separated from each other by *introns*—noncoding regions of base pairs.

- When a gene is transcribed into RNA, the entire stretch of DNA (exons plus introns) is transcribed into a primary RNA transcript. Enzymes modify this primary RNA transcript by *splicing* out the noncoding introns and bringing together all the coding exons. This yields a processed mature mRNA segment that is much shorter than the original transcript. This mRNA is translated into protein on ribosomes. Notice in Figure 6.1 that exons generally code for a discrete region of the protein, such as an extracellular *domain*, a transmembrane region, or a cytoplasmic tail. Thus proteins are assembled by putting together multiple functional regions, and each region is coded for by a separate gene segment.
- Genes coding for proteins expressed at the cell surface have a *leader sequence* (L exon) at the 5′ end. This codes for a sequence of about 10 mainly hydrophobic amino acids—the *signal peptide*—at the amino (NH_2) terminus of the protein. When the mRNA for a cell-membrane-associated protein is translated on ribosomes, the signal peptide directs the synthesis of the polypeptide chain to the endoplasmic reticulum. The nascent polypeptide chain is fed from the ribosomes into the interior of endoplasmic reticulum, where the signal peptide is cleaved off. The newly synthesized protein moves from the endoplasmic reticulum into the Golgi apparatus and then to the cell membrane.

The surface molecule depicted in Figure 6.1 is shown with its amino terminus and two domains outside the cell, a single transmembrane region, and a large carboxy-terminal region (COOH) inside the cell. The structure of a membrane Ig molecule expressed at the surface of a B cell has some similarities to the structure of the molecule depicted in Figure 6.1, especially the extracellular N-terminal domains and transmembrane region. However, membrane Ig also differs in important ways from the structure of the depicted molecule. First, Ig is a four-chain glycoprotein. To make a complete Ig molecule, the newly synthesized individual H and L chains must be assembled and glycosylated inside the cell before the four-chain molecule reaches the cell surface. Second, each Ig chain has a very short cytoplasmic tail.

Other molecules involved in the immune response are expressed at the cell surface with different configurations; for example, the carboxy-terminal region can be extracellular and the N-terminus intracellular. Other membrane molecules, such as CD81 expressed on B cells, loop multiple times through the membrane (see Chapters 7 and 10). Yet others, such as leukocyte function-associated antigen 1 (LFA-1; CD58) and decay-accelerating factor (DAF; CD55), are completely extracellular; they are linked to the surface of the cell via a covalent bond to an oligosaccharide, which in turn is bound to a phospholipid (phosphatidylinositol) in the membrane. Thus these molecules are referred to as glycosylphosphatidylinositol (GPI)-linked membrane molecules. (The functions of LFA-1 and DAF are discussed in Chapters 10 and 13, respectively.)

GENETIC EVENTS IN SYNTHESIS OF Ig CHAINS

Organization and Rearrangement of Light-Chain Genes

As we saw in Chapter 4, each κ and λ L-chain polypeptide consists of two major domains, a variable region and a constant region (V_L and C_L). The V_L is the approximately 108-residue amino-terminal portion of the light chain. V_L is coded for by two separate gene segments: *a variable (V) segment*, which codes for the amino-terminal 95 residues, and a small *joining (J) segment*, coding for about 13 residues (96–108) at the carboxy-terminal end of the variable region. One V gene and one J gene are brought together in the genome to create a gene unit that, together with the C-region gene, codes for an entire Ig L chain. This unique *gene rearrangement* mechanism—referred to as *V(D)J recombination*—is used only by genes coding for Ig L and H chains and genes coding for TCRs. D gene segments are discussed below with H-chain genes.

The complex, tightly regulated sequence of molecular events involved in gene rearrangement is only just beginning to be understood, but we do know that defects in the mechanism or regulation of V(D)J recombination can lead to disease (see Chapter 17). Many of the steps in the process appear to be common to both B and T cells. An enzyme complex, known as *V(D)J recombinase*, mediates the rearrangement of receptor genes in B and T cells. As their name implies, the products of two recombination-activating (RAG) genes *RAG-1* and *RAG-2* are critical in initiating recombination in lymphocyte precursor cells. Both RAG-1 and RAG-2 proteins are required in the first stages of cutting Ig and TCR DNA: mice lacking either of these genes ("RAG knockout mice") are deficient in both B and T cells. The V(D)J recombinase complex includes genes that are involved in the repair of DNA strands in all cells; by contrast, RAG-1 and RAG-2 gene products are expressed exclusively in developing lymphocytes.

κ-Chain Synthesis. We will first examine the synthesis of κ light chains. Figure 6.2 shows the set of human genes coding for κ chains—referred to as the κ *locus*—that is found on chromosome 2. The top line of the figure shows the arrangement of κ genes in the germline—that is, in *any* cell in the body: There are approximately 40 different Vκ genes, each of which can code for the N-terminal 95 amino acids of a κ variable region. The Vκ genes are arranged linearly in the genome, separated by noncoding DNA. Each Vκ gene has its own L (leader) sequence, which, for simplicity, has been omitted from the figure. A series of five Jκ gene segments is found downstream (i.e., $3'$) of this region. Each Jκ gene segment can encode the remaining 13 amino acid residues (96–108) of the κ variable region. An intron separates the Cκ gene segment—the gene coding for the single constant region of the κ chain—from the Jκ gene segments.

To make a κ chain, cell early in the B-lymphocyte lineage selects one of the Vκ genes from its DNA and physically joins it to one of the Jκ segments (in Fig. 6.2, V_2 rearranges to J_4). The V(D)J recombinase mediates the joining; it recognizes *recombination recognition sequences* that are located at the ends of the V and J gene segments. (These recombination recognition sequences are "conserved" among all V, D, and J gene segments used by Ig and TCR genes.) The mechanism of selection of V and J genes is unknown, but it is probably a random process. Figure 6.3 shows this V_2-to-J_4 rearrangement in more detail; note that the rearranged DNA in this early B cell still contains the unrearranged gene segments V_1 and J_5. In most cases the intervening DNA is looped, cut out, and ultimately degraded.

Figure 6.2 also indicates that after the DNA of a cell in the B-cell lineage is rearranged, a primary RNA transcript is made. This transcript is then spliced to remove all introns, bringing the Vκ, Jκ, and Cκ exons together in a mature mRNA. At the cell's rough endoplasmic reticulum, the mRNA is translated into the κ polypeptide chain.

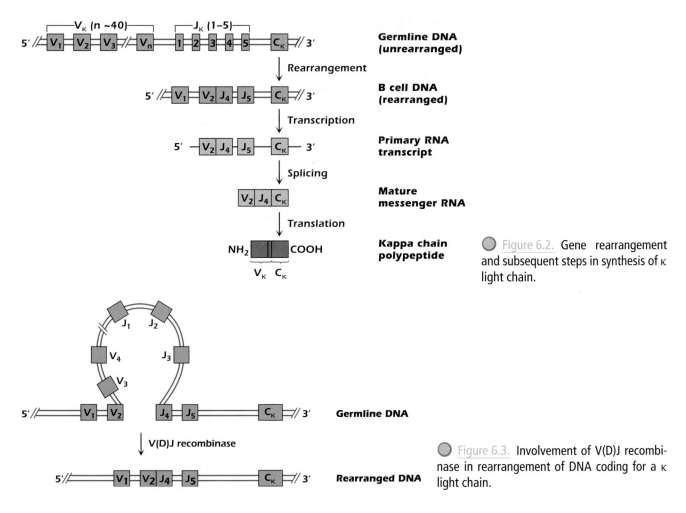

Figure 6.2. Gene rearrangement and subsequent steps in synthesis of κ light chain.

Figure 6.3. Involvement of V(D)J recombinase in rearrangement of DNA coding for a κ light chain.

The κ chain then moves into the lumen of the endoplasmic reticulum where the signal peptide (encoded by the leader sequence) is cleaved off, and the κ chain can now associate with a newly synthesized H chain to form an Ig molecule.

λ-Chain Synthesis.   The λ genes are found on chromosome 22 in the human—that is, on a chromosome distinct from the κ genes and the H-chain genes. Like κ chains, the synthesis of λ chains involves rearrangement of DNA, which joins a V_λ gene (coding for the N-terminal region of a λ variable region) with a Jλ segment (coding for the remaining 13 amino acids of the λ variable region). The human λ locus comprises about 30 Vλ and 4 Jλ genes. The organization of the λ gene locus is slightly different from the organization of the κ gene locus, which contains only one Cκ gene: By contrast, each Jλ is associated with a different Cλ gene. Thus, each λ chain will have one of four possible Cλ regions.

Organization and Rearrangement of Heavy-Chain Genes

Genes coding for immunoglobulin heavy chains—*the heavy-chain locus*—are found on a chromosome distinct

from either L chain locus. Figure 6.4 shows the organization of genes coding for the H chain (located on chromosome 14 in humans) and illustrates the similarities and differences of this locus with the L-chain loci. In contrast to the variable region of a light chain, which is constructed from two gene segments, the variable region of a heavy chain is constructed from three gene segments: V_H, D_H, and J_H. Thus, in addition to V and J segments, genes coding for the variable region of an H chain also use a *diversity* **(D)** *segment*. The D and J segments code for amino acid sequences in the third hypervariable region or *complementarity-determining region* (CDR3) of the heavy chain (see Chapter 4). Figure 6.4 indicates that the human H-chain locus includes approximately 50 V_H genes, about 20 D_H gene segments, and 6 J_H gene segments.

The second key feature of the H-chain genes is the presence in the germline of multiple genes coding for the C region of the immunoglobulin. As described in Chapter 4, the C region determines the class and hence biologic function of the particular antibody. Humans have nine constant-region genes, one for each class or subclass, clustered at the 3′ end of the heavy-chain locus. The order of C genes in the human is shown in Figure 6.4. The C

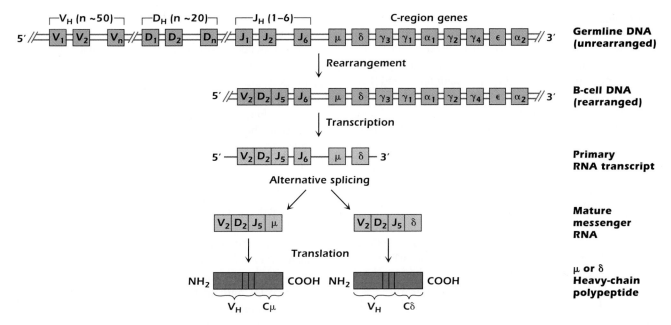

Figure 6.4. Gene rearrangements and subsequent steps in the synthesis of human heavy chains showing how alternative splicing in a B cell generates μ and δ chains of identical antigenic specificity.

genes closest to the V-region genes are μ and δ, which are transcribed first during B-cell development.

Heavy-chain synthesis uses the same mechanisms of rearrangement described for light chains—namely, the use of the V(D)J recombinase to mediate the joining of different gene segments. In the early stages of the life of a particular B cell, two rearrangements of germline DNA must occur. The first joins one D segment to one J segment. The second brings one V segment to the DJ unit ($V_2 D_2 J_5$ in Fig. 6.4), fixing the antigen specificity of the H chain. The rearranged DNA is then transcribed along with the closest C-region genes, $C\mu$ and $C\delta$. This primary transcript can be spliced in two different ways (*alternative splicing*) to yield either a VDJ-μ or a VDJ-δ mRNA: one B cell synthesizes both mRNAs. The two mRNAs may then be translated in rough endoplasmic reticulum to yield either a μ or δ polypeptide. The μ and δ polypeptides combine inside the cell with a κ or λ light chain to form IgM and IgD, respectively, which traffic to the cell membrane. In this way, an individual resting B cell may express at its surface both IgM and IgD with identical antigenic specificity.

Alternative splicing of the heavy-chain primary transcript also generates membrane and secreted forms of a heavy-chain polypeptide. Additional short exons (not shown in Fig. 6.4) are found at the $3'$ end of each C_H gene, for example at the $3'$ end of $C\mu$. These exons code for (a) the transmembrane plus cytoplasmic tail of the membrane form of the molecule and (b) the C-terminal end of the secreted form of the molecule. All the exons are transcribed into the primary transcript, but alternative RNA splicing results in mRNA for either the membrane form or the secreted form of the heavy-chain polypeptide.

Regulation of Ig Gene Expression

Theoretically, any one B cell has many genes from which it can synthesize an Ig molecule: multiple V, D, and J genes to form the variable regions and different genes for the κ and λ light chains. In reality, each B cell expresses one rearranged heavy-chain locus and one rearranged light-chain locus, either κ or λ. As a result, one B cell produces an immunoglobulin of a single antigenic specificity.

Furthermore, because a given B cell has two sets of chromosomes—one set from each parent—theoretically, Ig genes located on both chromosomes could synthesize Ig molecules. This does not occur. In contrast to almost all other gene products, which are derived from genes from both parental chromosomes, Ig chains are coded for by only one set of genes, from either the maternal or the paternal chromosome. For example, the H chain may be coded for by genes on the paternal chromosome and the L chain (either κ or λ) by genes on the maternal chromosome. This phenomenon of using genes from only one parental chromosome is known as *allelic exclusion*.

Although all of the control mechanisms are not yet completely clear, the steps in rearrangement, allelic exclusion, and synthesis of a complete Ig molecule are very tightly controlled. If a successful or *productive* rearrangement of V, D, and J gene DNA occurs on one of the parental chromosomes and an H-chain polypeptide is produced, the other parental H-chain locus stops rearranging as a result of some kind of suppressive mechanism. If the attempt to rearrange the V, D, and J genes on the first parental chromosome is unsuccessful (i.e., if it fails to produce a polypeptide chain), then the second parental chromosome continues H-chain locus rearrangement. The same process then occurs with the L-chain loci, first with the κ- and then with the λ-chain genes. Productive rearrangement resulting from the joining of a V segment to a J segment of any one of these genes causes the others to remain in germline form. In this way, the cell progresses through some or all of its chromosomal copies until it has successfully completed the productive rearrangement of genes for one H and one L chain. These chains then become the basis of the antibody specificity of that particular B cell.

In summary, only one H chain and one L chain are functionally expressed in a B cell, even though every B cell contains two chromosomes (paternally and maternally derived) that could code for the heavy chain and two chromosomes that could code for the light chain. This phenomenon of allelic exclusion ensures that an individual B cell expresses an Ig molecule (IgM, IgD, IgG, IgA, or IgE) on its cell surface of only one single antigen specificity; similarly, the antibody molecule synthesized and secreted by that B cell will be specific for a single antigenic epitope.

CLASS OR ISOTYPE SWITCHING

As we have described above, one B cell makes antibody of a single specificity that is fixed by the nature of VJ (L-chain) and VDJ (H-chain) rearrangements. These rearrangements occur in the absence of antigen in the early stages of B-cell differentiation. We have also described how a single B cell can synthesize IgM and IgD with the same antigenic specificity. In the paragraphs that follow, we show how an individual B cell can switch to make a different class of antibody, such as IgG, IgE, or IgA. This phenomenon is known as *class* or *isotype switching*. Class

switching changes the effector function of the B cell but does not change the cell's antigenic specificity.

Class switching occurs in antigen-stimulated mature B cells synthesizing IgM and IgD (discussed in Chapter 7) and involves further DNA rearrangement, juxtaposing the rearranged VDJ genes with a different heavy-chain C-region gene (see Fig. 6.5). Class switching is dependent on the presence of both antigen and factors known as *cytokines* secreted by T cells (see below and further discussion in Chapters 10 and 11). There is little or no class switching by B cells in the absence of T-cell-derived cytokines.

Figure 6.5 shows the mechanism by which mature B cells undergo class switching, known as *class switch recombination*. At the 5′ end of every H-chain C-region (C_H) gene, apart from Cδ, is a stretch of repeating base sequences called a *switch* (S) *region*. This S region permits any of the C_H genes (other than Cδ) to associate with the VDJ unit; in the figure, only the C_H genes γ_3, γ_1, and α_2 are shown, but other C_H genes may also be used. Under the stimulating influence of antigen and T-cell-derived cytokines, a B cell with a VDJ unit linked to Cμ and Cδ further rearranges its DNA to link the VDJ to an S region in front of another C_H-region gene (γ_1 in Fig. 6.5). After a primary RNA transcript is made from the rearranged DNA, the introns are spliced out to give an mRNA coding for the IgG_1 H chain. In so doing, the intervening C-region DNA, including the switch regions, is removed. Thus, at this stage, the cell loses its ability to revert to making a class of antibody whose C-region gene has been deleted (IgM, IgD, or IgG_3 in this example).

Class switch recombination is unique to the Ig heavy-chain locus. It allows an antibody with a particular antigenic specificity to associate with a variety of different constant-region chains and thus have different effector functions. For example, an antibody with a VDJ unit specific for a bacterial antigen may be linked to Cγ to produce an IgG molecule; this IgG antibody interacts with

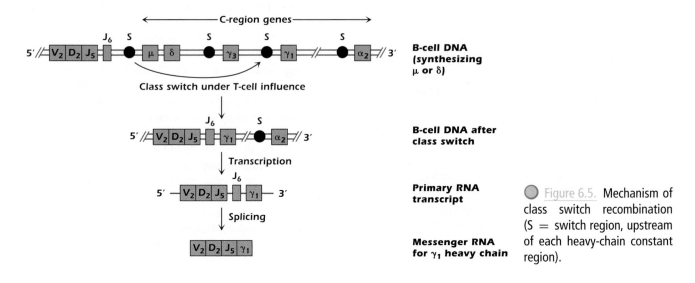

Figure 6.5. Mechanism of class switch recombination (S = switch region, upstream of each heavy-chain constant region).

cells such as macrophages that express receptors for Fcγ. Alternatively, the same VDJ unit may be linked to Cε to produce an IgE molecule; IgE antibody interacts with cells such as mast cells that express receptors for Fcε. As we indicated above, isotype switching does not affect the antigen specificity of this B cell because Ig V region gene usage is not modified.

T-cell-derived cytokines present when antigen activates B cells play a key role in C_H gene selection during isotype switching. For example, in the presence of the cytokine interferon-γ, the B cell can rearrange its VDJ to the $C\gamma_3$ heavy chain, and the cell switches to IgG_3 synthesis. By contrast, in the presence of the cytokine IL-4, a B cell can rearrange its VDJ to $C\gamma_4$ or Cε, and the cell switches to IgG_4 or IgE synthesis, respectively. (Cytokines influence which constant region is used during class switch recombination by providing signals that result in the accessibility of a particular switch region to the "switch recombinase" proteins.) The role of T-cell-derived cytokines in isotype switching is discussed further in Chapter 10.

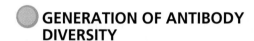

GENERATION OF ANTIBODY DIVERSITY

Thus far we have described the unique genetic mechanisms involved in generating an enormous variety of antibodies from a relatively small amount of DNA to cope with a multitude of antigens. Still more mechanisms exist for generating diversity, some of which are discussed briefly below.

Presence of Multiple V Genes in the Germline

The number of different genes for the V region in the germline constitutes the baseline from which antibody is derived and represents the minimum number of different antibodies that can be produced.

VJ and VDJ Combinatorial Association

As we have already described, any V gene segment can associate with any J gene segment to form an L-chain variable region. Similarly, any V gene segment can associate with any D or J gene segments in H-chain gene rearrangement. All of these distinct segments contribute to the structure of the variable region. As there are about 40 Vκ and 5 Jκ genes coding for the κ-chain variable region, assuming random association, then 40×5 or 200 κ chains can be formed; with 30 Vλ and 4 Jλ genes, 120 λ chains can be formed. Similarly, if there are about 50 V genes, 20 D genes, and 6 J genes that can code for an H-chain variable region and these may also associate in any combination, $50 \times 20 \times 6$ or 6000 different heavy chains can be formed.

Random Assortment of H and L Chains

In addition to VJ and VDJ combinatorial association, any H chain may associate with any L chain. Thus, a total of 1.2×10^6 different κ-containing Ig molecules (200×6000) and 0.72×10^6 (12×6000) λ-containing molecules can be generated from just 155 different genes (adding up all the H, κ, and λ segments)! This illustrates very effectively how a limited set of genes can generate a large number of different antibodies.

Junctional Diversity

The exact positions at which the genes for the V and J (or V, D, and J) segments are joined are not constant. Imprecise DNA recombination can lead to changes in the amino acids at these junction sites. Because imprecise recombination occurs in parts of the Ig hypervariable region where complementarity to antigen is determined, it leads to deletions or changes of amino acids that affect the antigen-binding site (*junctional diversity*). In addition, small sets of nucleotides may be inserted at the V–D and D–J junctions. The major mechanism for inserting nucleotides into the DNA sequence is mediated by the enzyme terminal deoxynucleotidyltransferase (TdT). The additional diversity generated is termed *N-region diversity*.

Somatic Hypermutation

Mutations that occur in V genes of heavy and/or light chains during the lifetime of a B cell also increase the variety of antibodies produced by the B-cell population. Generally, antibodies of low affinity are produced in the primary response to antigen. DNA and polypeptide sequencing of antibodies formed in the primary response indicates that the sequences closely match the sequences encoded by germline DNA. As the response matures, however, and especially after secondary stimulation by the antigen, the antibodies' affinity for antigen increases; the amino acid sequences of these antibodies diverge from those coded for in the germline DNA.

This divergence results predominantly from point mutations in the VDJ recombined unit of antibody V genes, which result in changes in individual amino acids. This phenomenon is referred to as *somatic hypermutation* because it occurs at a rate at least 10,000 times higher than the normal rate of mutation. As a consequence of this fine tuning of the immune response, somatic hypermutation increases the variety—as well as the affinity—of antibodies produced by the B-cell population. The evidence suggests that there is a narrow window of opportunity for somatic hypermutation—it occurs after antigenic stimulation in the germinal centers of lymph node and spleen (see Chapter 7).

Somatic Gene Conversion

The paradigm that Ig diversity is generated by VDJ recombination and somatic hypermutation evolved from studies of mouse and human B cells. However, subsequent studies in other species, most notably in birds and rabbits, revealed that these animals use a different mechanism, known as *somatic gene conversion*, to generate a wide variety of diverse B-cell specificities. Somatic gene conversion involves the nonreciprocal exchange of sequences among genes: Part of the donor gene or genes is "copied" into an acceptor gene, but only the acceptor gene is altered. The precise mechanism by which this occurs is currently not clear. Figure 6.6 shows the chicken H-chain locus, which includes a single functional V_H gene that rearranges in all B cells, along with approximately 20 *pseudogenes*—gene segments that have mutations that prevent them from synthesizing a polypeptide. The bottom line of the figure shows that in this particular B cell a diversified variable gene unit is generated by incorporating two short sequences from pseudogene 3 and one from pseudogene 8 into the rearranged VDJ gene. Somatic gene conversion can also generate L-chain diversity.

Many species other than humans and mice rely on somatic gene conversion and somatic hypermutation to generate diversity within the *primary* Ig repertoire—that is, before antigen stimulation. For example, chickens use somatic gene conversion as a major mechanism to generate the primary repertoire, and sheep use somatic hypermutation. Other species, such as rabbit, cattle, and swine, use very limited VDJ recombination plus somatic gene conversion and somatic hypermutation to generate their primary Ig diversity.

Receptor Editing

Under some circumstances, a cell in the B-cell lineage can undergo a second rearrangement of its L-chain variable gene segments, after it has formed a recombined VJ

unit. This process, known as *receptor editing*, is described in more detail in Chapter 7. The mechanism of receptor editing can be understood by looking at Figure 6.3. The rearranged DNA of this particular B cell contains the unrearranged elements V_1 and J_5, which can be used in a second rearrangement. Receptor editing can occur when a B cell with a receptor specific for a self-antigen interacts with that self-antigen. One outcome of this interaction is that the V and J genes of the B cell undergo a second rearrangement, which may generate a VJ recognition unit specific for a foreign, rather than a self, antigen. Thus, receptor editing may increase the diversity of the overall response to foreign antigens.

All these mechanisms contribute to the formation of a huge library or *repertoire* of B lymphocytes that contains all the specificities required to deal with the multitude of diverse epitopes that antibodies could encounter. Estimates of the number of total Ig specificities that can be generated in an individual are on the order of 10^{15}, which is increased even more by somatic hypermutation.

Role of Activation-Induced Cytidine Deaminase in Generating Antibody Diversity

In the last few years scientists have identified an enzyme, *activation-induced cytidine deaminase (AID)*, that plays a key role in initiating class switch recombination, somatic hypermutation, and gene conversion, the three major pathways that generate diversity of antibodies. As its name implies, AID removes cytidine groups from the DNA in activated B cells to form uridine. This generates U:G base pairs in DNA; the mismatched base pairs are then removed by one of several different enzymes. This, in turn, results in changes in the DNA, primarily in Ig V-region genes. Why AID interacts preferentially with Ig V-region genes is not currently well understood. The role of AID in class switch recombination and somatic hypermutation in the germinal center is discussed further in Chapter 7.

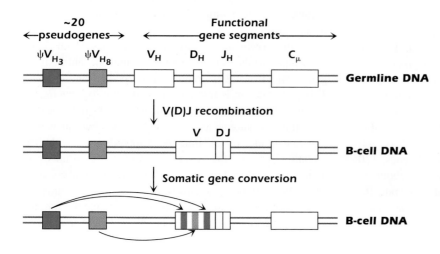

Figure 6.6. Somatic gene conversion generates diversity in the Ig genes of several species. The figure illustrates the phenomenon in the chicken Ig heavy-chain locus: short sequences of DNA from one or more pseudogenes (3 and 8 in the figure) are copied into the rearranged B-cell VDJ unit.

SUMMARY

1. Every individual synthesizes an enormous number of different Ig molecules, each of which can act as a receptor on the B-cell surface, specific for a particular epitope.

2. The variable region of the H chain in an Ig molecule is coded for by three separate genes, referred to as V_H (variable), D_H (diversity), and J_H (joining) gene segments. A distinct gene segment codes for the constant region of the heavy chain, C_H. The variable region of the L chain is coded for by two gene segments, V_L and J_L, distinct from the gene segments used for heavy-chain synthesis. DNA from every cell in the body (the germline) contains multiple V, D, and J gene segments for Ig H- and L-chain synthesis.

3. In the course of differentiation, a B cell rearranges its H chain DNA to join one V_H gene segment to one D_H gene segment and one J_H gene segment. The joined VDJ unit codes for the entire variable region of the heavy chain. These gene rearrangements put the VDJ unit close to the H chain constant-region genes, $C\mu$ and $C\delta$.

4. The same type of rearrangement produces a gene unit coding for the entire V region of an Ig L chain; one V_L gene segment is joined to one J_L segment, putting the VJ unit close to an L-chain constant-region gene. In a B cell committed to making a κ chain, the VκJκ unit is juxtaposed to the Cκ gene; in a B cell committed to making a λ chain, the VλJλ unit is juxtaposed to a Cλ gene.

5. Primary RNA transcripts are made from the rearranged DNA of heavy and light chain genes. Noncoding RNA is spliced out of the primary transcripts, resulting in mRNA. The mRNA is then translated into a light chain or a heavy chain. Alternative splicing of the heavy-chain primary transcript results in either a μ or δ chain; thus, the resulting IgM and IgD molecules have identical antigenic specificity.

6. In a B cell, the H chain is coded for by the H-chain gene segments found on either the maternally-derived chromosome or the paternally-derived chromosome; the L chain is also coded for by the L-chain gene segments found on only one of these two chromosomes. This phenomenon, called allelic exclusion, ensures that a particular B cell produces an immunoglobulin of a single antigenic specificity.

7. After antigenic stimulation, a B cell can further rearrange its H-chain DNA. The VDJ unit, which has joined to the $C\mu$ and $C\delta$ genes, can rearrange to join another C-region gene, such as $C\gamma$, $C\alpha$, or $C\varepsilon$. This phenomenon is known as class switch recombination. As a result, the B cell that was synthesizing IgM and IgD can now synthesize antibody of a different isotype (IgG, IgA, or IgE) but with the same antigenic specificity.

8. Diversity in antibody specificity is achieved by the following:
   - Multiple inherited genes for the V regions of both L and H chains.
   - Rearrangement of V, D, and J segments in different combinations and random assortment of H and L chains.
   - Junctional diversity at the sites of V, D, and J gene segment joining caused by imprecise joining, deletions, and TdT-mediated nucleotide insertions.
   - Somatic hypermutation, which occurs after stimulation by antigen, leading to selection for mutations that endow the antibody with higher affinity for the antigen.
   - Somatic gene conversion in species other than the human or mouse: Short DNA sequences from non-rearranging genes are copied into a rearranged VDJ gene unit.

These mechanisms allow a small number of genes to generate a vast number of antibody molecules with different antigenic specificities. One enzyme, activation-induced cytidine deaminase (AID), plays a key role in initiating class switch recombination, somatic hypermutation, and gene conversion—the three major pathways that generate diversity of antibodies.

REFERENCES

Chaudhuri J, et al (2007): Evolution of the immunoglobulin heavy chain class switch recombination mechanism. *Adv Immunol* 94:157.

Di Noia JM, Neuberger MS (2007): Molecular mechanisms of antibody somatic hypermutation. *Annu Rev Biochem* 76:1.

Dudley DD, Chaudhuri J, Bassing CH, Alt FW (2005): Mechanism and control of V(D)J recombination versus class switch recombination: Similarities and differences. *Adv Immunol* 86:43.

Odegard VH, Schatz DG (2006): Targeting of somatic hypermutation. *Nat Rev Immunol* 6:573.

Petersen-Mahrt S (2005): DNA deamination in immunity. *Immunol Rev* 203:80.

Schatz DG, Spanopoulou E (2005): Biochemistry of V(D)J recombination. *Curr Top Microbiol Immunol* 290:49.

 REVIEW QUESTIONS

For each question, choose the ONE BEST answer.

1. The DNA for an H chain in a B cell making IgG_2 antibody for diphtheria toxoid has the following structure: $5'-V_{17}D_5J_2$ $C\gamma_2-C\gamma_4-C\epsilon-C\alpha_2-3'$. How many individual rearrangements were required to go from the embryonic DNA to this B-cell DNA?
   A) 1
   B) 2
   C) 3
   D) 4
   E) none

2. If you had 50 V, 20 D, and 6 J regions able to code for a heavy chain and 40 V and 5 J-region genes able to code for a light chain, you could have a maximum repertoire of:
   A) $76 + 45 = 121$ antibody specificities
   B) $76 \times 45 = 3420$ specificities
   C) $(40 \times 5) + (50 \times 20 \times 6) = 6200$ specificities
   D) $(40 \times 5) \times (50 \times 20 \times 6) = 1,200,000$ specificities
   E) more than 1,200,000 specificities

3. The antigen specificity of a particular B cell:
   A) is induced by interaction with antigen
   B) is determined only by the L-chain sequence
   C) is determined by H + L-chain variable-region sequences
   D) changes after isotype switching
   E) is determined by the heavy-chain constant region

4. If you could analyze at the molecular level a plasma cell making IgA antibody, you would find all of the following *except*:
   A) a DNA sequence for V, D, and J genes translocated near the $C\alpha$ DNA exon
   B) mRNA specific for either κ or λ light chains
   C) mRNA specific for J chains
   D) mRNA specific for μ chains
   E) a DNA sequence coding for the T-cell receptor for antigen

5. The ability of a single B cell to express both IgM and IgD molecules on its surface at the same time is made possible by:
   A) allelic exclusion
   B) isotype switching
   C) simultaneous recognition of two distinct antigens
   D) alternative RNA splicing
   E) use of genes from both parental chromosomes

6. Which of the following statements concerning the organization of Ig genes is correct?
   A) V and J regions of embryonic DNA have already undergone a rearrangement.
   B) Light-chain genes undergo further rearrangement after surface IgM is expressed.
   C) V_H gene segments can rearrange with $J\kappa$ or $J\lambda$ gene segments.
   D) The VDJ segments coding for an Ig V_H region may associate with different heavy-chain constant-region genes.
   E) After VDJ joining has occurred, a further rearrangement is required to bring the VDJ unit next to the $C\mu$ gene.

7. Which of the following does not contribute to the antigen-binding site diversity of B-cell antigen receptors?
   A) multiple V genes in the germline
   B) random assortment of L and H chains
   C) imprecise recombination of V and J or V, D, and J segments
   D) inheritance of multiple C-region genes
   E) somatic hypermutation

8. Which of the following statements regarding a B cell expressing both IgM and IgD on its membrane is incorrect?
   A) The light chains of the IgM and IgD have identical amino acid sequences.
   B) The constant parts of the heavy chains of the IgM and IgD have different amino acid sequences.
   C) The IgM and IgD have different antigenic specificities.
   D) If it is triggered by antigen and T-cell signals to proliferate and differentiate, it may differentiate into a plasma cell that may secrete IgG, IgE, or IgA antibodies.
   E) The IgM on the surface will have either κ or λ light chains, but not both.

9. Which of the following plays a role in changing the antigen binding site of a B cell *after* antigenic stimulation?
   A) junctional diversity
   B) combinatorial diversity
   C) germline diversity
   D) somatic hypermutation
   E) differential splicing of primary RNA transcripts

CASE STUDY

As a member of a research team studying a newly discovered rodent found in a remote region of New Guinea, you make the astonishing discovery that these animals have only two V genes for the L chain and three V genes for the H chain of immunoglobulins.

Nevertheless, all the animals you examine seem healthy and able to resist the large number of pathogenic organisms endemic to the area. Suggest how this might be accomplished.

ANSWERS TO REVIEW QUESTIONS

1. *C* Three DNA rearrangements are required. First, $D_5 \rightarrow J_2$ rearrangement occurs, followed by $V_{17} \rightarrow D_5 J_2$. This permits synthesis of IgM and IgD molecules using $V_{17} D_5 J_2$. The third rearrangement is the class switch of $V_{17} D_5 J_2 C\mu C\delta$ to $V_{17} D_5 J_2 C\gamma_2$, leading to the synthesis of IgG_2 molecules.

2. *E* While 1,200,000 would be the product of all possible combinations of genes, many more antibody specificities are likely to be generated as a result of junctional diversity at the sites of V, D, and J gene segment joining (caused by imprecise joining, deletions, and nucleotide insertions) and somatic hypermutation.

3. *C* The antigenic specificity is determined by the sequences and hence the structure formed by the combination of heavy- and light-chain variable regions.

4. *D* As a consequence of the rearrangement of the VDJ to $C\alpha$ in the IgA-producing cell, the $C\mu$ gene will have been deleted. The other DNA sequences and mRNA species will be found in the cell.

5. *D* The simultaneous synthesis of IgM and IgD is made possible by the alternative splicing of the primary RNA transcript $5'$–VDJ–$C\mu$–$C\delta$–$3'$ to give either $VDJC\mu$ or $VDJC\delta$ mRNAs.

6. *D* The association of VDJ segments coding for an Ig V_H region with different heavy-chain constant-region genes is the basis of isotype or class switching.

7. *D* The presence of multiple C_H-region genes does provide the basis for functional diversity of Ig molecules but does *not* contribute to the diversity of antigen-specific receptors.

8. *C* The IgM and IgD expressed on a single B cell use the same heavy- and light-chain V(D)J gene units and therefore have the same antigenic specificity.

9. *D* Of the mechanisms described for generating diversity of Ig molecules, only somatic hypermutation affects the antigen binding site *after* antigen stimulation.

ANSWER TO CASE STUDY

Despite their paucity of V-region genes, this newly discovered rodent has presumably retained other mechanisms for generating diversity of its antibody genes. These mechanisms include the presence of multiple J and D gene segments in the germline,

junctional diversity due to deletion or insertion of bases at joining sites, random assortment of H and L chains, and somatic hypermutation. Thus, even with its limited V-gene repertoire, this animal generates sufficient diversity of antibody specificity to survive.

BIOLOGY OF THE B LYMPHOCYTE

 INTRODUCTION

This chapter describes the biology of **B lymphocytes**, the cells that synthesize antibody in response to antigen. In Chapter 6 we described the mechanisms by which B lymphocytes develop a vast repertoire of different antigenic specificities. These mechanisms help to explain two of the key features of the adaptive immune response that were initially described in the clonal selection theory section of Chapter 2: **diversity**, the ability to respond to many different antigenic determinants—**epitopes**—even if the individual has not previously encountered them; and **specificity**, the ability to discriminate among different epitopes. Thus, it can almost be guaranteed that every person contains one or more clones of B cells able to interact with measles virus, one or more clones of B cells able to interact with flu virus, and so on.

In this chapter we focus on the critical steps in B-cell development and describe how B cells acquire other features associated with the adaptive immune response: discrimination between self and nonself and memory. **Discrimination between self and nonself** is the ability to respond to those antigens that are "foreign," or nonself, and to prevent responses to those antigens that are part of self. **Memory** is the ability to recall previous contact with a particular antigen, so that a subsequent exposure leads to a quicker, more effective immune response than the response to the first exposure.

DEVELOPMENT OF B LYMPHOCYTES

Overview

B lymphocytes acquired their name from early experiments in birds: The synthesis of antibody was shown to require the presence of an organ called the bursa of Fabricius (an outpouching of the cloacal epithelium). Surgical removal of the bursa prevented antibody synthesis. Thus the cells that developed into mature, antibody-forming cells were called **bursa-derived** or **B cells**.

In contrast to birds, mammals do not appear to have a bursa; rather, B-cell differentiation occurs in a restricted number of critical sites, which will be described below. Our understanding of B-cell differentiation has been facilitated by the study of different animals in which the early embryonic stages can be easily manipulated. For this reason, B-cell differentiation is particularly well characterized in chickens and in mammals. Many of the differentiation steps are common to humans, chickens, and mice.

Figure 7.1 illustrates the key stages in the B-cell differentiation pathway, which will be explained further in the subsequent sections. Many of these stages are defined by specific Ig gene rearrangements that were described in Chapter 6. As we will describe below, many of these stages represent **developmental checkpoints**, following which the cell develops along one or another alternative pathway.

Immunology: A Short Course, Sixth Edition, By Richard Coico and Geoffrey Sunshine
Copyright © 2009 John Wiley & Sons, Inc.

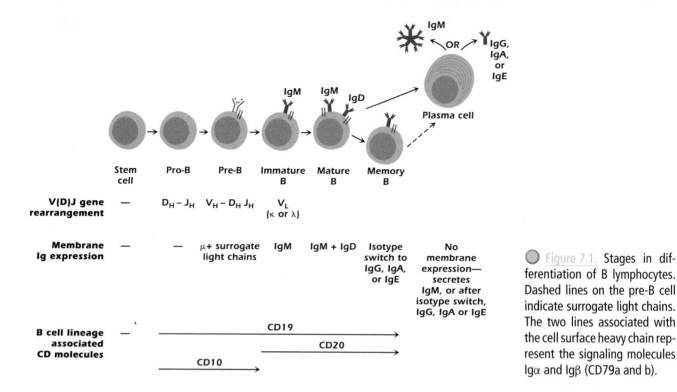

Figure 7.1. Stages in differentiation of B lymphocytes. Dashed lines on the pre-B cell indicate surrogate light chains. The two lines associated with the cell surface heavy chain represent the signaling molecules Igα and Igβ (CD79a and b).

Similar checkpoints are also found in the differentiation of the T-cell lineage.

In Chapter 5 we referred to the **CD nomenclature** for cell surface molecules: several stages of B-cell differentiation are characterized by the expression of different CD molecules. We will describe the most important B-cell developmental markers in this chapter; others are shown in Figure 17.9, which correlates the expression of CD molecules on B cells at different stages of normal development with different B-cell tumors.

Sites of Early B-Cell Differentiation

In mammals, precursors of the B-cell lineage are found early in fetal development, at sites including the fetal liver. Later in fetal development and after birth, the bone marrow is the primary site of B-cell differentiation. Studies suggest that B-cell differentiation occurs more or less throughout life, so the B-cell repertoire is continuously replenished. The bone marrow is therefore considered the **primary lymphoid organ** for B-cell differentiation in adult humans and other mammals (see Chapter 2).

Early Stages of B-Cell Differentiation: Pro-B and Pre-B Cells

B lymphocytes arise from **hematopoietic stem cells**. Adhesive interactions with the bone marrow **stroma**, the nonlymphoid cells that make up the framework or matrix of the marrow, and the actions of cytokines provide signals that promote the survival and enhance proliferation of cells early in the B-cell lineage. Figure 7.1 depicts the earliest distinguishable cell in the B lineage, the **pro-B cell**, which shows the first rearrangement of Ig genes: at the heavy-chain locus, a D_H gene segment rearranges to a J_H gene segment. Pro-B cells express **CD19**, and CD19 is expressed in all stages of B-cell development up to and including the mature B cell (but not the plasma cell). Only a few other, rare populations of cells express CD19, so expression of CD19 is a useful marker of all cells in the B-cell lineage up to the plasma cell. Pro-B cells also express **CD10**.

In the next stage of B-cell differentiation, the **pre-B cell**, a heavy-chain V_H gene segment rearranges to join the rearranged $D_H J_H$ segments, forming a VDJ unit. This rearranged VDJ is thus put close to $C\mu$ (see Fig. 6.4), and the pre-B cell synthesizes a μ chain. Pre-B cells express CD10 (in addition to CD19). Because CD10 is not expressed by B cells at later stages of development, it is a marker of early stages of B-cell differentiation.

The Ig gene rearrangements that occur during these early phases of B-cell differentiation follow an ordered sequence, which we described in Chapter 6: The heavy-chain locus rearranges first, initially joining a D gene segment to a J gene segment to form a DJ unit. A second rearrangement event then rearranges a V_H gene to the DJ and results in a VDJ unit. If this VDJ rearrangement is productive, that is, capable of being properly transcribed and translated into a μ chain, further rearrangement of heavy-chain gene segments is shut down. If the V-DJ rearrangement is not productive on the first of the two parental

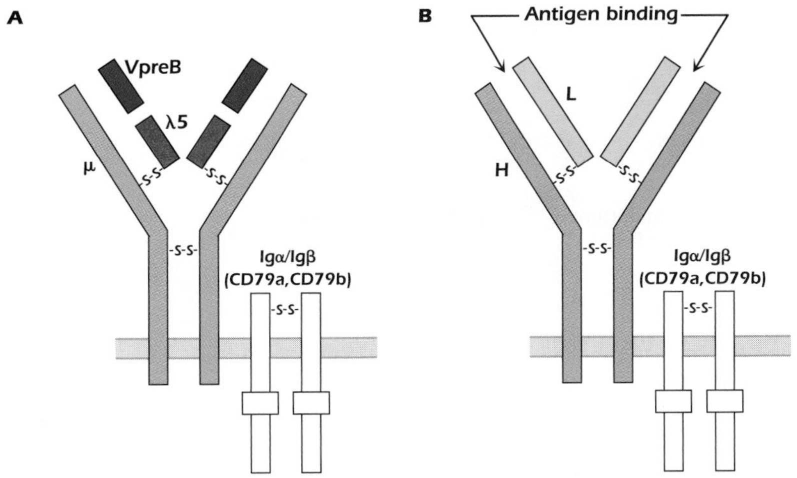

A

VpreB

λ5

μ

-S-S- -S-S-

-S-S-

Igα/Igβ
(CD79a,CD79b)

-S-S-

B

Antigen binding

L

H

-S-S- -S-S-

-S-S-

Igα/Igβ
(CD79a,CD79b)

-S-S-

Figure 7.2. (A) Pre-B-cell receptor (pre-BCR). (B) B-cell receptor. The heavy chain of the pre-BCR is a μ chain; the heavy chain of the BCR may be a μ, δ, γ, α, or ε chain. The immunoreceptor tyrosine-based activation motif (ITAM, discussed later in this chapter) is depicted as a rectangle in the Igα and Igβ polypeptides.

chromosomes, rearrangement takes place on the second chromosome. If rearrangement on the second chromosome is productive, then *this* chromosome makes a μ chain. If neither of these rearrangements is productive, the cell dies by *apoptosis*, also known as *programmed cell death*.

A key characteristic of the pre-B cell is that it expresses the μ chain as a transmembrane molecule at the cell surface in conjunction with the products of two nonrearranging genes, called λ5 and **VpreB**, which together function as *surrogate light chains* (shown as dashed lines in Fig. 7.1 and in more detail in Fig. 7.2). Figure 7.2A shows that the μ chain and surrogate light chains of the pre-B cell are expressed at the cell surface with two closely associated transmembrane molecules known as *Igα (CD79a)* and *Igβ (CD79b)*. Igα and Igβ are disulfide linked to each other. The complex of μ and surrogate light chains in conjunction with Igα and Igβ is referred to as the *pre-B-cell receptor (pre-BCR)*.

Igα and Igβ are associated with membrane Ig molecules on all cells in the B-cell lineage, from the pre-B cell to the memory B cell (see Fig. 7.1). The complex of Igα and Igβ associated with membrane Ig molecules of more mature cells in the B-lymphocyte lineage, known as the *B-cell receptor*, is depicted in Figure 7.2B. Igα and Igβ do not bind antigen. Their function is to transmit signals to the cell nucleus, leading to a change in the pattern of genes expressed; for this reason, Igα and Igβ are referred to as *signal transduction molecules* associated with the pre-BCR and the BCR. As we discuss in Chapters 9 and 10, signal transduction molecules are also associated with the antigen-specific receptor expressed at different stages of T-lymphocyte development.

On mature B cells, the role of Igα and Igβ in the BCR is to transmit signals after antigen binds to the variable domains of surface Ig (discussed in more detail in Chapter 10). There is no evidence that the pre-BCR binds antigen. Rather, studies suggest that Igα and Igβ associated

with the pre-BCR instruct the cell that it has successfully rearranged its Ig H-chain genes and has made a functional μ chain. As a result of this signaling through the pre-BCR, the pre-B cell further differentiates: It proliferates, shuts down surrogate light-chain synthesis, starts L-chain gene rearrangement, and stops further H-chain gene rearrangement.

Like heavy-chain gene rearrangements, light-chain gene rearrangement in the later phases of pre-B-cell development is sequential: the κ-chain genes rearrange first, but if neither of the chromosomes coding for κ chains successfully rearranges, λ gene rearrangement takes place. (If no productive L-chain gene rearrangement occurs, the cell dies.) As we pointed out in Chapter 6, the biological consequence of this use of genes from only one chromosome to make an H chain and genes from one chromosome to make an L chain—*allelic exclusion*—ensures that on its cell surface an individual B cell expresses an Ig molecule with a single antigenic specificity.

Bruton's tyrosine kinase (Btk) is an enzyme involved in intracellular signaling from the pre-BCR to the nucleus of the pre-B cell. Btk plays a crucial role in the transition of pre-B cells to the next stage in B-cell differentiation because boys with mutations in the *Btk* gene develop the immunodeficiency condition, *X-linked agammaglobulinemia*, in which B-cell differentiation is arrested at the pre-B-cell stage (discussed in Chapter 17.)

X-Linked Agammaglobulinemia

Immature B Cells

At the next stage of B-cell differentiation, L chains pair with μ chains to form monomeric IgM, which is inserted in the membrane and is expressed in association with Igα/Igβ. The cell bearing only monomeric membrane

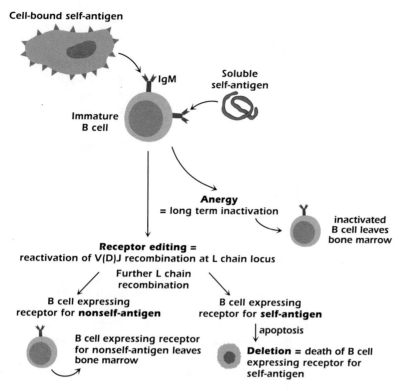

Cell-bound self-antigen

IgM

Soluble self-antigen

Immature B cell

Anergy = long term inactivation

inactivated B cell leaves bone marrow

Receptor editing = reactivation of V(D)J recombination at L chain locus

Further L chain recombination

B cell expressing receptor for **nonself-antigen**

B cell expressing receptor for **self-antigen**

B cell expressing receptor for nonself-antigen leaves bone marrow

apoptosis

Deletion = death of B cell expressing receptor for self-antigen

Figure 7.3. Responses of an immature B cell to self-antigens in the bone marrow: Interaction with cell-bound antigen reactivates V(D)J recombinase and receptor editing. Generation of a receptor reactive to self-antigen results in deletion of the B cell; generation of a receptor reactive to nonself-antigen allows the B cell to leave the bone marrow. Interaction of the immature B cell with soluble self-antigen results in anergy, long-term inactivation.

IgM as its antigen-specific receptor is referred to as an *immature B cell*. Immature B cells express *CD20*, which is also expressed by cells in the next stage of B-cell differentiation, the IgM+IgD+ B cell; thus, CD20 is a marker for the later stages of B-cell development.

Figure 7.3 shows that the immature B cell can respond to self-antigens expressed on the surface of bone marrow cells (such as MHC molecules). The interaction with self-antigen activates the pathway known as *receptor editing*, which we introduced in Chapter 6. In receptor editing, the cell's original Ig heavy chain is paired with a new light chain. As a result, the immature B cell synthesizes an Ig molecule with a different antigen specificity.

Receptor editing involves the reactivation of the cell's V(D)J recombinase, which acts on the cell's Ig light-chain genes. The light-chain genes then undergo a secondary rearrangement of unrearranged V or J segments. For example, in the rearrangement of the B cell's κ locus, shown in Figure 6.3, V₁ and J₅ are unrearranged gene segments that may be rearranged during receptor editing.

The recombination events that occur during receptor editing may generate an Ig specific for either a self- or a nonself- (foreign) molecule (Fig. 7.3). If receptor editing generates a specificity for a self-molecule, the immature B cell is *deleted* via apoptosis. In this way, B cells with the potential for high reactivity to self-molecules are prevented from exiting the bone marrow into the blood and tissues of the body. The interaction of self-molecules with developing B and T cells that results in the deletion of self-reactive cells is known as *negative selection*, a critical feature of

central tolerance—the establishment of tolerance to self that develops in the primary lymphoid organs. (Deletion and self-tolerance in the development of T cells are discussed in Chapters 9 and 12.)

Alternatively, if receptor editing generates an Ig molecule that is specific for a nonself-molecule, the immature B cell is "rescued" from deletion, the cell leaves the bone marrow, and it becomes part of the repertoire of B cells responsive to nonself-antigens.

Figure 7.3 also indicates an alternative fate for an immature B cell exposed to a self-antigen. If, as has been described in some experimental systems described in Chapter 12, the self-antigen is soluble—that is, nonmembrane—the immature B cell may become *anergic*, that is, functionally inactivated for a long period. These anergic B cells also leave the bone marrow. The factors determining the alternative fates of the immature B cell after encounter with self-antigen are likely to involve molecules on the cell surface other than immunoglobulin (such as the coreceptors described later in this chapter) and differences in intracellular signaling pathways. They are the subject of intense research interest.

Mature B Cells

The next step in the B-cell differentiation pathway is the development of the *IgM+ IgD+ mature B cell*. The membrane IgM and membrane IgD expressed on a single mature B cell have identical antigenic specificities; this results from the alternative splicing of a single RNA species transcribed from VDJ plus $C\mu$ and $C\delta$ genes (discussed in Chapter 6). In addition, both membrane IgM and membrane IgD on a single cell have BCR function. As discussed in Chapter 4, the function of IgD on the mature B cell is not well understood.

The signals that drive the differentiation of the IgM^+ B cell to the IgM^+ IgD^+ mature B-cell stage are not known, but they are thought to occur outside the bone marrow. In contrast to the inactivation and receptor-editing mechanisms that occur when antigen interacts with an immature IgM^+ B cell described earlier, the interaction of antigen with the mature IgM^+ IgD^+ B cell generally results in activation. (Under some conditions, described in Chapter 12, interaction of the mature B cell with antigen can result in the development of anergy.)

As we mentioned at the beginning of this chapter, the pathway of B-cell differentiation generates a large repertoire of antigen specificities, more or less guaranteeing a response to any antigen that a person may encounter. (As we describe below in the section on B-cell subsets, very young children may lack B cells specific for some bacterial antigens, but these B cells develop by about two years of age.) However, most mature B cells in the vast B-cell repertoire do not interact with antigen during their lifetime (estimated to be four to five months for a mature B cell found in the spleen) but remain as resting unstimulated (*naïve*) IgM^+ IgD^+ cells.

Antibody Synthesis: Plasma Cells. Activation of IgM^+ IgD^+ cells by antigen results in antibody synthesis. ***Plasma cells*** (depicted on the far right of Fig. 7.1) are the terminally differentiated stage of B-cell development that synthesize and secrete Ig molecules. An individual plasma cell secretes antibody of a single antigenic specificity—the same antigenic specificity as the immunoglobulin on the surface of the B cell that was initially triggered by antigen—and of a single isotype: IgM, IgG, IgA, or IgE. The plasma cell does not express a membrane form of immunoglobulin and does not express the CD molecules we referred to earlier in the chapter—CD10, CD19, or CD20—that characterize cells at earlier stages of B-cell development.

In responses to the major set of antigens known as ***thymus dependent***—because they require ***helper T cells***, described more fully in Chapter 10—plasma cells are generated in the ***germinal center*** of lymph nodes and spleen. (The events involved in antibody synthesis in the germinal center and responses of B cells outside germinal centers are described later in the chapter.) IgG- and IgA-secreting plasma cells produced in germinal centers of peripheral lymph nodes (that is, outside the mucosa) migrate primarily to the bone marrow, where they may live for years. These long-lived plasma cells synthesize high levels of IgG and monomeric IgA that provide protection in blood against a second or subsequent exposure to infectious agents such as viruses and bacteria.

Plasma cells that synthesize the dimeric IgA that protects mucosal surfaces (see Fig. 4.13) in the gastrointestinal and respiratory tracts, salivary and tear glands, and lactating mammary glands develop in the lymphoid tissue associated with mucosa (MALT). In a subsequent section of this chapter, we describe how B cells committed to IgA synthesis develop in MALT and subsequently further differentiate into IgA-secreting plasma cells.

In Chapter 5 we described how plasma cells can be transformed and "immortalized" in cell culture and used to generate monoclonal antibodies—antibodies specific for a single antigen epitope—that have a wide range of clinical and diagnostic functions. Neoplasms of plasma cells—particularly multiple myeloma—are discussed further in Chapter 17.

Plasma Cell Neoplasms

Memory B Cells. Antigen activation in the germinal center may also result in the development of ***memory B cells*** (shown in Fig. 7.1 as an alternative pathway in mature B-cell differentiation). Memory B cells are nonproliferating, generally long-lived B cells that can be activated for a subsequent (***secondary***) and more rapid response to antigen. They express isotypes other than IgM (IgG, IgA, or IgE) on their surface but do not express IgD. Human memory cells can be identified by their expression of ***CD27***.

How memory B cells develop in the germinal center of the lymph node is currently not well understood, but they do not appear to develop from plasma cells. Memory B cells leave the lymphoid organ in which they were generated and move into tissues.

B-Lymphocyte Traffic: Anatomical Distribution of B-Cell Populations

As we have described above, B cells at different stages of differentiation are found in different anatomical locations around the body. Naïve mature B cells circulate throughout the blood to secondary lymphoid organs, primarily peripheral lymph nodes, and GALT such as Peyer's patches of the intestine (see Chapter 2). The circulation time of about 12 hours quickly brings a B cell with the "correct" antigenic specificity in contact with antigen, if it is present. The ability of naïve B and T cells to circulate throughout the body and through secondary lymphoid organs is critical, because naïve lymphocytes do not have access to tissues such as the skin, the lungs, and the gastrointestinal tract, the points of entry for many pathogens.

If the B cell in a secondary lymphoid organ does not interact with antigen, it either leaves the lymphoid organ via the lymphatic vessels and continues to circulate or it dies in the organ. If the B cell does interact with antigen and helper T cells in the lymphoid organ, a *germinal center reaction* (see below) develops in which memory cells and plasma cells are generated. Antigen-activated memory and plasma cells take different routes through the body than naïve cells: As described above, memory B cells move out of the lymphoid organ and into tissues; plasma cells that develop in peripheral lymph nodes migrate through the lymphatic system, predominantly to the bone marrow. IgA-secreting plasma cells are also found in mucosal tissue (discussed later in the chapter).

The migration of naïve B cells into secondary lymphoid organs and the *"homing"* of antigen-activated memory and plasma cell populations into tissues are governed by expression at the B-cell surface of *adhesion molecules* and *chemokine receptors*. (As we discuss more fully in Chapter 11, chemokines are small cytokines produced by many types of cells that influence the movement of many types of leukocytes including B and T lymphocytes.) The pattern of B-cell (and T-cell) expression of adhesion molecules and chemokine receptors changes depending on the stage of development and whether or not the cell has been exposed to antigen.

Naïve B-cells express the chemokine receptor *CCR7* and the adhesion molecules *L-selectin* (CD62L) and *α4β7*. α4β7 is an *integrin*, a member of a family of two-chain molecules expressed by B cells, T cells, and many other cell types. L-Selectin and α4β7 bind to glycoprotein molecules expressed by endothelial cells in a specialized region of the vascular endothelium (HEV) at the boundary of lymph nodes. L-Selectin binds to HEV at the entrance to peripheral nodes (nonmucosal sites), and α4β7 binds to HEV in GALT. Thus naïve B-cell expression of both L-selectin and α4β7 ensures that these cells circulate through *all* lymph nodes. Activated B cells down-regulate L-selectin but B cells activated in GALT continue to express α4β7 so these cells still have access to mucosal sites. B cells activated in peripheral nodes down-regulate expression of α4β7 so they do not have access to GALT, but they express other integrins, which allow plasma cells that develop in peripheral nodes to home to the bone marrow. Activation also changes the pattern of expression of chemokine receptors.

● SITES OF ANTIBODY SYNTHESIS

Most antigens, especially proteins, are known as *thymus-dependent (TD) antigens* because they require *T helper cells* (described in more detail in Chapter 10) in order for B cells to synthesize antibody. Antibodies synthesized in TD responses are generally high affinity. The early phase of the primary response to TD antigens, which begins a few days after initial exposure, generates IgM antibodies; later primary and subsequent responses are characterized by the synthesis of antibody classes other than IgM (i.e., IgG, IgA

or IgE; see Fig. 4.12). TD antibody responses are also characterized by the development of long-lived memory B cells and plasma cells, which in many cases provide long-lasting protection against reinfection by infectious pathogens such as bacteria and viruses.

An important and distinct subset of antigens is referred to as *thymus independent (TI)* because the responding B cells do not require T helper cells to synthesize antibody. The polysaccharide components of bacterial capsules are one clinically important set of TI antigens. Responses to TI antigens are generally rapid (within a few days after exposure to antigen) and almost exclusively involve synthesis of IgM antibodies, which can agglutinate the antigen and activate the complement system. Thus, the IgM response to TI antigens provides crucial early protection against many bacterial infections, even in people who lack T cells (a topic discussed further in Chapter 17).

In this section we describe the sites in the body at which antibody responses to TD and TI occur and describe the pathways that result in antibody synthesis.

Thymus-Dependent Antibody Synthesis in the Germinal Center

T Cell–B Cell Interactions in the Lymph Node: Early Events. The B cells that participate in responses to TD antigens, which occur primarily in lymph nodes, are referred to as *follicular B cells* because they circulate between blood and the lymphoid follicle, the B-cell-rich region of the lymph node (shown in Fig. 2.10A). As described in Chapter 2, antigen that penetrates into tissues is carried to the lymph node draining the tissue. Figure 7.4 shows that if the antigen interacts in the lymph node follicle with a B cell expressing a receptor specific for that antigen, the B cell moves toward the boundary of the follicle with the T-cell region of the node. Figure 7.4 also shows that T helper cells specific for the same antigen that have been activated by the antigen bound to dendritic cells (described further in Chapter 10) also move to this boundary region from the T-cell area of the node. Contact between a T helper cell and a B cell specific for the same antigen takes place over several hours, resulting in the activation of both cells. Synthesis of antibody of the IgM class, the class of antibody that is synthesized earliest in the response, starts approximately 48 hours after the initiation of T- and B-cell interaction. Some antigen-activated B and T cells migrate back into the B-cell follicle and develop a germinal center, which we describe in the next section.

Events in the Germinal Center: Somatic Hypermutation, Class Switch Recombination, and Development of Plasma Cells and Memory B Cells. Figure 7.5 shows the critical roles played by the germinal center in the synthesis of antibody in TD responses. In

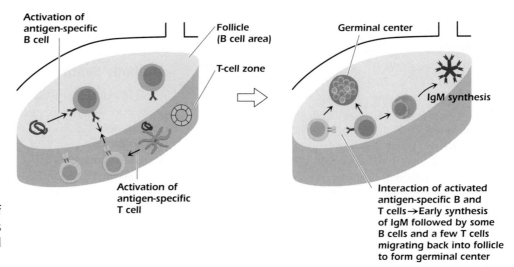

Figure 7.4. Interaction of antigen-specific B and T cells in development of germinal center in lymph node.

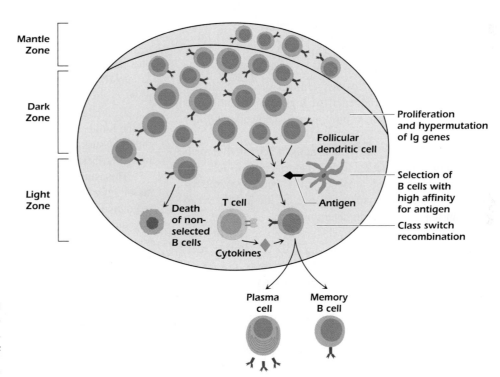

Figure 7.5. Key events in germinal center: somatic hyper-mutation and class switch recombination and development of plasma cells and memory B cells.

the germinal center the B cell undergoes (1) *somatic hypermutation* (described in Chapter 6), in which B cells with Ig variable-region genes that synthesize antibody with *higher affinity* for the activating antigen are selected, and (2) *class switch recombination*, in which an IgM$^+$IgD$^+$ B cell switches to synthesis of IgG, IgA, or IgE (see also Fig. 6.5). Plasma cells and memory B cells also develop as a consequence of the events in the germinal center. As noted in Chapter 6, the enzyme AID is critical in both somatic hypermutation and class switch recombination; AID is expressed in germinal center B cells and operates preferentially on DNA of Ig variable-region genes. In the

paragraphs that follow and in Figure 7.5 the events in the germinal center are described in more detail.

Figure 7.5 indicates that antigen-activated B cells proliferate rapidly in an area of the germinal center known as the *dark zone*. (B cells that do not proliferate in the germinal center are pushed out of the area of proliferation and form a *mantle zone* around the proliferating cells.) During this huge expansion of the B-cell population, B cells with mutations in their Ig variable-region genes are generated at a much higher rate than normal. This somatic hypermutation (referred to in Chapter 6) results in Ig heavy- and light-chain variable-region genes that synthesize Ig molecules with altered affinities for antigen.

Following somatic hypermutation, B cells enter another area of the germinal center, "the light zone". B cells are programmed to die in the light zone unless they receive survival signals from two different cell types: T helper cells specific for the antigen that initiated the response and antigen-bearing *follicular dendritic cells*. Follicular dendritic cells bind antigen in *antigen–antibody complexes* (antigen bound to antibody and complement components; see Chapter 13), retain it on their surface for long periods, and present it to B cells in the germinal center. As their name implies, follicular dendritic cells are characterized by long processes; they are unrelated to the family of dendritic cells we describe in Chapters 8–10, which play a major role in presenting antigen to T cells.

B cells in the light zone compete for the antigen presented by follicular dendritic cells: B cells with Ig variable-region genes mutated to synthesize antibody with the *highest affinity* for the activating antigen are clonally selected and expanded. B cells with mutations that result in lower affinity antibodies and B cells without mutations in their variable regions are *not* selected and die. Thus, somatic hypermutation in the germinal center results in an increase in the production of high-affinity antibodies to a particular antigen, a phenomenon known as *affinity maturation*.

Figure 7.5 also shows that antigen-activated B cells in the light zone interact with T helper cells, which synthesize cytokines that influence class switch recombination. The pattern of cytokines made by the T helper cell plays an important role in determining the isotype of antibody synthesized by the B cell (see Chapter 10). In class switch recombination, the IgM$^+$IgD$^+$ B cell further rearranges its DNA, juxtaposing its VDJ genes with a different heavy-chain constant-region gene (see Chapter 6 and Fig. 6.6). Regardless of the isotype of the immunoglobulin produced, all daughter cells will have the same antigenic specificity.

In addition, Figure 7.5 shows that a B cell activated by antigen and T helper cells in the germinal center may differentiate to become either a plasma cell or a memory B cell. The mechanisms that lead to the production of one or the other are currently unclear. As mentioned earlier in the chapter, plasma cells produced in germinal centers may be very long-lived (up to years); they migrate to other lymphoid organs, particularly the bone marrow where they continue to synthesize antibody. The antibodies secreted by the plasma cells in the bone marrow are thought to produce the bulk of the IgG and monomeric IgA found in serum; these antibodies have a protective function after re-exposure to antigen, that is, in a secondary response.

Memory B cells are generally long-lived and nonproliferating; re-exposure to antigen (usually requiring T cells) activates a secondary response to antigen that is more rapid than the primary response. Memory B cells differentiate into plasma cells that generally secrete isotypes other than IgM—namely, IgG, IgA, or IgE.

Antibody Synthesis in Mucosal Tissue

In our discussion of plasma cells earlier in the chapter, we referred to the synthesis of dimeric IgA in MALT and the role IgA plays at mucosal surfaces like those in the respiratory and gastrointestinal tracts. Protection of these areas is vital because they are the sites of exposure to multiple airborne, food-borne, and water-borne pathogens. The respiratory and gastrointestinal tracts occupy an enormous surface area within the body that is covered in most locations by a single layer of epithelial cells. Thus, mucosal tissue is particularly vulnerable to infection. In addition to exposure to pathogens in food and water, the gut also harbors several strains of *commensal bacteria* that generally live there without harming the host but are capable of inducing immune responses.

We described in Chapter 4 and showed in Figure 4.13 that plasma cells close to the epithelial basement membrane of mucosal tissue in the gastrointestinal and respiratory tracts, salivary and tear glands, and lactating mammary glands synthesize and secrete dimeric IgA. This IgA acts on the luminal side of the epithelial cell layer to protect the mucosal surfaces from the many pathogens that enter the body via these routes of exposure.

The synthesis of IgA in MALT differs from the synthesis of IgG, IgA, and other isotypes in the germinal center reaction described in the section above. The key differences are shown in Figure 7.6, which illustrates the induction and synthesis of IgA in the lymphoid tissue associated with the gut mucosa (GALT). In summary, antigen activation of B cells takes place at an *inductive site*, where antigen-activated B cells *commit* to synthesizing IgA and express IgA on their surface. An activated, IgA-committed B cell leaves the inductive site via the afferent lymphatics and enters the bloodstream; it then homes back to an *effector site* that may be somewhere else in MALT, where it completes its differentiation to an IgA-secreting plasma cell. These plasma cells secrete the dimeric IgA that is transported across epithelial cells to protect the luminal surface of the intestine (as described in Chapter 4).

Figure 7.6 shows some of the major features of GALT. It lies beneath and is closely associated with intestinal epithelium in an area of connective tissue known as the *lamina propria*. GALT comprises organized structures—*Peyer's patches*, the major inductive sites in GALT—as well as scattered lymphocytes throughout the lamina propria and within the epithelial layer. Some of the lymphocytes in the lamina propria are IgA-secreting plasma cells. Peyer's patches contain T- and B-cell areas and thus resemble other secondary lymphoid organs. *M cells*, specialized cells interspersed in the epithelial layer that covers the Peyer's patches, capture antigens in the

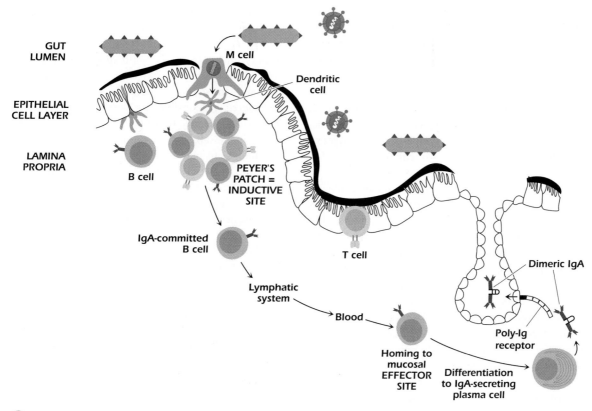

Figure 7.6. IgA antibody synthesis in GALT showing inductive and effector sites.

gut lumen and transport them through the cell into the area that contains T and B cells. Cells known as *dendritic cells*—not to be confused with the follicular dendritic cells that we described in the germinal center—present the transported antigens to T and B cells in GALT. (We describe the critical role of dendritic cells in other immune responses in Chapters 8–10.) Dendritic cells in GALT have also been shown to directly "sample" antigens on the luminal side of epithelium by pushing their processes between cells of the epithelial layer, without disturbing the integrity of the epithelial layer.

Cytokines produced by activated T cells and by other cells in the intestinal milieu promote B-cell class switching to IgA. Activated IgA$^+$ B cells—and T cells—in the gut migrate out of the lamina propria via draining lymphatics and eventually enter the circulation. These IgA-committed lymphocytes "home" back to GALT using the combination of adhesion molecules and chemokine receptors expressed on the cell surface that we described earlier in the chapter. (Recent evidence suggests that dendritic cells in GALT play a key role in inducing the expression of MALT-specific B-cell homing molecules.) IgA-committed B cells then complete their differentiation into IgA-secreting plasma cells at an effector site that may be in a completely different part of the GALT or even a non-GALT area of MALT.

Thymus-Independent Antibody Responses at Different Sites

In the section above we described the sites in the body and the pathways by which antibody is synthesized in response to TD antigens. These responses require T helper cells and B cells that both circulate to secondary lymphoid organs. In this section we turn our attention to responses of TI antigens. TI antigens do not require T helper cells for B cells to synthesize antibody. As we stated earlier in the chapter, responses to TI antigens are generally rapid, synthesize predominantly IgM antibody, and provide crucial early protection against infectious agents such as bacteria and viruses. Because these responses synthesize IgM, memory cells are not generated. As we also describe in the next paragraphs, TI responses are carried out by subsets of B cells at anatomical sites in the body that are distinct from the sites where TD responses take place.

Marginal-Zone B Cells. In Chapter 2 we described the spleen as a highly efficient organ for trapping and concentrating foreign substances carried in the blood: Blood-borne agents are filtered out by macrophages in the marginal zone of the spleen, a specialized area that separates the regions containing T and B lymphocytes from the red pulp. Macrophages in the marginal zone of lymph nodes play a similar filtering role for materials in lymph, for example, after subcutaneous exposure to a pathogen.

Marginal-zone B cells are a long-lived, sessile (remaining in the marginal zone for long periods) population of B cells distinct from the follicular B cells described earlier in the chapter. Marginal-zone B cells can participate in TD antigen responses and switch isotypes, but their key function is participation in the very earliest, TI synthesis of IgM in response to blood- or lymph-borne pathogens, particularly bacteria (and their polysaccharide components) and viruses.

The importance of these responses is underscored in very young children, who lack fully developed marginal-zone B cells until they are about one to two years old. Compared to older childern and adults, very young childern are particularly vulnerable to infection with bacteria such as *Haemophilus influenzae* b, which can cause pneumonia and meningitis. The capsular polysaccharides of this bacterium produce a strong TI IgM response. As we described above, TI IgM responses do not generate memory and thus vaccination (to generate memory cells) of very young children against this and similar clinically important pathogens expressing polysaccharide antigens used to be difficult. This problem has now been largely circumvented by the use of *conjugate vaccines*, in which the polysaccharide is conjugated to a protein (see Chapter 20). Injection of the conjugate generates a protective TD response involving follicular B cells. The mechanism by which conjugate vaccines generate a TD response is discussed in Chapter 10.

B-1 Cells. B-1 cells are a subpopulation of B cells that predominate in the peritoneal and pleural cavities of many species and are a minor population in spleen and lymph node. How exactly B-1 cells relate to the other B cells described so far has not been fully elucidated.

In adults, B-1 cells synthesize predominantly low-affinity IgM *polyspecific* antibodies (those that are reactive with many different antigens) early in the TI primary response to many bacteria. In addition, B-l cells are considered responsible for synthesizing most "natural" antibody, generally IgM antibodies that are detected in the blood in the absence of antigen priming. Thus, B-1 cells are thought to play a role as a first line of defense against systemic bacterial and viral infections. In mice, B-1 cells also produce a significant amount of the IgA that is found in serum and at mucosal surfaces. B-1 IgA synthesis is unusual because the switch to IgA synthesis occurs in the absence of T cells.

B-1 cells use a limited set of V gene segments to form their repertoire. Most B-1 cells are characterized by the surface expression of the molecule CD5, which is not expressed on other sets of B cells. CD5$^+$ B-1 cells are the predominant cell type in chronic lymphocytic leukemia (see Chapter 17).

Chronic Lymphocytic Leukemia

B-CELL MEMBRANE PROTEINS

In the following paragraphs and in Figure 7.7 we briefly describe some of the membrane proteins that characterize B cells at different stages of maturity.

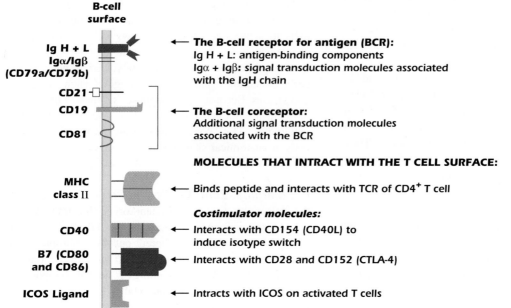

Figure 7.7. Important molecules expressed at the surface of B cells.

Stage-Specific Markers

Earlier in the chapter and in Figure 7.1 we described the expression of molecules expressed at different stages in B-cell development—CD10, CD19, CD20, and CD27; in addition, CD5 characterizes the B-1 subset of B cells. We describe the function of CD19 below.

Antigen-Binding Molecules: Membrane Immunoglobulin

The quintessential property of the B-lymphocyte lineage is the expression of Ig chains at the cell surface. (Note, however, that the pro-B cell—the most immature cell in the lineage—and the plasma cell—the end-stage cell of B-cell differentiation that secretes Ig—do not express immunoglobulin on their surfaces.) Because membrane-associated immunoglobulin binds antigen, the expression of surface immunoglobulin can be used both to identify B-cells and to separate them from other lymphocytes and mononuclear cells.

Signal Transduction Molecules Associated with Membrane Immunoglobulin

The function of key signal transduction molecules associated with the BCR is described in more detail in Chapter 10, in the section on intracellular events in B-cell activation. Here, we identify some of these molecules and briefly outline their function.

Igα and Igβ. Ig H and L chains have very short intracellular domains and do not transmit a signal directly into the B cell after antigen binding. Instead, the activation signal is transmitted into the interior of the B-cell by Igα (CD79a) and Igβ (CD79b). These molecules, which we mentioned earlier in the chapter, are noncovalently associated in the membrane of B cells with Ig H and L chains (see Fig. 7.2) and are also found in association with the pre-BCR.

The cytoplasmic regions of Igα (CD79a) and Igβ contain sequences of amino acids known as *immunoreceptor tyrosine-based activation motifs* (*ITAMs*). These sequences are referred to as *motifs* because they are found in a number of other signal transduction molecules expressed on cells of the immune system (such as those associated with the TCR; see Chapter 9). After antigen binds to the BCR, one of the earliest events in B-cell activation is the phosphorylation of tyrosine residues—the addition of a phosphate group—in the ITAMs by enzymes known as protein tyrosine kinases.

B-Cell Coreceptor. In addition to Igα and Igβ, other molecules on the B-cell membrane influence the signal that is transmitted through the BCR. *CD19, CD81* (also known as TAPA-1), and *CD21* are noncovalently associated in a complex that is known as the *B-cell coreceptor*. The coreceptor functions to reduce the threshold of B-cell

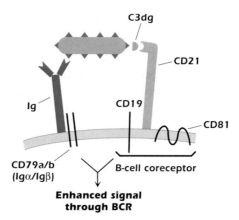

Figure 7.8. Activation via B-cell coreceptor CD19/CD21/CD81 lowers threshold for antigen needed to activate B cell. Simultaneous binding of antigen to Ig on the B-cell surface and complement component C3dg bound to CD21 of the coreceptor enhances the activation signal delivered through the BCR alone.

activation in response to an antigen. Estimates indicate that the amount of antigen needed to stimulate an antibody response is 100–1000 times less if the coreceptor is activated with BCR compared to BCR activation alone.

The role of the BCR coreceptor has been characterized best in the response to microbial antigens, which is shown in Figure 7.8. CD21 is the receptor for the complement component *C3dg* that is generated in plasma early in the response to microbial pathogens (see Chapter 13). C3dg coats or "tags" the pathogen; thus, as shown in Figure 7.8, the pathogen bound to C3dg becomes attached via CD21 to the B cell. The figure also shows the bacterium simultaneously binding to the immunoglobulin of a B cell expressing the appropriate Ig receptor. This simultaneous binding of pathogen to both the coreceptor and immunoglobulin enhances the signal to the B cell compared to the signal transmitted through the immunoglobulin alone. As a result, the B-cell coreceptor plays a major role in augmenting B-cell responses to pathogens that activate the complement pathway. Coreceptors with similar but not identical function, CD4 and CD8, are associated with the TCR (see Chapter 9).

Negative Regulation of B-Cell Signaling. Some molecules expressed on the B-cell surface have a *negative* effect on B-cell signaling. These include *CD22*, which negatively regulates the CD19, CD81, and CD21 coreceptors, as well as *CD32*. CD32 is the low-affinity receptor for the Fc region of IgG (FcγRIIb), expressed on virtually all mature B cells. CD32 binds IgG when it aggregates in the absence of antigen (see Chapter 4) and when the IgG is present in the form of an antigen–antibody complex. CD32 plays an important role in *antibody feedback*, the inactivation of B cells by antibody, by delivering a negative signal to the B cell (see Chapter 10).

Molecules Involved in T Cell–B Cell Interactions

Earlier in the chapter we referred to production of antibody in responses to TD antigens. In these responses, interactions between pairs of molecules on the B cell and T helper cell surfaces are critical. As we describe more fully in Chapter 10, the B cell not only synthesizes immunoglobulin but also presents antigen and activates the helper (CD4$^+$) T cell in these responses. Thus, B cells, and activated B cells in particular, share several important characteristics with the set of cells known as antigen-presenting cells that present antigen to CD4$^+$ T cells. First, B cells express on their surface proteins known as *major histocompatibility complex class II molecules* (see Chapter 8), which bind peptides derived from protein antigens and present them to CD4$^+$ T cells. MHC class II molecules are expressed on all cells in the B-cell lineage except pro-B cells.

Second, activated B cells also express high levels of *costimulatory molecules* (so called because they are required, along with antigen, to activate naïve T cells). All these costimulatory molecules are discussed in more detail in Chapter 10.

One of the key costimulatory molecules expressed by B cells is *B7*, now recognized as a family comprising several different molecules. *CD40* is another important costimulatory molecule expressed by B cells. CD40 interacts with CD40 ligand (CD40L or CD154) expressed on activated T cells. This interaction activates B cells and plays a critical role in isotype switching. The importance of the CD40–CD154 interaction is underscored by a condition known as human X-linked hyper-IgM syndrome. Boys who have a mutation in their CD154 gene and whose activated T cells either do not express CD154 or have a nonfunctional version of the gene make only IgM antibodies; their B cells cannot undergo isotype switching. *Inducible costimulatory (ICOS) ligand (ICOSL)* is another important costimulatory molecule expressed by B cells. The interaction of ICOSL with ICOS expressed by activated T cells appears critical for the formation of the germinal center: People who lack functional ICOSL or ICOS make very low levels of IgG, IgA, and IgE.

SUMMARY

1. In mammals, the early stages of B-cell differentiation take place in the bone marrow and throughout the life of an individual.

2. Different CD molecules are expressed at different stages of B-cell development.

3. The earliest recognizable cell in the B-cell lineage is the pro-B cell, in which the first stage of Ig H-chain gene rearrangement takes place: A D_H gene segment rearranges to a J_H gene segment.

4. The next stage is the pre-B cell, in which a V_H gene segment rearranges to the joined DJ segments to form a VDJ unit, putting the rearranged VDJ close to the Cμ gene. The pre-B cell synthesizes a μ chain that is expressed on the surface in association with nonrearranging surrogate light chains plus the signal transduction molecules Igα (CD79a) and Igβ (CD79b). The complex of μ and surrogate light chains in conjunction with Igα/β is referred to as the pre-B-cell receptor.

5. In the next stage of differentiation, L-chain genes start to rearrange; surrogate light-chain synthesis is shut down; and a κ or λ chain is formed that associates with the cell's μ chain. This cell, the immature B cell, expresses an IgM molecule in association with Igα/β on the surface of the cell. The complex of IgM and Igα/β is referred to as the B-cell receptor.

6. If the immature B cell interacts with cell-bound self-antigen, it undergoes receptor editing, in which unrearranged light-chain gene segments undergo further rearrangement. If the cell generates a receptor that is specific for a nonself molecule, the cell is "rescued" and differentiates further. If the cell generates a receptor that is still reactive to a self-molecule, the cell is deleted. The deletion of immature B cells with potential reactivity to self is an important feature of central tolerance in the B-cell lineage. Interaction of the immature B cell with soluble antigen in the bone marrow is thought to lead to long-term inactivation (anergy).

7. In the next phase of B-cell differentiation, the mature B cell expresses IgM and IgD—with identical antigenic specificity—on the cell surface.

8. Further development of the mature B cell occurs predominantly outside the bone marrow as a result of exposure to antigen. Activation of the B cell leads to proliferation and differentiation into plasma cells, the cells that synthesize and secrete antibody. Some activated B cells differentiate into memory cells, which make more rapid responses and synthesize non-IgM isotypes in subsequent responses to antigen.

9. Thymus-dependent antigens require T-cell help to induce B-cell antibody synthesis. In the early phase

of the response, IgM is synthesized, but in the later phases of the response other isotypes—IgG, IgA, or IgE—are synthesized.

10. The interaction of T and B cells takes place predominantly in the germinal centers of secondary lymphoid organs. The germinal center reaction involves (a) *somatic hypermutation* of genes coding for antibody V regions, resulting in affinity maturation, and (b) *class switch recombination*, in which a B cell that was synthesizing IgM and IgD switches to synthesizing antibody of a different isotype (IgG, IgA, or IgE) with the same antigenic specificity. Cytokines synthesized by T cells influence the isotype of antibody synthesized by the B cell.

11. B cells selected in the germinal center can develop into memory B cells or plasma cells. Memory cells "home" to different tissues; plasma cells home predominantly to bone marrow where they continue to synthesize antibody for a long time.

12. In mucosa-associated lymphoid tissue, IgA-committed B cells develop at an *inductive site*, migrate out of the lymphoid tissue and home back via the blood to a different mucosal *effector site*, where they complete their differentiation to IgA-secreting plasma cells.

13. B-cell responses to thymus-independent antigens involve other sets of B cells—marginal-zone B cells and B-1 cells—and generate almost exclusively IgM.

14. Expression of membrane Ig is unique to B cells. CD10, CD19, CD20, and CD27 expression defines stages of B-cell differentiation. B cells also express a coreceptor, CD19/CD21/CD81, that enhances signals through the B-cell receptor and lowers the threshold for the level of antigen required to activate the B cell after binding to Ig.

15. Mature and activated B cells also express an array of surface molecules that play a vital role in interactions with other cells, particularly T cells. These include MHC class II molecules and the costimulatory molecules B7, CD40, and ICOSL.

REFERENCES

Allen CD, Okada T, Cyster JG (2007): Germinal-center organization and cellular dynamics. *Immunity* 27:190.

Amanna IJ, Carlson NE, Slifka MK (2007): Duration of humoral immunity to common viral and vaccine antigens. *New Engl J Med* 357:1903.

Corthésy B (2007): Roundtrip ticket for secretory IgA: Role in mucosal homeostasis? *J Immunol* 178:27.

Kunkel EJ, Butcher EC (2002): Chemokines and the tissue-specific migration of lymphocytes. *Immunity* 16:1–4.

McHeyzer-Williams LJ, McHeyzer-Williams, MG (2005): Antigen-specific memory B cell development. *Annu Rev Immunol* 23:487–513.

Martin F, Kearney JF (2000): B cell subsets and the mature preimmune repertoire: Marginal zone and B1 B cells as part of a "natural immune memory." *Immunol Rev* 175:70.

Mora JR, Iwata M, et al. (2006): Generation of gut-homing IgA-secreting B cells by intestinal dendritic cells. *Science* 314:1157–1160.

Salmi M, Jalkanen S (2005): Lymphocyte homing to the gut: Attraction, adhesion, and commitment. *Immunol Rev* 206: 100–113.

● REVIEW QUESTIONS

For each question, choose the ONE BEST answer.

1. The earliest stages of B-cell differentiation:
   A) occur in the embryonic thymus
   B) require the presence of antigen
   C) involve rearrangement of κ-chain gene segments
   D) involve rearrangement of surrogate light-chain gene segments
   E) involve rearrangement of heavy-chain gene segments

2. Which of the following is expressed on the surface of the mature B lymphocyte?
   A) CD40
   B) MHC class II molecules
   C) CD32
   D) IgM and IgD
   E) all of the above

3. Which of the following statements is incorrect?
   A) Antibodies in a secondary immune response generally have a higher affinity for antigen than antibodies formed in a primary response.
   B) Somatic hypermutation of variable-region genes may contribute to changes in antibody affinity observed during secondary responses.

C) Synthesis of antibody in a primary response to a thymus-dependent antigen occurs predominantly in the blood.
D) Isotype switching occurs in the presence of antigen.
E) Predominantly IgM antibody is produced in the primary response.

4. Immature B lymphocytes:
A) have rearranged only D and J gene segments
B) are progenitors of T as well as B lymphocytes
C) express both IgM and IgD on their surfaces
D) are at a stage of development where contact with antigen may lead to receptor editing and deletion
E) must go through the thymus to mature

5. Antigen binding to the B-cell receptor:
A) transduces a signal through the antigen-binding chains
B) invariably leads to B-cell activation
C) transduces a signal through the Igα and Igβ molecules
D) results in macrophage activation
E) leads to cytokine synthesis, which activates T cells

6. Which of the following would not be found on a memory B cell?
A) Igα and Igβ
B) γ heavy chains
C) ε heavy chains
D) surrogate light chains
E) κ light chains

7. Germinal centers found in lymph nodes and spleen:
A) support the development of immature B and T cells
B) function in the removal of damaged erythrocytes from the circulation
C) act as the major source of stem cells and thus help to maintain hematopoiesis
D) are sites where antigen-activated mature B cells proliferate and differentiate
E) are the sites of T cell differentiation

ANSWERS TO REVIEW QUESTIONS

1. *E* The earliest events in B-cell differentiation take place in fetal liver and bone marrow in the adult and involve rearrangement of heavy-chain V, D, and J gene segments.

2. *E* All the molecules are expressed on the surface of the mature B cell.

3. *C* Antibody synthesis in the primary response to TD antigens occurs predominantly in secondary lymphoid organs—the spleen lymph nodes, and mucosal-associated lymphoid tissue.

4. *D* In immature B cells, which express only IgM, contact with cell-bound self-antigen initiates receptor editing—secondary rearrangement of light chain genes. If receptor editing results in a receptor specific for self, the B cell is deleted.

5. *C* The molecules Igα and Igβ, which are associated with the surface Ig molecule, transduce a signal following antigen binding to surface Ig.

6. *D* Surrogate light chains are expressed only at the pre-B-cell stage of B-cell differentiation.

7. *D* Germinal centers are the areas of lymph node and spleen in which antigen-activated B cells proliferate, undergo somatic hypermutation and class switch recombination, and ultimately differentiate into memory or plasma cells.

8

ROLE OF THE MAJOR HISTOCOMPATIBILITY COMPLEX IN THE IMMUNE RESPONSE

INTRODUCTION

So far we have focused on the development and function of one set of lymphocytes (B cells), their receptor for antigen (immunoglobulin), and the mechanisms by which B cells generate a huge array of clonally distributed receptors. Antibodies, the antigen-specific products of B cells, play a critical role in interacting with antigens *outside* cells, such as viruses or bacteria encountered in blood (IgG) or at mucosal surfaces (IgA). Many pathogens, such as viruses, bacteria, and parasites, invade host cells and live at least part of their life cycle inside them. Antibodies do not enter cells, so once a pathogen gains entry to a host cell, antibodies are an ineffective defense. The phase of the immune response to pathogens—and many "harmless" antigens—inside host cells is the domain of T cells and their products.

Antibodies bind to all types of antigens, regardless of whether the antigens are protein, carbohydrate, nucleic acid, or lipid. By contrast, T cells respond almost exclusively to proteins, or more precisely small peptides derived from the catabolism of proteins. Proteins are major constituents of pathogens such as bacteria, viruses, and parasites, and most other antigens are protein in nature. Proteins are also the products of viral infection. (Later in the chapter we describe that some T cells react with lipid components of certain bacteria.) Thus, T cells play a critical role in the response to nearly all potentially harmful agents and myriad other antigens to which an individual is exposed.

Because T cells interact with antigens inside cells, they use an antigen recognition system distinct from the one used by B cells: T cells interact with antigens expressed on the surface of host cells. Like B cells, T cells express an antigen-specific receptor, the *T-cell receptor (TCR)*, whose properties are discussed in greater detail in Chapter 9. Figure 8.1 shows that the TCR interacts with two components expressed at the surface of a host cell: a linear fragment of peptide derived from a protein antigen; and a protein to which the peptide is bound, a *major histocompatibility complex (MHC) molecule*, often referred to as an *MHC antigen*.

The critical role played by MHC molecules in T-cell responses is referred to as the *MHC restriction of T-cell responses*. Before we discuss T-cell function and the TCR (Chapter 9), we will focus in this chapter on the structure and function of MHC molecules and describe how they interact with peptides and different sets of T cells. We will also discuss the characteristics of the genes that code for MHC molecules and the enormous diversity of MHC genes and their products in the population.

HOW THE MHC GOT ITS NAME

The term *major histocompatibility complex* derives from research in transplantation that started in the mid-twentieth century. These experiments provided insight into the rules governing the acceptance or rejection of tissues—literally, *histocompatibility*—when tissues were transplanted between different members of the same species (generally mice; see Chapter 18 for more discussion). Researchers interpreted their early findings to indicate that rapid

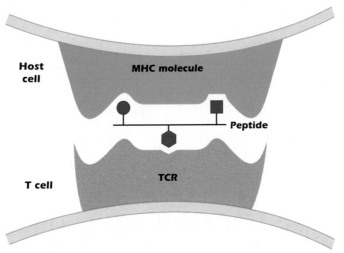

Figure 8.1. Interaction of an MHC molecule expressed on the surface of a host cell with bound peptide and a TCR.

rejection of such transplants was determined by a single gene, which they called the *major histocompatibility gene.* Because later studies indicated that this "gene" was actually a *complex*, a set of closely linked genes inherited as a unit, it became known as the major histocompatibility complex. We know now that every vertebrate species has an MHC containing multiple genes. The human MHC is known as *HLA (human leukocyte antigen)*.

Other early studies of transplantation in mice indicated that T cells played an important role in the rejection response (see Chapter 18 for more details). Taken together, these transplantation studies demonstrated an important but not well-understood connection between the MHC and T-cell responses. Because individuals do not normally undergo transplants, the function of the MHC in "everyday" T-cell responses became the focus of intense investigation. In the sections that follow, we will describe our understanding of the role of MHC molecules in T-cell responses that has emerged over the last 30 years.

DIFFERENT MHC MOLECULES INTERACT WITH DIFFERENT SETS OF T CELLS

In brief, the key functions of MHC molecules are twofold: (1) to bind peptides that are produced when proteins are catabolized—**processed**—inside cells of the host and (2) to **present** peptides to T cells with the appropriate TCR. Presentation of peptides derived from pathogens or other types of antigen triggers T-cell responses. Thus, we can say that MHC molecules "sample" the internal environment of the host cell and help T cells to identify whether a particular host cell has been infected or contains some "foreign" component requiring a response.

Figure 8.2 shows that two major sets of MHC molecules, *MHC class I molecules* and *MHC class II molecules*, play a key role in T-cell responses. MHC class

I molecules interact with the molecule CD8, whose expression defines the subset of T cells called **CD8$^+$ T cells**. The main function of CD8$^+$ T cells is cytotoxic, particularly toward pathogen-infected host cells. Thus, to expand on the expression introduced earlier in the chapter, *the responses of CD8$^+$ T cells are restricted by MHC class I molecules*.

MHC class I molecules are expressed on all nucleated cells (thus, they are not expressed on red blood cells). As will be described in more detail later in the chapter, MHC class I molecules bind peptides derived from proteins in the **cytoplasmic** compartment of the cell. Peptides derived from virus replication, from bacteria (such as *Mycobacterium tuberculosis*), and from parasites (such as single-celled protozoa that cause leishmaniasis and toxoplasmosis) that live inside host cells are all found in the cytoplasm. Thus, MHC class I molecules and CD8$^+$ T cells play critical roles in the responses to many pathogens; they also respond to tumors and transplanted tissue. Later in the chapter we also describe how MHC class I molecules interact with

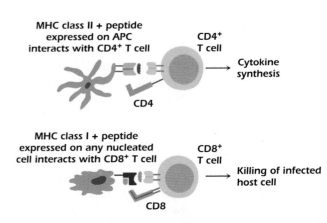

Figure 8.2. Cells expressing MHC class I interact with CD8$^+$ T cells, which kill infected host cells; cells expressing MHC class II interact with CD4$^+$ T cells, which synthesize cytokines.

cells other than CD8$^+$ T cells: They participate in a critical interaction with NK cells that prevents NK cells from killing normal host cells.

MHC class II molecules interact with the molecule CD4 expressed on the surface of the subset of T cells called **CD4$^+$ T cells**; thus, *the responses of CD4$^+$ T cells are said to be restricted by MHC class II molecules*. CD4$^+$ T cells synthesize an extensive array of cytokines, which affect many different cell types. The characteristics of the CD4$^+$ and CD8$^+$ sets of T cells are described in more detail in Chapter 9 and in many other chapters.

MHC class II molecules have a more limited distribution than class I molecules: They are expressed *constitutively* (i.e., under baseline conditions) only on (*antigen-presenting cells*, **APC**): cells that present antigen to T cells. In humans, the principal APC are dendritic cells, macrophages, B lymphocytes, and thymic epithelial cells. In the absence of inducing factors, most cells express MHC class I but not MHC class II molecules; APC constitutively express *both* MHC class I and class II molecules.

The expression of both classes of MHC molecules can be affected by many factors. Cytokines released during the response to infectious agents enhance the expression of MHC molecules: Interferons α, β, and γ upregulate MHC class I expression, and interferon γ (IFN-γ) upregulates MHC class II expression. As a consequence of this upregulation, MHC class II expression is *induced* on cells such as fibroblasts and endothelial cells that do not normally express it, and *increased* on APC. Induction and increased expression of MHC class I and II thus enhance T-cell responses to infectious agents. We will discuss the regulation of expression of MHC class molecules in greater detail later in this chapter.

As we also describe later in the chapter, MHC class II molecules bind peptides derived from proteins that are taken up from outside the cell into the *acidic* compartments (lysosomes and enodosomes) of the cell. APC are the predominant cell type in which this occurs. Thus, MHC class II molecules and CD4$^+$ T cells play critical roles in the responses to the protein constituents of pathogens and other types of antigen that are taken into APC.

VARIABILITY OF MHC CLASS I AND MHC CLASS II MOLECULES

Before discussing the detailed structures of MHC class I and II molecules, we note an important point: MHC class I and class II molecules differ from individual to individual and these differences are genetically determined; that is, MHC-distinct individuals express MHC molecules with somewhat different sequences. We will return to this feature of MHC molecules later in the chapter.

These differences in MHC molecule structure arise from two sources: polygenicity and polymorphism. First, the MHC is *polygenic*, meaning that MHC class I and II molecules are coded for by multiple independent genes. In humans, three independent genes—**HLA-A, HLA-B,** and **HLA-C**—code for MHC class I molecules expressed at the cell surface. Because each cell has two sets of chromosomes (one paternally derived and one maternally derived), every nucleated cell may express up to six different HLA class I molecules, each capable of binding peptides. (We explain later in the chapter why fewer than six different MHC class I molecules may be expressed.) Similarly, because human cells have genes that code for three different MHC class II molecules—known as **HLA-DP, HLA-DQ,** and **HLA-DR**—human APC may express up to six different HLA class II molecules.

Second, the MHC is highly *polymorphic*, meaning that multiple stable forms of each MHC gene exist in the population. Other important examples of genetic polymorphism in humans are the different forms of the red blood cell antigens (A, B, and O) and of hemoglobin molecules. However, the MHC is the most highly polymorphic gene system in the body and hence in the population: In humans hundreds of slightly different versions—*alleles*—of a gene that codes for the MHC class I molecule HLA-B have been identified.

The extensive polymorphism of human MHC genes makes it very unlikely that two random individuals will express identical sets of HLA class I and class II molecules. As we describe in Chapter 18, the enormous diversity of MHC molecules and the genes that code for them is a major barrier to successful transplantation of organs and tissues. Later in this chapter we discuss why we believe the MHC evolved to be so diverse.

Note that the mechanisms used to generate the diversity of MHC structures differ from the mechanisms used to generate the diversity of B-cell antigen receptors we described in Chapter 6. Generation of diversity among antigen-specific B-cell receptors arises from *gene recombination*, which produces one type of receptor per cell. (As we describe in Chapter 9, diversity among TCRs is also generated by gene recombination.) In contrast, although MHC molecules are diverse within the population, each cell in a particular person (liver, kidney, lymphocytes, etc.) expresses the same set of HLA class I and class II molecules.

STRUCTURE OF MHC CLASS I MOLECULES

Parts A–D of Figure 8.3 show different ways to represent the key features of the structure of a typical MHC class I molecule and how it interacts with peptide and a TCR. At the cell surface an MHC class I molecule is

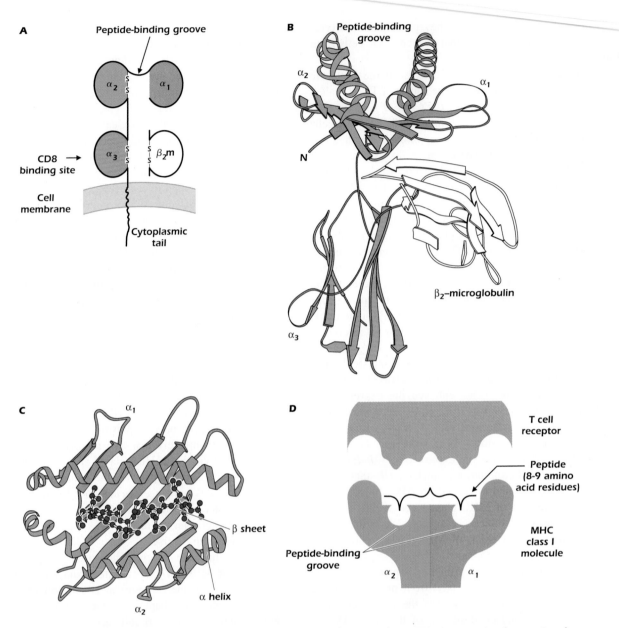

Figure 8.3. Different depictions of MHC class I molecule. (A) Cartoon of an MHC class I molecule associated at the cell surface with β_2m. (B) Side view of MHC class I molecule with β_2m, showing peptide-binding groove. (C) Top view of peptide-binding groove, showing bound peptide. (D) Diagram of interaction of T-cell receptor with MHC class I molecule and peptide bound in peptide-binding groove. (Parts B and C adapted from Bjorkman et al., 1987, with permission; part D adapted from Rammensee et al., 1993.)

a transmembrane glycoprotein (molecular weight approximately 43 kDa), expressed in noncovalent association with a small *invariant* (identical on all cells) polypeptide called **β_2-microglobulin** (**β_2m;** molecular weight 12 kDa). β_2m is encoded by a gene on a separate chromosome from the MHC. The MHC class I molecule is referred to as the α, or heavy, chain and comprises three extracellular Ig-like domains—α_1, α_2, and α_3. β_2m has a structure homologous to a single Ig domain; indeed, β_2m and MHC class I are members of the Ig superfamily described in Chapter 4. At

the cell surface, MHC class I plus β_2m has the appearance of a four-domain molecule—α_1 paired with α_2 on the exterior of the MHC class I molecule and α_3 and β_2m paired closer to the membrane.

Figure 8.3B shows the most striking feature of all MHC class I molecules that have been examined by X-ray crystallography: a deep groove or cleft in the part of the molecule farthest from the membrane that is composed of parts of the α_1 and α_2 domains. As its name implies, the **peptide-binding groove** is the binding site for peptides. As shown in Figure 8.3C, the groove resembles a basket with an irregular floor (made up of amino acids in a β-pleated sheet structure) surrounded by walls (formed by α helices). The groove holds peptides eight to nine amino acids long in a linear array (see also Fig. 3.5).

Figure 8.3D illustrates that peptide bound in this cleft and parts of the MHC class I molecule interact with the TCR. The center of the bound peptide—the only part of the peptide not buried in the MHC molecule—interacts with the TCR, which suggests that a small number of contacts with amino acids in the center of the peptide are critical for recognition by the TCR.

Selectivity of Peptide Binding to MHC Class I Molecules

We referred above to the tremendous variability of MHC class I molecules within the population. Looking at differences in sequence among MHC class I molecules, we find that most of the differences in amino acids are confined to a limited region in the extracellular α1 and α2 domains, and particularly in the floor and walls of the peptide-binding groove (see Figure 8.3C). These differences in amino acid sequence and hence structure of the binding groove play a critical role in determining which peptides bind to a particular MHC molecular. (The pockets forming the floor of the groove also help to align peptides so they can be recognized by specific T-cell receptors.)

Thus, binding of an MHC class I molecule to peptide is *selective:* One MHC molecule will bind with high affinity to only certain peptides. A single MHC class I molecule can bind to a variety of peptides but binds preferentially to peptides with certain *motifs*, invariant or closely related amino acids at certain positions (*anchor residues*) in the eight- or nine-amino-acid sequence; those at the other positions may vary. In this way, one MHC molecule can bind to a large number of peptides with different sequences. This helps explain why (with very few exceptions) T-cell responses are made to at least one epitope from almost all proteins and why failure to respond to a protein antigen is so rare.

CD8 Binding to Invariant Region of MHC Class I Molecules

Outside the peptide-binding cleft the sequences of different MHC class I molecules are very similar. Thus an individual class I molecule can be divided into a *polymorphic* or *variable region* (sequence unique to that molecule) in the area in and around the peptide-binding groove, and a *nonpolymorphic* or *invariant region* that is similar in all MHC class I molecules. CD8, the molecule that characterizes the CD8+ T-cell subset, binds to the invariant region of all MHC class I molecules, specifically in the α3 domain (see Fig. 8.3A).

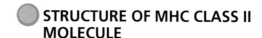

STRUCTURE OF MHC CLASS II MOLECULE

Figure 8.4 shows different ways to represent the key features of a typical MHC class II molecule. Figure 8.4A shows that an MHC class II molecule is a transmembrane glycoprotein comprising two chains, α and β (molecular weight of approximately 35,000 and 28,000 Da, respectively). Like MHC class I molecules, every MHC class II molecule is expressed at the cell surface as a four-domain structure: the α1 domain is paired with β1, and α2 with β2. α and β have cytoplasmic tails and extracellular Ig-like domains; they are also members of the Ig superfamily.

Like the MHC class I molecule, the MHC class II molecule contains a peptide-binding groove at the top of the molecule (shown in most detail in Figs. 8.4B and C), which is structurally analogous to the MHC class I groove. However, in the MHC class II molecule the groove is formed by interactions between the α1 and β1 domains. Figure 8.4C indicates that the floor and walls of the MHC class II cleft have the same β-pleated sheet and α-helical structures found in the MHC class I molecule.

In contrast to the 8- to 9-amino-acid peptides that bind to the cleft in the MHC class I molecule, the MHC class II groove binds peptides varying in length from 12 to approximately 17 linearly arranged amino acids, with the ends of the peptide outside the groove. Figure 8.4D shows that the TCR contacts the peptide bound in the groove of the MHC class II molecule and parts of the MHC class II molecule. As with MHC class I molecules, MHC class II molecules bind to peptides with specific motifs; because the lengths of the peptides that bind to MHC class II molecules are more variable than those that bind to MHC class I molecules, the motif is generally seen in the central region of the peptide, the region that fits inside the peptide-binding groove.

Like MHC class I molecules, MHC class II molecules are composed of variable or polymorphic regions and invariant or nonpolymorphic regions. CD4, the molecule that characterizes the CD4+ T-cell subset, binds to the invariant region of all MHC class II molecules, specifically in the β2 domain (see Fig. 8.4A).

ANTIGEN PROCESSING AND PRESENTATION: HOW MHC MOLECULES BIND PEPTIDES AND CREATE LIGANDS THAT INTERACT WITH T CELLS

In the previous sections we described the structure of MHC class I and II molecules at the cell surface and showed each molecule's peptide-binding site. In this section we describe how peptides are generated from proteins inside

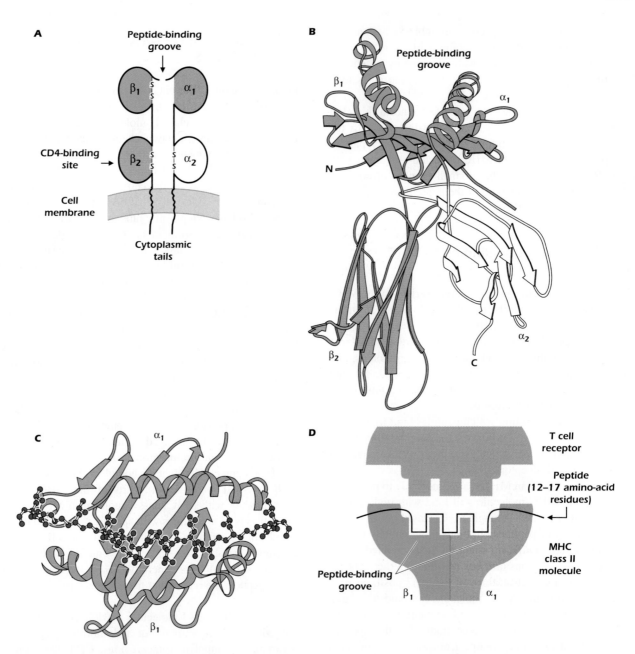

Figure 8.4. Different depictions of MHC class II molecule. (A) Cartoon of MHC class II molecule at cell surface. (B) Side view of MHC class II molecule showing peptide-binding groove. (Adapted from Stern and Wiley, 1994, with permission.) (C) Top view of peptide-binding groove. (Adapted from Stern et al., (1994), with permission.) (D) Diagram of interaction of T-cell receptor with MHC class II molecule and peptide bound in peptide-binding groove. (From Rammensee et al., 1993.)

cells, where in the cell peptides bind to MHC molecules, and how complexes of MHC and peptide interact with the TCR of a specific T cell.

Collectively, the pathways that create peptide ligands that activate T cells are known as the *processing and presentation* of protein antigens. We will focus on the processing and presentation of two different sets of protein antigens—known as *exogenous* and *endogenous antigens*—and show how peptides derived from these two types of antigens associate with MHC class II

and MHC class I molecules, respectively. The different peptide–MHC complexes interact with different sets of T cells: peptide + MHC class II with CD4[+] T cells and peptide + MHC class I molecules with CD8[+] T cells.

Exogenous Antigens and Generation of MHC Class II–Peptide Complexes

As the term implies, exogenous antigens are antigens that come from *outside* a host cell and are taken inside, normally by endocytosis or phagocytosis (see Fig. 2.2). Exogenous

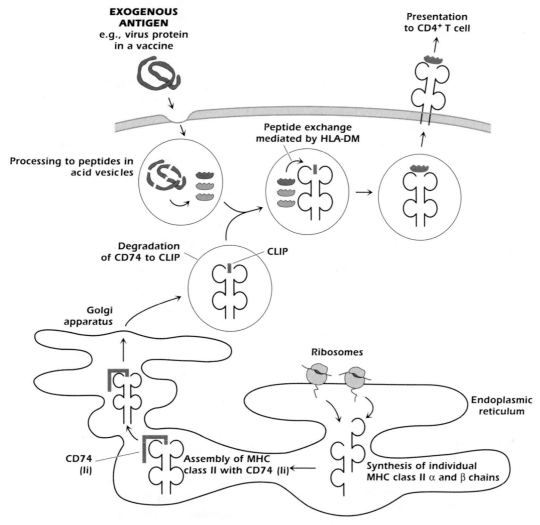

EXOGENOUS ANTIGEN
e.g., virus protein in a vaccine

Presentation to CD4⁺ T cell

Processing to peptides in acid vesicles

Peptide exchange mediated by HLA-DM

Degradation of CD74 to CLIP

CLIP

Golgi apparatus

Ribosomes

Endoplasmic reticulum

CD74 (Ii)

Assembly of MHC class II with CD74 (Ii)

Synthesis of individual MHC class II α and β chains

Figure 8.5. Processing of exogenous antigen in MHC class II pathway, (Ii = invariant chain; CLIP = fragment of Ii bound to MHC class II groove.)

antigens can be derived from pathogens (such as bacteria or viruses) or from foreign proteins (such as vaccines) that do not injure the host but activate an immune response. APC—predominantly dendritic cells, macrophages, and B cells—take up exogenous antigens. As we noted earlier in the chapter, these APC express MHC class II molecules constitutively.

Figure 8.5 shows the processing and presentation of a typical exogenous antigen, a protein injected as a component of an inactivated or "dead" virus vaccine. The protein is internalized, contained in an intracellular vesicle that fuses with endosomal or lysosomal vesicles that are highly acidic (pH approximately 4.0). These vesicles contain an array of degradative enzymes, including proteases and peptidases. Proteases known as cathepsins, which function at low pH, cut proteins into peptides in these vesicles. Catabolism of a typical protein antigen yields several peptides (only three are shown in Fig. 8.5).

Figure 8.5 also illustrates that the acid vesicles containing peptides intersect inside the cell with vesicles containing MHC class II molecules that have been synthesized on ribosomes of the rough endoplasmic reticulum. The MHC class II α and β chains are synthesized individually in the endoplasmic reticulum and are assembled there with **CD74, invariant chain (Ii)**. CD74 binds to the groove of the newly formed MHC class II molecule, preventing the binding of peptides that may be present in the endoplasmic reticulum, such as peptides derived from the processing of endogenous antigens (see below).

CD74 also acts as a **chaperone** for the newly synthesized MHC class II chains; that is, interaction with CD74 allows the MHC class II α and β chains to leave the endoplasmic reticulum and enter the Golgi complex; from there they proceed into the acid vesicle endocytic pathway. Removal of CD74 from the complex occurs in stages. Initially, CD74 is degraded proteolytically, leaving a fragment known as CLIP (Class II-associated Invariant Polypeptide) bound to the MHC class II groove. Vesicles containing MHC class II bound to CLIP then fuse with the acid vesicles (endosomes or lysosomes) containing peptides derived from the catabolism of exogenous antigens. In this compartment, a molecule known as HLA-DM catalyzes peptide exchange between the MHC class II–CLIP complex and peptides derived from the exogenous antigen. In this way, a peptide–MHC class II complex is generated, which moves to the cell surface where it can interact with—that is, be presented to—a CD4$^+$ T cell expressing the appropriate antigen receptor.

Although catabolism of a typical protein yields several peptides, not all the peptides formed bind to MHC molecules because MHC binding to peptides is selective. Figure 8.6 shows the situation with three of the many peptides that are derived from the catabolism of a larger protein. Peptides 35–48 and 110–122 bind to two different HLA class II molecules HLA-DR4 and HLA-DP2, expressed in this individual. Only these peptides have the potential to induce a T-cell response in this particular person to this protein antigen. Because peptide 1–13 does not bind to the MHC class II molecules, it does *not* trigger a CD4$^+$ T-cell response. We say that peptides 35–48 and 110–122 are the *immunodominant* CD4$^+$ T-cell epitopes of this protein in this particular person. Peptide 1–13 quite probably is an immunodominant epitope of this protein in a different person expressing a completely different set of MHC molecules. Thus, we can say that, almost without fail, every person will make a T-cell response to this viral protein; however, because of the selectivity of peptide–MHC binding, individuals who express different MHC molecules respond to different parts of the same protein.

Endogenous Antigens: Generation of MHC Class I–Peptide Complexes

Endogenous antigens are synthesized *inside* a cell and are generally derived from pathogens (such as viruses, bacteria,

and parasites) that have infected a host cell. Figure 8.7 illustrates the processing and presentation of a typical endogenous antigen, a viral protein synthesized after a cell has been infected by a virus. Processing occurs in the cytoplasm: The major mechanism for generating peptide fragments is via a giant cytoplasmic protein complex known as the *proteasome* that cleaves proteins into peptides about 15 amino acids in length. Cytosolic enzymes (aminopeptidases) remove even more amino acids from the peptides. Some peptides are destroyed, but some, 8–15 amino acids in length (such as the three shown in Fig. 8.7), are selectively transported into the endoplasmic reticulum by a peptide transporter; the peptide transporter is the product of the expression of two genes, *TAP-1* and *TAP-2*.

Peptides transported from the cytoplasm into the endoplasmic reticulum bind to newly synthesized MHC class I molecules. Figure 8.7 also shows that MHC class I and β_2m chains are synthesized separately in the rough endoplasmic reticulum and associate in this cellular compartment. As with the synthesis of MHC class II molecules, chaperones stabilize the structure of the assembled MHC class I with their β_2m chains in the endoplasmic reticulum and direct transport of the complex through the cell.

As indicated earlier, MHC class I molecules preferentially bind peptides eight to nine amino acids in length. The normal fate of peptides that reach the endoplasmic reticulum is degradation by an aminopeptidase, which removes amino acids one at a time until the peptides are completely degraded; peptides with the appropriate binding characteristics are "rescued" from this fate by binding to a newly synthesized MHC class I molecule.

A peptide that binds to an MHC class I molecule in the endoplasmic reticulum moves via the Golgi apparatus to the cell surface, where it is presented to a CD8$^+$ T cell expressing the appropriate antigen receptor. As described above for the interaction of peptides with MHC class II molecules, only those peptides that bind to MHC class I molecules trigger CD8$^+$ T-cell responses. These are the immunodominant epitopes for the CD8$^+$ T-cell response specific for that antigen; one such immunodominant epitope

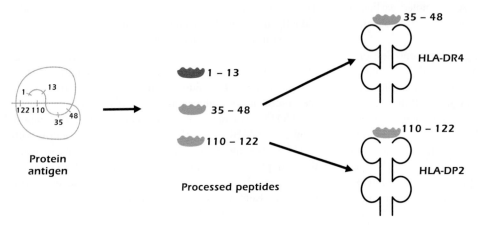

Figure 8.6. Selective binding of processed peptides by different MHC molecules. The numbers refer to positions of amino acids in the sequence of the protein antigen.

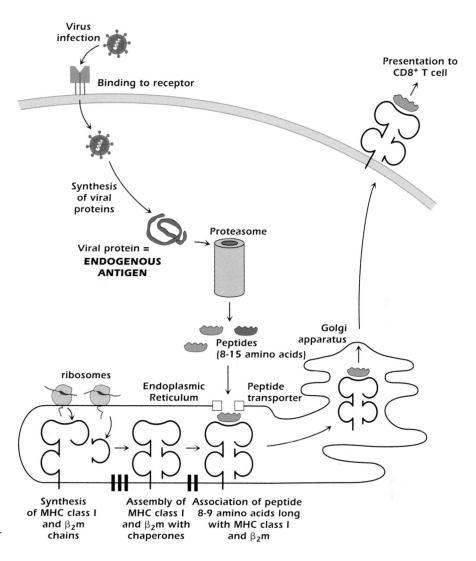

Binding to receptor

Presentation to CD8+ T cell

Synthesis of viral proteins

Proteasome

Viral protein = **ENDOGENOUS ANTIGEN**

Peptides (8-15 amino acids)

Golgi apparatus

ribosomes

Endoplasmic Reticulum

Peptide transporter

Synthesis of MHC class I and β₂m chains

Assembly of MHC class I and β₂m with chaperones

Association of peptide 8-9 amino acids long with MHC class I and β₂m

Figure 8.7. Processing of endogenous antigen in MHC class I pathway.

is the green peptide derived from the catabolism of a virus protein shown in Figure 8.7.

Because MHC class I molecules are expressed on all nucleated cells, the processing and presentation of endogenous antigens can occur in *every* cell in the body. Because pathogens can infect almost any cell in the body, CD8+ T cells "scan" MHC class I and peptide combinations expressed on any nucleated host cell to identify whether it has been infected.

Decreased MHC Class I Expression in Virus-Infected and Tumor Cells

Earlier in the chapter we mentioned that factors such as cytokines synthesized in responses to infectious agents induce or increase expression of MHC class I and class II molecules. This leads to enhanced immune responses to the pathogen that induced the response. In contrast, some viruses (such as the herpes simplex virus, adenovirus, and cytomegalovirus) synthesize proteins that interfere with steps in the pathway shown in Figure 8.7: they inhibit

the synthesis of MHC class I molecules or interrupt the transport of peptide–MHC class I complexes to the cell surface. In this way the virus *decreases* expression of MHC class I molecules and so decreases the CD8+ T-cell response to the virus. In addition, tumor cells frequently show decreased expression of MHC class I compared to normal cells, subverting a potential CD8+ T-cell response.

Although the decrease in MHC class I expression decreases the CD8+ T-cell response, it may also act as a trigger of NK-cell responses to the virus-infected cell or tumor cell. As shown in Figure 2.5, MHC class I molecules are negative regulators of NK-cell activity; that is, an MHC class I expressed on a normal host cell interacts with a Killer-inhibitory receptor (KIR) expressed on an NK cell and so prevents the NK cell from killing the host cell. If a host cell does not express MHC class I (as in the case of tumors or virus-infected cells) and the KIR–MHC class I interaction does *not* occur, NK cells are activated and kill the MHC-deficient cells.

Cross-Presentation: Exogenous Antigens Presented in the MHC Class I Pathway

In addition to their ability to process exogenous antigens in the MHC class II pathway, Figure 8.8 shows that APC—and particularly dendritic cells—have a unique pathway, called ***cross-presentation***, for generating peptides derived from exogenous protein antigens and presenting them to CD8$^+$ T cells. The dendritic cell takes up exogenous antigens (such as those derived from a virus-infected or dying cell) by either phagocytosis or pinocytosis. How peptides intersect with MHC class I molecules inside the cell is not completely understood; one mechanism appears to involve transferring antigen from acid compartments into the cytosol for processing in the MHC class I pathway.

Cross-presentation is believed to play an important role in activating CD8$^+$ T cells to respond to tissue cells infected by some viruses that are not taken up by APC (see Chapter 10). It is also thought to play a role in the response to dying cells.

Table 8.1 summarizes the characteristics of MHC class I and II molecules that we have described so far.

Which Antigens Trigger Which T-Cell Responses?

We have described how exogenous protein antigens are taken up by APC, processed in acid compartments that intersect with the MHC class II pathway, and presented to CD4$^+$ T cells. Thus, proteins from bacteria, most viruses, allergens, and completely harmless antigens all trigger CD4$^+$ T-cell responses. In contrast, only infectious pathogens, particularly viruses, create epitopes via the endogenous or cross-presentation pathways presented by MHC class I molecules, so they are the only types of antigen that activate CD8$^+$ T cells. Generally, but not always, infectious agents activate both CD4$^+$ T cells and CD8$^+$ T cells because these agents are taken up by APC; however, as we describe in Chapter 10, some viruses evoke responses by CD8$^+$ T cells almost exclusively.

Note that the processing pathway, rather than inherent properties of the antigen, determines whether a protein is presented to CD4$^+$ or CD8$^+$ T cells. This is illustrated by the cross-presentation pathway described above, in which an exogenous antigen ends up being processed in the MHC class I pathway and presented to CD8$^+$ T cells.

As described in detail in Chapter 18, transplantation responses—in which host T cells respond to nonself MHC molecules expressed on cells of the graft—generally activate both CD4$^+$ and CD8$^+$ T-cell responses. Immune responses to tumors are generally mediated by CD8$^+$ cells.

Binding of Peptides Derived from Self-Molecules by MHC Molecules

The phenomena of antigen processing and presentation described above—the catabolism of proteins and movement of products from compartment to compartment inside a cell—are all aspects of normal cell physiologic

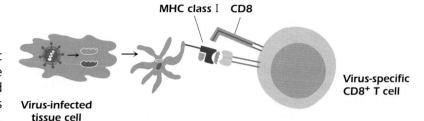

⬤ Figure 8.8. **Cross-presentation.** A dendritic cell takes up an exogenous antigen, for example derived from a virus-infected cell, but processed peptides associate with MHC class I molecules inside the cell and are presented to CD8$^+$ T cells.

⬤ TABLE 8.1. Comparison of Properties and Function of MHC Class I and II Molecules

Characteristic	MHC Class I	MHC Class II
Structure	α chain +β$_2$m	α + β chains
Cellular expression	All nucleated cells; upregulated on many cell types by interferons.	Constitutively on APC (dendritic cells, macrophages, B cells, thymic epithelial cells); inducible on many cell types by factors such as IFN-γ
Peptide-binding groove	Binds peptides 8–9 amino acids in length; formed by α$_1$ and α$_2$ domains	Binds peptides 12–17 amino acids long; formed by α$_1$ and β$_1$ domains
Binds peptides derived from	(1) Endogenous antigens catabolized in the cytoplasm or (2) cross-presentation	Exogenous antigens catabolized in acid compartments
MHC–peptide complex interacts with	CD8$^+$ T cells, NK cells	CD4$^+$ T cells

pathways. Thus, the proteins normally found inside cells—self-proteins—"turn over" and are catabolized using the same pathways described for the processing of protein antigens. For example, ribosomal and mitochondrial proteins are broken down inside cells and peptides derived from these molecules can associate with MHC molecules. Indeed, MHC molecules extracted from cells nearly always contain peptides derived from such self-proteins. From our description of protein processing above, proteins from inside host cells are expected to associate with MHC class I molecules, and indeed this is observed. In addition, recent studies indicate that some self-constituents also bind to MHC class II molecules. This occurs as a result of *autophagy*, an intracellular pathway in which proteins in the cytoplasm are transported into lysosomes for degradation. Self-peptides bind to MHC class II in these acid vesicles.

However, self-peptides bound to MHC molecules do not normally activate T cells. One reason is that T cells reactive to many self-molecules are removed or inactivated during differentiation in the thymus (a process discussed more fully in Chapter 9). However, we know that mature T cells with the potential to react with self-molecules are detectable outside the thymus (see Chapter 12). Why are these T cells not activated? Equally important, since an individual's cells are bathed in a sea of self-proteins that they are continually processing and binding to their MHC molecules, how can a person respond to a tiny amount of foreign protein? These are critical issues; a T cell must be able to distinguish between a normal host cell, to which no response is required, and a cell that has been infected by a pathogen.

The answer appears to be that pathogens induce effects that activate the immune response over and above their ability to generate peptides for binding to MHC molecules. The major effect induced by pathogens is *costimulator function*—also referred to as *second signals*—in the specialized APC that present antigen to T cells (this concept is discussed further in Chapter 10). Costimulator signals are required to activate naïve T cells (T cells that have not previously encountered antigen). By contrast, peptides derived from self-molecules generally encounter T cells on normal tissue cells (such as those of the liver or pancreas), which do not express costimulator function; thus, T cells are not activated. Even if peptides derived from a self-molecule are presented by an APC in the tissue, T cells are not activated because, in the absence of foreign antigen or an inflammatory response, APC in tissue do not express costimulator signals (see Chapter 10). This signaling requirement ensures that T cells do not normally respond to peptides derived from self-components but do respond to peptides derived from nonself, potentially harmful, antigens.

This also helps to explain why the induction of T-cell responses to even some "foreign" antigens, such as harmless antigens or some vaccines, can be difficult. To develop strong T-cell (and antibody) responses, such antigens are frequently administered with an *adjuvant* (literally, adding to the response). Adjuvants are generally products that activate APC such as dendritic cells, macrophages, and B cells.

Inability to Respond to an Antigen

As described in the preceding sections, limited numbers of different MHC class I and II molecules are expressed on the cells of any one person. For an antigen to generate a T-cell response, at least one peptide derived during processing must bind to one of these MHC molecules. A peptide that does not bind to an MHC molecule does not activate a T-cell response; thus, if an entire antigen fails to generate a single peptide able to bind to an MHC molecule, the individual will not mount a T-cell response to that particular antigen.

Naturally occurring pathogens are generally large and complex and contain multiple epitopes that stimulate responses by both T and B cells; thus, some sort of response to a pathogen is more or less certain. However, unresponsiveness to a large antigen can occur in the case of synthetic polymers of amino acids that contain a very limited number of epitopes. Another important situation is in the response to a small peptide, such as a vaccine comprising a single, small peptide. As described earlier in the chapter, because a population expresses many different types of MHC molecules, the MHC molecules expressed in some people may not bind this particular peptide. In vaccination this problem has been circumvented by coupling the peptide to a large protein, a *carrier*, which enhances the response to the peptide (described further in Chapter 10).

● OTHER TYPES OF ANTIGEN THAT ACTIVATE T-CELL RESPONSES

Figure 8.9A shows the key characteristics of the set of protein antigens known as *superantigens*; in humans, these are predominantly bacterial exotoxins, such as staphylococcal enterotoxin. Superantigens are not processed, but the intact molecule binds to MHC class II molecules outside the peptide-binding groove. The key biologic feature of superantigens is that they activate up to 10% of a person's total CD4$^+$ T cells: This is a huge number compared to the triggering of a few T-cell clones by a peptide–MHC class II complex from a conventional antigen. As we describe in Chapters 10 and 11, the activation of so many T cells can have clinical consequences; for example, it is responsible for inducing the shocklike syndrome of toxic shock.

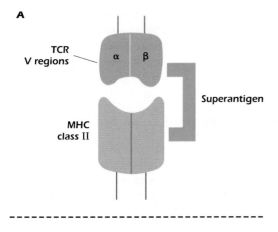

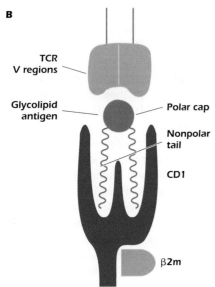

Figure 8.9. Interaction of TCRs with nonpeptide antigens: (A) superantigens bind outside MHC class II peptide-binding groove and interact with TCR Vβ; (B) CD1 presents glycolipid antigens.

LIPIDS AND GLYCOLIPIDS PRESENTED BY CD1 TO NKT CELLS

Some T cells can recognize lipids and glycolipids found in the cell walls of pathogens such as *Mycobacterium tuberculosis* that live inside macrophages; these T cells also respond to many host glycolipids. Figure 8.9B shows that lipids and glycolipids are presented by a family of molecules known as **CD1** (CD1a through CD1d) expressed by APC such as macrophages and dendritic cells. CD1 molecules are cell surface glycoproteins coded for outside the MHC region; like MHC class I molecules, they are expressed on the surface of APC in association with β₂m. As Figure 8.9B shows, the structure of a CD1 molecule is similar to that of an MHC class I molecule, but CD1

contains a larger binding groove with a deep cavity. The cavity binds the hydrophobic backbone of a lipid antigen, exposing the polar region of the lipid or glycolipid for binding to the T-cell receptor. Binding of lipid antigens to CD1 is believed to take place in acidic cellular compartments, similar to the loading of exogenous peptides onto MHC class II molecules. Like the binding of some viruses to components of the MHC class I–peptide processing pathway described earlier, recent evidence indicates that herpes simplex virus 1 down-regulates expression of CD1d, inhibiting glycolipid antigen presentation.

CD1a, b, and c present lipids to T cells that use an αβ TCR, but CD1d present lipids and glycolipids to a subset of T cells, NKT cells, which express both NK- and T-cell characteristics (NKT cells are discussed further in Chapters 9 and 10).

GENES OF THE HLA REGION

Polymorphic MHC Class I and II Genes

As stated at the beginning of the chapter, scientists have recognized for a long time that MHC genes are a **complex**, a group of tightly linked genes passed down as a unit. Figure 8.10 shows a simplified view of the region of the chromosome (chromosome 6) that contains the human MHC genes, HLA. It includes two regions: the class I and class II regions. The class I region contains three independent genes that code for the polymorphic MHC class I molecules, HLA-A, HLA-B, and HLA-Cw; the product of the *HLA-C* gene is called "Cw" to distinguish it from complement components that are designated C3, C5 and so on (see Chapter 13). The β₂m that is expressed at the cell surface with the MHC class I molecule is coded for outside the MHC.

Figure 8.10 also shows that the class II region includes pairs of genes that code for the polymorphic MHC class II molecules HLA-DP, HLA-DQ, and HLA-DR. Each of these MHC class II subregions contains an A gene and a B gene; these code for the α and β chain, respectively, of the two-chain MHC class II molecule. Thus, for example, the *HLA-DPA1* gene codes for DPα of the HLA-DP molecule and the *HLA-DPB1* gene codes for the other chain, DPβ, of the HLA-DP molecule. Some people have more than one DRB gene (*DRB1, DRB2*, etc.) that may be used to code for the DRβ chain, so they can express more than one pair of DRα and β chains.

Nomenclature of Polymorphic MHC Molecules

Originally, HLA molecules were characterized by serology, that is, using antibodies specific for different HLA class I or II molecules. This approach gave rise to a terminology that established differences among HLA antigens, for example, HLA-A2 differing from HLA-A25, HLA-B18

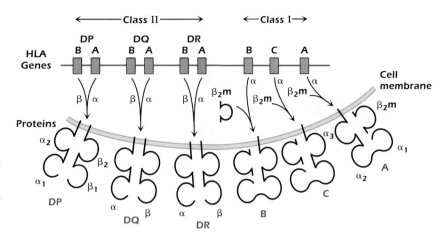

Figure 8.10. Simplified depiction of the human MHC, HLA, showing regions and genes coding for polymorphic MHC class I and II molecules expressed at the cell surface; β_2m encoded outside MHC.

from HLA-B27, and HLA-DR14 from HLA-DR16. The advent of PCR technology has provided a much more detailed description of differences among HLA molecules. For example, current terminology refers to *HLA-DRB1*1301*, in which the letters to the left of the asterisk specify the HLA gene, in this case *DRB1*, and the four (or, in some cases, six or eight) numbers to the right of the asterisk define the particular allele. This more extensive and precise characterization of HLA alleles has been invaluable in trying to match transplant donors and recipients and for identifying individuals who may be at risk for different autoimmune conditions (see Chapters 19 and 12, respectively). Important examples of specific alleles associated with human autoimmune conditions are given in Table 12.1.

REGULATION OF EXPRESSION OF MHC GENES

Codominant Expression

Figure 8.10 shows the HLA region of a single chromosome. However, as indicated earlier in the chapter, MHC class I and II molecules are *codominantly expressed*, that is, every cell expresses MHC molecules transcribed from both the maternal and paternal chromosomes. Thus, every nucleated cell of a particular person expresses up to six different HLA class I and six different HLA class II molecules. Some individuals may express fewer than six different class I or class II molecules because they are *homozygous* for a particular allele (both paternal and maternal chromosomes expressing the same allele).

Coordinate Regulation

Expression of MHC molecules is *coordinately regulated*, meaning that all class I molecules and all class II molecules are expressed at the same time on a single cell. Thus, factors such as IFN-γ enhance expression of all class I molecules

and induce all class II molecules on a particular cell. As the foregoing discussion has emphasized, MHC class I and II genes are regulated separately, because MHC class I molecules can be expressed in the absence of MHC class II molecules.

Rare people with *bare lymphocyte syndrome* lack the ability to express either HLA class I or class II molecules or both (see Chapter 17). Individuals who do not express HLA class II molecules have the most profound immunodeficiency, characterized by defective presentation of antigens to CD4+ T cells and decreased numbers of CD4+ T cells. These individuals have a mutation in one of the factors that controls the transcription of MHC class II genes.

Inheritance of MHC Genes

Figure 8.11 shows that the set of HLA class I plus class II genes expressed on an individual chromosome—referred to as a *haplotype*—is passed on to offspring as a unit. In this example, the cells of the father express HLA class I and II molecules coded for by his paternal and maternal chromosomes (haplotypes 1 and 2) and the cells of the mother express HLA class I and II molecules coded for by both her chromosomes (haplotypes 3 and 4). Because of the diversity of HLA genes and molecules in the population, it can almost be guaranteed that the HLA haplotypes 1 and 2 contributed by the father will differ from the haplotypes 3 and 4 contributed by the mother (represented by the different colors of the chromosomes in the figure).

Figure 8.11 also shows that the HLA haplotypes of a son or daughter differs from the haplotypes of his or her parents: Each parent expresses one HLA haplotype different from each child, and each child one HLA haplotype different from each parent. The figure also shows that every child in the family expresses a different set of HLA haplotypes, but there is a 1 in 4 chance that any two siblings will have identical HLA haplotypes. However, individuals within a family do not usually express identical MHC molecules, and as we described earlier in the chapter, the likelihood

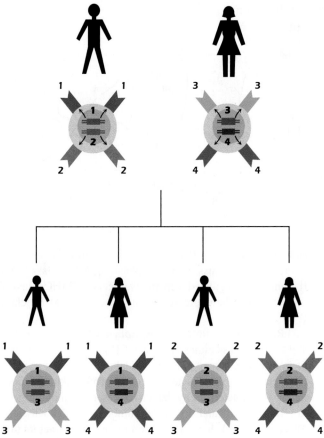

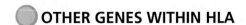

Figure 8.11. HLA genes are passed on as a unit from parent to child. Because HLA is highly polymorphic, it is likely that any two adults will have four distinct HLA haplotypes (father: 1 and 2, mother: 3 and 4). The children of these parents express four different haplotypes (1/3, 1/4, etc.). The different-colored structures expressed on the cell surface represent the combined set of HLA class I plus II molecules expressed by all the cells in that individual.

of finding individuals in the general population who are matched at all HLA alleles is extremely small.

OTHER GENES WITHIN HLA

The MHC of the human and the mouse have both been mapped and shown to contain many more genes and pseudogenes than the polymorphic MHC class I and class II molecules focused on in this chapter. The region between the class I and class II genes contains **MHC class III genes** that code for serum complement components C2, C4, and factor B (described in Chapter 13). In humans, this region also contains several different genes: the cytokines TNF-α and TNF-β heat-shock proteins hsp 70-1 and 70-2 (activated when cells are stressed), and 21-hydroxylase (an enzyme involved in steroid metabolism).

Additional human MHC class I genes—including **HLA-E, HLA-F,** and *HLA-G*—have been identified in the class I region. These genes and their products are much less polymorphic than the class I genes described in this chapter. The functions of the products of *HLA-E, HLA-F,* and *HLA-G* are not well understood but are thought to be involved in the presentation of antigens to NK cells. The expression of HLA-G by placental trophoblast cells

has been suggested as a potential mechanism preventing rejection of the fetus by the maternal host.

The MHC class II region also includes *HLA-DM* (which codes for a molecule described earlier in the chapter that is involved in peptide exchange in the MHC class II pathway); and genes coding for molecules involved in the MHC class I pathway: the peptide transporter molecules TAP-1 and TAP-2, and the major subunits of the proteasome. Why all these genes are linked in a complex that is passed down as a unit with genes coding for molecules responsible for crucial cell interactions is currently unknown.

MHC IN OTHER SPECIES

As indicated earlier in the chapter, every vertebrate species has an MHC. Generally, the names of the MHCs of other species are similar to the human MHC, HLA; for example, BoLA for the bovine system and SLA for swine. The mouse MHC, known as **H-2**, has been studied in great detail. The name H-2 differs because it was derived from the early studies of histocompatibility genes involved in transplantation responses. Intensive interest in H-2 developed because mice can be selectively bred to create **inbred strains** in which all members of the strain are genetically identical (a topic discussed in more detail in Chapter 5). Studies taking advantage of the genetic identity of inbred strains of mice and the identity of their MHC molecules have helped answer many fundamental immunologic questions that could not be addressed easily in humans. The genes and protein products of the human and mouse MHCs show a high degree of homology, indicating a common ancestral origin.

Figure 8.12 depicts H-2, located on mouse chromosome 17. Unlike the single MHC class I region of human HLA, mouse MHC class I genes are found at both ends of H-2. Three independent genes—*K, D*, and *L*—code for the murine MHC class I molecules, which are expressed at the cell surface in association with β_2m. H-2 contains a class II region that contains two pairs of genes (rather than the three found in humans) that code for the polymorphic MHC class II molecules, *I-A and I-E;* each of these comprises an α chain and a β chain. In mice, H-2 haplotypes are given superscript letters. For example, in the mouse strain H-2^b all the MHC class I and II genes and products are of type b (K^b, I-A^b, etc.), and in the MHC-distinct strain H-2^d all the MHC I and II genes are of type d (K^d, I-A^d etc.).

DIVERSITY OF MHC MOLECULES: MHC ASSOCIATION WITH RESISTANCE AND SUSCEPTIBILITY TO DISEASE

The extensive polymorphism of MHC genes and molecules is a great impediment to the acceptance of tissue transplanted between individuals, because it is highly unlikely that two random individuals are genetically identical (the topic of transplantation is discussed more fully in Chapter 18). Because nearly every vertebrate species has developed a similarly diverse array of MHC genes and molecules, the maintenance of MHC diversity must have some major benefit to the species.

The most likely explanation is that the diversity of MHC molecules is the species' protective response to the surrounding array of pathogenic organisms. Presumably, the variety of MHC molecules in the population enhances the probability that some pathogen-derived set of peptides will bind to MHC and activate a T-cell response in at least some individuals. To illustrate this point, imagine the extreme case if there were only one MHC molecule in the population. If a pathogen prevented the expression of this single MHC molecule (a situation we described earlier in the chapter that is a feature of the response to some viruses), no T-cell response would be mounted, and the entire species could be wiped out. Maintaining a large number of MHC genes and molecules in the species would greatly reduce the risk of such an event.

It is also apparent that the expression of a specific MHC allele is one of the important factors associated with susceptibility or resistance to different infectious agents. In humans, expression of specific HLA alleles has been associated with either susceptibility or resistance to a number of different infectious diseases, such as human T lymphotropic virus 1 (HTLV-1), hepatitis B, leprosy, malaria, tuberculosis, and rapid progression to AIDS. Similar MHC associations have been shown in infectious diseases afflicting other species. These include Marek's disease (a viral disease in chickens) and bovine leukemia virus infection in cows. In addition, as discussed in more detail in Chapter 12, individuals with certain HLA alleles have a higher risk of developing certain autoimmune or inflammatory diseases, although other genes and their products contribute to the development of these diseases.

Definitive mechanisms linking possession of a particular MHC gene or molecule with the onset or progress of disease have not been established for almost any of these diseases or conditions. Nonetheless, the onset and progression of many of these diseases are likely to be related in some way to the presentation of certain peptides by particular MHC molecules and the activation of "inappropriate" T-cell responses.

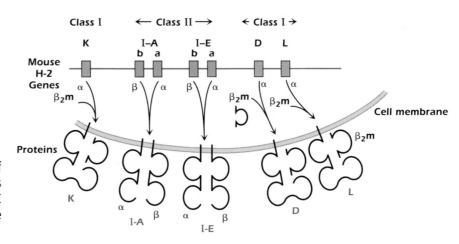

Figure 8.12. Simplified depiction of the mouse MHC, H-2, showing regions and genes coding for polymorphic MHC class I and II molecules expressed at the cell surface; β_2m encoded outside MHC.

SUMMARY

1. MHC molecules play a crucial role in the response of T cells to antigens that are taken into or live inside cells of the body: MHC molecules bind peptides derived from protein antigens and present them to T cells with the appropriate receptor. Thus, T-cell responses are said to be MHC restricted.

2. The MHC is a complex, a set of genes inherited as a unit. The MHC codes for two major categories of cell surface transmembrane molecules, MHC class I and MHC class II:
   - *MHC class I* is expressed on all nucleated cells in association with a small invariant peptide, β_2-microglobulin; peptide bound to MHC class I interacts with the TCR of a CD8$^+$ T cell, so responses of CD8$^+$ T cells are MHC class I restricted.
   - *MHC class II* is expressed constitutively only on cells that present antigen to T cells—APC such as dendritic cells, macrophages, and B cells. Peptide bound to MHC class II interacts at the cell surface with the TCR of a CD4$^+$ T cell. Thus, the response of CD4$^+$ T cells is MHC class II restricted.

3. The expression of MHC molecules is inducible on many cell types, particularly in response to cytokines generated in the response to infectious agents. This induction of expression enhances T-cell responses directed against the pathogen. Viruses inhibit MHC class I expression and so subvert the T-cell response directed against them.

4. Within one individual, the same MHC class I and II molecules are expressed on all cells of the body. Different individuals express different MHC class I and II molecules. This diversity arises because different individuals within a species have a huge range of inherited forms of MHC class I and II genes (genetic polymorphism), the most genetically diverse system in the population. Because of the extensive polymorphism of MHC genes, every individual has an almost unique array of inherited MHC genes.

5. The outer region of every MHC class I and II molecule contains a deep cleft called the peptide-binding groove that binds peptides derived from the catabolism (processing) of protein antigens.

The binding of peptides to MHC molecules is selective; that is, each MHC molecule favors the binding of peptides with particular motifs.

6. MHC class I and II molecules bind peptides derived from proteins processed in different compartments inside the cell.
   - *MHC class I* molecules bind peptides 8-9 amino acids long derived from proteins catabolized in the cytoplasm ("endogenous antigens"); peptides are transported into the endoplasmic reticulum where they interact with newly synthesized MHC class I and β_2-microglobulin chains.
   - *MHC class II* molecules bind peptides 12–17 amino acids long derived from proteins taken into cells ("exogenous" antigens) and catabolized in acid vesicles in APC.
   - Dendritic cells have a unique pathway—cross-presentation—in which antigen taken into the cell associates with MHC class I molecules and peptides are presented to CD8$^+$ T cells.

7. Because proteins are generally structurally complex, they usually generate at least one peptide able to bind to an MHC molecule, ensuring that a T-cell response is made to at least some part of a foreign antigen.

8. MHC class I molecules also interact with receptors on NK cells. This interaction prevents NK cells from killing normal cells of the host. Decreased expression of MHC class I, for example, after infection by certain viruses and in some tumors, results in NK cell killing of the host cell.

9. MHC molecules bind peptides derived from self-components as well as from foreign antigens, but self-components do not normally activate a T-cell response. This is because under normal conditions self-molecules do not generate the costimulator (second) signals needed to activate naïve T cells. The T-cell response is focused on the response to foreign (nonself) molecules, particularly components of pathogens, which induce these costimulator signals.

10. Susceptibility and resistance to many autoimmune and inflammatory conditions are associated with the expression of a particular MHC molecule.

REFERENCES

Bjorkman PJ, Saper MA, Samraoui B, Bennett WS, Strominger JL, Wiley DC (1987): Structure of the human class I histocompatibility antigen, HLA-A2. *Nature* 329:506–512.

Boyton RJ, Altmann DM (2007): Natural killer cells, killer immunoglobulin-like receptors and human leucocyte antigen class I in disease. *Clin Exp Immunol* 149:1–8.

Cresswell P, Ackerman AL, Giodini A, Peaper DR, Wearsch PA (2005): Mechanisms of MHC class I-restricted antigen processing and cross-presentation. *Immunol Rev* 207:145.

Rammensee HG, Falk K, Rötzschke O (1993): MHC molecules as peptide receptors. *Curr Opin Immunol* 5:35–44.

Rock KL, Shen L (2005): Cross-presentation: Underlying mechanisms and role in immune surveillance. *Immunol Rev* 207: 166.

Stern LJ, Brown JH, Jardetzky TS, Gorga JC, Urban RG, Strominger JL, Wiley DC (1994): Crystal structure of the human class II MHC protein HLA-DR1 complexed with an influenza virus peptide. *Nature* 368:215–221.

Stern LJ, Wiley DC (1994): Antigenic peptide binding by class I and class II histocompatibility proteins. *Structure* 2:245–251.

Trombetta ES, Mellman I (2005): Cell biology of antigen processing *in vitro* and *in vivo*. *Annu Rev Immunol* 23:975.

Trowsdale J (2005): HLA genomics in the third millennium. *Curr Opin Immunol* 17:498.

Villadangos JA, Schnorrer P, Wilson NS (2005) Control of MHC class II antigen presentation in dendritic cells: A balance between creative and destructive forces. *Immunol Rev* 207:191–205.

 # REVIEW QUESTIONS

For each question, choose the ONE BEST answer.

1. All the following are characteristics of both MHC class I and II molecules except:
   A) They are expressed codominantly.
   B) They are expressed constitutively on all nucleated cells.
   C) They are glycosylated polypeptides with domain structure.
   D) They are involved in presentation of antigen fragments to T cells.
   E) They are expressed on the surface membrane of B cells.

2. MHC class I molecules are important for which of the following?
   A) binding to CD8 molecules on T cells
   B) presenting exogenous antigen (e.g., bacterial protein) to B cells
   C) presenting intact viral proteins to T cells
   D) binding to CD4 molecules on T cells
   E) binding to Ig on B cells

3. Which of the following is *incorrect* concerning MHC class II molecules?
   A) B cells may express different allelic forms of MHC class molecules on their surface.
   B) MHC class II molecules are synthesized in the endoplasmic reticulum of APC.
   C) Genetically different individuals express different MHC class II alleles.
   D) MHC class II molecules are associated with β₂-microglobulin on the cell surface.
   E) A peptide that does not bind to an MHC class II molecule will not trigger a CD4⁺ T-cell response.

4. Products of *TAP-1* and *TAP-2* genes:
   A) bind β₂-microglobulin
   B) prevent peptide binding to MHC molecules
   C) are part of the proteasome
   D) transport peptides into the endoplasmic reticulum for binding to MHC class I
   E) transport peptides into the endoplasmic reticulum for binding to MHC class II

5. Which of the following statements about HLA genes is *incorrect*?
   A) They code for complement components.
   B) They code for both chains of every HLA class I molecule expressed.
   C) They code for both chains of every HLA class II molecule expressed.
   D) They are associated with susceptibility and resistance to different diseases.
   E) The total set of HLA alleles on the chromosome is known as the HLA haplotype.

6. Which of the following is found on the surface of every B cell, T cell and pancreatic cell?
   A) MHC class II molecules
   B) a rearranged antigen-specific receptor
   C) immunoglobulin
   D) MHC class I molecules
   E) CD19

7. After a virus infects a boy's liver cells, which of the following about the processing and presentation of virus-derived proteins is correct?
   A) All the peptides derived from the processing associate with his HLA class I molecules.
   B) Processing occurs exclusively in acid vesicles.
   C) The virus-derived peptides that bind to his HLA class I molecules also bind to his sister's HLA class I molecules.
   D) Some virus-derived peptides are presented to CD8⁺ T cells.
   E) His HLA class I molecules preferentially bind virus-derived peptides 12–17 amino acids long.

ANSWERS TO REVIEW QUESTIONS

1. *B* MHC class I molecules are expressed on all nucleated cells, but the constitutive expression of MHC class II molecules is limited to APC such as B cells and dendritic cells. MHC class II expression can be induced on other cell types such as endothelial cells and fibroblasts by cytokines.

2. *A* The interaction of CD8 expressed on the T cell and an invariant region of an MHC class I molecule expressed on a host cell plays a critical role in the triggering of CD8$^+$ T cells (see also Chapters 9 and 10).

3. *D* The MHC class I molecule, not the MHC class II molecule, associates with β_2-microglobulin.

4. *D* The products of the *TAP-1* and *TAP-2* genes selectively transport peptides generated in the cytoplasm into the endoplasmic reticulum where peptides 8-9 amino acids long they may bind to a newly synthesized MHC class I molecule.

5. *B* HLA class I molecules are expressed at the cell surface with β_2-microglobulin; the gene coding for β_2-microglobulin is located outside the MHC, on a different chromosome.

6. *D* MHC class I molecules are expressed on these cells, and all nucleated cells. MHC class II molecules are expressed constitutively on APC such as B cells, but not on T cells or pancreatic cells. T cells and B cells express an antigen-specific receptor (see also Chapter 9) but pancreatic cells do not. Ig and CD19 are expressed by B cells (Chapter 7).

7. *D* Because of the selectivity of binding of peptides to MHC molecules, some but not all of the peptides derived from processing the virus proteins are likely to associate with the boy's HLA class I molecules and activate a virus-specific CD8$^+$ T-cell response. The peptides that bind to HLA class I molecules are eight to nine amino acids long. Because the boy's sister is expected to have a different HLA haplotype, a distinct set of virus-derived peptides will bind to her HLA class I molecules.

9

BIOLOGY OF THE T LYMPHOCYTE

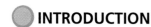

INTRODUCTION

Earlier chapters focused on the characteristics of B lymphocytes and their receptor for antigen, immunoglobulin. In Chapter 8 we introduced the role of immune responses involving T lymphocytes (T cells) and discussed the key roles of MHC molecules and peptides in these responses.

The focus of this chapter is the characteristics of T cells. As described in the previous chapter, we believe that T cells evolved to deal with the crucial phase of the response to pathogens—such as viruses, bacteria, and parasites—that takes place inside host cells. Because proteins are either major components of pathogens or are synthesized by pathogens, T cells play a critical role in the response to nearly all the harmful agents—and "harmless" antigens—to which an individual is exposed.

First we describe the T cell's receptor for antigen—*the TCR*—and compare its characteristics with those of Ig, and then we will describe other important molecules on the T-cell surface. Next we explain the key steps in T-cell development in the thymus, the organ in which a developing T cell acquires its TCR, and describe the critical role played by MHC molecules during T-cell development in the thymus.

THE ANTIGEN-SPECIFIC T-CELL RECEPTOR

Molecules That Interact with Antigen

Like B cells, T cells express an antigen-specific receptor that is *clonally distributed*; every clone of T cells expresses a TCR with a unique sequence. The huge repertoire of TCR molecules, calculated to be on the order of 10^{18} different possible structures, is generated by the same V(D)J gene rearrangement strategies described for Ig molecules in Chapter 6. The unique aspects of TCR gene rearrangement are discussed in more detail later in the chapter.

The left side of Figure 9.1 shows the form of the TCR expressed on the majority of mature T cells in humans and many other species. It comprises two disulfide-linked polypeptide chains, α and β. The TCR α and β are transmembrane glycoproteins with short cytoplasmic tails; because of differences in expression of carbohydrate, the molecular weights of the chains vary between 40 and 60 kDa. The TCR α and β chains comprise variable (V) and constant (C) regions, analogous to the V and C regions of Ig molecules (see Fig. 4.3 and 4.14). Each TCR V and C region folds into an Ig-like domain. In addition, like Ig,

Immunology: A Short Course, Sixth Edition, By Richard Coico and Geoffrey Sunshine
Copyright © 2009 John Wiley & Sons, Inc.

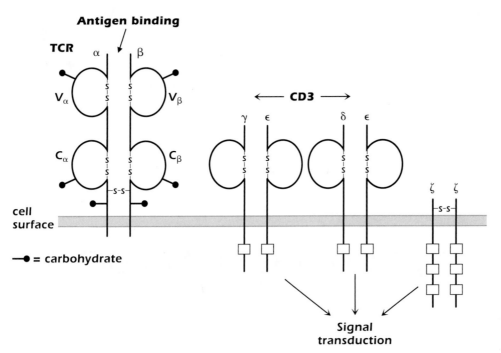

Figure 9.1. TCR complex: α and β antigen-binding chains with associated signal transduction complex, CD3 (γ, δ, and ε chains) plus ζ. ITAMs are indicated by rectangular boxes.

the TCR Vα, and Vβ regions contain three hypervariable or complementarity-determining regions (**CDR1**, **CDR2**, **and CDR3**; see Fig. 4.4) that come together in the three-dimensional structure to form the antigen-binding site.

The similarities between the structures of the TCR and Ig and the organization of the genes that code for these molecules (to be discussed later in the chapter) suggest that the TCR and Ig evolved from a common ancestral gene. As we described in Chapter 4 and illustrated in Figure 4.14, these genes are said to belong to the *Ig gene superfamily*, and the molecules are referred to as members of the *Ig superfamily*.

Although the structures of the TCR and Ig are similar, they differ in several important ways.

Valence and Conformation. The TCR is a two-chain structure that forms a single binding site for antigen; in other words, the TCR is monovalent and resembles the monovalent Fab fragment of an antibody. The TCR has a rigid conformation, unlike the four-chain Ig molecule with its hinge and two antigen-binding sites. These properties give the Ig molecule a flexibility that allows it to bind bivalently to antigens of different shapes and sizes. As described below, the rigid conformation of the TCR is appropriate for binding to the surface of other host cells, and the flexibility of Ig molecules facilitates binding to antigens either at the surface of the B cell or in solution.

Antigen Recognition. In Chapters 3 and 4 we described how Ig binds to many different types of antigen

(carbohydrates, DNA, lipids, and proteins), which it encounters in fluids such as serum. Ig can also respond to linear *and* conformational epitopes in an antigen; thus, both the three-dimensional shape and the sequence of an antigen are important in eliciting antibody responses. By contrast, as described in Chapter 8, the TCR interacts predominantly with small fragments of proteins called peptides, which are expressed on the surface of a host cell in association with a MHC. (In Chapter 8 we noted that the TCR of some T cells can recognize lipids.) Consequently, in contrast to the variety of structures and shapes recognized by Ig molecules, the antigen recognized by the TCR is generally a combination of MHC molecule (either MHC class I or II) and a small linear peptide (8–9 amino acids long for peptides bound to MHC class I or 12–17 amino acids long for peptides bound to MHC class II).

As noted in Chapter 8, the TCR makes critical interactions with both the MHC molecule and the peptide. The hypervariable region formed by the Vα and Vβ in the center of the TCR interacts with the two or three amino acids in the center of the peptide (see Fig. 9.2). This hypervariable region (known as the third hypervariable loop) is in CDR3 of the TCR. As we describe later in the chapter, CDR3 is the most variable region of the TCR. Thus, the variability of sequences among CDR3s in different TCRs appears critical in ensuring that different TCRs react specifically with only certain peptides.

Secretion of Receptor. Unlike Ig, the TCR does not exist in a specifically secreted form and is not secreted as a consequence of T-cell activation. Thus, unlike Ig, the

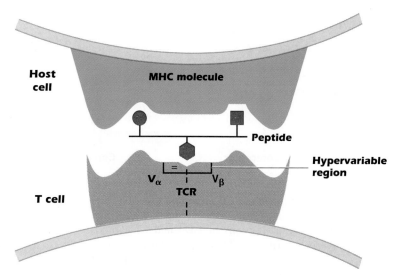

Figure 9.2. Interaction of TCR with prototypical MHC molecule (class I or II) and bound peptide expressed on the surface of a host cell.

TCR does not have an "effector" function. Rather, as we describe in Chapter 10, T-cell activation results in cytokine secretion and/or the killing of infected host cells. By contrast, after antigen binds to membrane Ig and activates the B cell, the B cell differentiates into a plasma cell that secretes Ig with the same antigenic specificity expressed by the B cell that initially bound the antigen (see Chapter 7).

No Change in TCR During Response to Antigen.

As we discussed in Chapters 6 and 7, over the course of a response to antigen, Ig molecules undergo *somatic hypermutation* (with associated affinity maturation) and *isotype switching*, the linking of one set of genes coding for a particular V region to different C region genes. These mechanisms are unique to B cells: The TCR does not change during the response to antigen.

T-Cell Receptor Complex

Figure 9.1 shows that the antigen-recognizing α and β chains of the TCR are also expressed on the surface of T cells in tight, noncovalent association with the molecule *CD3* and with two identical ζ (*zeta*) chains (*CD247*, molecular weight 16 kDa). CD3 and ζ do not bind antigen. They are *signal transduction molecules* activated after antigen binding to the α and β chains of the TCR and are analogous to the Igα and Igβ molecules associated with Ig at the surface in the B-cell antigen-specific receptor complex described in Chapter 7. The combination of the TCR α and β chains plus CD3 and ζ is referred to as the *TCR complex*.

CD3 comprises the three distinct polypeptides γ, δ, and ε (molecular weights 25, 20, and 20 kDa, respectively). All of these molecules contain a characteristic Ig-fold loop structure and are members of the Ig superfamily. Because CD3 plays a "chaperone" role in transporting the newly synthesized TCR molecule through the cell to the cell surface, it is always associated with the TCR. CD3 is *invariant* (the same) on all T cells; because it is expressed exclusively on T cells it can be used as a marker to distinguish T cells from all other cells.

Each chain of the CD3 complex also contains one tyrosine-containing sequence referred to as an *immunoreceptor tyrosine-based activation motif*—also found in Igα and Igβ—and the ζ chain contains three. As will be discussed in more detail in Chapter 10, after antigen binds to the α and β chains of the TCR, the ITAMs of the CD3 and ζ chains play important roles in the early phases of T-cell activation.

Coreceptor Molecules

On mature T cells, the TCR is expressed on the T-cell surface in association with another transmembrane molecule referred to as a *coreceptor*. The T-cell coreceptor does not bind antigen but enhances the ability of antigen to activate T cells; in other words, expression of the coreceptor *lowers the threshold* for antigen responses in ways that will be described below. In this way the T-cell coreceptor is analogous to the B-cell coreceptor—the complex of CD19, CD21, and CD81—that was described in Chapter 7.

Figure 9.3 shows that the coreceptor on mature T cells is either *CD4* or the two-chain molecule *CD8*, both of which are members of the Ig superfamily. As we describe later in this chapter, only immature T cells differentiating in the thymus express *both* CD4 and CD8. CD4 and CD8 are more or less specifically expressed on T cells; expression of the coreceptor splits the T-cell population into two major subsets, referred to as CD4$^+$ T cells and CD8$^+$ T cells. In healthy people, the ratio of CD4$^+$ T cells to CD8$^+$ T cells in the circulation is approximately 2 : 1, but in conditions with depleted levels of CD4$^+$ T cells, such as AIDS, this ratio is decreased (see Chapter 17).

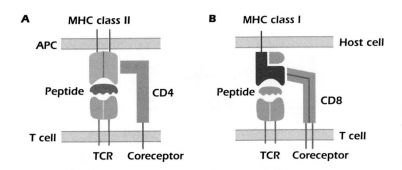

Figure 9.3. TCR coreceptors and their interaction with MHC molecules expressed on host cells: (A) CD4 with MHC class II expressed on APC; (B) CD8 with MHC class I expressed on all nucleated cells.

CD4 and CD8 have several important functions:

- The extracellular portions of CD4 and CD8 bind to the invariant portions of MHC molecules expressed on the surface of host cells. Figure 9.3A shows that CD4 binds selectively to cells expressing **MHC class II molecules**; as we described in Chapter 8 and will discuss further in this chapter and Chapter 10, MHC class II molecules are expressed constitutively on APC: dendritic cells, macrophages, B cells, and thymic epithelial cells. Thus, CD4⁺ T cells interact with host cells expressing antigen bound to MHC class II.

  Figure 9.3B shows that CD8 binds selectively to cells expressing **MHC class I molecules**, which are expressed on the surface of all nucleated cells in the body. Thus, CD8⁺ T cells interact with cells expressing antigen associated with MHC class I.

- The binding of CD4 or CD8 to MHC molecules expressed on the APC helps to tighten the binding of T cells to APC. Thus, CD4 and CD8 act as **adhesion molecules** in T-cell interactions with APC.

- CD4 and CD8 are involved in **signal transduction** after antigen binding to the TCR. Specifically, the intracellular portions of CD4 and CD8 are linked to enzymes, known as protein tyrosine kinases, which are important early components of the T-cell activation pathways. This concept will be discussed more fully in Chapter 10.

- A unique characteristic of the CD4 molecule is that it binds to HIV. This allows the virus to infect cells expressing CD4, eventually leading to the disease AIDS (see Chapter 17). In humans, CD4 is expressed at low levels by macrophages and dendritic cells as well as T cells; thus, all of these types of cells may be infected by HIV.

Other Important Molecules Expressed on the T-Cell Surface

In the following paragraphs and in Figure 9.4 we describe molecules in addition to those associated with the TCR complex and the T-cell coreceptors that play important roles in T-cell function.

Costimulatory Ligands. In order to be activated, **naïve T cells**, those T cells that have not previously encountered antigen, need more than the **first signal** interaction between peptide and MHC expressed on the APC and the TCR expressed by the T cell. In addition, naïve T cells need **second signals**, also known as **costimulatory interactions**, for full T-cell activation. These costimulatory interactions enhance the signal delivered by the TCR complex.

Multiple pairs of such costimulatory molecules have been defined on the T cell and APC surfaces. The best understood costimulatory interaction is between **CD28** expressed on the mature T cell and the **B7 family** of molecules expressed on APC. This interaction, which we will discuss in more detail in Chapter 10, is critical for antigen-activated T cells to synthesize the cytokine IL-2, a T-cell growth factor, which is required for the proliferation of T cells. T cells also express **CD40 ligand (CD40L or CD154)**, which interacts with CD40 expressed on macrophages, dendritic cells, and B cells. This interaction enhances the B7-CD28 costimulatory interaction. The CD40–CD40 ligand interaction also plays a critical role in T-cell-dependent isotype switching in B cells.

It is now apparent that the interaction of some costimulator pairs has effects distinct from activation of T cell, including *negative* signaling. **CTLA-4 (CD152)**, a molecule closely related to CD28, is expressed on activated T cells and interacts with B7 molecules to impart a negative signal to the activated T cell, which helps to terminate the response.

Molecules Involved in Adhesion and Homing. **CD2**, like CD4 and CD8, has adhesive and signal transduction properties. CD2 is expressed almost exclusively on T cells and is expressed by nearly all mature T cells. In humans, CD2 interacts with **CD58 (LFA-3)** expressed on many different cells.

T cells also express surface molecules associated with **homing**, the preferential entry of different types of lymphocytes into different tissues. Like B-cell homing (described in Chapter 7), T-cell homing is tightly regulated by the expression pattern of adhesion molecules and chemokine receptors (described below); their pattern of expression changes with the activation state of the cell.

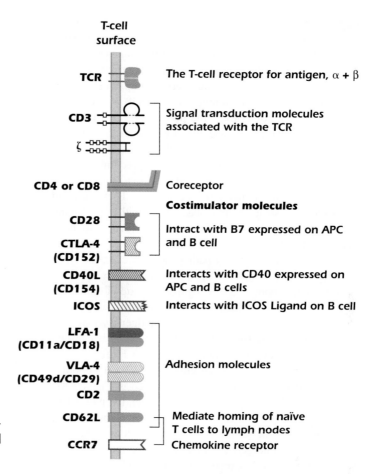

Figure 9.4. Important molecules expressed at T-cell surface. Hatched bars indicate expression induced on activated cell.

Naïve T cells, like naïve B cells, circulate through peripheral and mucosal lymph nodes. This enhances their ability to interact with antigen because naïve lymphocytes are not normally found in tissues, where an individual is likely to be exposed to pathogens. Entry of naïve T lymphocytes to lymph nodes is mediated by the expression of the same set of adhesion molecules and chemokine receptors expressed by naïve B cells. The critical adhesion molecules are *CD62L (L-selectin)* for entry to peripheral nodes (those outside the intestine) and the integrin α4β7 for nodes in the mucosa. These adhesion molecules bind to glycoproteins known as *addressins*, which are expressed on cells of the high endothelial venules, the specialized region of the vascular endothelium at the boundary of the nodes. Naïve T cells also express the chemokine receptor *CCR7*, which binds chemokines expressed by high endothelial venules of peripheral and mucosal nodes. Binding of the appropriate combination of adhesion molecule and chemokine receptor to their ligands expressed by high endothelial venules allows naïve T cells to leave the circulation and enter a particular lymph node. The mechanisms by which lymphocytes enter tissues from the bloodstream are similar to those described for other leukocytes in Chapter 11.

As will be described in more detail in Chapter 10, once T cells are activated in the nodes, the resulting *effector cells* and *memory T cells* change their patterns of expressing adhesion molecules and chemokine receptors and migrate out of the nodes and home to specific tissues. The expression pattern of adhesion molecules and chemokine receptors provides a "homing signature" or "address code" that identifies the tissue to which the T cell migrates. Generally, this homing takes the effector or memory T cell back to the region in which the T cell was originally activated; for example, cells that were initially activated in nodes draining the gut will home back to the gut.

LFA-1 (CD11aCD18) is another member of the two-chain integrin family expressed on a broad range of T cells. LFA-1 interacts with several ligands, including *ICAM-1(CD54)*, expressed on endothelial cells and APC such as macrophages and dendritic cells.

γδ T Cells. Most human T cells use αβ as their TCR but a minor population expresses a distinct two-chain TCR known as γδ; the cells expressing this receptor are referred to as *γδ T cells*. The γδ TCR is expressed in association with CD3 and ζ. (Note that the γδ chains of the TCR are different from the γ and δ chains of CD3.) Generally, γδ cells lack the CD4 and CD8 coreceptor molecules found on αβ-expressing T cells, but γδ cells found in the intestine express CD8. As we describe later in this chapter, the αβ and γδ lineages diverge early in intrathymic development.

γδ T cells are found predominantly at mucosal epithelial sites such as the skin, gut, and lung but are found at proportionately much lower numbers than αβ T cells in the circulation of normal adult humans. γδ T cells are present in all mammals at some level; the peripheral blood of ruminant species, which include the cow and deer, can have higher circulating levels of γδ T cells than αβ T cells.

Because γδ TCR cells are found predominantly at mucosal sites they are considered to provide a first line of defense against invading pathogens. They respond to pathogens such as mycobacteria, rapidly producing cytokines, particularly interferon gamma; they also have cytotoxic function. Thus, γδ TCR cells provide a first line of defense against invading pathogens. However, the types of antigens with which γδ T cells interact differ from the peptide–MHC complexes recognized by αβ T cells; γδ T cells respond to phospholipids and other small non-protein molecules, known as phosphoantigens, as well as *heat-shock proteins* (proteins that form in cells when they are heated or stressed in different ways). γδ T cells interact with these antigens presented either by CD1 or nonpoly-morphic MHC class I molecules (discussed in Chapter 8).

As we will describe in the next section, the number of possible structures that can be generated by recombination of Vγ and Vδ gene segments is as high or higher than the number that can be generated by recombination of Vα and Vβ gene segments. For reasons that are not clear, however, there is much less variability in the γδ TCR repertoire than in the αβ T-cell repertoire. γδ cells found at different sites in the body appear to use distinct but limited combinations of Vγ and Vδ gene segments.

GENES CODING FOR T-CELL RECEPTORS

The organization of the human gene loci coding for the α, β, γ and δ TCR chains is shown in Figure 9.5. Note the following features:

- The α and γ chains are constructed from V and J gene segments, like Ig light chains, but β and δ chains are constructed from V, D, and J gene segments, like Ig heavy chains.

- Gene segments of the α and δ TCR loci are interspersed on the same chromosome; in fact, genes coding for the δ chain of the TCR are flanked on both the 5′ and 3′ sides by genes coding for the α chain. Gene rearrangement mechanisms at the α and δ loci ensure that α and δ are not expressed on the same T cell.

- The β and γ TCR loci are each found on different chromosomes.

- There are many more Vα and Vβ genes (approximately 50 and 70, respectivley) than Vγ and Vδ genes (5–10) in the germline. In addition, there are two different Cβ genes ($C\beta_1$ and $C\beta_2$), but these genes and their products are virtually identical and have no known functional differences. Thus, they should not be confused with antibody isotypes, in which the Ig heavy-chain constant genes and products differ considerably and have different effector functions: the TCR C regions do not have effector function.

GENERATION OF T-CELL RECEPTOR DIVERSITY

The mechanisms for generating diversity in TCRs are very similar to the mechanisms of generating diversity in BCRs. The same fundamental principles of gene rearrangement described in Chapter 6 for Ig apply in the synthesis of the V and C regions of each chain of TCRs α, β, γ and δ. *Recombinases* and *joining sequences* are used to link up a VJ or a VDJ unit, generating the variable-region specificity of a particular TCR polypeptide chain. The same enzymes are involved in the recombination events in both B and T cells. As described in Chapters 6 and 7, the two genes known as *recombination activation genes (RAGs)*, *RAG-1* and *RAG-2*, play a crucial role in activating the recombinase

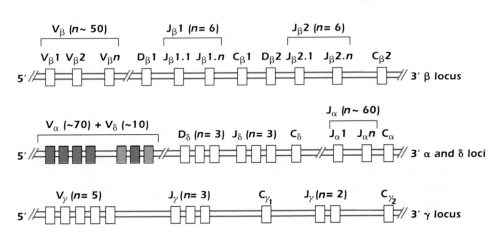

Figure 9.5. Organization of human α, β, γ and δ genes coding for TCR.

genes in both early B cells and early T cells. In addition, like B cells (see Chapter 6), defects in V(D)J recombination, which involve breakage and rejoining of DNA segments, can lead to disease, particularly malignancy, in the T-cell lineage (see also Chapter 17).

In summary, as in the generation of Ig diversity, TCR diversity is generated by (1) multiple V genes in the germline, (2) random combination of chains, and (3) junctional and insertional variability. However, earlier in the chapter we pointed out one important difference between the generation of diversity in TCRs and Ig molecules: Following antigenic stimulation Ig undergoes somatic hypermutation, but the TCR does not.

The theoretical number of different TCR structures that can be generated for $\alpha\beta$ and $\gamma\delta$ TCRs is approximately 10^{13}, the repertoire of $\alpha\beta$ T cells found in an individual is smaller, and, as noted earlier in the chapter, the number of $\gamma\delta$ T cells is still smaller. Junctional and insertional variability, which are important contributors to TCR diversity, result in an enormous number of different sequences for the part of the hypervariable region of the TCR known as CDR3. (The sequences of the TCR CDR1 and CDR2 are not generated by rearrangement but are coded for by the V genes found in the germline.) CDR3 is the region of the $\alpha\beta$ TCR binding site that makes contact with amino acids in the center of a peptide bound to an MHC molecule (see Fig. 9.2). The large number of different TCR CDR3 sequences ensures that TCR binding to the peptide portion of the peptide–MHC complex is highly specific.

In Chapter 6 we also described how Ig genes show allelic exclusion, which ensures that a single B cell makes a receptor with specificity for a single antigen. TCRβ and TCRγ genes also show allelic exclusion.

T-CELL DIFFERENTIATION IN THYMUS

As described in Chapter 2, the *thymus*, located above the heart, is the primary lymphoid organ for the development of T cells; it is here that precursor cells acquire the TCR as well as other characteristics of T cells. (As discussed in Chapter 7, the bone marrow is the primary organ for mammalian B-cell development.) Some children are born with a thymus that fails to develop correctly *in utero* (DiGeorge syndrome; see also Chapter 17); mice in which the thymus does not develop are called **nude mice** because they also lack hair. In both these cases mature T cells do not develop and T-cell responses are defective.

DiGeorge Syndrome

T-cell differentiation in the thymus occurs throughout the life of the individual but diminishes significantly after puberty. The size of the thymus decreases with the onset of puberty in mammals (*thymic involution*), presumably because of the increased synthesis of steroid hormones. In some species, particularly the mouse, the mature T-cell population is drastically depleted if the thymus is removed within a few days after birth. Indeed, these were the pioneering observations that established the crucial role of the thymus in T-cell responses. Removing the thymus later in the development of the animal has much less impact on the mature T-cell population.

T-cell differentiation in the thymus is a complex multistep process. As with the early phases of B-cell differentiation, most of the information about the early phases of T-cell differentiation in the thymus derives from work in nonhuman species such as the mouse. The paragraphs that follow and Figures 9.6 and 9.7 will focus on critical checkpoints in T-cell development, including descriptions of the interactions of developing T cells with nonlymphoid cells of the thymus, the sequence of TCR gene rearrangements, the differing pattern of expression of the coreceptor molecules CD4 and CD8, and thymic selection.

Interactions of Developing T Cells with Nonlymphoid Cells of Thymus

Figure 2.8 shows the detailed structure of the thymus and the cells within it. Developing T lymphocytes in the thymus (*thymocytes*) are in contact with, and interact with, a mesh formed by the thymic nonlymphoid cells, the most important of which are (1) epithelial cells in the *cortex* and *medulla* (the outer and inner regions of the thymus, respectively) and (2) dendritic cells, found predominantly at the junction of the cortex and medulla. Thymic dendritic cells are derived from bone marrow and are members of the same family of cells that present antigens to T cells in other tissues and organs (see Chapter 10). Thymic epithelial cells and thymic dendritic cells express MHC class I *and* II molecules, a characteristic of APC.

The nonlymphoid cells provide critical cell surface interactions required for thymic selection, which will be described shortly. The nonlymphoid cells also produce the cytokine *IL-7*, which induces proliferation and survival of cells in the early stages of T-lymphocyte development. Indeed, the thymus is a site of intense proliferation of developing T cells; however, the vast majority of these cells—calculated to be around 95% of the cells produced daily—dies in the thymus for reasons that will be described in subsequent sections of this chapter.

The pathways of T cell development in the thymus are illustrated in Figure 9.6 and in the paragraphs that follow.

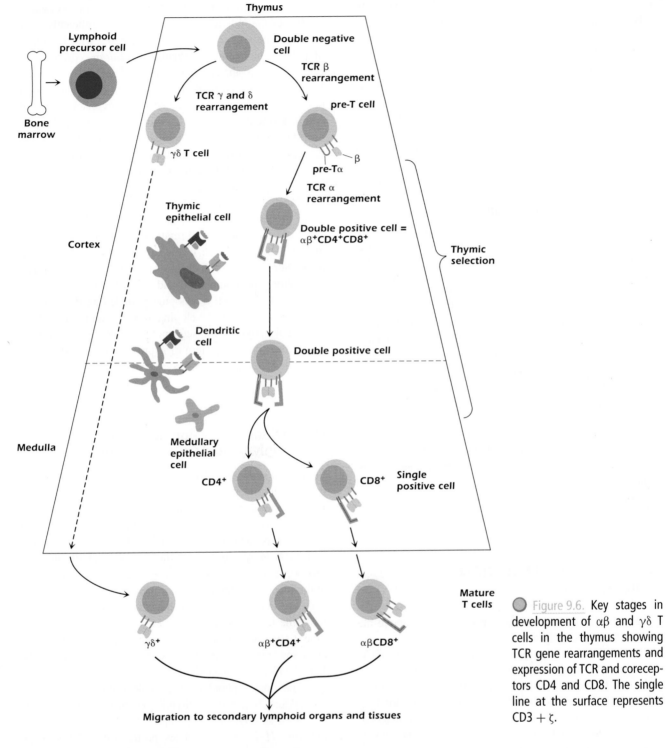

Figure 9.6. Key stages in development of αβ and γδ T cells in the thymus showing TCR gene rearrangements and expression of TCR and coreceptors CD4 and CD8. The single line at the surface represents CD3 + ζ.

Early T-Cell Receptor Gene Rearrangements: Double-Negative Cells and Splitting Off of γδ T Cells

Bone marrow-derived precursor cells enter the thymus through the blood at the junction of the cortex and medulla. As we describe later in the chapter, these precursors are not fully committed to the T-cell lineage; other cell types may also develop from these very early thymic precursor cells. These early thymic precursors have their TCR genes in an unrearranged (germline) configuration.

TCR γ, δ, and β-chain genes then start to rearrange more or less simultaneously in the thymic cortex; these cells do not express either the CD4 or CD8 coreceptor and so are referred to as *double-negative cells*. The decision

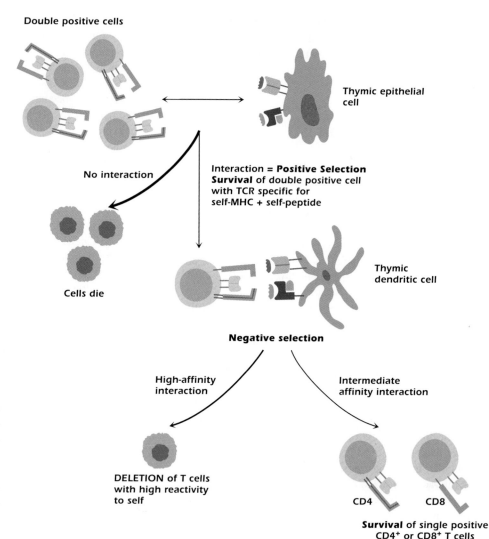

Figure 9.7. Positive and negative thymic selection: positive selection, showing interaction of $\alpha\beta TCR^+CD4^+CD8^+$ double-positive cell with cortical epithelial cells; negative selection, showing double-positive cell interacting with thymic dendritic cell.

whether to become an $\alpha\beta$ or a $\gamma\delta$ T cell occurs at the double-negative stage, but the signals that determine the pathway chosen are not well understood. Double-negative cells that productively rearrange both a γ and a δ gene shut down β-gene rearrangement and express TCR γ and δ chains on the cell surface in association with CD3 and ζ. These $\gamma\delta$ TCR-expressing cells exit the thymus and form the pool of peripheral $\gamma\delta$ T cells. Cells expressing $\gamma\delta$ as their TCR $\gamma\delta$T cells arise early in development of the individual but are later swamped by the development of $\alpha\beta$ T cells.

Pre-T Cells

Double-negative cells that productively rearrange a β gene express the TCR β chain on the surface of the cell in association with an invariant molecule known as *pre-Tα*. These cells are referred to as ***pre-T cells***. The combination of β chain and pre-Tα (together with CD3 and ζ) constitutes the ***pre-T cell receptor (pre-TCR)***, analogous to the pre-B-cell receptor expressed by pre-B cells that we discussed in Chapter 7.

Signaling through the pre-TCR, like signaling through the pre-B-cell receptor, is a critical checkpoint in the development of cells expressing α and β as their TCR. Signaling through the pre-TCR stops further rearrangement of TCRβ genes, ensuring that it expresses only one type of β chain (allelic exclusion). In addition, expression of pre-Tα is down-regulated, *RAG1* and *RAG2* genes are reactivated, and α genes start to rearrange. As noted above, gene segments of the α and δ TCR loci are interspersed on the same chromosome, so rearrangement of the α focus on a particular chromosome also deletes the δ locus. The α genes do not show allelic exclusion, so rearrangement of α genes may occur on both chromosomes.

Double-Positive Cells

Signaling through the pre-TCR also initiates cell proliferation and the expression of CD4 and CD8. Thus, the next cell in the T-cell differentiation sequence expresses an $\alpha\beta$ TCR (together with CD3 and ζ) and both CD4 and CD8 coreceptor molecules on its surface. This $\alpha\beta^+CD3^+CD4^+CD8^+$

thymocyte, referred to as a CD4+CD8+ or ***double-positive cell***, comprises the biggest population of thymocytes (over 80%) in the young mammalian thymus. Double-positive cells are found in the cortex but not the medulla of the thymus.

 THYMIC SELECTION

Double-positive thymocytes undergo the critical process known as ***thymic selection*** that is shown in Figure 9.7. As its name implies, thymic selection ensures that double-positive thymocytes with only specific characteristics are selected to develop further. The double-positive cells that survive thymic selection—a very small percentage of the initial double-positive population—differentiate further and leave the thymus to form the populations of mature CD4+ and CD8+ T cells.

Thymic selection comprises two major stages: positive selection and negative selection. In both stages the TCR complex plus CD4 and CD8 expressed by double-positive cells makes critical interactions with MHC molecules plus peptides expressed by thymic nonlymphoid cells. These interactions determine the fate of the double-positive cell. Because most studies suggest that positive and negative selection take place on different thymic nonlymphoid cells found in different parts of the thymus, this is the scenario that we describe in the subsequent paragraphs.

In the first stage, ***positive selection***, double-positive cells interact with MHC class I and II molecules expressed by epithelial cells in the thymic cortex. This interaction results in the survival of the double-positive cell. A double-positive cell that does not make this interaction dies. Our understanding of the mechanisms of thymic selection is still incomplete, but current evidence indicates that the ***affinity*** of these interactions determines the outcome. Thus, to survive and be positively selected, the double-positive T cell must have some affinity for ***self-MHC***, the MHC molecules that are expressed by the individual's thymic epithelial cells. As described in Chapter 8, MHC molecules expressed on the surface of cells have peptides bound in their peptide-binding groove and this is true for thymic epithelial cells, which have peptides bound to both MHC class I and II molecules at the cell surface; these peptides are derived from self-molecules found in the thymus. Thus, we can say that positive selection is the recognition by the double-positive cell of a combination of ***self-MHC and self-peptide***.

If the double-positive cell has a receptor with no affinity or very low affinity for self-MHC, then it is not selected and dies by apoptosis. This appears to be the case for the vast majority of double-positive cells generated in the thymus (more than 90%); presumably, the random generation of TCRs by gene recombination results in the development of many double-positive cells with TCRs that have very low affinity for the MHC and peptide combinations expressed by thymic cortical epithelial cells.

Positive selection also results in the down-regulation of *RAG-1* and *RAG-2* gene expression, so no further gene rearrangement occurs. This stops further attempts at rearrangement by the TCR α genes. Consequently, even if a cell expresses two different α chains in combination with a β chain (as appears to be the case in some human and mouse T cells), positive selection of a developing T cell on one MHC–peptide complex ensures that only one of the expressed TCR αβ-chain combinations is functional.

Although a double-positive T cell needs to have some affinity for self-MHC to be positively selected, allowing T cells with too high a reactivity to self-MHC to leave the thymus could result in undesirable autoimmune responses in tissues. This is prevented by ***negative selection***: double-positive cells with too high a reactivity to self-MHC are removed.

Negative selection is thought to occur primarily when the double-positive cell interacts with dendritic cells at the interface of the cortex and medulla, but recent evidence, described below, suggests that epithelial cells in the medulla also play a role. A double-positive cell that reacts with too high an affinity to the combination of MHC and peptide is deleted by apoptosis. Thus, negative selection removes T cells expressing TCRs with high reactivity to self-components; in other words, negative selection prevents T-cell reactivity to self-components. This is a critical feature of the development of ***central tolerance*** in T cells, analogous to the development of central tolerance in B cells described in Chapter 7 (see also Chapter 12).

To summarize the selection process, we can say that double-positive cells with affinity that is either *too low* or *too high* for self-MHC do not survive thymic selection. Only double-positive cells with some *intermediate* affinity for self-MHC survive thymic selection.

As we mentioned above, several questions remain about the mechanisms involved in thymic selection. The central issue is to understand how the signals delivered by the same pairs of molecules (MHC plus peptides and TCR plus coreceptors) differ in positive versus negative selection. The nature of the intracellular signals involved and the identification of thymic nonlymphoid cells involved in different stages of selection are areas of intense research activity. Another key question is whether the peptides expressed by thymic nonlymphoid cells differ in positive versus negative selection. Some evidence supports this possibility, but further studies will be needed to resolve the issue.

Role of AIRE Gene Product in Negative Selection

We described above that negative selection involves the presentation of peptides derived from self molecules by dendritic cells in the thymus. As a consequence, developing T cells potentially responsive to molecules found in the thymus are deleted. How do we develop self-tolerance to molecules normally found outside the thymus? Studies indicate that at least some self-molecules normally synthesized by tissues outside the thymus, including insulin (the pancreas), thyroglobulin (thyroid), and myelin basic protein (central nervous system), are expressed by epithelial cells in the thymic medulla.

These studies suggest that the medullary epithelial cells—and more specifically, the product of the *autoimmune regulator* or *AIRE* gene expressed by these cells—also plays a role in negative selection (see also Chapter 12). The AIRE gene product codes for a protein that at least partly controls the expression of self-molecules in thymic medullary epithelial cells. If the AIRE gene product is lacking, deletion of autoreactive T lymphocytes is impaired and autoimmune responses develop: the rare individuals who do not make a functional product of the *AIRE* gene suffer from a condition called autoimmune polyendocrinopathy-candidiasis-ectodermal dystrophy syndrome (APECED), in which multiple endocrine organs are targeted.

Single-Positive Cells

Double-positive cells that survive negative selection down-regulate expression of either CD4 or CD8, resulting in either *CD4$^+$* or *CD8$^+$* *("single-positive") T cells*, which are found in the thymic medulla. The precise mechanism by which a double-positive cell down-regulates the expression of one of its coreceptors is currently unclear. Single-positive T cells are the endpoint of the complex pathway of αβ TCR differentiation in the thymus; from studies in mice it has been determined that this process takes approximately three weeks.

CD4$^+$ and CD8$^+$ T cells leave the thymus via the bloodstream. As mentioned earlier in the chapter, these naïve T cells express a pattern of adhesion molecules and chemokine receptors that allows them to circulate through all secondary lymphoid organs, where a cell with the appropriate receptor may encounter and respond to antigen. Naïve T cells may live for a long time (up to years) in a resting state without encountering antigen; recent studies suggest that mature T cells in the periphery that have not encountered antigen need signals (including the cytokine IL-7) to keep them alive.

Generation of the T-Cell Repertoire

Thymic differentiation of T cells expressing αβ as their TCR generates a huge repertoire of mature CD4$^+$ T cells and CD8$^+$ T cells in the periphery, that is, outside the thymus, that the individual uses to respond to the universe of nonself- (foreign) antigens. As we described in the section of Chapter 2 on the clonal selection hypothesis, T-cell clones with the appropriate receptor for self-MHC plus peptide exist in the repertoire prior to exposure to antigen. As with B cells, the appropriate T-cell clone may never be triggered because the person may never be exposed to that particular virus or bacterium. Nonetheless, it can almost be guaranteed that the T cell (or B cell) with the "right" receptor is present; under the conditions described in Chapter 10, this receptor will be triggered by foreign antigen.

Characteristics of αβ T Cells Emerging from Thymus

As noted above, the thymus is a site of intense proliferation but also of the death of the overwhelming majority of developing thymocytes. The single-positive CD4$^+$ and CD8$^+$ T cells that emerge from the thymus are the survivors of many critical steps in the differentiation pathways. The surviving single-positive T cells have two important characteristics:

1. *T cells are self-MHC restricted*: Positive selection gives rise to a population of T cells that respond to antigen *only* when associated with the MHC molecule(s) that the developing T cell interacted with in the thymus. This interaction gives T cells a sense of immunological "self": The MHC molecules that the developing T cell encounters define "self-MHC" for the rest of the life of the surviving T cell. In the previous chapter, we referred to the MHC restriction of T-cell responses. More specifically, we say that T-cell responses are *self*-MHC-restricted; mature CD4$^+$ and CD8$^+$ T cells respond to a combination of self-MHC and peptide.

2. *T cells are self-tolerant*: Negative selection prevents the emergence from the thymus of T cells with too high a reactivity to self-molecules (such as molecules made by the liver or pancreas). Thus, mature CD4$^+$ and CD8$^+$ T cells do not respond to self components.

Note that a developing T cell that survives thymic selection has been selected as a result of an interaction with self-MHC + *self*-peptide, that is, a peptide derived from a self-molecule expressed in the thymus. Nonetheless, the same T cell responds as a mature T cell to self-MHC + *nonself*-peptide, that is, derived from a "foreign" antigen. How does the same TCR respond to both self- and nonself-peptides? As described in Chapter 8, the most likely explanation is that a single MHC molecule may bind different peptides; studies suggest that an MHC molecule's peptide-binding properties are flexible enough to allow peptides derived from self- *and* nonself-proteins to bind.

Further Differentiation of CD4$^+$ and CD8$^+$ T Cells Outside Thymus

As will be described more fully in Chapter 10 and later chapters of the text, once a CD4$^+$ T cell or a CD8$^+$ T cell has been triggered by antigen, it differentiates into an **effector** T cell; CD4$^+$ effector cells predominantly synthesize cytokines that affect the activity of a vast array of cell types. CD8$^+$ effector cells predominantly kill host cells infected with viruses. A small fraction of antigen-activated T cells become **memory** cells, long-lived cells that play a key role in the second or subsequent responses to antigen and help provide protection in second and subsequent exposures to many pathogens. It is not currently clear whether memory cells differentiate from effector cells or whether memory and effector cells diverge early after activation. As described earlier in the chapter, effector and memory T cells use the same types of "address codes" of adhesion molecules and chemokine receptors that are used by activated B cells (see Chapter 7) to home to tissues to combat infection, particularly to sites such as the skin and mucosa.

Differentiation of Other Sets of Cells in Thymus

This chapter has focused on the development of the two major subsets of T cells, CD4$^+$ and CD8$^+$ T cells, which use α and β chains as their TCR. We also described the properties and differentiation in the thymus of T cells that use $\gamma\delta$ as their TCR. The following are other sets of cells that develop in the thymus and are found outside the thymus.

NK Cells.   NK cells develop in the thymus from the same bone marrow precursor that gives rise to the T-cell lineage. However, because NK cells split off from the T-cell lineage at an early stage of double-negative cells before TCR genes start to rearrange, they do not express a TCR. NK cells, which are involved in the early phase of the immune response and are considered part of the innate immune defenses, kill virus-infected and tumor cells (see Chapter 2). NK cells express the molecules CD16 and CD56, which may be used to distinguish them from other cell types.

NKT Cells.   NKT cells are a small subset of T cells (about 1% of peripheral blood mononuclear cells in people) that express both a TCR and a surface molecule, NK1.1 (CD161c in humans) characteristic of NK cells. NKT cells respond to glycolipid antigens presented by CD1d, rather than MHC molecules. NKT cells regulate the function of other sets of T cells and are thought to have key roles in regulating conditions including autoimmunity, cancer, and infection. NKT cells arise in the thymus when the recombination events in the developing T cell generate a T cell with a TCR that interacts, by chance, with CD1d expressed by thymic nonlymphoid cells. Because most NKT cells use only one type of TCR Vα gene and a limited number of Vβ genes, their TCR usage is referred to as *semi-invariant*. Consequently, they are thought not to respond to a wide variety of antigens. Because of these characteristics, NKT cells are considered to have features of both the innate and adaptive immune defenses.

T$_{reg}$ Cells.   T$_{reg}$ cells are a subset of CD4$^+$ T cells (approximately 10% of peripheral CD4$^+$ T cells) that inhibit the actions of other sets of T cells. They characteristically express the molecule CD25 and the transcription factor Foxp3 (discussed further in Chapters 11 and 12). T$_{reg}$ cells that develop in the thymus are autoreactive; that is, they are T cells that recognize combinations of self-peptide and self-MHC but have survived negative selection in the thymus. Some T$_{reg}$ cells also develop outside the thymus. T$_{reg}$ cells play a role in inhibiting responses to both self *and* foreign antigens; in this way, they help to maintain and regulate self-tolerance and limit potentially damaging host responses to pathogens in tissues (see Chapter 12).

SUMMARY

1. T cells express a unique, clonally distributed receptor for antigen, known as the T-cell receptor. The same V(D)J recombination strategies and recombinase machinery used by B cells to generate Ig diversity are also used to generate a huge repertoire of T cells with different TCRs.

2. On the majority of human and mouse T cells, the TCR is a two-chain transmembrane molecule, $\alpha\beta$. The TCR comprises V and C regions, analogous to those of Ig molecules. The extracellular portion of the TCR resembles the Fab fragment of an antibody.

3. An $\alpha\beta$ TCR interacts with peptide bound to an MHC molecule on the surface of a host cell. The antigen-binding $\alpha\beta$ chains are expressed on the surface of the T cell in a multimolecular complex (the TCR complex) in association with CD3 and ζ polypeptides, which act as a signal transduction unit after antigen binding to $\alpha\beta$.

6. Coreceptor molecules are associated with the $\alpha\beta$ TCR. On mature T cells the coreceptor is either CD4 or CD8, dividing T cells into two major subsets, either $\alpha\beta^+$ CD4$^+$ or $\alpha\beta^+$ CD8$^+$. The functions of these coreceptor molecules are (a) to bind to the invariant portion of an MHC molecule on a host cell (CD4 with MHC class II and CD8 with MHC class I); (b) to tighten the adherence between the T cell and the host cell and (c) to play a role in signal transduction after activation of the TCR.

5. The T cell also expresses molecules on its surface with important costimulatory and adhesion properties. These include CD28, CTLA-4 (CD152), the integrins LFA-1 (CD11aCD18) and VLA-4 (CD49dCD29), and CD2. The pattern of expression of adhesion molecules and chemokine receptors plays a key role in homing of T cells at different stages of differentiation to different tissues.

6. $\gamma\delta$ is the TCR on a minor population of human T-cells found predominantly at mucosal epithelial sites such as the intestine and skin. $\gamma\delta$ is expressed on the surface of the T cell in association with CD3 and ζ. Most $\gamma\delta^+$ T cells do not express CD4, but some express CD8. The functions of $\gamma\delta^+$ T cells are not as well understood as those of $\alpha\beta^+$ T cells, but they are thought to have a role as a first line of defense against pathogens.

7. The thymus is the organ in which developing T cells acquire a TCR. The thymus is a site of intense proliferation and differentiation of developing T cells but most die there. The few mature T cells that emerge give rise to the mature population of T cells found in the circulation and tissues outside the thymus.

8. TCR gene rearrangement starts in early "double-negative" thymocytes in the thymus. $\alpha\beta$ and $\gamma\delta$ T cells diverge at the double-negative stage. If $\gamma\delta$ T cells are formed, they exit the thymus.

9. Alternatively, thymocytes that express a rearranged β chain express it on the surface in association with a nonrearranged molecule, pre-Tα, in the pre-T cell. The next stage of $\alpha\beta^+$ T cells development is a "double-positive" cell, expressing an $\alpha\beta$TCR (in association with CD3 and ζ) and both coreceptor molecules, CD4 and CD8.

10. The double-positive cell undergoes thymic selection, mediated by interactions of the TCR and CD4 and CD8 on the developing T cell with MHC molecules and peptides expressed by the thymic nonlymphoid cells. *Positive selection* on cortical epithelial cells "educates" the developing T cell: as a mature cell, it responds to antigen only when presented by a cell that expresses the same MHC molecules that the T cell interacted with during differentiation in the thymus (self-MHC restriction of the T-cell response). *Negative selection* on dendritic cells and medullary epithelial cells removes T cells with potential reactivity to self-molecules, ensuring self-tolerance. Thus, $\alpha\beta$TCR$^+$ T cells that emerge from the thymus are self-MHC restricted and self-tolerant.

11. $\alpha\beta$TCR$^+$CD4$^+$ and $\alpha\beta$ TCR$^+$ CD8$^+$ T cells that survive negative selection, together with $\gamma\delta^+$ T cells, leave the thymus. These cells constitute the repertoire of peripheral T cells in blood, secondary lymphoid organs, and tissues that respond to nonself- (foreign) antigen. After antigen activation, a T cell differentiates into an effector cell; some activated T cells become memory CD4$^+$ or CD8$^+$ cells.

12. In addition to $\alpha\beta$ and $\gamma\delta$ T cells, NK cells, NKT cells, and T$_{reg}$ cells also develop in the thymus.

REFERENCES

Anderson G, Lane PJ, Jenkinson EJ (2007): Generating intrathymic microenvironments to establish T-cell tolerance. *Nature Rev Immunol* 7:954.

Gallegos AM, Bevan MJ (2006): Central tolerance: Good but imperfect. *Immunol Rev* 209:290–296.

Kronenberg M, Engel I (2007): On the road: Progress in finding the unique pathway of invariant NKT cell differentiation. *Curr Opin Immunol* 19:186–193.

Laky K, Fowlkes BJ (2005): Receptor signals and nuclear events in CD4 and CD8T cell lineage commitment. *Curr Opin Immunol* 17:116–121.

Lauritsen JP, Haks MC, Lefebvre JM, Kappes DJ, Wiest DL (2006): Recent insights into the signals that control $\alpha\beta/\gamma\delta$-lineage fate. *Immunol Rev* 209:176–190.

Mathis D, Benoist C (2007): A decade of AIRE. *Nature Rev Immunol* 7:645.

Rodrigo Mora J, von Andrian UH (2006): Specificity and plasticity of memory lymphocyte migration. *Curr Top Microbiol Immunol* 308:83–116.

Rudolph MG, Stanfield RL, Wilson IA (2006): How TCRs bind MHCs, peptides, and coreceptors. *Annu Rev Immunol* 24:419.

REVIEW QUESTIONS

For each question, choose the ONE BEST answer.

1. Which of the following statements concerning T-cell development is correct?
   A) Progenitor T cells that enter the thymus from the bone marrow have already rearranged their TCR genes.
   B) Interaction with thymic nonlymphoid cells is critical.
   C) Maturation in the thymus requires the presence of foreign antigen.
   D) MHC class II molecules are not involved in positive selection.
   E) Mature, fully differentiated T cells are found in the cortex of the thymus.

2. The development of self-tolerance in the T-cell compartment is important for the prevention of autoimmunity. Which of the following results in T-cell self-tolerance?
   A) allelic exclusion
   B) somatic hypermutation
   C) thymocyte proliferation
   D) positive selection
   E) negative selection

3. Which of the following statements is correct?
   A) The TCR chains transduce a signal into a T cell.
   B) A cell depleted of its CD4 molecule would be unable to recognize antigen.
   C) T cells with fully rearranged TCR chains are not found in the thymus.
   D) T cells expressing the TCR are found only in the thymus.
   E) CD4$^+$ CD8$^+$ T cells form the majority of T cells in the thymus.

4. Which of the following is *incorrect* regarding mature T cells that use αβ as their antigen-specific receptor?
   A) They coexpress CD8 on the cell surface.
   B) They may be either CD4$^+$ or CD8$^+$.
   C) They interact with peptides derived from nonself-antigens.
   D) They can further rearrange their TCR genes to express γδ as their receptor.

E) They circulate through blood and lymph and migrate to secondary lymphoid organs.

5. Which of the following statements is *incorrect* concerning TCR and Ig genes?
   A) In both B- and T-cell precursors, multiple V-, D-, J-, and C-region genes exist in an unrearranged configuration.
   B) Rearrangement of both TCR and Ig genes involves recombinase enzymes that bind to specific regions of the genome.
   C) Both Ig and TCR are able to switch C-region usage.
   D) Both Ig and the TCR use combinatorial association of V, D, and J genes and junctional imprecision to generate diversity.

6. Which of the following statements is *incorrect* concerning antigen-specific receptors on both B and T cells?
   A) They are clonally distributed transmembrane molecules.
   B) They have extensive cytoplasmic domains that interact with intracellular molecules.
   C) They consist of polypeptides with variable and constant regions.
   D) They are associated with signal transduction molecules at the cell surface.
   E) They can interact with peptides derived from nonself-antigens.

7. Which of the following is correct concerning the characteristics of T cells that exit the thymus?
   A) do not express CD4 or CD8 but express a TCR that has high affinity for MHC plus self-antigen
   B) express CD4 and CD8 but no TCR and have low affinity for MHC plus self-antigen
   C) express either CD4 or CD8 with a TCR that has high affinity for MHC plus self-antigen
   D) express either CD4 or CD8 with a TCR that has low to moderate affinity for MHC plus self-antigen
   E) express CD4, CD8, and a TCR that has high affinity for MHC plus self-antigen

ANSWERS TO REVIEW QUESTIONS

1. *B* Interaction of thymocytes with thymic nonlymphoid cells—cortical epithelial cells, dendritic cells and medullary epithelial cells—is critical in T-cell development.

2. *E* Negative selection removes developing T cells with potential reactivity to self-molecules.

3. *E* CD4$^+$ CD8$^+$ T cells form the majority of cells in the thymus.

4. *D* The genes of T cells that use αβ as their receptor cannot further rearrange to use γδ as their receptor; TCR δ gene segments are interspersed with the α locus and are deleted when the α locus rearranges.

5. *C* The ability to change the heavy-chain constant region while retaining the same antigen specificity is a property unique to Ig. The other features are common to both the TCR and Ig.

6. *B* Both the TCR and Ig have short cytoplasmic tails. The signal transduction molecules associated with the antigen-binding chains interact with intracellular molecules.

7. *E* T cells that use αβ as their TCR and emerge as the end stage of differentiation in the thymus express either CD4 or CD8 (as well as a TCR) and, as a result of thymic selection, have a low to intermediate affinity for self-antigen associated with self-MHC (the MHC molecules expressed by the individual's thymic non-lymphoid cells.)

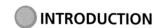

ACTIVATION AND FUNCTION OF T AND B CELLS

 INTRODUCTION

In this chapter we describe the events that follow the interaction of antigen with mature T and B cells that express the appropriate receptor. The events are broadly similar in both sets of lymphocytes: T and B cells are activated, they proliferate, and further differentiate into *effector cells*. A small fraction of the expanded cell population becomes *memory cells*. The effector functions of T and B cells are completely different, however: Effector CD4$^+$ T cells secrete an array of cytokines that affect many different cell types; and effector CD8$^+$ T cells are directly cytotoxic to infected cells of the host. By contrast, the activation and differentiation of B cells results in the synthesis of antibody of different isotypes. This chapter will focus on how T and B cells are activated, how they exert their effector functions, and how they interact.

ACTIVATION OF CD4$^+$ T CELLS

Specialized Cells Present Antigen to Naïve CD4$^+$ T Cells

As described in Chapter 8, specialized, or "professional", APC—dendritic cells, macrophages, and B cells—process protein antigens and present selected catabolized linear fragments of the protein (peptides) to T cells. Antigens can enter the body by several different routes—especially the airways, gastrointestinal tract, or skin—and APC are found at all of these entry sites as well as in lymphoid organs and other tissues throughout the body.

Dendritic cells, a heterogeneous family of cells found in the circulation and many tissues, are the principal APC for initiating *primary T-cell responses*—that is, the first activation of naïve mature T cells by foreign antigen. In Chapter 9 we discussed the role of dendritic cells in negative selection of developing T cells in the thymus, a key feature of the establishment of central tolerance in the T cell population. Thus, dendritic cells play a critical role in both the activation and tolerization of T cells. As we describe in more detail below, dendritic cells are a key example of the influence of cells of the innate immune system on responses of the adaptive immune system.

Two major subsets of dendritic cells—"myeloid" and "plasmacytoid"—have been distinguished based on expression of surface molecules and function. *Plasmacytoid dendritic cells* synthesize the interferons α and β in the early phases of an immune response and are major contributors to the innate phase of the response to pathogens such as viruses. In the paragraphs below, in Figure 10.1, and in subsequent chapters we focus on *myeloid dendritic cells* because they have a major role in the induction of T-cell responses.

Figure 10.1 shows some of the key characteristics of dendritic cells that contribute to their effectiveness as APC for CD4$^+$ T cells, in this case in the response to a Gram-negative bacterium that has infected a tissue. First,

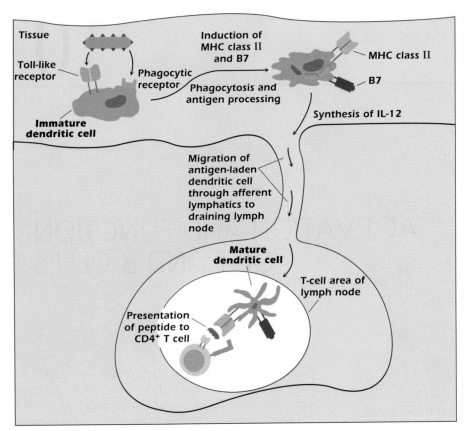

Figure 10.1. Dendritic cell maturation in response to pathogen: The immature cell interacts with a bacterium in a tissue; processes bacterial proteins; up-regulates the expression of MHC class II and costimulatory molecules, and migrates to the T-cell area of the lymph node draining the tissue.

dendritic cells are found in many tissues in addition to the thymus; dendritic cells are also found in tissues close to the entry sites for antigen as well as secondary lymphoid organs such as the lymph nodes and spleen.

Second, as shown on the left of Figure 10.1, dendritic cells found in tissues (referred to as *immature dendritic cells*) typically express many different *pattern recognition receptors* (*PRR*) that interact with components of several types of infectious microorganisms, particularly bacteria and viruses (described in Chapter 2). Among these PRR are the Toll-like receptors (TLRs), a family of predominantly cell surface molecules that interact with bacterial DNA, lipoprotein, and lipopolysaccharide, as well as viral RNA and DNA. In Figure 10.1, the cell wall of a Gram-negative bacterium contains lipopolysaccharide, which interacts with TLR-4 expressed on the dendritic cell. Immature dendritic cells in tissues also express phagocytic receptors, which enhance uptake of the bacterium into the cell.

Once inside the cell, the immature dendritic cell is also very efficient at catabolizing (processing) the protein components of the bacterium into peptides in the acid vesicle, MHC class II pathway of the cell that we described in Chapter 8. The uptake and processing of a pathogen by a dendritic cell also induce the expression of high levels of MHC class II and costimulatory molecules, particularly of the B7 family that we referred to in

Chapter 7; we will describe the function of MHC class II and costimulatory molecules further in this chapter. The dendritic cell's interaction with bacterial pathogens also results in the synthesis and secretion of many cytokines. One of the most important of these is IL-12; the function of IL-12 in shaping the response of T cells is described later in this chapter and in Chapter 11. The dendritic cell also upregulates the expression of the chemokine receptor CCR7 (see Chapter 11). Because the ligand for CCR7 is expressed by high endothelial venules at the entrance to lymph nodes, the antigen-stimulated dendritic cell leaves the tissue where it encountered the pathogen and migrates via the lymphatics to the lymph node "draining" the tissue.

The migration of an antigen-bearing dendritic cell to the draining node, combined with the ability of naïve T cells to recirculate through lymph nodes (Chapters 2 and 9), increases the likelihood that the rare T cell expressing the "correct" TCR—estimated to be about 1 in 10^5–10^6 of the total T-cell population—interacts with an antigen-bearing dendritic cell. The lower part of Figure 10.1 shows that the interaction of the now *mature dendritic cell* with a naïve CD4+ T cell takes place in the T-cell area of the node. The mature dendritic cell presents the combination of MHC class II and peptide on its cell surface to a CD4+ T cell with the appropriate TCR. The interaction between the antigen-bearing dendritic cell and the CD4+ T cell generally occurs in vivo within 8–10 hours of exposure to antigen.

In the last few years researchers have developed new approaches to visualize the events that occur in an intact (mouse) lymph node during the response to antigen. Multiphoton intravital microscopy is one such technique; it uses lasers that penetrate deep into tissues, different fluorescent "tags" to identify different cell types, and a camera to record events over several hours. Researchers can now visualize the early events that occur in the development of T- and B-cell responses in an intact lymph node for a period of several hours after antigen is administered. This technique has been used to visualize the activation of CD4+ T cells by dendritic cells, the development of the germinal center, and the activation of CD8+ T cells. These techniques should help to shed light on critical cellular interactions in the induction of many different immune responses.

Note that in the absence of signals induced by pathogens immature dendritic cells express low levels of costimulatory and MHC class II molecules. Thus, antigens that do not induce high levels of costimulator function do not activate naïve T cells. This is why it is believed that the encounter of a dendritic cell with self-molecules in normal tissue does not lead to activation of the dendritic cell or of T cells—costimulator function is not induced (see Chapter 8). Similarly, as pointed out in Chapters 3 and 8, T-cell and antibody responses to many "harmless" foreign antigens (e.g., injection with peptides or even small proteins that are found in some vaccines) may evoke little or no response unless administered with an *adjuvant*. One of the key features of an adjuvant—and those used in nonhuman species frequently include bacteria or synthetic bacterial components—is the activation of APC, in particular to express costimulatory molecules.

Paired Interactions at the Surface of APC and CD4+ T Cells

Figure 10.2 and the paragraphs in this section describe the key interactions that take place between the surfaces of the dendritic cell (and other types of APC) and the CD4+ T cell in the T-cell area of the lymph node, which lead to activation of the CD4+ T cell.

Peptide/MHC and TCR. The interaction between peptide + MHC class II molecule expressed on the APC and the variable regions, Vα + Vβ, of the T-cell's TCR is the critical antigen-specific *first signal* for the activation of the CD4+ T cell. Recent studies indicate that the TCR can detect very small number of foreign peptides—as

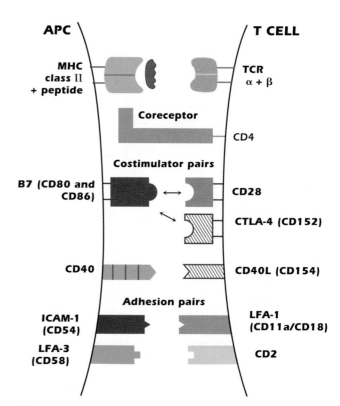

Figure 10.2. Paired interactions at the surface of an APC and a CD4+ T cell that lead to T-cell activation, cytokine synthesis, and proliferation. Hatching indicates expression upregulated by activation.

low as four peptide molecules out of the thousands of peptides expressed on a particular APC—so the T cell is very sensitive to foreign antigen. However, because this interaction is of low affinity, it is necessary but not sufficient for the activation of naïve CD4+ T cells. The paired interactions described below enhance the affinity of the interaction between the TCR and the peptide–MHC.

MHC Class II with CD4 Coreceptor. The interaction of the nonpolymorphic region of an MHC class II molecule (the region outside the peptide-binding groove) with the coreceptor CD4 greatly enhances the ability of the T cell to respond to antigen and hence lowers the T-cell antigen stimulation threshold. It has been estimated that the CD4–MHC class II interaction makes a cell 100-fold more responsive to antigen than in the absence of the interaction. In addition, CD4 plays an important role in T-cell signal transduction, which is described in more detail below under "Intracellular Events in CD4+ T-Cell Activation."

Costimulator Pairs. Earlier in the chapter we described how the interaction with pathogen induces *costimulator* molecules on the surface of dendritic cells. Costimulator pairs at the surface of the dendritic cell (and other APC) and the CD4+ T cell deliver *second signals* that enhance and sustain signals delivered by the first signal, the MHC–peptide–TCR interaction. The mechanisms thought to be responsible are described later in the chapter.

The best characterized costimulator interactions are between a family of molecules known as *B7*, expressed on professional APC (dendritic cells, macrophages, and activated B cells) and *CD28*, expressed constitutively on T cells. The B7–CD28 interaction is a critical positive signal in $CD4^+$ T-cell activation: As we discuss further in Chapter 12, in the absence of the B7–CD28 signal, the first signal alone not only is insufficient to activate the naïve $CD4^+$ T cell but also results in T-cell inactivation (anergy).

Within the B7 family, most is known about *B7.1* and *B7.2* (CD80 and CD86, respectively), both of which bind to CD28. It is currently not clear if B7.1 and B7.2 have distinct functions. Figure 10.2 also shows that B7.1 and B7.2 interact with *CTLA-4* (*CD152*), which is induced by T cell activation. As we discuss later in the chapter, the B7–CTLA-4 interaction plays a role later in T-cell activation to turn off the response.

A further important costimulatory interaction occurs between *CD40* expressed by APC and *CD40 ligand* (*CD40L*, or *CD154*) expressed on activated T cells. The interaction of peptide–MHC with the TCR upregulates T-cell expression of CD40L, which in turn induces increased expression of CD40 on the APC. This CD40–CD40L interaction further increases B7 expression on the APC, enhancing the B7–CD28 interaction between the APC and the T cell. The interaction of CD40 ligand on activated T cells with CD40 expressed on B cells has an additional critical role in T cell–B cell interactions that we will describe later in the chapter.

Recent studies have expanded the number of molecules in the B7 family as well as their paired ligands on the surface of the activated T cell (not shown in Fig. 10.2). Inducible costimulatory molecule (*ICOS*) is induced on $CD4^+$ T cells by TCR activation and interacts with its ligand, *ICOSL*, expressed on APC, particularly B-cells, and many other types of cells. The ICOS-ICOSL interaction has an important role in T-cell-B-cell interactions that we describe later in the chapter. The costimulator function of other molecules in the B7 and CD28 families is currently being evaluated.

Adhesion Molecules. Pairs of adhesive interactions strengthen and stabilize the interaction of the APC and T cell over the several hours that the cells need to be in contact to ensure T-cell activation. These are (1) *intercellular adhesion molecule 1 (ICAM-1, CD54)* expressed on the APC and the integrin *leukocyte function-associated antigen 1 (LFA-1, CD11a/CD18)* expressed on the T cell (molecules expressed on multiple cell types) and (2) *CD58* (*LFA-3*) expressed on the human APC and *CD2*

expressed on the T cell. These adhesive interactions are also thought to slow down the movement apart of the APC and T cell after the cells first interact. This allows more time for the TCR to "scan" the APC for the appropriate MHC class II–peptide.

Intracellular Events in $CD4^+$ T-Cell Activation

Figure 10.3 and the following paragraphs describe the intracellular pathways in $CD4^+$ T-cell activation. Although the focus of the discussion is the activation of $CD4^+$ T cells, the pathways described are very similar for the activation of $CD8^+$ T cells and B cells as well.

In brief, the recognition of antigen at the cell surface triggers multiple intracellular cascades that spread in an ordered manner from the surface of the cell through the cytoplasm and into the nucleus. As a consequence of activation, the T cell also reorganizes the structure of both its internal cytoskeleton and its cell membrane. Some events occur within seconds, others within minutes, and yet others within hours of the initial interaction. As a result of these events, the T cell changes its pattern of gene expression from a resting or quiescent state to an activated state; the cell proliferates and expands the initial clone size and differentiates into an effector cell able to carry out the major T-cell functions.

Understanding the intracellular pathways of T-cell activation also provides insights into how T-cell activation may be blocked and the function of activated cells prevented. These concepts are critical in the treatment of many different conditions—including transplantation, autoimmunity, and allergy—in which T-cell activation is an undesirable but central features (further discussed in chapters 12 and 18).

In the paragraphs below, we outline the sequence of events in the activation of the $CD4^+$ T cell.

Initial Signal. The binding of peptide–MHC to the extracellular variable regions ($V\alpha + V\beta$) of the TCR transmits a signal via the tightly associated CD3 and ζ molecules into the interior of the T cell. The nature of the signal across the membrane is not currently clear: It may involve the aggregation of multiple TCR molecules in the cell membrane (similar to the initial steps in activation through the BCR, described later in the chapter) or a conformational change in the transmembrane region of the TCR chains.

Activation of Kinases, Phosphorylation of ITAMs, and Assembly and Activation of Signaling Complexes at the Cell Membrane. One of the earliest detectable events inside the T cell after binding to the TCR is the activation within seconds of tyrosine kinases, *Fyn* - associated with the cytoplasmic regions of CD3 and ζ - and *Lck*, associated with the cytoplasmic regions of CD4. Fyn and Lck belong to the Src (pronounced "sark")

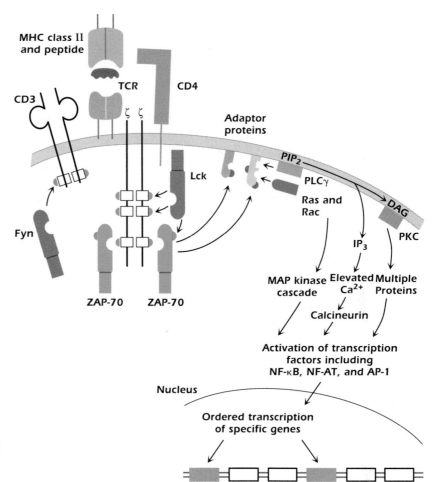

 Figure 10.3. Intracellular events in CD4+ T-cell activation. For simplicity, only one chain of CD3 and ζ and one phosphorylated ITAM are shown. Orange semicircles indicate phosphate groups added to activated molecules. The intracellular pathways that follow the B7–CD28 costimulator interaction are not shown; these result in enhanced transcription and increased stabilization of IL-2 mRNA.

family of tyrosine kinases, enzymes that activate proteins by adding phosphate groups to tyrosine residues. Fyn and Lck are activated by the membrane protein CD45 (not shown in Fig 10.2), a tyrosine phosphatase that removes inhibitory phosphate groups.

When Fyn and Lck are activated, they bind to regions of the CD3 and ζ chains that contain the previously described ITAMs and phosphorylate them. Because Lck is associated with CD4, this binding also pulls CD4 into close association with the TCR complex. The phosphorylated ITAMs in CD3 and ζ then act as docking sites for another tyrosine kinase, **ZAP-70** (belonging to a second tyrosine kinase family known as Syk). This step appears critical for T-cell activation, because T cells from the rare individuals who lack ZAP-70 do not respond to antigen; these individuals are profoundly immunodeficient (see Chapter 17) Because CD3 and ζ contain multiple ITAMs, more than one molecule of ZAP-70 is recruited into this complex of signaling proteins.

Lck activates ZAP-70 when it has joined the multiprotein signaling protein complex. Activated ZAP-70 phosphorylates multiple proteins inside the cell: Among the most important substrates of activated ZAP-70 are **adaptor** molecules—proteins that do not have enzymatic activity

but contain multiple binding domains for other proteins. Two adaptor molecules phosphorylated after T-cell activation are shown in Figure 10.3. The phosphorylated adaptors are recruited to the cell membrane, forming an even larger complex of signal transduction molecules at the immunologic synapse. In summary, a multiprotein complex of signal transduction molecules is assembled in sequence and activated on the cytoplasmic side of the T-cell membrane.

Formation of the Immunologic Synapse.

The interaction of APC and peptide with the CD4+ T cell forms an area of contact between the cells known as the **immunologic synapse**, by analogy with the area of contact between neurons and other cells. The immunologic synapse appears to be required for sustained intracellular signaling, lasting until the APC and T cell split apart after approximately 8 hours in contact. The synapses is also formed when CD4+ T cells interact with B cells, described later in the chapter. The synapse incorporates the MHC–peptide and TCR, CD4, and pairs of costimulatory and adhesion molecules. In addition, on the T-cell side, the synapse includes signaling molecules recruited from inside the T cell (described below) and cytoskeleton proteins.

The process of formation and development of the synapse is dynamic; its composition and structure change with time after the initial contact. For example, the paired adhesion molecules ICAM-1 and LFA-1 are found in different regions of the synapse at different times after initial contact between the cells. In addition, other molecules are included or excluded from the synapse at different times.

Several experiments suggest that the T cell reorganizes the structure of both its internal cytoskeleton and its cell membrane as a consequence of activation. In the T-cell membrane, the structure of the lipids is not homogeneous; instead, they form what are referred to as "microdomains" or lipid rafts, enriched in cholesterol and glycosphingolipids. When the T cell is activated, these lipid rafts—which had been dispersed throughout the membrane—are mobilized to the synapse and draw with them the intracellular signaling components described below. This redistribution also pushes those molecules not involved in the APC–T cell interaction out of the contact area.

Activation of Intracellular Signaling Pathways.

Activated adaptor molecules that are recruited to the immunologic synapse bind enzymes and other adaptors, activating several major intracellular signaling pathways. The adaptor molecules bind *phospholipase C-γ (PLC-γ)*; after being phosphorylated by ZAP-70, PLC-γ catalyzes the breakdown of the membrane *phospholipid phosphatidylinositol bisphosphate (PIP$_2$)*. PIP$_2$ is split into two components, *diacylglycerol (DAG)* and *inositol triphosphate (IP$_3$)*.

DAG activates the membrane-associated enzyme *protein kinase C (PKC)*, which in turn activates a cascade of kinases, ultimately leading to the activation

in the cytoplasm of a transcription factor, *NF-κB*. IP$_3$ increases intracellular free calcium levels. The increased calcium in turn activates the cytoplasmic molecule *calcineurin*, ultimately activating the transcription factor *NF-AT*. This pathway is clinically significant because the immunosuppressive agents cyclosporin A and tacrolimus (originally FK506)—used to prevent graft rejection when tissues are transplanted between genetically different individuals—bind to calcineurin and thereby inhibit the subsequent steps in T-cell activation (see Chapter 18).

In addition, activated adaptor molecules bind to and activate guanosine-nucleotide-binding proteins known as Ras and Rac, which in turn activate a cytoplasmic cascade of *mitogen-activated protein (MAP)* kinases, leading to the activation of the transcription factor AP-1.

IL-2 Synthesis and Proliferation.

The bottom part of Figure 10.3 shows that activated transcription factors NF-κB, NF-AT, and AP-1 enter the nucleus of the activated T cell and bind selectively to regulatory sequences of several different genes. Two of the most important genes that are transcribed and translated in the activated T cell (within 24 hours of the onset of activation) are the cytokine IL-2 and IL-2Rα (CD25), the α chain of the IL-2 receptor.

Figure 10.4 shows that the CD4$^+$ T cell that receives the first and second signals via the TCR and CD28, respectively, synthesizes and secretes IL-2. The critical role of the B7-CD28 second signal in the synthesis of IL-2 is discussed in the next section. IL-2 is a growth factor for T cells that can act on both the T cell that synthesized and secreted it and an adjacent T cell. Figure 10.4 also shows that the resting naïve CD4$^+$ T cell expresses two chains, β and γ, of the IL-2 receptor, which bind IL-2 with low to moderate affinity. The synthesis of the IL-2Rα chain as a consequence

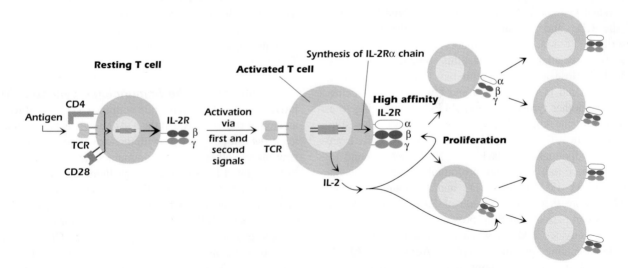

Figure 10.4. Activated CD4$^+$ T cell synthesizes and secretes IL-2 and synthesizes the IL-2 receptor α chain. The interaction of IL-2 and the high-affinity IL-2 receptor results in proliferation of CD4$^+$ T-cell clone.

of T-cell activation converts the IL-2 receptor on the surface of the activated T cell into a three-chain high-affinity receptor (a process described further in Chapter 11). Thus, the interaction of IL-2 and the high-affinity IL-2 receptor results first in enlargement of the CD4$^+$ T cell (to a *T-cell blast*) and then proliferation (within 48–72 hours after the initiation of activation).

IL-2 Synthesis and B7–CD28 and B7–CD152 Costimulator Interactions.

We referred earlier in the chapter to the interaction of B7 expressed on the APC and CD28 expressed on the naïve CD4$^+$ T cell providing a critical costimulatory or second signal in T-cell activation. The major mechanism by which this second signal augments T-cell activation is through the enhancement of IL-2 protein synthesis (calculated to be as much as 100-fold) over and above the IL-2 synthesis induced by signaling through the TCR alone. This enhancement results from both an increased rate of transcription of the IL-2 gene (via increased production of transcription factors) and an increase in the lifetime of IL-2 mRNA. In addition, the B7-CD28 interaction also mobilizes lipid rafts inside the T cell; this brings tyrosine kinases and other molecules involved in T-cell activation inside the T cell to the area of contact between the TCR and the APC. The B7–CD28 interaction is thought to initially activate a T-cell kinase, *phosphatidylinositol-3* (*PI*$_3$) kinase.

We previously mentioned the *negative* signal that results from the interaction between B7.1 and B7.2 and CTLA-4 (CD152), whose expression is induced on activated T cells. The interaction between B7 and CTLA-4 is of higher affinity than the interaction between B7 and CD28; consequently, the B7–CTLA-4 interaction turns off the production of IL-2 and thus ends T-cell proliferation, limiting the extent of the immune response. The mechanism of B7–CTLA-4's negative effect is not fully elucidated; like the B7–CD28 interaction, multiple biochemical pathways are probably involved. Recent studies suggest that CTLA-4 acts in the immunologic synapse by displacing critical components of the signaling complex and/or by limiting their function.

Clonal Expansion, Differentiation to Effector Cells, and Migration Out of the Lymph Node

As a consequence of the activation events we have described, CD4$^+$ T cells (and CD8$^+$ T cells if the antigen is an infectious organism) proliferate rapidly within a few days after initial exposure to antigen. This results in an enormous expansion of the original clone of antigen-specific cells: up to 10,000 times the original clone size in some virus infections. This expansion is noted as a swelling of the node in which the response occurs. Toward the end of this phase of rapid expansion,

the activated T cells differentiate into *effector T cells*, which now have the capability to carry out the effector function (synthesis of cytokines, killing of targets, etc.) of their particular subset of T cells. Effector cells generally exert their functions outside the node in which they were activated, particularly in tissues to which pathogens have gained access.

Activation of T cells in the node also results in a change in expression of adhesion molecules and chemokine receptors: Effector cells (and memory cells, described later in the chapter) migrate out of the node in which they were activated and move to different tissues. Effector cells down-regulate the adhesion molecule and chemokine receptor that allowed the naïve T cell to enter the node, L-selectin (CD62L) and CCR7, respectively. They upregulate adhesion molecules and chemokine receptors that allow them to migrate out of the node and move to different sites in the body, particularly to locations infected by pathogens (see also Chapter 9). For example, many effector cells upregulate the integrin VLA-4 (CD49CD29) and the chemokine receptor CCR10, which mediate homing to many tissues (except the skin) and sites of inflammation. Homing to skin is mediated by upregulation of CCR10 and the adhesion molecule, cutaneous lymphocyte antigen. Like that of activated B cells, migration of effector T cells to mucosal nodes is mediated by the integrin α4β7 and the chemokine receptor CCR9.

OTHER WAYS TO ACTIVATE CD4$^+$ T CELLS

In the preceding sections, we focused on how a peptide–MHC complex expressed on an APC activates a specific clone of T cells. Since naïve T cells expressing any one particular peptide specificity are rare, approximately 1 in 10^5–10^6 T cells (only a small fraction of the total T-cell pool) is activated by any one peptide–MHC complex. Detecting and studying the response to antigen of those rare antigen-specific cells in the total T-cell population have thus far proved challenging. To address questions about T-cell activation and function, immunologists have developed many tools for studying the responses of isolated antigen-specific T cells. These include growing clones of individual antigen-activated T cells *in vitro* and using transgenic mice that have T cells expressing only one TCR. These approaches have provided important information (see Chapter 5 for further discussion).

Some agents, however, can stimulate more than the rare clones of naïve CD4$^+$ T cells activated by peptide–MHC complexes. The agents we describe below activate multiple clones of T cells to produce cytokines and to proliferate.

Superantigens

Figure 8.9 showed the unique MHC–TCR binding properties of superantigens. In humans superantigens are predominantly bacterial toxins from disease-causing organisms, such as *Staphylococcus aureus*. Superantigens activate CD4$^+$ T cells expressing a particular Vβ molecule as one chain of its TCR. Since individual Vβ segments (such as Vβ$_3$ or Vβ$_{11}$) may be expressed in up to 10% of the T-cell population, a high percentage of T cells of various antigenic specificities may become activated when a superantigen interacts with an individual's T cells. The massive release of cytokines following superantigen action can result in injury to the host (see Chapter 11).

Plant Proteins and Antibodies to T-Cell Surface Molecules

Several naturally occurring materials have the ability to trigger the proliferation and differentiation of many if not all clones of T lymphocytes. These substances are referred to as polyclonal activators or **mitogens** because of their ability to induce mitosis of the cell population. The plant glycoproteins concanavalin A (Con A) and phytohemagglutinin (PHA) are particularly potent T-cell mitogens. These substances are **lectins**, molecules that bind to carbohydrate moieties on proteins. Both Con A and PHA are thought to act through the TCR. Because the T-cell response of healthy human blood to Con A and PHA falls in a well-defined range, a low response to Con A or PHA frequently indicates that a person is immunosuppressed. Another plant lectin, **pokeweed mitogen**, activates both T and B cells.

Some antibodies specific for CD3 have the ability to activate T cells. Since CD3 is expressed on all T cells in association with the T-cell receptor, these anti-CD3 antibodies thereby induce all T cells to proliferate.

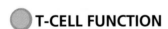 **T-CELL FUNCTION**

CD4$^+$ T Cells

As we wrote at the beginning of the chapter, the major effector function of CD4$^+$ T cells is the synthesis of a vast array of cytokines, which affect multiple cell types, including other sets of T cells, B cells, bone marrow precursor cells, and many effector cells of the innate immune response. The impact of cytokines synthesized by CD4$^+$ T cells on so many different cell types helps explain why the loss of CD4$^+$ T cells in AIDS is so devastating (see Chapter 17).

Many important functions of CD4$^+$ T cells will be discussed in subsequent chapters and the properties of cytokine receptors are discussed in detail in Chapter 11. This chapter will focus on the cytokines produced by CD4$^+$ T cells

and the interaction between CD4$^+$ T cells and B cells that results in the synthesis of antibody. Later in the chapter the function of CD4$^+$ T cells in the activation of CD8$^+$ T cells will be described.

Subsets of CD4$^+$ T Cells Defined by Cytokine Production and Effector Function

Until recently, the activated naïve CD4$^+$ T cell (T_H0) was described as differentiating into one of two major subsets of CD4$^+$ T cells, either T_H1 or T_H2, which differed in the cytokines they synthesized. Thus, each subset was characterized by the synthesis of a set of unique or "**signature**" cytokines, which are described below. Because each cytokine interacts with a specific receptor expressed on a particular effector cell (see Chapter 11), the cytokines synthesized by the different subsets of CD4$^+$ T cells interact with distinct sets of effector cells. These distinct sets of effector cells play different roles in the immune response.

The paradigm of subsets of CD4$^+$ T cells synthesizing differentiating cytokines that affect distinct effector cells still applies. (Some cytokines, including interleukin 3 and GM-CSF, are synthesized by both T$_H$1 and T$_H$2 subsets). Our understanding of the subsets of CD4$^+$ T cell has recently expanded and is reflected in Figure 10.5 and the following paragraphs. Figure 10.5 shows the four major subsets, which now include T_H17 and T_{reg} **cells** in addition to T$_H$1 and T$_H$2. The figure shows the signature cytokines that characterize all four subsets, the cells these cytokines interact with, and the types of effector functions in which they play a role. In the next section we describe how these different subsets of CD4$^+$ T cells are generated.

T$_H$1 cells synthesize IFN-γ macrophages; IL-2 and TNF-β (lymphotoxin). These cytokines activate CD8$^+$ T cells, and NK cells. Once these cells have been activated, they kill host cells that have been infected with viruses or intracellular bacteria such as listeria. These are the characteristic features of **cell-mediated immunity**, which will be described further in Chapters 16 and 18. In addition, as discussed later in this chapter, IFN-γ influences B-cell isotype switching to Ig isotypes that bind to pathogens, which in turn activates complement, and so enhances the phagocytosis of microbial pathogens by phagocytic cells (see also Chapter 13).

T$_H$2 cells synthesize IL-4, IL-5, and IL-13. IL-4 and IL-13 influence B-cell class switch to IgE and IgG$_4$ in humans and IL-5 activates eosinophils. These are characteristic features of the immune response to parasitic worms as well as to allergens (discussed in Chapter 14).

T$_H$17 cells are a recently characterized third subset of antigen-activated CD4$^+$ T cells. T$_H$17 cells synthesize and secrete the IL-17 family of cytokines (particularly IL-17A and IL-17F, described in Chapter 11) and IL-22. T$_H$17 cells and IL-17 and IL-22 are **proinflammatory**, that is, they promote inflammatory responses, particularly at mucosal sites. T_H17 cells and cytokines have been described in some human autoimmune inflammatory conditions, including rheumatoid arthritis, multiple sclerosis, and inflammatory bowel disease, and in the skin condition psoriasis (see Chapters 11 and 12).

Psoriasis

IL-17 stimulates many cells of the innate immune system (particularly recruiting and activating neutrophils to sites of inflammation) as well as other types of cells (endothelial cells and epithelial cells) to synthesize the cytokines IL-1, IL-6, and TNF-α that also result in inflammation. IL-22 acts on many cells in the skin and digestive system and activates inflammatory responses. In addition, IL-22 induces epithelial cells to produce antibacterial peptides, which play a protective role in responses to bacteria at mucosal surfaces.

Recent studies suggest that human and mouse T_H17 cells appear to differ in the synthesis of cytokines other than IL-17 and IL-22. Further experiments will be needed to confirm these findings.

Studies also suggest that the T_H17 subset is involved in responses to extracellular bacteria (such as the spirochete *Borrelia burgdorferi*) and fungi (such as the major human fungal pathogens *Candida albicans* and *Aspergillus fumigatus*). T_H1 and T_H2 subsets have little effect on these pathogens, suggesting that the T_H1, T_H2, and T_H17 subsets of CD4$^+$ T cells respond to different, nonoverlapping sets of pathogens.

T_{reg} cells are the fourth subset of CD4$^+$ T cells shown in Figure 10.5. T_{reg} cells inhibit or *suppress* the differentiation and function of other subsets of CD4$^+$ T cells; that is, T_H1, T_H2, and T_H17 cells. They also suppress the activation and proliferation of other cell types, including dendritic cells and B cells. T_{reg} cells, which generally express CD25, suppress immune responses directed at both self-molecules and foreign antigens. The importance of T_{reg} cells in responses to self is shown by the autoimmune inflammatory conditions that result from defective development or function T_{reg} cells. One example is immunue dysregulation, polyendocrinopathy, enteropathy, X-linked (IPEX) syndrome, in which Treg cells are lacking; it is characterized by autoimmune disease, allergy, and inflammatory bowel disease (see Chapter 12). T_{reg} cells' inhibitory actions are probably mediated by both direct cell contact and the secretion of the cytokines IL-10 and transforming growth factor β (TGF-β), both of which have suppressive functions described further in Chapters 11 and 12.

T_{reg} cells are heterogeneous in humans and mice, the two species in which they have been most studied. Some T_{reg} (natural T_{reg}) cells are autoreactive and develop in the thymus, as we described in Chapter 9. Other T_{reg} (induced T_{reg}) cells develop outside the thymus either by chronic antigenic stimulation or, as we describe in the next section, in the presence of TGF-β.

Note that a cytokine synthesized by one particular subset of CD4$^+$ T cells is not necessarily produced *only* by that subset of cells; for example, IL-4 is synthesized by T_H2 cells but is also made by mast cells and NKT cells, and IFN-γ is synthesized by T_H1 cells but also CD8$^+$ T cells.

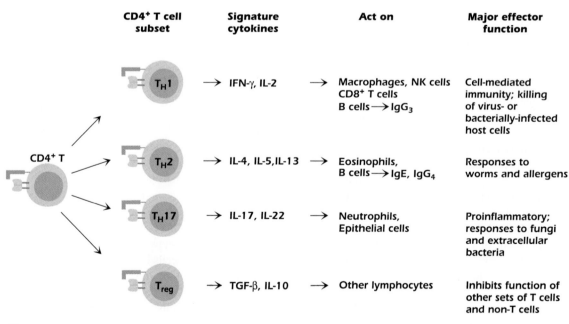

Figure 10.5. Major subsets of CD4$^+$ T cells: T_H1, T_H2, T_H17, and T_{reg}.

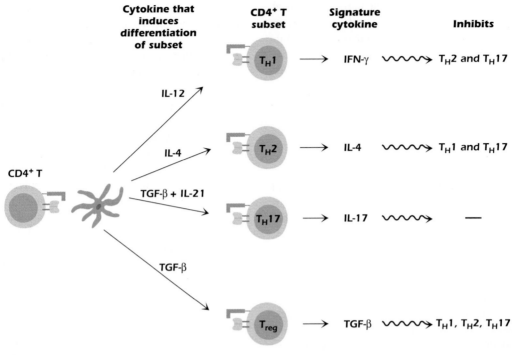

Figure 10.6. Cytokines influence the differentiation into a particular subset of CD4$^+$ T cells. Cytokines synthesized by one subset of CD4$^+$ T cells inhibit the development of other subsets. Wavy lines indicate inhibition. Cytokines synthesized by T$_H$17 cells are not known to inhibit the function or development of other subsets. Human T$_H$17 cells develop in the presence of IL-21 and TGF- but mouse T$_H$17 cells develop in the presence of IL-6 and TGF-β.

Nonetheless, the patterns of cytokines made by the subsets of CD4$^+$ T cells do appear to be unique and so are frequently useful in designating a particular response as "T$_H$1-type" or "T$_H$2-type" and so on.

Cytokines Influence Differentiation into a Particular Subset of CD4$^+$ T Cells.

Figure 10.6 indicates that the cytokines present during the activation of CD4$^+$ T cells drive the differentiation of the naïve CD4$^+$ T cell into a particular subset: T$_H$1, T$_H$2, T$_H$17, or T$_{reg}$. The cytokines that influence the differentiation of CD4$^+$ T cells are generally derived from cells of the innate immune system, particularly from dendritic cells. Thus, cells of the innate immune system have a critical role in shaping the pattern of the adaptive immune response. The critical role played by these cytokines is often referred to as a "***third signal***" that works in conjunction with the first (peptide–MHC–TCR) and second (costimulatory) signals in driving the differentiation of activated CD4$^+$ T cells. In Chapter 11 we describe how the development of each subset of CD4$^+$ T cells is associated with the activation of specific intracellular activation pathways and a "lineage-determining" transcription factor.

T$_H$1 cells develop in the presence of IL-12; as described at the beginning of this chapter, IL-12 is synthesized early in the immune response to bacteria and

viruses by dendritic cells and other cells of the innate immune system, including NK cells. T$_H$2 cells develop in the presence of IL-4. The source of this IL-4 is currently not clear; different studies have shown that several different cells—including mast cells, activated CD4$^+$ T cells, and NKT cells—are capable of synthesizing the IL-4 required to drive the differentiation of the T$_H$2 subset. Recent research suggests that T$_H$17 cells develop from naïve CD4$^+$ T cells in the presence of TGF-β and IL-21, a cytokine synthesized by activated CD4$^+$ T cells and NKT cells that drives the differentiation of NK cells; further studies will be needed to confirm these findings. The development of T$_H$17 cells in the mouse appears to require a different set of cytokines, TGF-β and IL-6, the latter synthesized by many cells of the innate immune system. T$_{reg}$ cells develop from naïve T cells in the presence of TGF-β.

Cross-Inhibition of CD4$^+$ T-Cell Subsets.

Figure 10.6 also shows that cytokines produced by one subset of CD4$^+$ T cells inhibit the function of other subsets. The key examples of this ***cross-inhibition*** are (1) IFN-γ synthesized by T$_H$1 cells inhibits the development and function of T$_H$2 cells; (2) IL-4 synthesized by T$_H$2 cells inhibits the development and function of T$_H$1 cells; and (3) IFN-γ and IL-4, the signature cytokines of the T$_H$1 and T$_H$2 subsets, respectively, also inhibit T$_H$17 cells; thus, the development of either T$_H$1 or T$_H$2 cells prevents the induction of the T$_H$17 subset. (4) As we noted above, T$_{reg}$ cells inhibit the development and function of all the other T-cell subsets. No evidence suggests that cytokines produced by T$_H$17 cells inhibit the function of any other subset of T cell.

As a result of the cross-inhibiting properties of different cytokines, the immune response to a particular antigen may end up "skewed" or *polarized* toward the production of only one subset of CD4$^+$ T cells, the production of one set of cytokines, and one type of effector responses. An important example is in the response to bacteria and viruses. Early in the immune response to these pathogens, cells of the innate immune system—dendritic cells and NK cells in particular—synthesize IL-12. This polarizes the response toward the development of T$_H$1 cells and the cytokine IFN-γ and away from T$_H$2 and T$_H$17 cells and cytokines they synthesize. This polarization toward T$_H$1 cells activates the effector cells that remove virus- or bacterially infected cells. By contrast, in the response to parasitic worms, IL-4 is synthesized early in the response, driving CD4$^+$ T cell differentiation toward T$_H$2 cytokines and the T$_H$2 set of responses and effector cells (IgE synthesis and eosinophil activation). Similarly, responses to allergens are dominated by the T$_H$2 – type pattern of IL-4 and IgE synthesis (see Chapter 14).

Furthermore, as Figure 10.6 shows and we noted above, exposure to a cytokine in addition to TGF-β—IL-21 in people (IL-6 in the mouse)—tips the balance between T$_H$17 and T$_{reg}$ cells towards T$_H$17 cells. Because IL-21 (and IL-6) is synthesized during the early phases of the response to an infectious agent or in an inflammatory response, the synthesis of these additional cytokines prevents the development of the inhibitory T$_{reg}$ subset and drives the development of T$_H$17 cells, which promote an inflammatory response.

The phenomenon of polarization also suggests potential therapies: for example, attempts have been made to skew the response *away* from T$_H$2 cell responses that dominate in allergic responses, either by trying to inhibit the function of T$_H$2 cells per se or by activating other subsets of CD4$^+$ T cells specific for the allergen (see Chapter 14). In addition, treatments that inhibit the function of T$_H$17 cells in conditions such as psoriasis or that expand the development of T$_{reg}$ cells in autoimmune inflammatory conditions may be clinically beneficial.

Although we indicated above that the designation of a response as T$_H$1 type or T$_H$2 type, for example, may be helpful, the response to infectious agents such as parasites is frequently complex; one subset of responses may dominate at a particular stage of the response, and another may dominate at another. Furthermore, responses to many harmless antigens do not show a skewed pattern of cytokines. Note too that other factors may influence the development of CD4$^+$ T cells into one subset or other and hence influence

the resulting effector responses. These include the route of administration of antigen (for example, oral or nasal administration of vaccines to develop mucosal immunity), the concentration of antigen, and the APC that initially activates the immune response.

T-Helper-Cell Function: Interaction of CD4$^+$ T Cells with B Cells to Synthesize Antibody

In Chapter 7 we described how the B-cell response in the germinal center to TD antigens requires helper T cells (T$_H$) to cooperate with B cells in the synthesis of antibodies of different isotypes and in the induction of memory cells. Acting as a T$_H$ is a key function of CD4$^+$ T cells. In Figures 10.7 and 10.8 and the paragraphs that follow, we describe the interactions between T and B cells that lead to antibody synthesis in the response to TD antigens.

As Figure 10.7 shows, the T$_H$ cell and B cell that cooperate in the response to a particular TD antigen must both be specific for that antigen. The T$_H$ and the B cell may respond to different epitopes in the antigen—the T$_H$ to an internal epitope generated during the processing of the antigen, the B cell to an external epitope. For the T$_H$ and B cells to cooperate effectively, the epitopes they recognize must be part of the same protein sequence. For this reason, T–B cooperation in the response to a TD antigen is also known as **linked recognition**, shown in Figure 10.7.

The B Cells Presents Antigen to the T$_H$. As shown in Figure 10.8, a critical initial step in the induction of an antibody response is the capture of "free" antigen by a B cell with the appropriate receptor. (This generally occurs in the B-cell area of a secondary lymphoid organ, such as a lymph node.) After the antigen binds to the membrane Ig, the complex of antigen and Ig is taken into the cell, and the antigen is processed in acid compartments. As described in Chapter 8, some of the peptides that

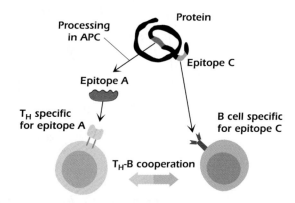

Figure 10.7. Linked recognition: For T helper cell–B cell cooperation in antibody synthesis, the epitopes recognized by the helper T cell (epitope A) and the B cell (epitope C) must be physically linked in the same antigen.

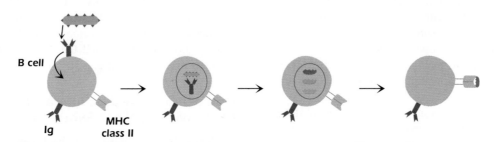

B cell captures antigen via antigen-specific receptor, Ig, and internalizes Ig-bound antigen

Antigen processed to peptides in acid vesicles

Processed peptide associates with MHC class II, traffics to B-cell surface

Figure 10.8. B cells present antigen to T helper cells. A B cell with the appropriate antigen-specific receptor captures a protein antigen via interaction with membrane Ig; the B cell processes the antigen and presents peptides associated with MHC class II molecules to a helper CD4$^+$ T cell with the appropriate receptor.

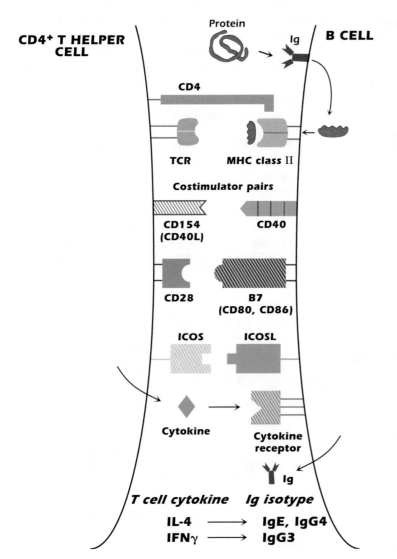

Figure 10.9. Key interactions involved in T helper–B cell cooperation. Hatching indicates expression of costimulator molecules upregulated by activation. T-cell-derived cytokines associated with switch to specific B-cell isotypes are also shown.

result from the catabolism of the antigen selectively bind to newly synthesized MHC class II molecules that link up with these acid compartments as they traffic through the B cell.

Peptide–MHC class II complexes at the B-cell surface can then be presented to a CD4+ helper T cell with the appropriate TCR. In this way, the B cell acts as an APC to the T helper cell (see top of Fig. 10.9). As we described in Chapter 7, this T_H–B interaction takes place in the lymph node follicle and ultimately leads to the formation of the germinal center.

Paired Interactions Activate Both T_H and B Cells. Figure 10.9 shows that the interaction of an antigen-presenting B cell with a T_H shares many of the same characteristics we described earlier in the chapter for dendritic cell activation of CD4+ T cells. Peptide–MHC on the B cell interacting with the TCR provides the critical antigen-specific first signal. The costimulatory pairs B7-CD28, CD40-CD40 Ligand (CD40L), and ICOS-ICOSL, play important roles in the mutual activation of the T_H and B cell, which we describe below. In addition, paired adhesion molecules (not shown in the figure) LFA-1 and ICAM-1 and CD2-CD58 help to maintain contact between the T_H and the B cell. The area of contact between the T_H and B cell also forms an immunologic synapse. Not only is this synapse required for sustained signaling, but the cells reorganize their internal structure so that the key interactions are localized to the area of contact between the cells.

B-cell presentation of peptide–MHC class II to the TCR upregulates CD40L expression on the T_H. Interaction of CD40L ligand with CD40 expressed on the B cell in turn upregulates low-level expression of the costimulatory molecule B7 on the B cell, which interacts with CD28 expressed on the T cell. (This enhanced expression of B7 by activated B cells helps to explain why activated B cells are efficient APC, whereas resting B cells are not.) The interactions between CD40 and CD40L and B7 and CD28, as well as the ICOS-ICOSL interaction, result in the activated T cell synthesizing cytokines that induce T-cell proliferation and also act on the activated B cell, which upregulates expression of receptors for the T-cell-derived cytokines.

Costimulator Pairs Are Critical in T_H-Dependent Antibody Synthesis and Isotype Switch. The CD40–CD40 ligand interaction appears critical in the activation of B cells in thymus-dependent antigen responses because it is required for the B cell to switch from the synthesis of IgM to other isotypes, such as IgG (isotype switch). In the absence of this interaction, only IgM is made. In the condition known as X-linked hyper-IgM syndrome (see Chapter 17), boys with a nonfunctional CD40L produce IgM antibody but no other isotype.

Hyper-IgM Syndrome

The ICOS–ICOSL interaction we mentioned earlier in the chapter and in Chapter 7 also appears to be an important T_H–B cell interaction. ICOS is induced on activated T cells and is expressed by T_H in the germinal center of the lymph node. People who lack a functional ICOS gene product (and ICOS knockout mice) do not develop normal germinal centers and are profoundly immunodeficient, with low levels of IgG, IgA, and IgE.

Thus, isotype switching by the B cell requires costimulator interactions between the Th and B cell and the synthesis of cytokines by the activated T cell. Figure 10.8 also shows that the cytokine produced by the T cell determines the particular antibody isotype synthesized by the B cell. If the T cell synthesizes IL-4, B cells switch to producing predominantly IgE and IgG_4; if the T cell synthesizes IFN-γ, B cells switch to producing IgG subtypes such as IgG_3 that activate complement (see Chapters 4 and 13). At mucosal sites, TGF-β and other cytokines including IL-4 and IL-5 are thought to be required to switch to IgA.

As described earlier in this chapter, naïve CD4+ T cells are most effectively activated by antigen processed and presented by dendritic cells in the T-cell area of the lymph node; the cytokines present when the naïve T cell is first activated influence the pattern of cytokines synthesized by the activated CD4+ T cell. For example, a T cell activated by a dendritic cells activated by T_H-type in the primary response is likely to differentiate in the presence of IL-12 to a T_H1–type response that synthesizes IFN-γ. If this T cell interacts with an activated B cell that has captured antigen through its surface Ig, IFN-γ will induce the B cells to switch antibody synthesis to IgG_3. IgG_3 antibodies are effective activators of the complement cascade (see Chapter 13). In general terms, each type of antigen induces a set of inter-connected responses that results in the removal of the antigen; in this example, the bacterium induces IL-12 synthesis by cells of the innate immune system, the development of CD4+ T cells T_H1 cells, synthesis of IgG3 antibody by B cells, and the activation of complement.

 ## ACTIVATION AND FUNCTION OF CD8+ T CELLS

We now turn our attention to the other major subset of T cells, CD8+ T cells, whose principal function is to kill cells that have been infected by viruses and bacteria. CD8+ T cells are also involved in killing transplanted foreign cells (graft rejection) and tumor cells (see Chapters 18 and 19).

For this reason, a CD8$^+$ T cell is referred to as a *killer T cell* or *cytotoxic T lymphocyte* (*CTL*). The cell killed by a CTL is known as a *target*; the target can be an APC such as a dendritic cell or any other cell in the body. In the paragraphs that follow we will describe how CD8$^+$ T cells are activated to become effector cells and how they kill their targets.

Generation of Effector CD8$^+$ T Cells

Much of our understanding of the activation of and generation of effector CD8$^+$ T cells is derived from studies of infectious agents in mice, particularly their responses to viruses and bacteria. These studies show that the population of CD8$^+$ T cells specific for a particular virus or bacterial epitope expands enormously—from a total of approximately 100 naïve cells to millions—within the first seven days after infection.

The activation of CD8$^+$ T cells to proliferate and differentiate into effector cells follows many of the same principles that we described above for the generation of effector CD4$^+$ T-cells: a first signal, peptide–MHC interacting with the TCR; second or costimulatory signals, particularly B7–CD28 and CD40–CD40L; and a third signal, cytokines, synthesized by cells of the innate immune response. IL-12 is considered critical in the activation of CD8$^+$ T cells, and interferons α and β are also thought to play a role. All these signals are required to provide maximal stimulation.

Figure 10.10 shows several pathways for the activation of CD8$^+$ T cells by viruses: Interactions with dendritic cells are considered to be critical. Figure 10.10A shows how a dendritic cell can present a virus-derived peptide associated with an MHC class I molecule and directly activate a CD8$^+$ T cell with the appropriate TCR. (As we described in Chapter 8, virus-derived peptides associated with the MHC class I molecules in this dendritic cell may have resulted from either infection of the cell or via processing in the cross-presentation pathway.) In this pathway, the dendritic cell provides the first and second signals, as well as IL-12, to activate the CD8$^+$ T cell. The combination of these signals results in the rapid proliferation of CD8$^+$ T cells; the CD8$^+$ T cell is thought to synthesize IL-2 that induces the proliferation of the activated CD8$^+$ T cells.

Many virus-specific CD8$^+$ T-cell responses require virus-specific CD4$^+$ T cells, and CD4$^+$ T cells seem to be critical for the induction of memory CD8$^+$ T cells. However, the precise way in which CD4$^+$ T cells are involved in the activation of naïve CD8$^+$ T cells and killer T-cell effector generation is not completely understood.

Figure 10.10B shows one pathway in which CD4$^+$ T cells play a role in the generation of CD8$^+$ effector T cells: A dendritic cell that has taken up virus as an exogenous antigen presents virus-derived peptides in association with MHC class II molecules to a virus-specific CD4$^+$ T cell. In conjunction with the costimulator interaction B7–CD28, the CD4$^+$ cell is activated to proliferate and synthesize IL-2. As described earlier in this section, however, the same dendritic cell may also present virus antigens to CD8$^+$ T cells via cross-presentation in the MHC class I pathway. Thus, the interaction of the CD8$^+$ T cell with virus-derived peptides presented by MHC class I expressed on the dendritic cell, in combination with IL-2 synthesized by the CD4$^+$ T cell, induces virus-specific CD8$^+$ T-cell proliferation and differentiation. In this pathway, the virus epitope that activates the CD4$^+$ T cell (red peptide) is different from the epitope that activates the CD8$^+$ T cell (green peptide).

Because the likelihood of two rare antigen-specific T cells (the virus-specific CD4$^+$ and CD8$^+$ T cells) interacting with the same APC is very low, until recently it was not clear whether this three-cell interaction could occur under physiologic conditions. Recent evidence suggests, however, that an initial dendritic cell–CD4$^+$ T-cell interaction can occur, with a CD8$^+$ T-cell joining this stabilized interaction later.

A variation of the activation pathway involving the dendritic cell and virus-specific CD4$^+$ and CD8$^+$ T cells has been suggested in a pathway referred to as *licensing*, in which the dendritic cell activation of the CD4$^+$ T cell and of the CD8$^+$ T cell are separate events. In the licensing pathway an immature dendritic cell interacts first with a CD4$^+$ T cell; the dendritic cell upregulates costimulator molecules (particularly CD40), and the CD4$^+$ T cell upregulates CD40L. The now mature dendritic cell, with upregulated CD40 and the ability to synthesize and secrete IL-12, can move away from the CD4$^+$ T cell to interact with and activate a naïve virus-specific CD8$^+$ T cell.

Whichever pathway is used to activate the CD8$^+$ T cell, the intracellular events in CD8$^+$ T-cell activation are similar to those described above for CD4$^+$ T-cell activation. Like CD4, CD8 is associated with the tyrosine kinase Lck; the same pairs of costimulatory and adhesion molecules described in the activation of CD4$^+$ T cells—CD28–B7, LFA-1–ICAM-1, and CD2–CD58—are also involved.

CD8$^+$ T-Cell Killing of Target Cells

Figure 10.10C indicates that, once activated, the CD8$^+$ T cell initiates killing by attaching to the target cell. Interactions between peptide associated with MHC class I molecules expressed by the target and CD8 and the TCR expressed by the CD8$^+$ T cell are critical; in addition, paired adhesion molecules expressed on the T cell and target cell surfaces (not shown in the figure) help to maintain contact between the cells for several hours.

The figure also shows the effector CD8$^+$ T cell contains granules formed when the CD8$^+$ T cell is activated. These granules contain proteins with cytotoxic function. The effector CD8$^+$ T cell also expresses the surface molecule Fas ligand (CD178). As we describe in the paragraphs that follow. The proteins contained in the granules and Fas ligand are critical in target cell killing: Both activate apoptosis (programmed cell death) of the target cell.

Killing by CD8+ T cells is thought to occur by two pathways. The first, and considered to be the predominant pathway for killing most target cells, involves the contents of the granules inside the CD8+ T cells. After attaching to the target cell, the CD8+ T cell reorganizes its internal structure so that these granules are close to the area of contact with the target cell. Figure 10.10C also shows that the CD8+ T cell releases the contents of the granules onto the target cell by a process known as exocytosis. The major constituents of the granules involved in target cell killing

are perforin and granzymes. **Perforin** forms pores in the target cell membrane. The resulting increase in permeability of the cell membrane contributes to the eventual death of the cell. The action of perforin on cell membranes is similar to that of the complement membrane attack complex described in Chapter 13. **Granzymes** are serine proteases that pass into the target cell through the pores created by perforin; granzymes interact with intracellular components of the target cell to induce apoptosis. **Granulysin** (not shown in the figure) is a small protein that also enters the target cell; it activates pathways that lead to the killing of intracellular pathogens such as *Listeria* and *Mycobacteria*, organisms that live inside macrophages and dendritic cells.

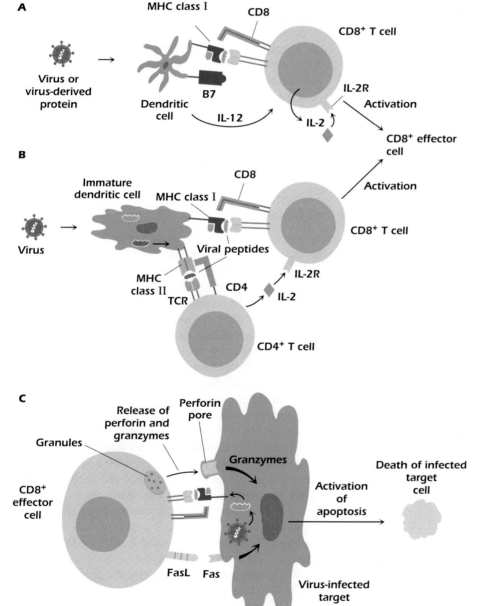

Figure 10.10. CD8+ T cells: Generation of effector cells and target cell killing. (A) dendritic cells activate CD8+ T cells directly. (B) One pathway for CD4+ T cells to activate CD8+ T cells. (C) Target cell killing by a CD8+ effector T cell.

A second pathway of target cell killing occurs via the interaction of the molecule Fas ligand on the CD8$^+$ T cell with Fas, a surface molecule expressed on many host cells. This interaction activates the apoptosis of the target cell via a sequential activation of caspases, a set of proteolytic enzymes, inside the target cell (see Chapter 12 for further details). As a result, the cell dies within hours. Since death by apoptosis does not result in the release of the cell's contents, killing infected cells by apoptotic mechanisms may prevent the spread of infectious virus into other cells.

Once the CD8$^+$ T cell has initiated these killing pathways, it detaches from the target cell to attack and kill additional target cells.

As the preceding paragraphs illustrate, activation of CD8$^+$ T cell and killing of the target cell are separate events. This can be demonstrated by preparing CD8$^+$ T cells from an individual who has been infected with a virus: The virus-specific cytotoxic cells are able to kill virus-infected targets outside the body. (The assay for CD8$^+$ T-cell killing of targets is described in Chapter 5.) In vitro killing of the infected target does not require additional factors.

MHC Restriction and CD8$^+$ T Cell Killer Function

We stress here the concept of MHC restriction of T-cell responses we referred to in previous chapters: A virus-specific CD8$^+$ CTL recognizes, and subsequently kills, a target cell expressing a specific combination of viral peptide and a particular MHC class I molecule. For example, this means that a CD8$^+$ CTL specific for a flu virus peptide and HLA-A2 kills a target cell expressing HLA-A2 that has bound the flu-derived peptide. In the absence of the flu peptide, this CTL does not kill uninfected or normal cells from an individual expressing HLA-A2. In addition, this virus-specific CD8$^+$ T cell does not kill targets expressing different combinations of peptides plus MHC molecules, such as a measles-virus-derived peptide bound to HLA-A2 or even the same flu peptide bound to a different HLA molecule. These findings, which earned Rolf Zinkernagel and Peter Doherty the Nobel Prize in 1996, established the concept of MHC restriction of T-cell responses, indicating that T cells recognize the combination of antigen plus MHC molecule rather than antigen alone.

In addition, the recognition of peptide–MHC class I by a CD8$^+$ T cell occurs regardless of the expression of any MHC class II molecule by the target cell. This has important biologic consequences; as described in Chapter 9, MHC class I molecules are expressed on almost every cell in the body. Since an infectious pathogen (such as a virus, parasite, or bacterium) may infect any nucleated cell in the body, a pathogen generates peptides that associate with MHC class I molecules expressed on the surface of

any nucleated host cell. Expression of the pathogen-derived peptide–MHC class I complexes at the cell surface leads to recognition by CD8$^+$ T cells, followed by the killing of the infected cell. Thus, killing by CD8$^+$ T cells provides a mechanism to eliminate any cell in the body that becomes infected with a pathogen. Clearly, elimination of the pathogen does result in the destruction of host cells, but this is the price the individual pays for removal of the source of infection.

To repeat and elaborate on a concept introduced in Chapter 8, generally, only intracellular pathogens such as viruses, parasites, and bacteria generate peptides that associate with MHC class I molecules and evoke CD8$^+$ T-cell responses. These pathogens also activate pathogen-specific CD4$^+$ T cells and induce antibody synthesis because they are taken up by APC such as dendritic cells and macrophages. In this way, CD4$^+$ T cells, CD8$^+$ T cells, and antibody, along with other cells such as $\gamma\delta$ T cells, are all likely to be involved in the host's protective immune response against a particular pathogen (see Chapter 20). In contrast, harmless or noninfectious antigens (such as a killed virus protein in a vaccine) do not generally trigger CD8$^+$ T-cell responses. These exogenous antigens are taken up into the acidic compartments of an APC, interact with MHC class II molecules, and activate CD4$^+$ T-cell and antibody responses.

Termination of the Response: Induction of Memory Cells

In previous sections we described how the interaction of antigen with naïve CD4$^+$ or CD8$^+$ T cells induces enormous proliferation of naïve cells to generate a very large effector cell population. Once the antigen has been eliminated or the infectious agent cleared, however, 99% of this pool of activated and effector cells die. This leaves a surviving population of memory T cells that is still expanded—generally 100- to 1000-fold—compared to the original naïve cell clone size.

The signals that govern the contraction of the expanded T-cell population and generate memory cells are not completely understood. Studies indicate that T cells are susceptible to apoptosis after they have been activated, particularly after repeated antigenic stimulation; the vast majority of activated T cells are eliminated by an apoptotic pathway known as activation-induced cell death, mediated by the interaction of Fas and Fas ligand. As we described earlier in this chapter, this interaction triggers apoptosis in target cells. Because activated T cells express *both* Fas and Fas ligand, however, the activated T cells use this interaction to kill each other once antigen has been removed.

The memory T cells that survive the phase of contraction of the clone size are generally long-lived, frequently with a lifetime of years. They are involved in protective responses after a subsequent exposure to many types of pathogen (see Chapter 20). Memory T-cell responses are also more rapid and effective than primary responses. One reason is that the clonal size of the memory population specific for a particular antigen is much larger than the size of the original clone in the naïve T-cell population. In addition, reinfection or restimulation with a particular antigen activates the proliferation and differentiation of memory T cells to effector cells so that the clone size is expanded even further.

We have previously referred to the fact that the circulatory properties of effector and memory T cells differ from those of naïve T cells. Unlike naïve cells, which can circulate only through lymph nodes, effector and memory cells can enter tissues. Different subsets of memory cells have been identified based on the tissues to which they circulate. As mentioned in previous chapters, their ability to enter specific tissues is governed by the expression of combinations of adhesion molecules and chemokine receptors. *Effector memory cells* down-regulate the adhesion molecules and chemokine receptors expressed by naïve cells (L-selectin and CCR7, respectively) and upregulate a different pattern of molecules that allows migration to peripheral tissues. One pattern allows the memory cells to move to the skin and another set permits movement to the mucosa—major sites in the body under threat from infectious organisms. Reexposure to antigen at these sites rapidly induces effector memory cells to become effector cells. *Central memory cells* express a pattern of adhesion molecules and chemokine receptors that is very similar to the pattern expressed by naïve T cells; thus, central memory cells recirculate through peripheral lymph nodes. Reexposure to antigen in the nodes induces effector function from central memory cells, although this generally occurs less rapidly than responses of effector memory cells.

It is not clear whether the persistence of memory cells requires the presence of antigen, even at some very low level; some studies indicate that in the absence of the priming antigen memory cells die. As we mentioned earlier in the chapter, the generation of memory CD8$^+$ T cells requires CD4$^+$ T cells. This suggests another reason why the loss of CD4$^+$ T cells in AIDS may be so devastating; their loss prevents the continuing development of memory CD8$^+$ T cells that might contain the infection.

FUNCTION OF NKT CELLS AND γδ T CELLS

Because CD4$^+$ and CD8$^+$ T cells are critical components of the adaptive, cell-mediated immune responses, this chapter has focused on their activation and provided an introduction to their effector function. Many other aspects of immune responses associated with these cells will be described in the remaining chapters of this book. Before leaving the subject of T cells, we turn our attention to two other subsets of T cells: NKT cells and γδ T cells. These subsets are thought of as somewhat more "primitive" than CD4$^+$ and CD8$^+$ and show characteristics of both the innate and adaptive immune responses.

NKT Cells

In Chapter 9, we briefly described the differentiation of the subset of T cells referred to as **NKT cells** because they expressed a T-cell receptor as well as the molecule NK1.1 and other molecules typical of NK cells. NKT cells recognize and respond to lipid and glycolipid antigens derived from infectious pathogens (such as *Sphingomonas* bacteria and *B. burgdorferi*) as well as glycosphingolipids expressed by host cells. Thus, NKT cells respond to both microorganisms and self-antigens. Most NKT cells use a "semi-invariant" TCR, one Vα with a restricted set of Vβ, which responds to antigen presented by CD1$^+$ APC, such as dendritic cells.

After stimulation by antigen, NKT cells very rapidly synthesize high levels of both T$_H$1- and T$_H$2-associated cytokines, particularly IL-4 and IFN-γ. Thus, NKT cells are thought to play an important role in the early clearance of bacteria. NKT cells have also been suggested as one source of the IL-4 that polarizes the differentiation of naïve CD4$^+$ T cells toward the T$_H$2 subset. In addition, NKT cells are thought to play a key role in regulating many different immune responses; defects in NKT cells have been associated with diseases that include autoimmunity and cancer.

γδ T Cells

In Chapter 9 we described the differentiation of the subset of T cells that use γδ rather than αβ as their two-chain antigen-recognizing TCR. γδ T cells, found predominantly at mucosal epithelial sites, are thought to provide a first line of defense against invading pathogens. They rapidly produce cytokines, particularly IFN-γ, in response to pathogens such as mycobacteria and have also been described to have cytotoxic function (using cytotoxic mechanisms similar to those of CD8$^+$ T cells). They also can respond to heat-shock proteins produced when host cells are shocked or stressed. γδ T cells do not generally respond to peptides associated with MHC molecules but do respond to phospholipids and other small nonprotein molecules, known as phosphoantigens.

B-CELL FUNCTION: ANTIBODY SYNTHESIS IN THE ABSENCE OF T-CELL HELP

So far in this chapter we have discussed the function of T cells and described how T helper cells cooperate with B cells in the response to thymus-dependent (TD) antigens.

An important and distinct group of antigens is called **thymus-independent (TI)** because B cell responses to these antigens do not require helper T cells. As their name implies, responses to TI antigens can occur in people or animals that lack a functional thymus or T cells.

TI antigens are divided into two classes, **TI-1** and **TI-2**. TI-1 antigens are mitogenic at high concentrations; that is, they are able to activate multiple B-cell clones to proliferate and produce antibody. Because of this antigen-nonspecific activation property, such antigens are called polyclonal B-cell activators. Lipopolysaccharide derived from Gram-negative bacteria such as *E. coli* are TI-1 antigens. In addition, the protein coats of some viruses such as the polio virus, which have a repeating structure, are also TI-1 antigens. TI-2 antigens include bacterial and fungal polysaccharides (e.g., dextrans and ficoll and the polysaccharide capsule of extracullular bacteria such as *Haemophilus influenzae* and *Streptococcus pneumoniae*); TI-2 antigens are not mitogenic at high concentrations.

TI responses have two biologically relevant features. First, unlike responses involving T-cell-dependent antigens, responses to TI antigens primarily generate IgM and do not give rise to memory cells. In other words, a second injection of a TI antigen leads to the same level of production of IgM as the first, with no increase in level, speed of onset, or class switch. This finding reinforces the importance of T-cell-derived cytokines in both the development of memory cells and the B-cell isotype switch. Second, even if an individual lacks T cells, an immune response can still be made against TI antigens. Thus, patients with T-cell immune deficiencies can still make protective

IgM responses against extracellular bacteria, even if they cannot make significant responses to T-cell-dependent viruses.

Conjugate Vaccines

In Chapter 7, we described how marginal-zone B cells synthesize early (within 2-3 days), protective IgM antibodies in response to many bacterial pathogens. We also noted that marginal zone B cells do not develop until a child is about 1 to 2 years old. Consequently, very young children are susceptible to infections from pathogens such as the bacterium *H. influenzae* b, which can cause pneumonia and meningitis.

As we noted in the preceding section, the capsular polysaccharide antigens of *H. influenzae* b induce a potent TI response, of limited usefulness for developing a vaccine. However, the introduction of **conjugate vaccines** (further discussed in Chapter 20) in the last 20 years has dramatically reduced diseases caused by organisms such as *H. influenzae* b and *S. pneumoniae*. Conjugate vaccines utilize the principle of **linked recognition** we described above to generate protective *thymus-dependent* response. This is illustrated in Figure 10.11: purified polysaccharide from the bacterium is conjugated, i.e. physically linked, to a **carrier** protein—tetanus toxoid is used in the *H. influenzae* b conjugate vaccine and many others. The carrier protein generates T-cell epitopes that activate T helper cells, and these T helper cells interact with B cells specific for the polysaccharide. As we described earlier, the resulting

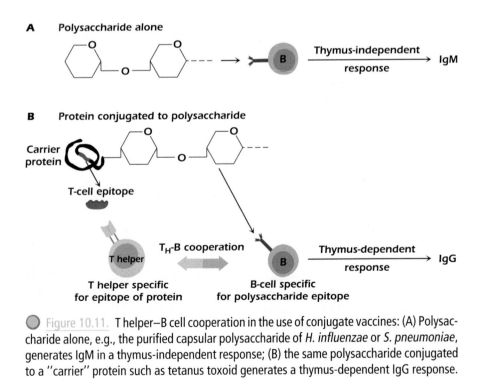

Figure 10.11. T helper–B cell cooperation in the use of conjugate vaccines: (A) Polysaccharide alone, e.g., the purified capsular polysaccharide of *H. influenzae* or *S. pneumoniae*, generates IgM in a thymus-independent response; (B) the same polysaccharide conjugated to a "carrier" protein such as tetanus toxoid generates a thymus-dependent IgG response.

thymus-dependent response involves switching to isotypes such as IgG and the development of long-term memory.

Intracellular Pathways in B-Cell Activation

In this section we describe the intracellular pathways involved in B-cell activation. Figure 10.12 shows that multivalent antigens with repeating epitopes, such as those found in many TI antigens, directly activate the B cell. Activation is initiated by *receptor cross-linking*, bringing together more than one BCR complex in the cell membrane. Like the antigen-binding chains of the TCR, Ig H and L chains have very short intracellular domains and do not play a direct role in signal transduction after they bind antigen.

Figure 10.12 indicates that cross-linking activates pathways inside the B cell that are very similar to the cascades that occur during CD4⁺ T-cell activation, which were described earlier in the chapter. These include the phosphorylation of kinases, assembly and activation of signaling complexes at the cell membrane, and activation of intracellular signaling pathways. However, the end result of B-cell activation is the transcription and translation of Ig and cytokine receptor genes, rather than the transcription and translation of cytokine genes that were key features of T-cell activation.

As in T-cell activation, one of the earliest events in B-cell activation is the activation of Src family tyrosine kinases—Lyn, Blk, Lck, and Fyn—associated with the BCR (see Fig. 10.12). These kinases are believed to be activated by the same CD45 described for T-cell activation. The activated kinases phosphorylate tyrosine residues in ITAMs of the Igα and Igβ molecules (CD79a and b) associated with Ig chains in the membrane. Phosphorylation of these ITAMs recruits another kinase (Syk) to the cluster of molecules, and Syk is phosphorylated and activated. Syk is in the same family of kinases as ZAP-70, which plays a central role in T-cell activation.

Activated Syk recruits and activates adaptor molecules, which in turn activate intracellular signaling pathways similar to those described for activated T cells. These include the following: the activation of PLC-γ, leading to the activation of protein kinase C, increases in intracellular calcium ion levels, and the subsequent activation of multiple cytoplasmic enzymes; and the activation of Ras and Rac, which in turn activate a cytoplasmic cascade of MAP kinases. As a result of this sequence of intracellular signaling pathways, transcription factors (including NF-AT, AP-1, and NF-κB) enter the nucleus of the B cell and promote the transcription of several genes, the most important of which are Ig and

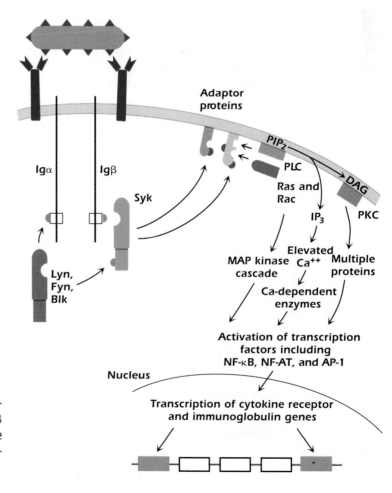

Figure 10.12. Intracellular events in B-cell activation. For simplicity, only one chain of Igα and Igβ associated with each Ig molecule is shown. Orange semicircles indicate phosphate groups added to activated molecules.

cytokine receptor genes. Approximately 12 hours after antigenic stimulation, the B cell increases in size (becoming a B-cell blast); the B-cell blast proliferates and differentiates into a cell that synthesizes and secretes Ig (a plasma cell). In the absence of T-cell cytokines, the B cell synthesizes IgM. As described earlier in the chapter and in Chapter 7, in the presence of antigen and T-cell-derived cytokines the B cell may switch isotypes and develop into a memory B cell or plasma cell that synthesizes Ig isotypes distinct from IgM.

Modulation of BCR Signal

Positive Modulation. Another feature shared by the BCR and the TCR is a coreceptor that enhances the signal through the antigen-binding receptor. For the T cell, the coreceptor is CD4 or CD8; these molecules enhance the binding of an APC or target to a T cell, thereby decreasing the amount of antigen needed to trigger the T cell. Figure 10.11 shows that the molecules CD19, CD81, and CD21 (discussed in Chapter 7)—which are noncovalently associated in the B-cell membrane function—play a similar role as coreceptors for the BCR. The BCR coreceptor role has been characterized best in the response to microbial antigens; estimates indicate that 100- to 1000-fold less antigen is needed to stimulate an antibody response by activating the B cell via the coreceptor plus BCR compared to activation via the BCR alone.

Figure 10.13 indicates how the coreceptor lowers the threshold for stimulating B-cell responses to microbial pathogens. Microbial pathogens activate the complement pathways found in plasma (see Chapter 13) and become coated or "tagged" with complement component C3dg. The receptor for C3dg is the B-cell coreceptor molecule CD21. Thus, the pathogen bound to C3dg becomes

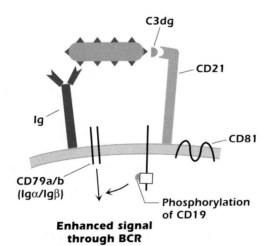

Figure 10.13. B-cell coreceptor CD19/CD21/CD81 and complement component C3dg enhance B-cell activation through B-cell receptor.

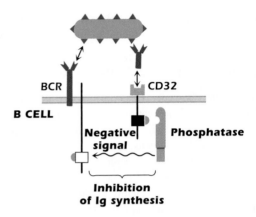

Figure 10.14. Antibody feedback inhibits B-cell activation. Simultaneous binding of the antigen and antibody components of an antigen–antibody complex to receptors on a B cell (antigen to the Ig, and the Fc portion of the antibody component to the FcR, CD32) results in a negative signal to the cell. The rectangle in the cytoplasmic region of CD32 represents the ITIM.

attached via CD21 to the B cell. The pathogen can also bind to IgM on the same B cell. This cross-linking of antigen via IgM and C3d on the B-cell surface delivers simultaneous activating signals to the B cell; CD19 in the coreceptor complex is phosphorylated and activates the ITAMs in Igα/Igβ (CD79a/b). Thus, activating the B cell via the coreceptor plus BCR augments the signal.

Negative Modulation. The signal through the BCR can also be modulated *negatively*. This occurs as a result of **antibody feedback** after an antibody has been synthesized in response to an antigen; the antibody produced inhibits a further B-cell response to that antigen. Antibody feedback can also be induced by injecting an antibody into an individual shortly before or during an immune response; the injected antibody shuts off the response to the antigen for which the antibody is specific. Antibody feedback has been used clinically to treat a condition in newborns in which antibody responses are made to the erythrocyte antigen Rh (see Chapter 15 for a fuller description of Rhesus incompatibility reactions).

One important way in which the presence of antibody inhibits B-cell function is by forming antigen–antibody complexes that interact with the low-affinity Fc receptor for IgG (FcRγIIb, CD32) expressed on the B cell. Figure 10.14 shows how this leads to negative signaling to the B cell: The Fc end of the antigen–antibody complex binds to CD32, while the antigen end of the complex simultaneously binds to the Ig on the same cell. This simultaneous binding to Ig and the FcR results in a negative signal to the B cell. Binding to the extracellular portion of CD32 recruits a phosphatase to an intracellular portion of CD32, which contains a tyrosine-containing sequence of amino acids. By analogy to the previously described ITAMs, the sequence in CD32 and other molecules is known as ***immunoreceptor tyrosine-based*** ***inhibitory motif*** (***ITIM***). The phosphatase that binds to the CD32 ITIM removes phosphate groups from tyrosine residues in the signal transduction polypeptides associated with the BCR. As a result, the activating signal through the BCR is inhibited.

SUMMARY

1. The dendritic cell is the principal, specialized APC to activate naïve $CD4^+$ T cells. On interaction with a pathogen in tissues immature dendritic cells mature, migrate to the draining lymph node, and present peptides associated with MHC class II to a $CD4^+$ T cell with the appropriate TCR.

2. Full activation of a naïve $CD4^+$ T cell requires multiple paired interactions at the surface of the APC and the T cell: a first signal (peptide+MHC class II with the TCR); MHC class II with the coreceptor, CD4; a second or costimulatory signal (B7–CD28 and CD40–CD40 Ligand); and paired adhesion molecules.

3. T-cell activation involves a cascade of events spreading from the area of contact between the APC and the T cell (the immunologic synapse) through the cytoplasm and into the nucleus. The critical pathways include the phosphorylation of kinases, the assembly and activation of signaling complexes at the cell membrane, the activation of intracellular signaling pathways, and the activation of multiple transcription factors that selectively activate the transcription of genes.

4. Among the most important genes transcribed and translated in the activated $CD4^+$ T cell are those coding for cytokines, particularly IL-2, and cytokine receptors, including one chain of the IL-2 receptor. Ultimately, activation results in the proliferation and expansion of the T-cell clone, differentiation to an effector T cell, and migration of the effector cell out of the node and to tissues or sites where pathogens have infiltrated.

5. As a consequence of activation by antigen, $CD4^+$ T cells secrete cytokines that affect multiple cell types. Four major subsets of $CD4^+$ T cells have been defined by their function and range of cytokines they produce; each subset produces a characteristic pattern of cytokines that interact with specific sets of effector cells.

6. T_H1 cells synthesize IL-2 and IFN-γ, which activate the effector cells of cell-mediated immunity. T_H2 cells synthesize IL-4, IL-5, and IL-13, which activate the effector cells involved in responses to parasitic worms and allergens. The recently characterized T_H17 subset synthesizes IL-17 family cytokines, which induce pro-inflammatory responses in many different cell types. T_H17 cells also respond to fungi and some extracellular bacteria. T_{reg} cells inhibit the function of the other subsets of $CD4^+$ T cells by cell contact and by the synthesis of inhibitory cytokines TGF-β and IL-10.

7. Cytokines produced by one subset of $CD4^+$ T cells in response to a specific antigen inhibit the development or function of other subsets and so skew the response toward one subset or another and hence one set of effector cells. Cytokines synthesized by cells of the innate immune system influence the differentiation into specific subsets of $CD4^+$ T cells.

8. $CD8^+$ T cells (CTL) interact with and kill target cells infected by microorganisms such as bacteria and viruses. The TCR of the $CD8^+$ T cell interacts with peptide derived from the pathogen bound to an MHC class I molecule on the surface of the target cell. A $CD8^+$ T cell must be activated and differentiate to an effector before it kills its target. The $CD8^+$ T cell can be activated by different pathways. $CD8^+$ T cells kill target cells by inducing apoptosis in the target via two main pathways: (1) action of cytotoxic materials contained in granules inside the $CD8^+$ T cell and secreted into the target cell, and (2) interaction of Fas expressed on the target with Fas ligand expressed on the $CD8^+$ T cell. Both pathways induce apoptosis in the target cell.

tissues migrate to the lymph nodes in response to the activity of these cytokines. There, they serve as potent APC to facilitate the adaptive immune responses needed to control infections.

The term *interferon* was coined because these cytokines interfere with viral replication, thus blocking the spread of viruses to uninfected cells. IFN-α and IFN-β, which are synthesized by many cell types following viral infection, are distinguished from another glycoprotein, IFN-γ, made by activated NK cells and effector T cells. In addition to their antiviral activities, IFN-α and IFN-β induce increased MHC class I expression on most uninfected cells, thus enhancing their resistance to NK cells and making newly infected cells more susceptible to killing by CD8 cytotoxic T cells. Finally, IFN-α and IFN-β activate NK cells, which contribute to early host responses to viral infections.

Cytokines that Regulate Adaptive Immune Responses

As discussed in Chapter 10, B- and T-cell activation in response to antigen stimulation is regulated by cytokines. Depending on the cytokines involved, regulation can be positive or negative and can impact cell proliferation, activation, and differentiation. Ultimately, cytokines regulate the intensity and duration of immune responses. A major feature of all adaptive immune responses is their antigen specificity. Given the potent immunoregulatory activities of cytokines, how does the immune system ensure that antigen-nonspecific B and T cells are not activated during an immune response? One mechanism to ensure the specificity of the immune response is the selective expression of functional cytokine receptors on lymphocytes that have been stimulated by antigen. As a consequence, cytokines tend to act only on antigen-activated lymphocytes. A second mechanism involves the need for cells to interact with each other through cell-to-cell contact, also known as *cognate* interaction. For example, cognate interactions that might occur between CD4$^+$ T helper cells and APC (e.g., dendritic cells, macrophages, B cells) generate high local concentrations of cytokines. In this way, only the target cell(s) participating in the interaction are affected by the cytokines produced. Finally, since the half-life of cytokines is very short, particularly in the bloodstream and extracellular spaces, the period of time during which they are able to act on other target cells is very limited.

Cytokines that Induce Differentiation of Distinct T-Cell Lineages

T_H1- and T_H2-Cell Lineages. It is now clear that certain cytokines play a key role in determining the fate of naïve T cells by staging the signaling events involved in lineage-specific differentiation. As discussed in earlier chapters, activated naïve CD4$^+$ T cells (T_H0 cells) differentiate into T_H1 cells under the influence of IL-12 produced by dendritic cells (DCs) and macrophages in the skin and mucosa (Fig. 11.2). Numerous studies illustrate the importance of this pathway by establishing that IL-12 is required for the development of protective innate and adaptive responses to many intracellular pathogens. Given the central role of this factor in the development of cell-mediated immunity, it is not surprising that IL-12 has also been implicated in the development of various autoimmune inflammatory conditions. The advent of bioinformatics tools and protein sequence databases led to the discovery of two IL-12-related cytokines that had already been named IL-23 and IL-27. Together, these cytokines constitute the IL-12 family of cytokines. As we shall see in the section that follows, these discoveries have provided a much deeper understanding of how our immune system responds to pathogenic challenges.

In contrast with T_H1-cell differentiation, the differentiation of naïve CD4$^+$ T cells into T_H2 cells is promoted by IL-4 produced by DCs and other innate cell populations (e.g., mast cells) (see Fig. 11.2). The type of antigen initiating the DC response appears to be a key factor in determining whether an IL-12 or IL-4 response will occur and, hence, whether the T_H1 or T_H2 lineage will develop. For example, intracellular bacteria (e.g., *Listeria*) and viruses activate DCs, macrophages, and NK cells to produce IL-12. In the presence of these cytokines, T_H0 cells tend to develop into T_H1 cells. The complex cell signaling and transcriptional events controlling these phenomena are beginning to emerge. Following activation, naïve CD4$^+$ T cells differentiate toward T_H1 in the presence of IL-12, which upregulates IFN-γ via Stat4; this leads to IFN-γ-mediated Stat1 activation and induction of the T_H1 lineage-determining transcription factor *T-bet*. By contrast, other pathogens (e.g., parasitic worms) do not induce IL-12 production but instead cause release of IL-4 by other cells (e.g., mast cells). IL-4 tends to promote the development of T_H0 cells into T_H2 cells as a result of its ability to activate Stat6, resulting in induction of the transcription factor known as GATA3. GATA3 expression results in chromatin remodeling at the T_H2 cytokine gene loci, leading to the signature cytokine profile associated with the T_H2 lineage.

The section that follows introduces a recently identified group of related cytokines (members of the IL-17 family). Their discovery preceded the identification of a new T-cell lineage, called the T_H17 T-cell lineage, that is a major cellular source of the IL-17 family of cytokines. Together, these two discoveries have provided fundamental new insights into the developmental pathways that promote the differentiation and function of CD4$^+$ T helper cells.

T$_H$17 T-Cell Lineage. The T$_H$1/T$_H$2 paradigm provides a framework for understanding T-cell biology and the interplay of innate and adaptive immunity. It is widely believed that T$_H$1 and T$_H$2 immunity evolved to enhance clearance of intracellular pathogens and parasitic helminths, respectively. What about T-cell responses to extracellular pathogens and fungi? The answer emerged recently, in part, with the discovery of the ***IL-17 family of cytokines*** and the subsequent discovery of a lineage of IL-17-producing T cells aptly called ***T$_H$17 cells***. T$_H$17 cells appear to have evolved as an arm of the adaptive immune system specialized for enhanced host protection against extracellular bacteria and some fungi, microbes probably not well covered by T$_H$1 or T$_H$2 immunity.

The IL-17 family of cytokines includes IL-17A, B, C, D, E, and F (Table 11.2). IL-17A was the name given to the founding member of the family. Because IL-17E had already been independently identified and given the name IL-25, that designation is commonly used instead. As a family, they share similar structural motifs and contain an unusual pattern of intrachain disulfide bonds.

The roles played by T$_H$17 cells and the IL-17 family of cytokines in host defense against pathogens are only beginning to emerge. IL-17 stimulates the mobilization and *de novo* generation of neutrophils by granulocyte colony-stimulating factor (G-CSF), thereby bridging innate and adaptive immunity. It has been suggested that this might constitute an early defense mechanism against severe trauma that would result in tissue necrosis or sepsis. Interestingly, we know less about their physiologic roles than we do regarding the pathologies in which they have been implicated. As discussed later in this chapter, IL-17 cytokines are key mediators in a diverse range of autoinflammatory disorders. The identification of T$_H$17 cells as the principal pathogenic effectors in several types of autoimmunity previously thought to be T$_H$1 mediated promises new approaches for therapies of these disorders, as does identification of IL-25 as a potentially important mediator of dysregulated T$_H$2 responses that cause asthma and other allergic disorders.

T$_H$17 T cells differentiate from naïve CD4$^+$ T cells in response to IL-6 and TGF-β. Signaling via IL-6 activates Stat3 and the lineage-determining transcription factor RORγt. The precise role of TGF-β in this differentiation process is not well understood although it is known that T cells defective in TGF-β receptor signaling cannot differentiate to T$_H$17 cells.

Cytokines that Inhibit Lineage-Specific T-Cell Differentiation

T$_H$1 and T$_H$2 subsets can also regulate one another's growth and effector functions. This phenomenon occurs as a result of the activity of cytokines produced by the subset that is being activated; its apparent purpose is to make it difficult to shift the response to the other subset. For example, production of IL-10 and TGF-β by T$_H$2 cells inhibits activation and growth of T$_H$1 cells. Similarly, production of IFN-γ by T$_H$1 cells inhibits proliferation of T$_H$2 cells. These effects permit either subset to dominate a particular immune response by inhibiting the outgrowth of the other subset.

As noted above, the T$_H$17 T-cell subset develops in response to IL-6 and TGF-β. This differentiation step is strongly inhibited by T$_H$1 or T$_H$2 cytokines. IL-27 is also a negative regulator of T$_H$17 differentiation. Interestingly, in the absence of IL-6, naïve T cells exposed only to TGF-β differentiate into regulatory T cells (T$_{reg}$).

Cytokines that Promote Inflammatory Responses

Many cytokines activate the functions of inflammatory cells and are therefore known as ***proinflammatory cytokines***. Examples of proinflammatory cytokines include IL-1, IL-6, IL-23, and TNF-α. During localized acute inflammatory responses, they cause increased vascular permeability, which ultimately leads to the swelling and

TABLE 11.2. IL-17 Family of Cytokines

Family Member	Alternate Names	Predicted Molecular Weight (kDa)	Percent Homology with IL-17A	Percent Homology with Human	Cellular Sources
IL-17A	IL-17 CTLA-8	35	100	62	T$_H$17 cells, CD8 T cells, NK cells, γδ T cells, neutrophils
IL-17B	CX1 NERF	41	21	88	T$_H$17 cells
IL-17C	CX2	43	24	75	T$_H$17 cells
IL-17D	IL-27	45	16	82	T$_H$17 cells
IL-17E	IL-25	38	16	76	T$_H$17 cells, T$_H$2 cells, eosinophils, mast cells
IL-17F	ML-1	34	45	54	T$_H$17 cells, CD8 T cells, NK cells, γδ T cells, neutrophils

redness associated with inflammation. As inflammatory mediators, they act in concert with the chemokines to ensure the development of physiologic responses to a variety of stimuli such as infections and tissue injury. Acute inflammatory responses develop rapidly and are of short duration. The short time span is probably related to the short half-lives of the inflammatory mediators involved as well as the regulatory influence of cytokines such as TGF-β, which limits the inflammatory response (see below). Typically, systemic responses accompany these short-lived responses and are characterized by a rapid alteration in levels of acute-phase proteins as described earlier in this chapter. Sometimes, persistent immune activation (as in chronic infections) can lead to chronic inflammation, which subverts the physiologic value of inflammatory responses and causes pathologic consequences.

The neutrophil plays a key role in the early stages of inflammatory responses (see Fig. 11.3). Within a few hours, neutrophils infiltrate the tissue area where the inflammatory response is occurring. Their migration from the blood to the tissue site is controlled by the expression of adhesion molecules on vascular endothelial cells—a mechanism regulated by mediators of acute inflammation, including IL-1 and TNF-α. Following exposure to these cytokines, vascular endothelial cells increase their expression of adhesion molecules (e.g., E- and P-selectin, ICAM-1; see Chapter 9), which in turn bind to selectin ligands (such as the sialyl Lewis moiety) expressed on the surface of neutrophils. The neutrophils attach securely to the endothelial cells and undergo a process of end-over-end rolling. Chemokines also activate the neutrophils and cause conformational changes in membrane integrin molecules. Figure 11.4 shows a schematic illustration of the conformational change in the heterodimeric (α- and β-chain) integrin molecule, LFA-1, which allows it to ligate ICAM-1. The change in conformation increases the affinity of neutrophils for the adhesion molecules on the endothelium.

Finally, the neutrophil undergoes transendothelial migration. This results in extravasation of the neutrophil, which is guided to the damaged or infected tissue site under the direction of chemokines in a process known as chemotaxis. It should be noted that lymphocytes and monocytes also undergo extravasation using the same basic steps as the neutrophil, although different combinations of adhesion molecules are involved. Other cytokines that play a significant role in inflammatory responses include IFN-γ and TGF-β. In addition to its role in activating macrophages to increase their phagocytic activity, IFN-γ has been shown to chemotactically attract macrophages to the site where antigen is localized. The migration of all of these cell types (neutrophils, lymphocytes, monocytes, macrophages) plus eosinophils and basophils, which are attracted to the site of tissue damage by complement activation, leads to clearance of the antigen and healing of the tissue. TGF-β plays a role in terminating the inflammatory response by promoting the accumulation and proliferation of fibroblasts and the deposition of extracellular matrix proteins required for tissue repair.

Cytokines that Affect Leukocyte Movement

The term chemokine is used to denote a family of closely related, low-molecular-weight chemotactic cytokines containing 70–80 residues with conserved sequences, which are known to be potent attractors for various leukocyte subsets, including neutrophils, monocytes, and lymphocytes. Table 11.3 lists some of the important chemokines among the 50 that have been identified. Structurally, this large superfamily consists of four subfamilies that display one of four highly conserved NH2-terminal cysteine amino acid residues: CXC, CC, C, and CX3C (where X represents a nonconserved amino acid residue). Most chemokines fall into the CXC and

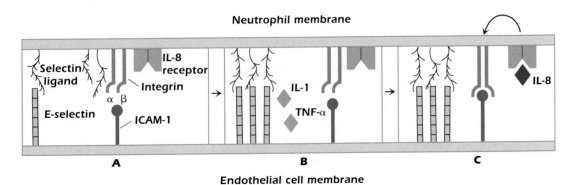

Figure 11.4. Cell membrane adhesion molecules and cytokine activation events associated with neutrophil transendothelial migration. (A) Weak binding of selectin ligands on neutrophil to E-selectin on endothelial cells. (B) IL-1 and TNF-α upregulation of E-selectin, which facilitates stronger binding. (C) Activation effects of IL-8 on neutrophils, which causes conformational change in integrins (e.g., LFA-1) to allow them to bind ICAM-1.

TABLE 11.3. Selected Chemokines and Their Functions

Chemokine	Produced By	Chemoattracted Cells	Major Functions
IL-8	Monocytes, macrophages, fibroblasts, keratinocytes, endothelial cells	Neutrophils, naïve T cells	Mobilizes and activates neutrophils; promotes angiogenesis
RANTES	T cells, endothelial cells, platelets	Monocytes, NK cells, T cells, basophils, eosinophils	Degranulates basophils; activates T cells
MCP-1	Monocytes, macrophages, fibroblasts, keratinocytes	Monocytes, NK cells, T cells, basophils, dendritic cells	Activates macrophages; stimulates basophil histamine release; promotes T_H2 immunity
MIP-1α	Monocytes, macrophages, T cells, mast cells, fibroblasts	Monocytes, NK cells, T cells, basophils, dendritic cells	Promotes T_H1 immunity; competes with HIV-1
MIP-1β	Monocytes, macrophages, neutrophils, endothelial cells	Monocytes, NK cells, T cells, dendritic cells	Competes with HIV-1 for chemokine receptor binding

^{a}IL, interleukin; MCP, monocyte chemotactic protein; MIP, macrophage inflammatory protein; NK, natural killer; T_H, helper T cell.

CC groups. As discussed above, chemokines function in concert with inflammatory mediators to regulate the expression and conformation of cell adhesion molecules in leukocyte membranes. Some cytokines have also been shown to induce respiratory burst, enzyme release, intracellular Ca^{2+} mobilization, and angiogenesis. The latter is a biologic function consistent with the important role some chemokines play in wound healing and tissue repair. Production of chemokines may either be induced or constitutive. Those chemokines capable of being induced or strongly upregulated in peripheral tissues in response to inflammation are primarily involved in wound healing and tissue repair mechanisms. By contrast, constitutively produced chemokines fulfill housekeeping functions and may be involved in normal leukocyte traffic.

IL-8, a member of the CXC subfamily, is among the most well characterized of the chemokines that have been identified to date. It is produced by many different cell types, including macrophages, T cells, endothelial cells, fibroblasts, and neutrophils. IL-8 plays a major role in inflammatory responses and wound healing, primarily because of its ability to attract neutrophils to sites of tissue damage. Another important function of IL-8 is its ability to activate neutrophils following their attachment to vascular endothelium (see Fig. 11.3).

A noteworthy characteristic of certain CC chemokines (e.g., RANTES, MIP−1α, and MIP−1β) is their ability to suppress infection of T cells *in vitro* with M-trophic HIV strains. These strains of HIV were named because of their ability to infect macrophage cell lines *in vitro*, although it is now known that M-trophic HIV strains can infect dendritic cells, macrophages, and T cells *in vivo* as well (Chapter 17). Lymphocyte-trophic HIV strains infect only $CD4^+$ T cells *in vitro*. The different variants of HIV and the cell types they infect are largely determined by the chemokine receptor they use as a required HIV coreceptor. For example, dendritic cells, macrophages, and T cells all express CCR5, and primary infections with M-trophic HIV variants use this chemokine receptor. Because CCR5 also binds to chemokines RANTES, MIP−1α, and MIP−1β, the addition of these chemokines to lymphocytes sensitive to HIV infection blocks the infection because of competition between the CC chemokines and the virus for the target cell coreceptor CCR5.

By contrast, the chemokine receptor that binds to certain members of the CXC subfamily (CXCR4) is the coreceptor responsible for entry of lymphocyte-trophic strains of HIV into target cells. The establishment of a heterotrimeric complex between the viral envelope protein gp120, CD4, and one of these chemokine receptors facilitates viral entry into cells. However, the molecular mechanisms associated with this phenomenon are only beginning to be understood.

Cytokines that Stimulate Hematopoiesis

As discussed in Chapter 2, myeloid and lymphoid cells are derived from pluripotent stem cells (see Fig. 2.1). Cytokines capable of inducing growth of hematopoietic cells *in vitro* were initially characterized using cultures of bone marrow cells grown in soft agar and thus are referred to as ***colony-stimulating factors (CSF)***. Several biochemically distinct CSFs have been identified by the particular lineage of hematopoietic cells that were stimulated to form colonies. These include ***macrophage CSF*** (M-CSF), which supports the clonal growth of macrophages, ***granulocyte CSF*** (G-CSF), which supports the clonal growth of granulocytes, and ***granulocyte–macrophage CSF*** (GM-CSF), which supports the clonal growth of both monocytes and macrophages. **IL-3** is another cytokine capable of stimulating clonal growth of hematopoietic cells; however, unlike the CSFs, IL-3 is capable of promoting proliferation of a large number of cell populations, including granulocytes, macrophages, megakaryocytes, eosinophils, basophils, and mast cells. Moreover, in the presence of ***erythropoietin***, a kidney-derived growth factor that has the ability to support the growth and terminal differentiation of cells of the erythroid lineage, IL-3 is also capable of stimulating development of normoblasts and red cells. IL-7, a cytokine produced largely by bone marrow and thymic stromal cells, induces differentiation of lymphoid stem cells into progenitor B and T cells. Like other functional categories of cytokines, the list of factors that are involved in hematopoiesis has grown significantly in recent years. Perhaps more than any other category of cytokines, CSFs have emerged as important therapeutic agents. For example, G-CSF is used to treat patients undergoing high-dose chemotherapy to reverse neutropenia. GM-CSF is used to boost clonal expansion of the granulocyte and macrophage populations in patients undergoing bone marrow transplantation.

CYTOKINE RECEPTORS

Cytokine Receptor Families

As you have already learned, cytokines can only act on target cells that express receptors for that cytokine. Often, cytokine receptor expression, like cytokine production itself, is highly regulated, so that resting cells either do not express a given receptor or express a low- or intermediate-affinity version of the receptor. The IL-2 receptor is an example of the latter; it can be expressed on the membranes of cells as either an intermediate-affinity dimer (β and γ chains) or a high-affinity trimer containing three subunit chains α, β, and γ (see below). IL-2 is

capable of activating cells expressing the high-affinity form of the IL-2 receptor—a property unique to T cells undergoing antigen stimulation. The relative importance of these receptor subunits in binding to IL-2 and signaling the target cell is discussed later in this chapter. For now what you need to know is that the regulation of the receptor level expressed on the target cell membrane and/or the receptor form expressed helps to ensure that only an activated target population will respond to the cytokine(s) within the local microenvironment.

Understanding how cytokines affect their target cells has been the subject of many recent studies. As discussed later in this chapter, knowledge about cytokine–cytokine receptor interactions may be useful in devising strategies to prevent cytokine activity in inflammatory responses such as rheumatoid arthritis or in immune responses such as transplantation rejection.

Receptors for cytokines can be divided into five families of receptor proteins (Fig. 11.5):

- Immunoglobulin superfamily receptors
- Class I cytokine receptor family
- Class II cytokine receptor family
- TNF receptor superfamily
- Chemokine receptor family

The **immunoglobulin superfamily** receptors contain shared structural features that were first defined in immunoglobulins; each has at least one Ig-like domain (see

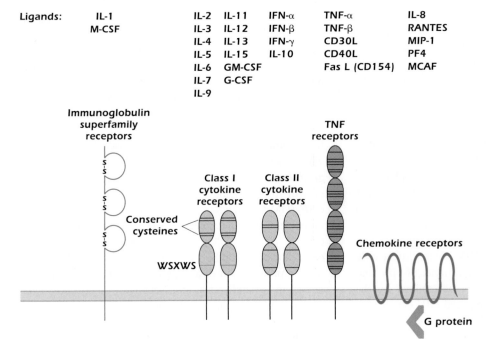

Figure 11.5. Structural features of five types of cytokine receptors. Many contain highly conserved cysteine residues.

Chapter 4). Examples of cytokines with immunoglobulin superfamily receptors include IL-1 and M-CSF. *Class I cytokine receptors* (also known as the hematopoietin receptor family) are usually composed of two types of polypeptide chains: a cytokine-specific subunit (α chain) and a signal-transducing subunit (β or γ chain). Important exceptions include the high-affinity receptors for IL-2 and the IL-15 receptor, both of which are trimers. Most cytokines identified to date utilize the class I family of cytokine receptors. *Class II cytokine receptors* are also known as the interferon receptor family because their ligands are interferons (e.g., IFN-α, IFN-β, and IFN-γ) or have biological activities that overlap with those of some interferons (e.g., IL-10). The *TNF receptor* (*TNFR*) *superfamily* is divided into three divergent subgroups that are classified by differences in their cytoplasmic tails: death receptors, decoy receptors, and activating receptors. Each of these subgroups contains similar extracellular ligand-binding domains. When TNFRs are activated, they mediate their intracellular signals through a set of adaptor proteins called *TNF-receptor-associated factors* (*TRAF*). TNFR ligands can be membrane associated or secreted proteins. For example, most effector T cells express membrane-associated forms, including TNF-α and TNF-β (also known as lymphotoxin-α). Both of these can also be released as secreted proteins. Other TNFRs include Fas, which contains the "death domain" in its cytoplasmic tail, and CD40, which is involved in such functions as B-cell proliferation, maturation, and class switching. In short, the TNFR and TNF superfamilies regulate the life and death of activated cells of the immune system. Finally, the *chemokine receptors* belong to a superfamily of so-called serpentine G-protein-coupled receptors, which get their name from a unique snakelike extracellular-cytoplasmic structural configuration and an association with G proteins, which mediate signal transduction (Fig. 11.5). A growing list of CC and CXC chemokine receptors have been cloned. Some of these have been found to be *promiscuous*, or capable of binding not only to chemokines but also to a

diverse set of pathogens. These pathogens include bacteria [such as *Streptococcus pneumonia*, which binds to the platelet activating-factor receptor (PAF)], parasites (such as *Plasmodium vivax*, which binds to the chemokine receptor known as Duffy blood group antigen), and certain viruses (such as T-tropic HIV-1 strains that use the CXCR4 chemokine receptor.

Common Cytokine Receptor Chains

As noted earlier in this chapter, it is common for different cytokines to have overlapping (redundant) functions; for example, both IL-1 and IL-6 induce fever and several other common biologic phenomena. Several cytokines use multichain receptors to mediate their effects on target cells and some of these receptors share at least one common receptor molecule called the *common γ chain* (see Fig. 11.6), an intracellular signaling molecule. The presence of a common receptor molecule helps to explain the functional overlap.

The high-affinity IL-2 receptor (IL-2R) consists of the common γ chain, an IL-2-specific α chain, and a β chain. In contrast, an intermediate-affinity IL-2 receptor is expressed as a dimer containing only the β and γ chains (Fig. 11.7). IL-2 is capable of activating cells expressing the high-affinity form of the IL-2 receptor, a property reserved for T cells undergoing antigen-specific activation. It is noteworthy that a defect in the common IL-2Rγ chain has been shown to cause a profound immune deficiency in males suffering from X-linked severe combined immunodeficiency disease (see Chapter 17). This defect abolishes the functional activity of multiple cytokines because of their shared use of the common γ chain.

Severe Combined Immunodeficiency Disease

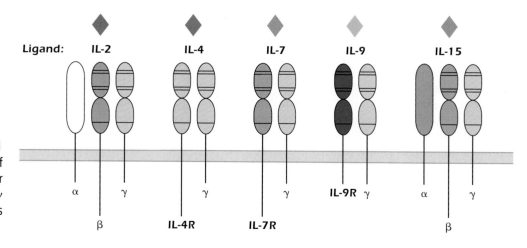

Figure 11.6. Structural features of members of class I cytokine receptor family that share common γ chain (*green*) that mediates intracellular signaling.

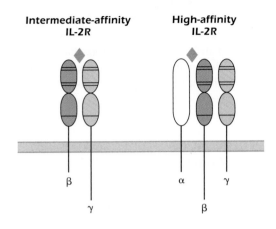

Intermediate-affinity IL-2R **High-affinity IL-2R**

Affinity constant: 10^{-9} M 10^{-11} M

Cell expression: NK cells resting T cells Activated T cells

Figure 11.7. Comparison of two forms of IL-2 receptors expressed on cells.

CYTOKINE RECEPTOR-MEDIATED SIGNAL TRANSDUCTION

We have already presented some of the signaling pathways that are selectively activated by specific cytokines to promote lineage-specific T-cell differentiation. In order for cytokines to mediate virtually all of their diverse biologic effects on target cells, they must generate intracellular signals that result in the production of active transcription factors and, ultimately, gene expression (Fig. 11.8). Binding of a cytokine to its cellular receptor induces dimerization or polymerization of receptor polypeptides at the cell surface. The mechanism illustrated applies to most, if not all, class I and class II cytokine receptor families. It is not clear how signal specificity is maintained when different cytokine receptors use the same cytoplasmic signaling pathways. In the case of the two receptor families illustrated in Figure 11.8, the dimerization/polymerization of receptor subunits juxtaposes their cytoplasmic tails, allowing the dimeric receptor to engage the intracytoplasmic signaling machinery. Signaling is initiated by the activation of *JAK kinases*, a family of cytosolic protein tyrosine kinases. JAK kinases interact with the cytoplasmic domains of the receptor, which results in the phosphorylation of tyrosine residues on the cytoplasmic domain and on a family of transcription factors known as *STATs* (signal transducers and activators of transcription). Once phosphorylated, the STAT transcription factors dimerize and subsequently translocate from the cytoplasm to the nucleus, where they bind to enhancer regions of genes induced by the cytokine.

The signaling events described above result in the biologic properties of the cytokine at the cellular level. However, at some point these signals must be terminated. Until recently, the mechanism responsible for down-regulation of cytokine-mediated signaling was poorly understood. Studies have now identified a family of intracellular proteins that plays a key role in the suppression of cytokine signaling. These *suppressor of cytokine signaling* (*SOCS*) proteins regulate signal transduction by direct interactions with cytokine receptors and signaling proteins and have a generic mechanism of targeting associated proteins for degradation. Given the central contribution of cytokines to many diseases, including the ones discussed in the next section, the deregulation of normal SOCS may play an etiologic role. The manipulation of SOCS function may provide potent therapeutic options in the future.

ROLE OF CYTOKINES AND CYTOKINE RECEPTORS IN DISEASE

Given the complex regulatory properties of cytokines, it is not surprising that overexpression or underexpression of cytokines or cytokine receptors have been implicated in many diseases. Here we discuss some examples of diseases with cytokine-associated pathophysiology.

Toxic-Shock Syndrome

Toxic-shock syndrome is initiated by the release of *superantigen* (enterotoxin) from certain microorganisms. For example, the toxins derived from *Staphylococcus aureus* or *Streptococcus pyogenes* cause a burst of cytokine production by T cells. The toxin accomplishes this by activating large numbers of CD4 T cells, which use certain Vβ segments as part of their TCR. The toxin cross-links the Vβ segment of the TCR with a class II MHC molecule expressed on APC (see Fig. 8.9). It has been estimated that

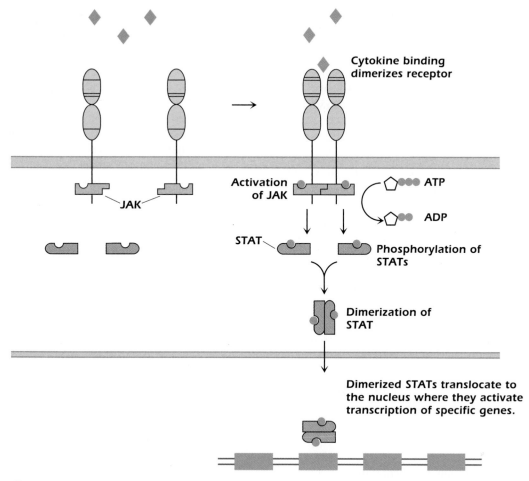

Figure 11.8. Model of cytokine receptor signaling using receptor-associated kinases to activate specific transcription factors.

one in every five T cells can be activated by superantigens. The activity of superantigen-activated T cells results in excessive production of cytokines that ultimately cause dysregulation of the cytokine network. Extremely high levels of IL-1 and TNF-α induce systemic reactions including fever, blood clotting, diarrhea, a drop in blood pressure, and shock. Sometimes these reactions are fatal.

Bacterial Septic Shock

Overproduction of cytokines is also associated with infections caused by certain Gram-negative bacteria, including *Escherichia coli, Klebsiella pneumonia, Enterobacter aerogenes, Pseudomonas aeruginosa*, and *Neisseria meningitidis*. Endotoxins produced by these bacteria stimulate macrophages to overproduce IL-1 and TNF-α, which causes an often fatal form of bacterial septic shock.

Cancers

Several lymphoid and myeloid cancers have been shown to be associated with abnormally high levels of cytokines and/or cytokine receptor expression. Perhaps the best example of an association between malignancy and overproduction of a cytokine and its receptor is adult T-cell leukemia disease that is strongly associated with the human T-cell lymphoma (HTLV-1) retrovirus. T cells infected with HTLV-1 constitutively produce IL-2 and express the high-affinity IL-2 receptor in the absence of activation by antigen. This results in autocrine stimulation of infected T cells, leading to their uncontrolled growth. Other examples include myelomas (neoplastic B cells), which produce large amounts of the autocrine IL-6, and follicular lymphoma, a lymphoma in which the reactive milieu is the result of abundant production of cytokines, particularly IL-5 (see also Chapter 17).

 Follicular Lymphoma

Autoimmunity and Other Immune-Based Diseases

A great deal of evidence suggests that T cells exert a controlling influence on the generation of autoantibodies and on the regulation of autoimmunity (see Chapter 12). Many of the observed phenomena are manifestations of the actions of cytokines, including IL-23, IL-12, IL-10, IFN-γ, IL-4, and members of the IL-17 family. Research has demonstrated the association of several abnormalities of cytokines and cytokine receptors with systemic autoimmune diseases. Some occur late in illness and are probably not causal, while others may be involved in dysregulation of immune responses and may help promote autoreactivity. For example, the autoimmune disease systemic lupus erythematosus (SLE) has been associated with elevated levels of IL-10. Recent studies of cytokines involved in autoimmune diseases have examined whether skewing of the T$_H$-cell subset phenotype contributes to disease initiation or disease progression. The importance of T$_H$2 cells in promoting systemic autoimmunity has been reported in research utilizing experimental animal models of autoimmune disease. Future studies will be needed to clearly elucidate the roles played by cytokines and cytokine receptors in autoimmune disease.

Systemic Lupus Erythematosus

Cytokines play a major role in the pathophysiology of other immune-based diseases, including allergy, asthma, and inflammatory diseases such as rheumatoid arthritis (RA). Many clinical features associated with these diseases are the result of cytokine receptor-mediated signaling and the biologic effects of such signaling (e.g., cell activation, cell death). Our understanding of the roles played by cytokines and cytokine receptors in the manifestation of these and other diseases continues to expand. The crucial interactions between cytokines and their receptors in many autoimmune diseases and other immune-based diseases warrants further investigation and could represent a unique opportunity to intervene successfully even after the onset of symptoms.

Asthma

In the next section we discuss the application of what we already know about cytokines and cytokine receptors to the development of treatments for some of these diseases.

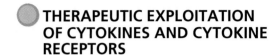

THERAPEUTIC EXPLOITATION OF CYTOKINES AND CYTOKINE RECEPTORS

Knowledge of the cellular and molecular components of immune responses to infectious microbes and, specifically, the roles played by cytokines in regulation and homeostasis of hematopoietic cells has opened opportunities for new therapies. The many opportunities for clinical uses of cytokines, soluble cytokine receptors (antagonists), cytokine analogs, and anticytokine or anti–cytokine receptor antibody therapies have sparked a great deal of commercial interest.

Cytokine Inhibitors/Antagonists

Several naturally occurring soluble cytokine receptors have been identified in the bloodstream and extracellular fluids. These act, *in vivo*, as **cytokine inhibitors**, or **antagonists**, and are released from the cell surface as a result of enzymatic cleavage of the extracellular domain of the cytokine receptor. Circulating soluble cytokine receptors maintain their ability to bind to a specific cytokine, thus neutralizing its activity. Examples of such inhibitors include those that bind to IL-2, IL-4, IL-6, IL-7, IFN-γ, and, last but not least, TNF. Experimental use of soluble TNF receptors has led to the development of a new class of biologic response modifier drugs called **TNF inhibitors**. TNF inhibitors have shown significant clinical utility in the treatment of RA. Patients with RA have increased levels of TNF and IL-1 in their joints—a phenomenon that leads to RA-associated pain, swelling, stiffness, and other symptoms. TNF inhibitors (**soluble TNF receptor molecules**) compete with endogenously produced TNF for binding to TNF receptors (Fig. 11.9). Most RA patients treated with TNF inhibitors show significant improvement of their symptoms, but approximately 30% are nonresponsive to this treatment.

Rheumatoid Arthritis

The soluble **IL-2 receptor** (IL-2R) has also been studied extensively. It is formed by the proteolytic release of a 45-kDa portion of the IL−2 α chain of the IL-2R. Chronic T-cell activation is associated with very high levels of soluble IL-2R in the bloodstream. Thus, IL-2R has been used as a clinical marker for chronic T-cell activation in patients with certain autoimmune diseases and those undergoing transplant rejection.

Another well-characterized cytokine antagonist is the naturally occurring **IL-1 receptor antagonist** (IL-1Ra). This protein also plays a role in regulating the intensity of

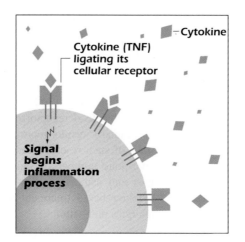

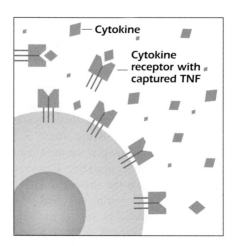

Figure 11.9. Soluble TNF receptors can interfere with inflammatory properties of TNF.

inflammatory responses by binding to the IL-1 receptor on CD4$^+$ T cells, thus preventing their activation. Binding of IL-1Ra to the IL-1 receptor does not mediate cell signaling through this receptor. IL-1Ra has been cloned and is currently under clinical investigation to determine whether it can be used as a therapeutic agent for chronic inflammatory diseases.

Reversing Cellular Deficiencies

Several cytokines, such as G-CSF and GM-CSF, have been used to treat acute events such as cellular deficiencies arising from chemotherapy or radiotherapy. As discussed earlier in this chapter, treatment with these hematopoietic growth factors escalates the rate of natural reconstitution of desired hematopoietic cell lineages.

Treatment of Immunodeficiencies

Cytokines have also been used to treat patients with immunodeficiency diseases, many of which are described in Chapter 17. For example, patients with X-linked agammaglobulinemia have been treated successfully with G-CSF to reverse their disease-associated neutropenia.

X-Linked Agammaglobulinemia

Patients suffering from a form of SCID due to adenosine deaminase (ADA) deficiency—a disease often associated with a profound IL-2 deficiency—have been treated with recombinant human IL-2. Finally, several leukocyte adhesion deficiency diseases characterized by recurrent or progressive soft tissue infection, periodontitis, poor wound healing, and leukocytosis have been successfully treated with recombinant IFN-γ to reduce the severity and frequency of infections, probably by increasing nonoxidative antimicrobial activity.

Treatment of Cancer and Transplant Patients

Patients with cancer have also benefited from the use of cytokines in passive cellular immunotherapies. Such therapies utilize **lymphokine-activated killer** (LAK) cells, as described in Chapter 19. Culturing populations of NK cells or cytotoxic T cells in the presence of high concentrations of IL-2 generates effector cells with potent antitumor activities. The availability of recombinant IL-2 in large quantities has made the LAK cell plus IL-2 therapy feasible, and some melanoma and renal carcinoma patients have shown objective responses. Another variation of passive cellular immunotherapy is the concurrent use of IFN-γ. Administration of IFN-γ enhances the expression of MHC and tumor-associated antigens on tumor cells, thereby making them more "visible" to the infused effector cells.

Cytokine receptor-specific antibodies have also proven useful in the treatment of certain cancers. The relative accessibility of certain cytokine receptor-positive leukemic cells has encouraged numerous trials with native as well as toxin-conjugated antibodies. In one subset of leukemia with leukemic cells that constitutively express the IL-2 receptor α chain (CD25) [adult T-cell leukemia/lymphoma (ATLL)], antibodies to CD25 (also known as anti-Tac antibodies) have been shown to induce therapeutic responses in approximately one-third of the patients treated.

Anti-CD25 therapy has also been used as part of a regimen of immunosuppressive therapy to treat patients receiving organ transplants. The rationale for such treatment is based on the chronic activation of alloreactive T cells caused by exposure to alloantigens expressed by the grafted tissue. Such activation induces the expression of CD25 by these cells. Anti-CD25 therapy is often used with other immunosuppressive drugs to dampen the host's immune response to the alloantigens, thus reducing the incidence of graft rejection. Chapter 18 contains additional information about immunotherapies used to treat patients who have received organ transplants.

Treatment of Allergies and Asthma

Our current understanding of T_H2 cells and the roles played by the cytokines they produce (e.g., IL-4, IL-13) in the pathophysiology of allergies and asthma suggests that therapies that target these cytokines or their receptors may prove to be effective in treating these conditions (Chapter 14). Given the cross-antagonistic effects of T_H1 and T_H2 cells, it may be possible to skew the production of antibody away from IgE in response to a given allergen using strategies that selectively silence the undesired T_H2 subset. At present, this remains an experimental goal which is being investigated aggressively in animal models. Promising results have emerged from clinical trials using a related strategy that specifically targets IL-4, the major cytokine responsible for promoting B-cell isotype class switching to IgE (see Chapters 10 and 14). Injection of antibodies specific for IL-4 has been shown to dramatically decrease IL-4 production in mice. Another related strategy involves the use of soluble IL-4 receptors, with promising, although again preliminary, results reported to date. The clinical applications of such research cannot be underestimated given the enormous number of individuals who suffer from allergies and asthma worldwide. Chapter 14 discusses other cytokine-based treatment strategies used in patients with allergies and asthma.

SUMMARY

1. Cytokines are low-molecular-weight antigen-nonspecific proteins that mediate cellular interactions involving immune, inflammatory, and hematopoietic systems.

2. Cytokines exhibit the properties of pleiotropy and redundancy and often display synergism or antagonism with other cytokines.

3. Cytokines are short-lived and may act locally—either on the same cell that secreted them (autocrine) or on other cells (paracrine)—or systemically (endocrine).

4. Cytokines have a wide variety of functional activities as illustrated by their ability to (a) regulate specific immune responses, (b) facilitate innate immune responses, (c) activate inflammatory responses, (d) affect leukocyte movement, and (e) stimulate hematopoiesis.

5. Subsets of CD4 T_H cells have been defined by the range of cytokines they produce. T_H1 cells secrete IL-2 and IFN-γ (as well as several other cytokines), but not IL-4 or IL-5. Cytokines produced by these cells also activate other T cells, NK cells, and macrophages (cell-mediated immune responses). By contrast, T_H2 cells secrete IL-4 and IL-5 (as well as other cytokines), but not IL-2 or IFN-γ, and predominantly affect antibody responses.

6. Knowledge regarding the new CD4 T-cell subset called Th17 T cells and the IL-17 family of cytokines is filling many gaps in our understanding of how immune responses are regulated. IL-17 stimulates the mobilization and generation of neutrophils, thereby bridging the gap between innate and adaptive immunity.

7. Cytokines can only act on target cells that express receptors for that cytokine. Cytokine receptor expression is highly regulated; resting cells either do not express a given receptor or express a low- or intermediate-affinity version of that receptor. Increased levels of cytokine receptor expression or expression of high-affinity forms of a given receptor predispose target cells to respond to a cytokine.

8. The common γ chain is a cytokine receptor subunit utilized by several cytokine receptors as the signal-transducing subunit, including IL-2, IL-4, IL-7, IL-9, and IL-15. This structural feature helps to explain the redundancy and antagonism often exhibited by some cytokines.

9. Ligation of cytokine receptors by cytokines generates intracellular signals that result in the production of active transcription factors and, ultimately, gene expression. Binding of a cytokine to its cellular receptor often induces dimerization or polymerization of receptor polypeptides at the cell surface and permits association of JAK kinases with the receptor cytoplasmic domain. This association activates the kinases and causes phosphorylation of tyrosine residues in STATs (signal transducers and activators of transcription). Once phosphorylated, the STAT transcription factors dimerize and subsequently translocate from the cytoplasm to the nucleus, where they bind to enhancer regions of genes induced by the cytokine. Suppression of cytokine signaling (SOCS) proteins down-regulate signal transduction and help terminate cytokine responses.

10. Overexpression and underexpression of cytokines or cytokine receptors have been implicated in several diseases, including bacterial toxic shock, bacterial sepsis, certain lymphoid and myeloid cancers, and autoimmunity.

11. Cytokine-related therapies offer promise for the treatment of certain immunodeficiencies, the prevention of graft rejection, and the treatment of certain cancers. The utility of cytokine-related therapies is best seen in the use of (a) hematopoietic growth factors (G-CSF, GM-CSF) to reverse certain cellular deficiencies associated with chemo- or radiotherapy, (b) the use of anti-IL-2 receptor therapy to help reduce graft rejection, and (c) the use of IL-2 to generate lymphokine-activated killer cells (NK and cytotoxic T cells) employed in the treatment of patients with certain cancers.

REFERENCES

Alexander WS (2002): Suppressor of cytokine signaling (SOCS) in the immune system. *Nature Rev Immunol* 2:411.

Campbell JJ, Butcher EC (2000): Chemokines in tissue-specific and microenvironment-specific lymphocyte homing. *Curr Opin Immunol* 12:336.

DeVries ME, Kelvin DJ (1999): On the edge: The physiological and pathophysiological role of chemokines during inflammatory and immunological responses. *Semin Immunol* 11:95.

Ezerzer C, Harris N (2007): Physiological immunity or pathological autoimmunity—A question of balance. *Autoimmun Rev* 6(7): 488.

Fernandez-Botran R, Crespo FA, Sun X (2000): Soluble cytokine receptors in biological therapy. *Expert Opin Biol Ther* 2:585.

Kisseleva T, Bhattacharya S, Braunstein J, Schindler CW (2000): Signaling through the JAK/STAT pathway, recent advances and future challenges. *Gene* 20:1.

Koch, AE (2007): The pathogenesis of rheumatoid arthritis. *Am J Orthop* 36:5.

Leonard WJ (2001): Cytokines and immunodeficiency diseases. *Nat Rev Immunol* 1:200.

Ma A, Koka M, Burkett P (2006): Diverse functions of IL-2, IL-15, and IL-7 in lymphoid homeostasis. *Annu Rev Immunol.* 24:821.

Matsuzaki G, Umemura M (2007): Interleukin-17 as an effector molecule of innate and acquired immunity against infections. *Microbiol Immunol* 51:1139.

McGeachy MJ, Cua DJ (2007): T cells doing it for themselves: TGF-β regulation of Th1 and Th17 cells. *Immunity* 26: 547.

Minami Y, Kono T, Miyazaki T, Taniguchi T (1993): The IL-2 receptor complex: Its structure, function, and target genes. *Annu Rev Immunol* 11:245.

Weaver CT, Harrington LE, Mangan PR, Gavrieli M, Murphy, KM (2006): Th17: An effector CD4 T cell lineage with regulatory T cell ties. *Immunity* 24:677.

 ## REVIEW QUESTIONS

For each question, choose the ONE BEST answer.

1. Polarization of naïve CD4$^+$ T-cell differentiation toward the T$_H$2 lineage is associated with which of the following cytokines?
   A) IL-1
   B) IL-4
   C) IL-6
   D) IL-23
   E) IL-25

2. A patient with active rheumatoid arthritis feels systemically ill with low-grade fever, malaise, morning stiffness, and fatigue. The protein(s) or cytokine(s) most likely to be responsible for these symptoms are:
   A) rheumatoid factor
   B) TNF and IL-1
   C) IL-4 and IL-10
   D) complement components 1–9
   E) altered gammaglobulin

3. When IL-2 is secreted by antigen-specific T cells activated due to presentation of antigen by APC, what happens to naïve antigen-nonspecific T cells in the vicinity?
   A) They proliferate due to their exposure to IL-2.
   B) They often undergo apoptosis.
   C) They begin to express IL-2 receptors.
   D) They secrete cytokines associated with their T cell phenotype.
   E) Nothing happens.

4. IL-1, IL-6, and TNF-α are proinflammatory cytokines that are known to:
   A) cause increased vascular permeability
   B) act in concert with chemokines to promote migration of inflammatory cells to sites of infection
   C) initiate acute-phase responses
   D) have endogenous pyrogen properties
   E) all of the above

5. Which of the following cytokines plays a role in terminating inflammatory responses?
   A) IL-2
   B) IL-4
   C) TGF-β
   D) IFN-α
   E) IL-3

6. Assuming there were no other compensatory mechanisms to replace IL-8 function, which of the following would be preserved as a functional activity in an IL-8 knockout mouse strain?
   A) activation of neutrophils
   B) attraction of neutrophils to sites of tissue damage
   C) wound healing
   D) extravasation of neutrophils
   E) reduction of cytokine production by T_H1 cells

7. Superantigens cause a burst of cytokine production by T cells due to their ability to cross-link:
   A) the Vβ segments of T-cell receptors with class II MHC molecules on APC
   B) the Vα segments of T-cell receptors with class II MHC molecules on APC
   C) T-cell receptors and CD3
   D) multiple cytokine receptors on a large population of T cells
   E) CD3

ANSWERS TO REVIEW QUESTIONS

1. *B* Activation of innate immune cells, such as mast cells, triggers the synthesis of several cytokines, including IL-4, which promotes T_H2-cell differentiation.

2. *B* Patients with rheumatoid arthritis have elevated levels of proinflammatory cytokines TNF and IL-1 in their joints, which play a key role in the pain, swelling, stiffness, and other symptoms associated with this disease.

3. *E* Cytokines secreted by antigen-activated T cells only regulate the activities of other cells involved in that immune response by binding to cytokine receptors (e.g., high-affinity IL-2R) expressed by these cells. Such cytokine receptors are upregulated only on antigen-activated T cells that bear the appropriate TCR for that antigen; because they are not upregulated on antigen-nonspecific T cells in the vicinity, these cells will not be activated by IL-2.

4. *E* The answer is self-explanatory.

5. *C* Among the cytokines listed, TGF-β plays a role in terminating inflammatory responses by promoting the accumulation and proliferation of fibroblasts and the deposition of extracellular matrix proteins required for tissue repair.

6. *E* IL-8 plays no role in regulation of cytokine production by T_H1 cells—a biologic property ascribed to IL-10 produced by T_H2 cells. Therefore, functional integrity of T_H1 would be predicted in IL-8 knockout mice. IL-8 chemotactically attracts and activates neutrophils and induces their adherence to vascular endothelium and extravasation (activities that should be deficient in IL-8 knockouts). Because these activities are important for wound healing, this phenomenon would also be predicted to be deficient in such mice.

7. *A* Superantigens bind simultaneously to class II MHC molecules and to the Vβ domain of the TCR, activating all T cells bearing a particular Vβ domain. Thus, they activate large numbers of T cells (between 5 and 25%), regardless of their antigen specificity, causing them to release harmful quantities of cytokines.

12

TOLERANCE AND AUTOIMMUNITY

Contributed by LINDA SPATZ

INTRODUCTION

The immune system functions to protect the host from invasion by foreign organisms. However, this protective response can cause damage to the host if it is directed against the individual's own antigens, which are often referred to as *self-antigens* or *autoantigens*. Therefore, the immune system has developed a series of checks and balances that enable it to distinguish dangerous from harmless signals and allow it to respond to foreign antigens but not self-antigens. Both the innate and adaptive immune responses have evolved to make this distinction. This chapter focuses on the adaptive immune responses that are the basis for tolerance to self-antigens.

One of the earliest experiments that demonstrated tolerance was performed by Ray Owens in 1945. He showed that dizygotic cattle twins, which share a common vascular system in utero, were mutually tolerant of skin grafts from one another as adults. Thus, "foreign" antigens expressed by cells of the other twin had produced long-lasting tolerance. These observations provided the basis for classic experiments by Peter Medawar and co-workers in the 1950s, for which they won the Nobel Prize. Medawar first showed that adult mice of strain A rejected skin grafts from mice of strain B; the difference between the two was the MHC molecules they expressed. However, mice of strain A that were injected within 24 h after birth with bone marrow

stem cells from strain B did *not* reject skin grafts from the donor B strain when they grew to adulthood. These results suggested that, unlike mature lymphocytes, when immature, developing lymphocytes are exposed to a foreign antigen, they fail to mount an immune response to the antigen. Rather the antigen is accepted as self and the immune system becomes tolerant to it. This phenomenon came to be known as *neonatal tolerance*.

Self-tolerance can be defined as a state of unresponsiveness to self-antigen. It occurs when the interaction of an autoantigen with self-antigen-specific lymphocytes results in signals that fail to activate the lymphocyte. As a consequence of the tolerizing interaction, the cell or the individual exposed to the antigen is said to be tolerant. There are several stages of development during which tolerance can be induced to provide added protection against the development of autoimmunity. Tolerance induced during the early stages of lymphocyte development is referred to as *central tolerance*; tolerance induced in mature lymphocytes is referred to as *peripheral tolerance*. Central tolerance occurs in the primary lymphoid organs (the bone marrow for B cells and the thymus for T cells) as part of the process known as *negative selection* (see Chapters 7 and 9). Negative selection in central lymphoid organs ensures that the majority of B and T cells that emerge in the periphery react only with foreign antigens. Nevertheless, this process is not perfect; some autoreactive cells inevitably escape to

Immunology: A Short Course, Sixth Edition, By Richard Coico and Geoffrey Sunshine

peripheral lymphoid organs such as the spleen and lymph nodes. If this happens, peripheral tolerance mechanisms may keep them under control.

A fundamental question in studies of tolerance and autoimmunity is how do lymphocytes distinguish self from nonself? As Medawar's early experiments demonstrated, self-antigens have no specific characteristics that distinguish them from foreign antigens. Thus, lymphocytes must rely on some other characteristics to make this distinction. The modern interpretation of Medawar's studies is that exposure of immature lymphocytes to antigen results in tolerance, exposure of mature lymphocytes to the same antigen results in activation. What conditions favor the development of tolerance rather than activation? One is that immature lymphocytes are much more sensitive than mature lymphocytes to strong signals delivered through their antigen receptors. This is the basis for negative selection of B cells in the bone marrow and T cells in the thymus. Another scenario that favors tolerance is continuous exposure of lymphocytes to high levels of antigen, which can lead to chronic antigen receptor signaling. Lymphocytes are continuously exposed to high levels of self-antigen, while exposure to foreign antigen is generally abrupt and short lived. Lymphocytes also learn to distinguish self from nonself by the context in which they encounter the antigen. If the antigen is encountered in the absence of costimulatory signals, then the lymphocytes are tolerized; if antigen is encountered in the presence of costimulatory signals, the lymphocytes are activated. Because foreign antigens such as infectious organisms are much more likely to come in contact with lymphocytes in the presence of costimulatory signals, they are more likely to activate lymphocytes than self-antigens.

The first part of this chapter will discuss the basic mechanisms of central and peripheral tolerance and how these mechanisms protect the host from harmful immune reactions to self. The second part of the chapter will discuss how mechanisms of tolerance can go awry, leading to the activation of autoreactive lymphocytes and the development of autoimmune disease.

CENTRAL TOLERANCE

The process of generating diversity in BCRs and TCRs inevitably generates receptors that can recognize self-antigens. This concept was initially proposed in the 1950s by Frank Macfarlane Burnet in his *clonal selection theory*. B and T cells with receptors for self-antigen are referred to as *autoreactive*. Burnet hypothesized that autoreactive lymphocytes pose a danger to the host and must be purged from the developing lymphocyte repertoire by deletion, thereby maintaining tolerance. We now know that there are several mechanisms of central tolerance that prevent the expansion of autoreactive lymphocytes in addition to deletion. These include anergy, receptor editing, and clonal ignorance. The

particular mechanism employed and the conditions under which it is implemented are explored below.

Anergy, Receptor Editing, Deletion, and Clonal Ignorance

Anergy is defined as the functional inactivation of a lymphocyte, resulting in unresponsiveness upon contact with self-antigen. Anergic B cells cannot be activated to proliferate and differentiate into antibody-secreting cells upon engagement of their BCRs with the autoantigen. Likewise, anergic T cells cannot be activated to proliferate and secrete cytokines following ligation of their TCR with self-antigen in the context of self-MHC.

Evidence for central B-cell anergy was first observed in 1980. Nossal and Pike (1980) demonstrated that when a cross-linking signal was delivered to immature B cells via their BCR, the B cells were anergized and were unable to mature or be activated. B-cell anergy has since been studied in transgenic mouse systems; antiself B cells are generated by introducing rearranged immunoglobulin genes into the germline of mice. The classic transgenic mouse system that first provided evidence for anergy came from the laboratory of Chris Goodnow. Goodnow and colleagues generated mice transgenic for the immunoglobulin heavy-chain (HC) and light-chain (LC) genes of an antibody to HEL. B cells in these mice were able to produce antibodies to HEL. However, when these mice were bred to mice expressing soluble HEL (sHEL) as autoantigen, the HEL-specific B cells were rendered anergic. Two other laboratories (under Betty Diamond and Martin Weigert) generated mice transgenic for the heavy chain of an anti-DNA antibody. In both of these transgenic models, the heavy-chain transgene could pair with the mouse's endogenous light chains to produce anti-DNA antibodies. Studies revealed that anti-DNA B cells present in these mice were anergic and unable to secrete transgenic anti-DNA antibody because of exposure to endogenous self-antigen. These anergic B cells were arrested in an immature stage of development and had a shortened life span.

There is evidence of T-cell anergy as a major mechanism for T-cell tolerance in the periphery, but there are few data supporting T-cell anergy in the thymus. Most negative selection of autoreactive T cells in the thymus appears to occur by deletion (see below).

Receptor editing is a major mechanism of central tolerance in B cells. This process of ongoing receptor gene rearrangement serves to alter or "edit" antigen receptor specificity. Following reexpression of *RAG-1* and *RAG-2* genes, the existing rearranged variable region is replaced with an upstream variable segment that rearranges to a more downstream J region (see Chapters 6 and 7). It has been postulated that receptor editing has evolved as a mechanism for averting autoreactivity, since it leads to a BCR with a new specificity that often lacks autoreactivity. However, the secondary rearrangement does not always eliminate autoreactivity. In this case, rearrangement will continue until all available upstream variable regions have been exhausted or until a non-autoreactive receptor is generated. Evidence for BCR editing was first observed in the bone marrow of mice transgenic for an antibody to an endogenous MHC class I molecule and in mice transgenic for an antibody to double-stranded DNA (dsDNA). In David Nemazee's laboratory, mice were made transgenic for the heavy and light-chain genes of an antibody to the MHC class I molecule H-2K^b. Two different strains of mouse, both transgenic for the heavy- and light-chain of the anti-H-2k^b antibody, were compared; one strain expressed H-2k^b as autoantigen and the other strain expressed H-2k^d. In mice expressing H-2k^d, B-cell development was normal and most B cells expressed the transgene-encoded receptor, which was specific for H-2k^b. However, in mice expressing H-2k^b, B cells underwent continuous rearrangement at the LC locus due to persistent encounter with the autoantigen (H-2K^b), resulting in transgenic B cells with edited BCRs.

In the laboratory of Martin Weigert, mice transgenic for the heavy and light chain of an antibody to DNA also demonstrated receptor editing. When the light-chain locus was analyzed in the B cells of these mice, preferential rearrangement to downstream Jκ regions, particularly Jκ$_5$, was observed, evidence of continued editing. In addition, a higher frequency of B cells expressing λC was observed. Rearrangements at the λ LC locus occurred after continuous rearrangements at the κ locus failed to eliminate autoreactivity.

In developing thymocytes, rearrangement at the TCR α locus occurs continuously on both chromosomes until the cell is positively selected (which requires recognition of self-peptide and self-MHC) or it dies. However, whether or not continuous rearrangement at the Vα locus plays a role in editing out autoreactive specificities that may arise in the TCR is unknown.

Deletion is a mechanism by which autoreactive B and T cells are eliminated from the repertoire by undergoing *apoptosis* (programmed cell death). Evidence for deletion of autoreactive B cells came from studies in the laboratory of Chris Goodnow using mice transgenic for both antibody to HEL and for membrane-bound HEL as autoantigen. When anti-HEL B cells came in contact with membrane HEL, they were deleted in the bone marrow. These results conflicted with previous studies in the Goodnow laboratory demonstrating that anti-HEL B cells were anergized when they came in contact with soluble HEL (see above discussion on anergy). It was then discovered that membrane HEL induces more extensive cross-linking of the BCR, thereby delivering a stronger signal to the B cell when it engages its receptor than soluble HEL. In summary, these studies revealed that encounter with a self-antigen that induces extensive cross-linking and delivers a strong signal induces deletion; encounter with a self-antigen that induces more moderate cross-linking and delivers a weaker signal induces anergy.

Central deletion is a dominant mechanism for negative selection of autoreactive T cells in the thymus. Double-positive T cells that bind with high affinity to self-antigens plus self-MHC in the thymus undergo rapid deletion. This prevents mature autoreactive T cells from exiting the thymus and moving out into the periphery. What puzzled immunologists for a long time was how T cells specific for nonthymic, tissue-specific self-antigens could be eliminated in the thymus since these self-antigens were not thought to be expressed in the thymus. The answer became apparent from studies to uncover the cause of *autoimmune polyendocrinopathy candidiasis ectodermal dystrophy (APECED)*, a disease in which patients suffer from a number of autoimmune symptoms including hypoparathyroidism, adrenal insufficiency, thyroiditis, type I diabetes, and ovarian failure. As described in Chapter 9, a gene known as *AIRE* (autoimmune regulator), which encodes a transcription factor regulator allowing peripheral tissue antigens to be expressed in the thymus, is defective in patients with APECED. *AIRE* is predominantly expressed in lymphoid organs, particularly the thymus, by thymic epithelial cells and dendritic cells. This gene is now known to facilitate the expression of peripheral self-antigens on thymic medullary cells and is therefore involved in the negative selection of self-reactive T cells. In *AIRE* gene knockout mice, autoreactive T cells escape thymic deletion and exit to the periphery, where they may induce autoimmune disease.

Clonal ignorance refers to autoreactive lymphocytes that have escaped tolerance mechanisms because they have a weak affinity for self-antigen or because the self-antigen is present in such a low concentration. Clonally ignorant B cells can mature and move out into the periphery; although they persist in the host in an unactivated state, they can be activated under certain conditions. For example, if the concentration of autoantigen is increased when heightened cell death results in the release of excessive amounts of intracellular self-antigens or when a strong costimulatory signal is delivered to the clonally ignorant cell during an infection, then clonally ignorant B cells may be activated. These autoreactive lymphocytes generally do not pose a threat to the host, but they may be precursors to autoreactive B cells that have undergone somatic mutation to acquire an even higher affinity for autoantigen.

What determines which of the spectrum of mechanisms leading to tolerance will govern the fate of seleted immature lymphocytes? It is currently believed that the threshold of receptor signaling is the major force that determines which mechanism of tolerance governs immature lymphocytes. The strength, or *avidity*, of interaction of the BCR or TCR with its autoantigen influences cell fate. Avidity with respect to B cells depends on the affinity of interaction between the BCR and its antigen, density of the surface

BCR, and the nature and concentration of the autoantigen. The higher the affinity of the antibody for its antigen and the more BCR expressed on the B-cell membrane, the greater the avidity of the antigen–antibody interaction. This correlates directly with the extent of immunoglobulin receptor cross-linking. The nature of the autoantigen also influences its ability to induce BCR cross-linking. For example, multivalent and membrane-bound antigens mediate more extensive receptor cross-linking than monovalent or soluble antigens. Initially a B cell with a high avidity for an autoantigen will undergo receptor editing in an attempt to avert autoreactivity. If continued editing fails to result in a non-autoreactive BCR, the B cell will undergo deletion. B cells with more moderate avidity for an autoantigen are targeted to anergy, while B cells with a weak avidity for autoantigen become clonally ignorant.

In the thymus, the affinity of the TCR for self-peptide plus self-MHC, the level of TCR on the surface of the T cell, and the level of MHC molecules expressed on the surface of the APC determine avidity and affect T-cell selection. In addition, the type of cell presenting self-antigen to the T cell seems to influence whether the T cell undergoes positive or negative selection. T cells that recognize peptide plus MHC expressed on epithelial cells in the cortex are positively selected. At the corticomedullary junction, T cells come in contact with self-antigen and MHC molecules expressed on dendritic cells. It is in this context that T cells with a high avidity for peptide plus MHC undergo negative selection and are deleted. Whether dendritic cells deliver different signals than epithelial cells, leading to negative rather than positive selection of self-reactive T cells, is unknown. Anergy and editing seem to play minor roles in central T-cell tolerance.

PERIPHERAL TOLERANCE

Occasionally, autoreactive B cells and T cells escape negative selection and enter the periphery. In addition, B cells sometimes acquire autoreactive specificities through somatic mutation in the periphery. Peripheral tolerance has evolved as a safety net to catch autoreactive B and T cells that escape to or arise in the periphery. Mechanisms of peripheral tolerance include anergy, Fas-mediated activation-induced cell death, and the induction of regulatory T cells. Although receptor editing has been shown to occur in peripheral B cells, it is not yet clear whether the objective of peripheral editing is to avert autoreactivity or to increase B-cell diversity. We discuss these mechanisms in the sections that follow.

ANERGY

In the late 1960s, Bretscher and Cohn hypothesized that B cells specific for T-dependent antigens require two signals to be activated: The first signal is provided by antigen, and the second signal is provided by T cells. They also hypothesized that B cells would be rendered unresponsive in the absence of the second signal. We now know that this second signal can be provided by the engagement of CD40 ligand (CD40L) on the surface of the T cell with CD40 expressed on the B cell. Studies in transgenic mouse systems have confirmed that B cells exposed to self-antigen become anergized in the absence of T-cell help (Fig. 12.1). Since autoreactive T cells usually get deleted in the thymus, they are generally not available in the periphery to provide costimulatory help to autoreactive B cells.

Anergic B cells cannot successfully compete for entry into B-cell follicles in the spleen and lymph nodes with nonanergic B cells. Instead they are arrested in development at the T cell–B cell border in a process known as *follicular exclusion* and soon die by apoptosis. It is now thought that follicular exclusion occurs because anergic B cells require higher concentrations of a B-cell factor known as BAFF (B-cell activating factor of the tumor necrosis factor family) for survival than naïve B cells; in an environment with a limited amount of BAFF, anergic B cells are at a

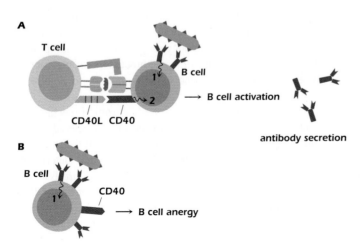

Figure 12.1. Lack of costimulation leads to B-cell anergy. (A) Two signals are required for B-cell activation by a T-dependent antigen. Signal 1 is provided by antigen binding to and cross-linking the BCR. Signal 2 is provided by the interaction of CD40L expressed on the T cell with CD40 on the B cell. (B) In the absence of this second, costimulatory signal, B cells fail to be activated and are anergized.

disadvantage and therefore undergo cell death instead of entering follicles.

T-cell anergy is believed to be a major mechanism of tolerance to self-antigens that are encountered in the periphery. T cells also require two signals to be activated (see Chapter 10). The first signal is provided by the MHC–peptide complex. The second signal must be provided by interactions between costimulatory molecules expressed on the APC and the respective ligands on the T cell. A major costimulatory signal is provided by the ligation of B7-1 (CD80) and/or B7-2 (CD86) expressed on the APC with CD28 expressed on the T cell. Delivery of signal 1 to the T cell leads to the induction of several transcription factors, one of which binds to the promoter region of the IL-2 gene, allowing for its transcription. If signal 1 is not accompanied by the costimulatory B7–CD28 interaction, then IL-2 mRNA is rapidly degraded, IL-2 protein is not made, and the T cell fails to be activated. Not all APC constitutively express costimulatory molecules. B cells, macrophages, and immature dendritic cells must be activated before they express costimulatory molecules (see Chapter 10). Hence, if an unactivated macrophage or immature dendritic cell presents an antigen to a T cell, then the T cell will be anergized because of the absence of a costimulatory signal (Fig. 12.2).

FAS–FASL INTERACTIONS

Fas-mediated apoptosis is thought to play a critical role in the removal of mature autoreactive B and T lymphocytes. **Fas**, a monomer expressed by activated lymphocytes, is a member of the TNF receptor family. The ligation of Fas by **Fas ligand (FasL)**, a member of the TNF family of membrane proteins, delivers an apoptotic signal to the cell expressing Fas. FasL is expressed by several cell

types, including activated T cells and certain epithelial cells. When FasL binds to Fas, it causes Fas to trimerize. This activates a "death" domain in Fas that interacts with the death domains of several cytosolic adaptor proteins, the most important of which is **FADD (Fas-associated death domain)**. This then triggers the activation of a series of cysteine proteases known as caspases, resulting in apoptosis of the cell (Fig. 12.3).

The importance of Fas–FasL interactions was initially established by studies of two mouse strains with an autoimmune condition that causes them to accumulate enormous numbers of lymphocytes in the spleen and lymph nodes. These mouse strains, known as **lpr** (for lymphoproliferative) and **gld** (for generalized lymphoproliferative disease), were observed to have mutations in Fas and FasL genes, respectively. These mutations prevent the mice from deleting autoreactive B and T cells, resulting in an elevated lymphocyte population. People with a mutated Fas gene have also been described; they have an autoimmune condition known as **autoimmune lymphoproliferative syndrome** (ALPS),

Autoimmune Lymphoproliferative Syndrome

with characteristics similar to those described for the mutant mice. Not only has Fas–FasL-mediated apoptosis been shown to play a role in eliminating autoreactive T cells in the periphery, but recent studies suggest that it may also play a role in the negative selection of T cells in the thymus. Anergic B cells, some of which express Fas, are also susceptible to Fas-mediated apoptosis. Interaction with CD4$^+$ T cells that express FasL leads to death of these self-reactive B cells.

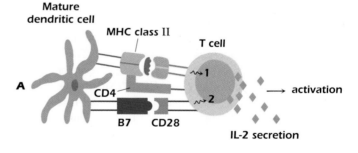

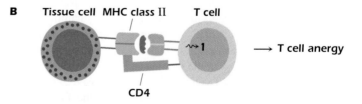

○ Figure 12.2. Antigen recognition in the absence of costimulation leads to T-cell anergy. (A) Two signals are required for T-cell activation. Signal 1 is provided by the recognition of peptide plus MHC. Signal 2 is provided by the interaction of the costimulatory molecule B7.1 or B7.2 expressed on the surface of an APC such as a mature dendritic cell with CD28 on the surface of the T cell. (B) If a T cell receives signal 1 in the absence of signal 2, it is anergized.

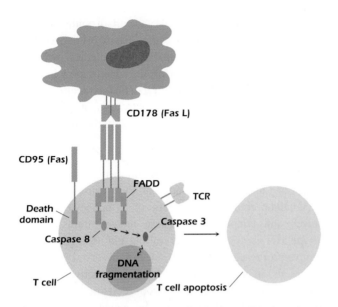

Figure 12.3. Fas-mediated apoptosis of T cells. The ligation of FasL to Fas causes Fas to trimerize. This activates the death domain in Fas, which then interacts with the death domain in FADD. A caspase cascade is then activated, which ultimately leads to apoptosis of the Fas-expressing cell.

REGULATORY/SUPPRESSOR T CELLS

In the early 1970s, experiments suggested that a specialized population of T cells suppressed the responses of other lymphocytes. However, the inability to isolate and clone a suppressor T-cell population led to skepticism about whether this population really existed. Renewed interest in *T suppressor cells* emerged in the 1990s with the identification of a population of CD4$^+$ T cells with the ability to down-regulate T-cell function. It was initially observed that neonatal thymectomy of mice resulted in autoimmunity, which could be prevented by transferring splenocytes from untreated mice back into the thymectomized mice. The suppressive activity in the splenocytes was eventually linked to a population of CD4$^+$ T cells that became referred to as suppressor or natural *regulatory T cells (T$_{reg}$)*. These T cells were observed to express CD25, the IL-2 receptor α chain, and became known as *CD4$^+$CD25$^+$ suppressor T cells*. CD25 is not unique to suppressor T cells and is also expressed on activated, effector CD4$^+$ T cells. This has made it difficult to isolate a pure suppressor T-cell subset for functional studies. Studies of the Scurfy disease in mice and immune dysregulation polyendocrinopathy enteropathy X-linked syndrome (IPEX) in humans led to the identification of a marker specific for T$_{reg}$, known as Foxp3 (forkhead box P3). Foxp3 is a transcription factor that is required for the development of T$_{reg}$ in the thymus and has been shown to induce nonregulatory T cells to acquire suppressive activity in the periphery. An X-linked mutation in the Foxp3

gene observed in Scurfy mice and in IPEX has been shown to lead to severe autoimmunity in affected males. Foxp3 is an intracellular marker for T$_{reg}$. More recently, a cell surface molecule known as GITR (glucocorticoid-induced TNF receptor family-related gene) has been shown to be expressed at high levels on T$_{reg}$ and is currently used as a marker for these cells.

As described in Chapter 9, natural CD4$^+$CD25$^+$ T$_{reg}$ cells represent a distinct lineage of T cells that is selected during T-cell development in the thymus. T$_{reg}$ cells constitute approximately 10% of peripheral CD4$^+$ T cells. Depletion of T$_{reg}$ in mice leads to organ-specific autoimmune diseases, such as thyroiditis, gastritis, and type I diabetes, any of which can be averted by T$_{reg}$ replacement. In addition to their role in self-tolerance, T$_{reg}$ can suppress graft versus host disease (discussed in Chapter 18); immune responses to tumor cells, allergens, and pathogens; and immune responses to organ transplants. T$_{reg}$ cells require IL-2 for their maintenance and activation and have been shown to utilize a diverse repertoire of TCRs. However, they seem to have an increased affinity for self peptide–MHC class II complexes. T$_{reg}$ cells require specific TCR engagement to be activated, but once activated, their *suppressive function is antigen nonspecific*. Thus, T$_{reg}$ can suppress autoreactive effector CD4$^+$ and CD8$^+$ T cells that are specific for different antigens than those recognized by the T$_{reg}$ themselves. T$_{reg}$ cells have also been shown to suppress B cells, dendritic cells, and NK cells. Many hypotheses have been proposed for the mechanism of suppression of T$_{reg}$ cells. Evidence suggests that CTLA-4, which is constitutively expressed on T$_{reg}$ cells, plays an important role in T$_{reg}$ suppression, since blockade of CTLA-4 results in organ-specific autoimmune

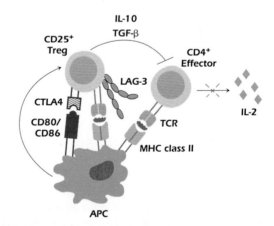

Figure 12.4. T-cell suppression. T$_{reg}$ receive a signal via CTLA-4 which induces their suppressive activity. T$_{reg}$ may also receive a signal triggering their suppressive activity following interaction of LAG-3 with an MHC class II molecule. T$_{reg}$ may then suppress the activation of CD4$^+$ T cells by secreting IL-10 and TGF-β.

disease. One hypothesis suggests that interaction of CD80 and CD86 on APC with CTLA-4 on T$_{reg}$ cells delivers a costimulatory signal to the T$_{reg}$ that induces their suppressive activity (Fig. 12.4). Lymphocyte activation gene 3 (*LAG3*), a CD4-associated adhesion molecule that binds MHC class II molecules, is expressed on the surface of T$_{reg}$ cells. Upon engagement with MHC class II molecules, *LAG3* is also thought to have a role in the suppressive activity of T$_{reg}$ cells. T$_{reg}$ may also induce down-regulation of CD80 and CD86 on dendritic cells, making them weaker activators of effector T-cells. Suppression of responder T cells involves inhibiting their proliferation and activation and preventing their production of IL-2. Several studies suggest that IL-10 and TGF-β are needed for T$_{reg}$ suppression, but this model remains controversial. Secretion of IL-10 by T$_{reg}$ cells in the lamina propria has been shown to control colitis by suppressing resident autoreactive T cells; however, blocking IL-10 *in vitro* fails to abrogate suppression. Involvement of cell surface expression of TGF-β by T$_{reg}$ cells has been reported in suppression mediated by cell contact. However, T$_{reg}$ cells isolated from mice deficient in TGF-β still have immunosuppressive activity. TGF-β may be more involved in the maintenance of T$_{reg}$ cells.

It is now becoming clear that CD4$^+$ CD25$^+$ T$_{reg}$ cells are clinically relevant. Enhancement of these T cells may be important for treating autoimmune diseases and for suppression of allograft rejection. In addition, depletion of these T cells may enhance immune responses to tumor vaccines and vaccines for infectious agents such as HIV.

Two other types of T cells that have suppressive activity, *type 1 T regulatory cells (Tr1)* and *T$_H$3 cells*, have been identified within the CD4$^+$ T-cell subset. These are known as *adaptive regulatory T cells* because they can be induced from naïve T cells by specific antigens in the context of a certain cytokine milieu. They have been shown to induce suppression through the release of inhibitory cytokines such as TGF-β and IL-10. These suppressor T cells appear to be either CD25$^-$ or CD25^{low} and are distinguished by their cytokine profiles. Tr1 cells are activated *in vitro* upon culture with IL-10. They produce high levels of TGF-β, which is responsible for their immunosuppressive function, and very little IL-2 and no IL-4. Tr1 cells seem to be involved in mediating protection against inflammatory bowel disease in mice and autoimmune diabetes in rats, but their role in protection against these autoimmune disorders in humans remains unclear. T$_H$3 cells were initially described in

---

Inflammatory Bowel Disease

---

studies on oral tolerance (see below). Feeding animals large amounts of antigen resulted in the expansion of T$_H$3

cells, which led to unresponsiveness to the fed antigen. T$_H$3 cells seem to reside in the mucosa, where they are involved in suppressing immune responses. Although they primarily produce TGF-β they also produce variable amounts of IL-10 and IL-4, which are responsible for their differentiation. The absence of T$_H$3 cells is associated with inflammatory bowel disease in humans.

Natural and adaptive regulatory T cells are involved in maintaining homeostasis between immune responsiveness and self-tolerance. The redundancy of these regulatory T-cell subsets, their specialized roles in dampening the immune response, and their relationship to one another remain areas of active research.

ORAL TOLERANCE

Oral tolerance is defined as the lack of a humoral or cellular immune response to ingested food antigens. It is mediated by T cells, and the mechanisms for establishing it are dependent on the dose of ingested antigen. A low dose of ingested antigen seems to induce T$_H$3 suppressor cells, while a high dose seems to induce T-cell anergy or deletion. Oral tolerance is first initiated when orally administered antigen encounters GALT, which includes the epithelial cells of the villi, intraepithelial lymphocytes, lamina propria lymphocytes, and lymphoid nodules of the Peyer's patches (PP). DCs, the major APC in the GALT, process and present most ingested antigens; however, other APC, such as macrophages, B cells, and epithelial cells, also play a role. When a large dose of food antigen is administered, not all of it is degraded by the time it reaches the small intestine; consequently, some food antigens get absorbed intact into the systemic circulation. The antigen is then processed and presented by peripheral APC in the absence of costimulatory interactions, which results in T-cell anergy.

Low-dose tolerance is induced locally, in the gut. The cytokine milieu of the GALT, which contains elevated levels of IL-4, IL-10, and TGF-β, promotes differentiation into T$_H$2 and T$_H$3 cells and inhibits differentiation into T$_H$1 cells. T$_H$3 cells, as previously discussed, mediate suppression via secretion of TGF-β. Triggering of T$_H$3 cells is antigen specific, but suppression induced by these cells is antigen nonspecific.

Several laboratory studies have demonstrated that low doses of oral antigen can suppress models of autoimmune diseases in animals. *Experimental autoimmune encephalomyelitis* (EAE) is a rodent model of *multiple sclerosis* (MS). Rats or mice immunized with myelin basic protein (MBP), or proteolipid protein (PLP) in complete Freund's adjuvant (CFA), develop cellular infiltration in the myelin sheaths of the central nervous system, which leads to demyelination and eventual paralysis. These symptoms mimic those observed in MS patients. Mice fed low doses of MBP prior to injection with MBP are presumably protected from developing EAE by the induction of regulatory T_H3 cells. Similarly, oral administration of type II collagen suppresses collagen-induced arthritis in susceptible rodent strains, and oral administration of thyroglobulin suppresses autoimmune thyroiditis in mice.

Studies using oral antigen to treat patients with autoimmune diseases have met with limited success. The cytokine environment and the presence of certain costimulatory molecules may influence the response to oral antigen. It has been reported that the cytokine milieu in the human gut may differ from that in the mouse gut. These differences will need to be characterized more carefully before oral tolerance can be used as an effective therapy for autoimmune diseases.

 IMMUNE PRIVILEGE

There are several sites in the body that do not develop immune responses to pathogens, tumor cells, or histoincompatible tissue transplants. These sites, known as *immune privileged sites*, include the *eye, testis, brain, ovary*, and *placenta*. The immune privilege of the eye is illustrated by the fact that corneal transplants in humans do not require tissue matching or immunosuppressive therapy. It was previously believed that immune protection in privileged sites was predominantly due to (1) lack of lymphatic drainage and (2) the blood barrier; both of these inhibit inflammatory cells from reaching antigens in the privileged sites. However, it is now known that other factors, such as the immunosuppressive cytokines IL-10 and TGF-β and expression of FasL, play important roles in establishing immune privilege. Studies have demonstrated that FasL is expressed on several types of cells found in immune privileged sites; the interaction of these FasL-expressing cells with infiltrating Fas-expressing inflammatory T cells leads to apoptosis of the T cells. Human retinal pigment epithelial (RPE) cells and corneal endothelial cells have been observed to express FasL and to induce apoptosis of inflammatory T cells. The success of corneal transplants in mice has been shown to be due to expression of FasL by cells of the graft, which prevent inflammatory damage to the graft by eliminating infiltrating Fas$^+$ T cells. When corneas from mice lacking functional FasL (gld mice) are transplanted into allogeneic recipients, the grafts are rejected because infiltrating Fas$^+$ lymphocytes cannot be eliminated by FasL-mediated apoptosis. Human RPE cells have also been shown to secrete soluble factors such as TGF-β that suppress infiltrating T cells.

AUTOIMMUNITY AND DISEASE

At the turn of the twentieth century, the German bacteriologist and immunologist Paul Ehrlich coined the term *horror autotoxicus* to describe a potentially toxic immune response to self. According to Erhlich, the body was incapable of producing an autoimmune response because of the "horror" this would inflict on the individual. We now know that autoreactive lymphocytes do arise both centrally and peripherally, but they are normally kept in check and prevented from expanding by mechanisms of tolerance that we described earlier in the chapter. However, sometimes these tolerance mechanisms go awry and autoreactive lymphocytes escape regulatory checkpoints. If they are then triggered to undergo activation, autoimmunity and autoimmune disease may ensue.

Unlike immunodeficiency diseases, which are usually caused by a single gene defect, autoimmune diseases are rarely caused by an anomaly of a single gene. Some rare exceptions are ALPS (caused by a mutation in the *Fas* gene), APECED (caused by an alteration in the *AIRE* gene), and IPEX (caused by a defect in the *FoxP3* gene) (see above). However, most autoimmune diseases are caused by a constellation of genetic and environmental factors. Although certain gene defects may predispose an individual to autoimmunity, exposure to an environmental factor may be necessary to precipitate disease. For example, overexpression of genes that promote lymphocyte survival may predispose to autoimmunity because this would enable autoreactive lymphocytes (which often have shortened life spans) to live longer. However, innate signaling provided by microbial pathogens may still be the trigger needed for activation of these autoreactive lymphocytes. In the following section we describe the multifactorial causes of autoimmune diseases, including genetic and environmental influences.

Genetic Susceptibility

The most common evidence for the existence of a *genetic predisposition* to autoimmune disease is the higher incidence of autoimmune disease among monozygotic twins and a lower but still increased incidence in dizygotic twins and family members when compared with an unrelated population. Although familial tendencies occur, the pattern of inheritance is generally complex and indicates that the disease is polygenic. This means that no individual gene is sufficient to elicit the disease; many genes may interact with one another. The fact that predisposing genes are usually common in the general population makes the study of genetic susceptibility even more difficult. In addition, many autoimmune diseases are genetically heterogeneous, and the same clinical disease may result from the combined effect of different genes.

One gene family associated with autoimmune disease that has been studied extensively is the *HLA complex*, the human MHC. This is not surprising, considering the importance of HLA molecules in shaping the TCR repertoire and their role in peptide presentation and recognition by the

⬤ TABLE 12.1. Autoimmune Diseases

Autoimmune Disease	MHC Association	Allele	Strength of Association
Class I			
Ankylosing spondylitis	B27	*B*2702, −04, −05*	Strong
Reiter syndrome	B27		Strong
Acute anterior uveitis	B27		Strong
Hyperthyroidism (Graves)	B8		Weak
Psoriasis vulgaris	Cw6		Intermediate
Class II			
Rheumatoid arthritis	DR4	*DRB1*0401, −04, −05*	Strong
Sjogren syndrome	DR3		Intermediate
SLE			
Caucasian	DR3		Weak
Japanese	DR2		Intermediate
Celiac disease	DR3	*DQA1*0501*	Strong
Pemphigus vulgaris	DR4, DR6		Strong
Type I diabetes mellitus	DR4	*DQB1*0302*	Strong
	DR3		Intermediate
Multiple sclerosis	DR2	*DRB1*1501*	Intermediate
Myasthenia gravis	DR3		Weak
Goodpasture syndrome	DR2		Intermediate

TCR. Some allele-specific MHC molecules may be better than others at presenting self-peptides to autoreactive T cells, thereby predisposing to autoimmunity. Susceptibility to specific autoimmune diseases is usually linked to MHC class II alleles, but association with MHC class I alleles is also observed. For example, SLE, myasthenia gravis, and type I diabetes are generally associated with class II DR3 alleles, rheumatoid arthritis is affiliated with a DR4 allele; ankylosing spondylitis is strongly associated with an MHC class I allele (B27) (Table 12.1). While susceptibility to an autoimmune disease may be linked to a specific MHC allele, eliciting the disease may require other genes or certain environmental triggers.

Studies in mice have shown that alterations in the expression of a variety of non-HLA genes can interfere with many different pathways of cellular function and contribute to autoimmunity. Overexpression or underexpression of genes involved in apoptosis and cell survival, cytokine expression, BCR or TCR signaling pathways, costimulatory interactions, and immune clearance of apoptotic cells and immune complexes have all been shown to lead to an autoimmune phenotype in mice. A deficiency in the pro-apoptotic molecules Fas or FasL or overexpression of anti-apoptotic molecules such as bcl-2 leads to diminished apoptosis and results in an increased number of autoreactive B and/or T cells and increased

autoantibody production, especially the production of anti-nuclear antibodies. Elevated levels of serum BAFF, a factor that promotes B-cell survival, have been observed in patients with Sjogren's syndrome and SLE. Overexpression of various proinflammatory cytokines such as TNF-α and IFN-α have been linked to autoimmune diseases such as inflammatory bowel disease and SLE, respectively. Interestingly, some patients treated for chronic viral infections with IFN-α have developed autoimmunity. Overexpression of receptor–ligand molecules involved in costimulatory activation of B cells or T cells (such as CD40 and CD40L or B7 and CD28, respectively) and decreased expression of inhibitors of T-cell activation (such as CTLA-4) have also been linked to autoimmunity. Lack of expression of molecules involved in negative regulation of BCR signaling (such as CD22, lyn, or SHP-1) and overexpression of molecules involved in positively modulating BCR signaling (such as CD19) have also been linked to autoantibody production and autoimmunity. Finally, reduced expression of proteins involved in clearance of apoptotic particles (such as C-reactive protein, serum amyloid protein, or the membrane tyrosine kinase c-mer) have been shown to lead to an autoimmune syndrome analogous to SLE.

Decreased clearance of immune complexes due to a deficiency of the complement components C1q, C2, C3, or C4 has been observed in many patients with autoimmune diseases (see also Chapter 13). In fact, SLE has been shown to occur in over 80% of individuals with complete deficiency of C1, C4, or C2. A deficiency in the split products C3b and C4b, which bind to immune complexes, or a decrease in the complement receptor CR1, which is expressed on the surface of macrophages, can also lead to impaired clearance of immune complexes. This can result in inappropriate deposition of immune complexes in the joints and various organs of the body, including the lungs, heart, and kidney, which can result in organ damage. Similarly, an abnormality in Fc-gamma receptors on macrophages can lead to inefficient clearance of immune complexes, thereby predisposing to autoimmunity.

Target organ damage in autoimmune disease may also be genetically determined. Murine models of autoimmune myocarditis reveal that disease susceptibility and cardiac damage is dependent on antigen display, which differs in different strains of mice.

Environmental Susceptibility

In addition to genetic predisposition, several environmental factors, both infectious and noninfectious, can trigger autoimmunity by (1) inducing the release of sequestered antigens, (2) molecular mimicry, or (3) polyclonal activation.

As described earlier in the chapter, a few autoantigens are protected (*sequestered*) from the immune system. Thus, even if some individuals possess autoreactive T and B cells, these cells will not be activated to initiate autoimmunity because they never come in contact with the autoantigen. The chondrocyte antigens in cartilage and some neuronal and cardiac antigens are examples of sequestered antigens. When they are exposed to the immune system—by a physical accident or infection—an autoimmune response may result. Autoimmune myocarditis has been observed to arise in some cases following a cardiac ischemic attack. It is believed that autoreactivity to cardiac antigens develops as a consequence of exposure of sequestered antigens when the heart is damaged.

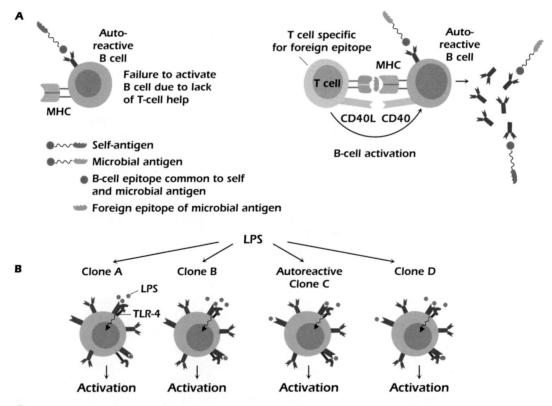

Figure 12.5. Possible mechanisms for triggering autoimmunity. (A) Molecular mimicry. A B cell specific for a self-antigen is not activated in the absence of T-cell help. However, this same B cell can be activated by a microbial antigen that has an epitope in common with the self-antigen. A T cell that recognizes a foreign epitope on the microbial antigen can provide help to the autoreactive B cell, activating it to secrete antibodies that bind to the foreign antigen and cross-react with the self-antigen. (B) Polyclonal B-cell activation. Mouse B-cell clones, including autoreactive clone C, may be activated nonspecifically via a polyclonal activator such as LPS (a component of the cell wall of Gram-negative bacteria). LPS binds to a receptor on the surface of the B cell, which associates with TLR-4. TLR-4 delivers an activating signal to the nucleus.

Autoimmunity may also arise when an antibody or T cell specific for a microbial antigen cross-reacts with a self-antigen (due to an epitope on the microbial antigen that is similar to an epitope present on the self-antigen). This phenomenon is referred to as *molecular mimicry*. Since autoreactive T cells are generally eliminated in the thymus, they may not be available in the periphery to activate autoreactive B cells to secrete antibody in response to a self-antigen. However, an antibody to a self-antigen may be elicited by a foreign antigen containing a homologous epitope if a nonself-determinant on the foreign antigen recruits T-cell help (Fig. 12.5A). Molecular mimicry is believed to play a role in the onset of rheumatic fever, which sometimes develops after a streptococcal infection. Rheumatic fever is an inflammatory disease in which the heart valve may become damaged. It is believed that autoantibodies to cardiac myosin that cross-react with the M protein of *Streptococcus pyogenes* are responsible for this heart damage. Viral infections can sometimes trigger autoimmunity because of T-cell cross-reactivity. A T cell specific for a viral peptide can cross-react with a peptide derived from an autoantigen. In type I diabetes mellitus, a T cell that recognizes a peptide from glutamic acid decarboxylase (GAD) (an antigen in β-islet cells) has been shown to cross-react with a peptide derived from coxsackievirus.

Figure 12.5B shows that microbial antigens can also induce autoimmunity by polyclonal activation. *Polyclonal activators* may nonspecifically activate all B or T cells; some of these may be autoreactive and trigger autoimmunity. Certain conserved, molecular structures found on a large group of microorganisms [*pathogen-associated molecular patterns (PAMPs)*], such as lipoteichoic acid (a component of the cell wall on Gram-positive bacteria) or LPS on Gram-negative bacteria, interact with signaling receptors such as TLRs expressed either on the surface of lymphocytes or intracellularly. LPS can polyclonally activate B cells (including autoreactive B cells) by interacting with a receptor on the cell surface that is associated with TLR-4.

Figure 12.6 illustrates that some PAMPs can activate autoreactive B cells by interacting with TLRs expressed intracellularly, in endosomes. However, in order to come in contact with the intracellular TLRs, they must first gain entry into the B cell via specific BCRs. For instance, hypomethylated CpG DNA sequences commonly found in bacterial DNA can be endocytosed by B cells following engagement with BCRs specific for DNA or proteins that form complexes with DNA. Once inside the B-cell endosome, the CpG DNA sequences can interact with TLR-9 and deliver a stimulatory signal. Similarly, RNA can activate anti-RNA-specific B cells because it is recognized by endosomal TLR-7 and TLR-8. An attractive hypothesis suggests that innate signaling through toll pathways may be a mechanism for activating anergic

B cells that are unresponsive to signaling via BCR cross-linking.

Drug and Hormonal Triggers of Autoimmunity

Noninfectious triggers of autoimmunity include hormones and drugs. The influence of hormones is illustrated by gender-specific factors that help trigger autoimmune diseases; for example, SLE is more common in women than in men and may be exacerbated by estrogen. Certain drugs can chemically alter the epitope of a self antigen to render it immunogenic, resulting in autoimmunity. For instance, penicillin may bind to a protein on the surface of red blood cells (RBCs); this entire complex may then act as an antigen, eliciting antibodies to the surface of the blood cell, causing lysis or phagocytosis of the RBC and leading to drug-induced hemolytic anemia. Another example of drug-induced anemia occurs in a small minority of patients using α-methyldopa, an antihypertensive drug. Clinical manifestations similar to those observed in SLE can also be induced by certain drugs. Chlorpromazine (used to treat schizophrenia), hydralazine (used to treat hypertension), and procainamide (used to treat arrhythmias) have all been observed to induce the production of antinuclear antibodies in some individuals and have been linked on rare occasions to drug-induced lupus. Generally, drug-induced autoimmune diseases are *self-limiting*: The disease disappears when the drug is discontinued.

● AUTOIMMUNE DISEASES

Traditionally, autoimmune diseases have been classified as B- or T-cell-mediated diseases. Because we now know that most B-cell responses are T-cell dependent and that B cells may be important APC for T-cell activation, this distinction

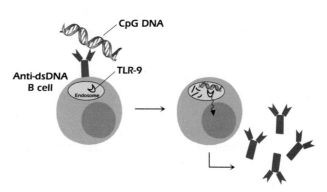

● Figure 12.6. Activation of an DNA-specific B cell via TLR-9 signaling. An anti-dsDNA B cell endocytoses DNA containing CPG-rich DNA sequences. Once in the endosome the CpG DNA engages TLR-9, which then delivers an activating signal to the nucleus. The activated B cell becomes an anti-dsDNA-secreting B cell.

TABLE 12.2. Autoimmune Diseases, Target Autoantigens, and Effector Cells

Autoimmune Diseases	Autoantigen	Effector Cells
Graves disease	TSH receptor	B cells/autoantibody
Myasthenia gravis	Acetylcholine receptor	B cells/autoantibody
Pernicious anemia	Gastric parietal cells; intrinsic factor	B cells/autoantibody
ANCA-associated vasculitis	Myeloperoxidase serine proteinase	B cells/autoantibody
Autoimmune hemolytic anemia	Rh blood group antigens	B cells/autoantibody
Idiopathic thrombocytopenic purpura	Platelet membrane protein, integrin	B cells/autoantibody
SLE	dsDNA histones; ribonucleo proteins (snRNPs)	B cells/autoantibody
Sjogren syndrome	Salivary duct antigens; SS-A, SS-B nucleoproteins	B cells/autoantibody
Scleroderma	Centromeric proteins in fibroblasts; nucleolar antigens; IgG; Scl-70	Unknown
Pemphigus vulgaris	Desmoglein 3	B cells; autoantibody
Goodpasture syndrome	Renal and lung basement membrane collagen type IV	B cells; autoantibody
Rheumatoid arthritis	Unknown cartilage antigen, IgG	CD4$^+$ T cells; CTLs; B cells/autoantibody
Hashimoto thyroiditis	Thyroid proteins (thyroglobulin, microsomal antigens, thyroid peroxidase)	CD4$^+$ T cells; B cells/autoantibody
Type I diabetes mellitus	Pancreatic β-islet cell antigen	CD4$^+$ T cells; CTLs; B cells/autoantibody
Multiple sclerosis	Myelin basic protein	CD4$^+$ T cells

no longer seems useful. In the past, autoimmune diseases were also classified as systemic or organ specific. Again, the classification no longer seems useful. In some diseases, the autoantigen is ubiquitous, but the damage is limited to a single tissue. Other autoimmune diseases previously thought to be caused by pathogenic manifestations of organ-specific immune responses are now recognized to involve multiple organs. We have therefore classified diseases by the effector mechanism that appears most responsible for organ damage: antibody or T cells. This also is not a perfect system, because all mechanisms are operative in many diseases. Table 12.2 lists many autoimmune diseases, their target autoantigen, and the effector cells that mediate them.

Autoimmune Diseases in Which Antibodies Play a Predominant Role in Mediating Organ Damage

Autoimmune Hemolytic Anemia. In *autoimmune hemolytic anemia*, antibodies to antigens on the surface of RBCs are responsible for destroying these RBCs. This results in *anemia*, a reduced number of RBCs in the circulation. The destruction of the red cells can be attributed to two mechanisms. One involves the activation of the complement cascade and eventual lysis of the

cells. The resultant release of hemoglobin may lead to its appearance in the urine (*hemoglobinuria*). The second mechanism is the opsonization of RBCs facilitated by antibody and the C3b component of complement (see Chapter 13). In the latter case, the RBCs are bound to and engulfed by macrophages with receptors for Fc and C3b that attach to the antibody-coated RBCs.

It is customary to divide the antibodies responsible for autoimmune hemolytic anemia into two groups on the basis of their physical properties. The first group consists of the *warm autoantibodies*, so-called because they react optimally with RBCs at 37°C. The warm autoantibodies belong primarily to the *IgG class*, and some react with Rh antigens on the surface of the RBCs. Because activation of the complement cascade requires the close alignment of at least two molecules of IgG and Rh antigens are sparsely distributed on the surface of the erythrocyte, complement-mediated lysis does not occur. Instead, IgG antibodies to these antigens are effective in inducing immune adherence to macrophages and facilitating phagocytosis. Individuals with autoimmune hemolytic anemia can be identified by a Coombs test (see Chapter 5), which is designed to detect bound IgG on the surface of RBCs.

A second type of antibody, the *cold agglutinins*, attach to RBCs only when the temperature is below 37°C and dissociate from the cells when the temperature rises above 37°C. Cold agglutinins belong primarily to the *IgM class* and are specific for I or i antigens present on the surface of RBCs. Because the cold agglutinins belong to the IgM class, they are highly efficient at activating the complement cascade and causing lysis of the attached erythrocytes. Nevertheless, hemolysis is not severe in patients with autoimmune hemolytic anemia due to cold agglutinins as long as body temperature is maintained at 37°C. When the arms, legs, or skin are exposed to cold and the temperature of the circulating blood is allowed to drop, severe attacks of hemolysis may occur. Sometimes, cold agglutinins appear after infection by *Mycoplasma pneumoniae* or viruses, implicating an infectious disease trigger in genetically susceptible individuals.

Myasthenia Gravis. Another autoimmune disease implicating antibodies to a well-defined target antigen

Myasthenia Gravis

is *myasthenia gravis*. The target self-antigen in this disease is the acetylcholine receptor at neuromuscular junctions. Figure 12.7A shows that the autoantibody acts as an antagonist that blocks the binding of acetylcholine (ACh)

to the receptor. This inhibits the nerve impulse from being transmitted across the neuromuscular junction, resulting in severe muscle weakness, manifested by difficulty in chewing, swallowing, and breathing and eventually death from respiratory failure. Myasthenia gravis affects individuals of any age, but the peak incidence occurs in women in their late twenties and men in their fifties and sixties. The female-to-male ratio is approximately 3 : 2. Some babies of myasthenic mothers have transient muscle weakness, presumably because they received sufficient amounts of pathogenic IgG by transplacental passage.

The development of myasthenia gravis appears to be linked to the thymus; many patients have concurrent *thymoma* (hypertrophy of the thymus), and removal of the thymus sometimes leads to regression of the disease. Molecules cross-reacting with the ACh receptor have been found on various cells in the thymus, such as thymocytes and epithelial cells, but whether these molecules are the primary stimulus for the development of the disease is unknown. There is a genetic component to the disease; myasthenia gravis is associated with HLA-DR3 alleles (see Table 12.1).

The disease can be experimentally induced in animals by immunization with ACh receptors purified from torpedo fish or electric eel, both of which are homologous to mammalian receptors. In the experimental disease, which results from the formation of antibodies against the foreign receptors, the antibodies cross-react with the mammalian receptors and mimic almost exactly the natural form of

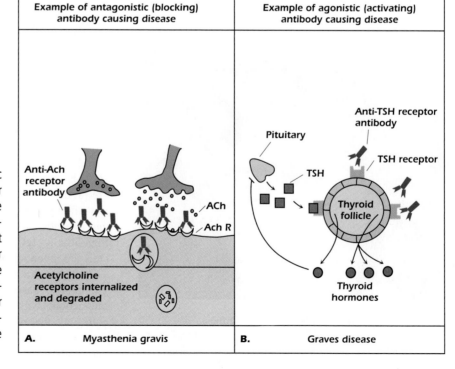

Figure 12.7. Autoantibodies specific for cell surface receptors can be either receptor agonists or antagonists. (A) The antibody to the Ach receptor in myasthenia gravis acts as an antagonist that blocks binding of ACh to the receptor and prevents transmission of the nerve impulse across the neuromuscular junction. (B) The antibody to the TSH receptor in Graves disease acts as a receptor agonist and induces chronic stimulation of the thyroid to release thyroid hormones.

the disease. The disease may be passively transferred with antibody.

Graves Disease. One of the main manifestations of ***Graves disease*** is a hyperactive thyroid gland (***hyperthyroidism***). Graves disease is an example of an autoimmune disease in which antibodies directed against a hormone receptor act as agonists and activate the receptor rather than interfere with its activity. For reasons not yet understood, patients with this disease develop autoantibodies against thyroid cell surface receptors for thyroid-stimulating hormone (TSH). Figure 12.7B shows that the interaction of autoantibodies with the TSH receptor activates the cell in a manner similar to TSH activation, thereby stimulating excess production of thyroid hormone. Normally, TSH produced by the pituitary binds to TSH receptors on the thyroid gland, activating the gland to produce and secrete thyroid hormones. When the level of thyroid hormones get too high, the production of TSH and thus the production of thyroid hormones is shut down via a negative-feedback loop. However, in Graves disease the autoantibodies continuously stimulate the TSH receptors, resulting in continuous production of thyroid hormone, which leads to hyperthyroidism. One of the main symptoms of hyperthyroidism is an increase in metabolism. Other signs and symptoms include heart palpitations, heat intolerance, insomnia, nervousness, weight loss, hair loss, and fatigue. In addition, patients with severe disease may develop eye problems, including inflammation of the soft tissue surrounding the eye, bulging of the eye, and double vision. Some patients with Graves disease develop an enlarged thyroid gland known as a goiter.

The indirect evidence that Graves disease is an autoimmune disease includes familial predisposition, genetic association with HLA class II genes, and correlation of disease severity with antibody titer to TSH receptors. However, the best evidence is that transmission of thyroid-stimulating antibodies from a thyrotoxic mother cross the placenta, causing ***transient neonatal hyperthyroidism*** until the maternal IgG is catabolized. The disease most commonly affects women in their thirties and forties; the female to male ratio is about 8 : 1. A susceptibility gene for Graves disease has been identified on chromosome 20 (20q11.2).

Systemic Lupus Erythematosus. ***Systemic lupus erythematosus (SLE)*** is an autoimmune disease that is nine times more common in women of childbearing age than in men and three times more common in African Americans, Caribbean Americans, and people of Asian and Hispanic descent than in Caucasians. The disease gets its

Systemic Lupus Erythematosus

name (which literally means "red wolf") from a reddish rash on the cheeks ("malar"), a frequent early symptom. However, the distribution of the rash resembles the wings of a butterfly rather than the face of a wolf (Fig. 12.8). The term systemic is quite appropriate, because the disease affects many organs of the body. It is mediated by autoantibodies and immune complexes, which often deposit in the skin, joints, lungs, blood vessels, heart, kidney, and brain. Symptoms include fever, skin rashes, joint pain, and damage to the central nervous system, heart, lungs, and kidneys. The pathophysiology of the kidney lesions is the primary cause of mortality from SLE.

The origin of this disease is still a mystery, but details of the immunologic mechanisms responsible for the pathology are partially known. Patients with SLE produce antibodies against several nuclear components of the body [antinuclear antibodies (ANAs)], notably against native dsDNA. Antibodies may also be produced against denatured, single-stranded DNA, ribonucleoproteins, and nucleohistones, but clinically, the presence of anti-dsDNA correlates best with the pathology of renal involvement in SLE (see below). Antibodies to single-stranded DNA are produced in normal individuals, but they are generally low-affinity IgM antibodies. However, isotype switching and somatic mutation can result in the production of high-affinity IgG antibodies to dsDNA, provided the B cells are given appropriate T-cell help.

Double-stranded DNA may become trapped in the glomerular basement membrane through electrostatic interactions with constituents of the membrane such as collagen, fibronectin, or laminin. The bound dsDNA may then trap circulating IgG anti-dsDNA antibodies and lead to the formation of immune complexes. These

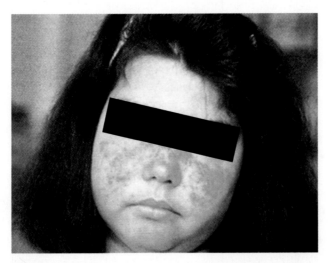

Figure 12.8. Typical reddish, butterfly or malar rash on the face of a young girl with SLE (Courtesy of L. Steinman, Department of Pathology, Stanford University School of Medicine.)

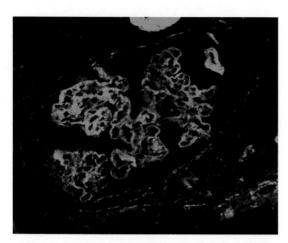

Figure 12.9. Antibody deposition in the kidney of a patient with SLE. Fluorescent-labeled antibody to human IgG, used to immunostain a kidney section, shows deposits of IgG antibody in glomeruli. (Courtesy of H. Rennke, Department of Pathology, Brigham and Women's Hospital, Boston.)

complexes may activate the complement cascade and attract granulocytes. Alternatively, anti-dsDNA antibodies may cross-react with glomerular antigens. Deposition of IgG antibodies in the kidneys of lupus patients can be demonstrated by immunostaining a tissue section from the kidney with a fluorescently labeled antibody to human IgG (Fig. 12.9). In the kidney, the extent of the inflammatory reaction forms the basis of classifying kidney pathology. Damage to the kidneys (***glomerulonephritis***) leads to leakage of protein (***proteinuria***) and sometimes hemorrhage (***hematuria***), with symptoms waxing and waning as the rate of formation of immune complexes rises and falls. As the condition becomes chronic, inflammatory CD4$^+$ T cells enter the site and attract monocytes, which further contribute to the pathologic lesions.

Although the antigen that initiates production of these antibodies is unknown, infectious agents, including the Epstein Barr virus (EBV), have been proposed to play a role in the etiology of the disease. Antibodies to viral antigens in EBV have been shown to cross-react with some nuclear antigens. Another environmental factor that may influence SLE is UV light. UV rays from the sun have been shown to exacerbate disease, presumably by enhancing cell death, which results in an increase in the release of target nuclear autoantigens. Evidence for genetic predisposition to SLE includes the increased risk of developing SLE among family members, the higher rate of concordance (25%) in monozygotic twins when compared with dizygotic twins (<3%), linkage with HLA class II genes, and the presence of an inherited deficiency of an early complement component in 6% of SLE patients. Hormones also play a role in lupus; estrogen seems to exacerbate disease symptoms.

SLE is often very difficult to diagnose because the symptoms are nonspecific and not all patients share the same symptoms. Symptoms such as fever, weight loss, joint pains, and fatigue are also characteristic of many other disorders. In addition, the laboratory test used to diagnose the presence of ANAs (the ANA assay) is not specific for lupus, because ANAs sometimes arise in other disorders. Hence, a diagnosis of SLE may take many years of careful review of a patient's history. It is based on a combination of positive ANA tests, patient's symptoms, and examination results.

Animal models of lupus have been very useful for understanding disease development and pathogenesis. The NZB/W F1 hybrid mouse strain, generated by crossing New Zealand Black (NZB) with New Zealand White (NZW) mice, and the MRL/lpr/lpr mouse strain both develop autoantibodies to dsDNA and lupuslike symptoms, including glomerulonephritis. NZB/NZW F1 mice more closely resemble human lupus; the incidence of disease is greater in female mice than males, and kidney pathology is similar to that observed in human patients. Furthermore, the defect appears to be polygenic. As previously described, the defect in MRL/lpr/lpr mice is due to a mutation in the *Fas* gene; these animals have more of a lymphoproliferative syndrome than observed in lupus patients.

Hashimoto's Thyroiditis. *Hashimoto's thyroiditis* is an autoimmune disease of the thyroid gland named after the Japanese physician Hashimoto Hakaru, who first described it in 1912. This disease, most commonly found in middle-aged women, is characterized by the production of antibodies to two major thyroid proteins: thyroid peroxidase and the hormone thyroglobulin. These autoantibodies play a major role in the destruction of the thyroid gland, eventually causing a decline in the output of thyroid hormones resulting in hypothyroidism. Symptoms of hypothyroidism include dry skin, brittle hair and nails, cold intolerance, weight gain, muscle cramps, depression, and extreme fatigue.

T_H1 cells also contribute to the destruction of the thyroid gland in Hashimoto's thyroiditis. Histologic findings show that there is an infiltration of large numbers of B and T lymphocytes and macrophages into the thyroid gland (Fig. 12.10). As it attempts to regenerate, the thyroid often more closely resembles a lymphoid follicle with proliferating germinal centers than a gland with epithelial cells lining the follicles. In some patients the gland may become enlarged, causing a ***goiter*** (Fig. 12.11).

There is strong evidence for genetic susceptibility to Hashimoto's thyroiditis. Family members of patients with this disease have a greater incidence of developing Hashimoto's thyroiditis as well as other autoimmune diseases than the normal population. Treatment for Hashimoto's thyroiditis is thyroid hormone replacement therapy.

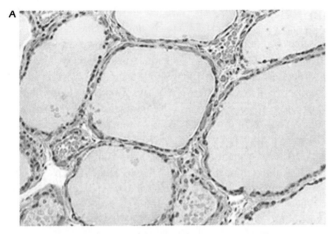

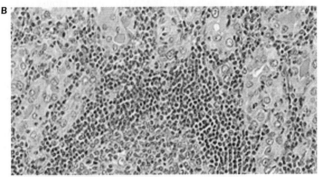

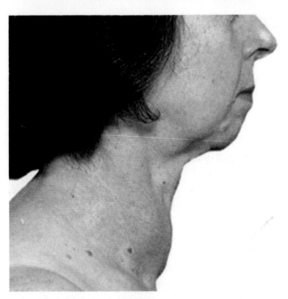

Figure 12.10. Thyroid sections from control subject and patient with Hashimoto's thyroiditis. (A) Light micrograph of normal thyroid gland showing follicular epithelial cells lining a follicle. (B) Thyroid gland from patient with Hashimoto's thyroiditis in which normal thymic architecture of thyroid has been replaced by intense lymphocyte proliferation and infiltration. [Reprinted with permission from RA Goldsby, TJ Kindt, and BA Osborne (eds) (2000): *Kuby Immunology*, 4th ed. New York: Freeman.]

Figure 12.11. Formation of goiter in patient with Hashimoto's thyroiditis. [Reprinted with permission from IM, Roitt J Brostoff, and DK Malem (eds) (1989): *Immunology*, 2nd ed. New York: Grower Medical.]

Autoimmune Diseases in Which T Cells Play A Predominant Role in Organ Damage

Multiple Sclerosis. Multiple sclerosis (MS) is an inflammatory, T-cell mediated autoimmune disease characterized by the demyelination or destruction of the myelin sheaths surrounding central nervous system (CNS; brain and spinal cord) nerve axons. This results in lesions in the white matter. The disease may take two courses: a relapsing–remitting course or a chronic

Multiple Sclerosis

progressive paralytic course. In the relapsing–remitting form of MS, sudden attacks may be followed by months or years of remission of disease activity. The CNS lesions in MS resemble the cellular infiltrates associated with T_H1

cells reminiscent of delayed-type hypersensitivity (see Chapter 16). There are a host of symptoms associated with MS, including changes in sensation (**hypoesthesias**), muscle weakness and or muscle spasms, difficulties with coordination and balance (**ataxia**), visual problems such as double vision or blindness, problems in speech (**dysarthria**) or swallowing (**dysphagia**), depression, and cognitive impairment.

It is not clear whether the autoimmune response is due to the release of sequestered myelin antigens following trauma to the CNS or molecular mimicry to a neuroepitope following a viral infection. EBV is one virus that has been implicated in MS. Much of the evidence that MS is an autoimmune disease has relied on the EAE rodent model described earlier in the chapter. Animals with EAE develop many of the same characteristics as patients with MS. CD4$^+$ T-cell clones specific for MBP or proteolipid protein can transfer the EAE disease. Circumstantial evidence for the autoimmune nature of MS includes the HLA class II association with disease susceptibility and the finding of a higher T-cell response to myelin components in cerebrospinal fluid of MS patients than in control subjects.

One area of study has established the ability of T cells to penetrate the blood–brain barrier, which ordinarily prevents cells and macromolecules from entering the CNS. Permeability of the blood–brain barrier may be compromised during viral infections, thus enabling T cells to penetrate the brain. In addition, integrins are upregulated in activated T cells, which may allow the T cells to adhere to the vessels near the brain. Activated T cells can produce metalloproteinases, which disrupt the collagen in the basal lamina, allowing T cells to accumulate in the CNS. Once in the brain T cells must undergo antigenic stimulation (perhaps via microglia, the macrophage-like APC present in the brain) to persist there. Autoreactive T_H1 cells are stimulated to secrete inflammatory cytokines such as IFN-γ and TNF-α which activate macrophages. The release of chemokines and cytokines by macrophages attracts inflammatory cells to the site. This results in the accumulation of not only additional T cells and macrophages but also neutrophils and mast cells. Recent studies also suggest that the proinflammatory cytokine IL-17 is made in MS lesions, and thus that CD4$^+$$T_H17$ cells may play a role in MS. (T_H17 cells have been implicated in EAE, the animal model of MS.) All these cells contribute to tissue injury. Antibodies are also frequently present in these inflammatory regions, although their role in the disease is unclear. The inflammatory process induces upregulation of Fas expression on oligodendrocytes, making them targets for T cells and microglia that express FasL; programmed cell death is consequently induced in the oligodendrocytes.

Familial aggregations occur in MS, with a high concordance rate among identical twins (25–30%) as compared with dizygotic twins (2–5%). MS is twice as common in females as in males and has its peak incidence at age 35.

Genetic studies suggest that approximately 12 regions of the human genome may be important for susceptibility to MS. Identifying these genes and determining how they relate to the immune system will aid in understanding the underlying defect and immunopathogenesis of MS.

Type I Diabetes Mellitus. *Type I diabetes mellitus (TIDM)*, also referred to as insulin-dependent diabetes or juvenile diabetes, is a form of diabetes that involves chronic inflammatory destruction of the insulin-producing β cells in the islets of Langerhans of the pancreas. This results in little or no insulin production. Insulin facilitates the

Diabetes Mellitus

entry of glucose into cells, where it is metabolized for energy production. In the absence of insulin, levels of blood glucose rise, resulting in increased hunger, frequent urination, and excessive thirst. Other symptoms include weight loss, nausea, and fatigue. A major concern is the development of **ketoacidosis**, the production of ketoacids, which lowers blood pH. This occurs when cells begin to break down proteins and fatty acids to meet metabolic demands in the absence of glucose.

In TIDM, the major contributors to β-cell destruction are cytotoxic CD8$^+$ T cells. However, inflammatory infiltrates in the islets of Langerhans include CD4$^+$ T cells and macrophages along with the cytokines they secrete, such as IL-1, IL-6, and IFN-α. Many patients with TIDM also develop autoantibodies to insulin and other islet antigens such as glutamic acid decarboxylase (GAD). It is thought that these autoantibodies arise as a consequence of β-cell destruction and are not the initial cause of the destruction.

Genetic factors predisposing to TIDM include several genes in the MHC class II region, the insulin gene on chromosome 11, and at least 11 other non-HLA-linked diabetes susceptibility genes. Some HLA class II haplotypes predispose to the disease, and others are protective. For example, approximately 50% of TIDM patients are HLA-DR3/DR4 heterozygotes, in contrast to 5% of the normal population. On the other hand, individuals with HLA-DQB1*0602 rarely develop the disease. Viruses are among the environmental agents that have been linked to TIDM, suggesting that molecular mimicry may be involved. TIDM has been observed to occur occasionally after infection with coxsackievirus; a protein in this virus shares some homology to GAD.

An experimental animal model, the nonobese diabetic (NOD) mouse, shares many key features with the human disease, including the destruction of pancreatic β-islet cells by infiltrating lymphocytes (Fig. 12.12), the association with MHC susceptibility genes, and the transmission by T cells.

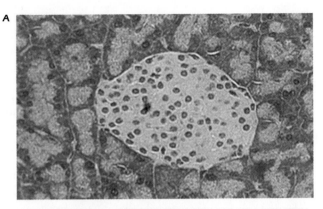

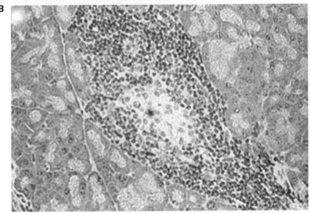

Figure 12.12. Light micrograph of islets of Langerhans. (A) Pancreas of a normal mouse. (B) Pancreas of NOD mouse with IDDM-like disease, revealing infiltration of lymphocytes in islets of Langerhans (insulitis). (Courtesy of M. Atkinson, Department of Pathology, University of Florida College of Medicine, Gainsville.)

Rheumatoid Arthritis. *Rheumatoid arthritis (RA)* is an autoimmune disease that causes chronic inflammation of the joints, resulting in pain, swelling, and stiffness.

Rheumatoid Arthritis

Other symptoms include fatigue, low-grade fever, and loss of appetite. RA is characterized by chronically inflamed *synovium* (soft tissue that lines the joints), densely crowded with lymphocytes, which results in the destruction of cartilage and bone. In RA the inflamed synovial membrane, usually one cell thick, becomes so cellular that it mimics lymphoid tissue and forms new blood vessels. The synovium is densely packed with dendritic cells, macrophages, T and B cells, NK cells, and plasma cells. In some cases the synovium develops secondary follicles.

It was previously thought that the inflammatory process in RA was initiated by autoantibody (generally IgM), specific for a determinant on the Fc portion of IgGs. This anti-IgG antibody is called rheumatoid factor (RF). When RF binds to IgG, the resulting immune complexes can deposit in the joints, where they recruit complement and establish an inflammatory process. However, while autoantibodies play an important role in this disease, it is unlikely that RF is the common initiator of RA;

30% of RA patients do not have detectable levels of RF. Autoreactive $CD4^+$ T_H1 cells play a dominant role in the development of RA and recent studies also suggest that $CD4^+T_H17$ cells and the cytokines they produce have a role in the bone destruction that is characteristic of RA. The production of IFN-γ and IL-17 by the T cells induces activation of synovial macrophages and fibroblasts. These cells secrete proinflammatory cytokines, such as TNF-α and IL-1, which mediate tissue damage by secreting degradative enzymes and toxic radicals that destroy the integrity of the cartilage. The macrophages continue to secrete proinflammatory cytokines, which drive the inflammatory process. In addition, ***chondrocytes***, the cells of the cartilage, become exposed to the immune system and perpetuate the damage, not only by serving as potential targets but also by releasing cytokines and growth factors. Synovial fluid often accumulates in the joints of RA patients and contains large numbers of neutrophils. After repeated bouts of inflammatory insults, fibrin is deposited, cartilage is replaced by fibrous tissue, and the joint fuses (***ankylosis***). Although the joints are the primary targets of inflammatory processes in RA, organs such as the skin, heart, lungs, blood vessels, and eyes may be involved as well. Patients with RA frequently develop ***Sjogren's syndrome***, an autoimmune disease characterized by inflammation of the glands of the eyes and mouth, which can lead to severe dryness. Autoantibodies to ribonucleoproteins are common in this syndrome.

RA affects women three times more often than men; the age of onset is usually during the fourth and fifth decades of life. The association of various genes in RA has been examined in family studies for many different populations. The association of HLA-DR4 alleles and RA has been confirmed in many of them, although the subtype varies. For example, the HLA–DRB1 association for North American Caucasians is *0401 and *0404. For Israelis, it is *0102 and *0405, and for Yakima Indians, it is *1402. In other ethnic populations, there is no association of RA with DR4 genes. DNA sequencing of all these class II MHC molecules shows that they share a segment of the outermost domain of the HLA-DR β chain called the **shared epitope**. Other genes strongly associated with RA include those encoding TNF-α and heat-shock proteins. A mouse model of RA, induced by injection of collagen II into mice, suggests that collagen II may be an important autoantigen in human disease pathogenesis. It has also been suggested that viral and bacterial infections may trigger RA. Viruses that have been linked to RA include EBV, rubella, and influenza viruses.

Therapeutic Strategies

For many years, the major approach to the treatment of most autoimmune diseases has been the elimination of autoreactive cells. Because it is not routinely possible to distinguish an autoreactive B or T cell from one that will protect against microbial infection, broadly ablative therapies have been used. Therapeutic agents often include cytotoxic drugs such as **cyclophosphamide** or **azathioprine**, which interfere with DNA replication and indiscriminately destroy the body's white blood cells (WBC). In addition, drugs like **cyclosporin A** or **FK506** block intracellular signaling pathways and prevent cellular activation (see Chapter 18).

More recently, **anticytokine therapies** have proven very successful against several diseases. Blockade of TNF-α by antibody or soluble receptor is an important therapeutic option in RA and inflammatory bowel disease. Inhibition of IL−1β by soluble receptor also seems a useful strategy in RA. Although these immunomodulatory agents prevent an inflammatory response and appear to curtail the disease process, they also render the host immunosuppressed. Thus, infections represent a major complication of the treatment of many autoimmune diseases. Some autoimmune diseases may be treated by removing or administering a cytokine; for example, IFN-β is used in the treatment of multiple sclerosis. How this cytokine exerts its therapeutic effect is not understood.

Recently, more targeted approaches to therapy have been explored. A nondepleting **monoclonal antibody to CD3** is being tested in new-onset autoimmune diabetes. A monoclonal antibody (rituximab) to a surface molecule expressed on human B cells is being used to treat patients with RA. Its mode of action is unclear, but it is thought to promote B-cell apoptosis and ADCC. Costimulatory blockade to prevent the interaction of B7 molecules with CD28 appears promising in RA and psoriasis. These new approaches have demonstrated efficacy, but it is likely that they will interfere with protective as well as pathogenic immune responses and thus be immunosuppressive. Additional information about the mechanisms of action of these and other immunosuppressive drugs is presented in Chapter 18.

There are some antigen-specific approaches to therapy that may eliminate autoreactivity without causing global immunosuppression. Altered peptide ligands, peptides that bind to the MHC groove but are not capable of activating a given T cell, have been used to induce tolerance in rodent models of disease but have not demonstrated efficacy in humans. Oral antigen has also been used to induce tolerance in animal models, but clinical trials with oral collagen and MBP in rheumatoid arthritis and multiple sclerosis, respectively, have not demonstrated efficacy. In ongoing studies, TCRs have been administered to patients as an immunogen in an effort to raise clonotype-specific cytolytic T cells.

The recent recognition of multiple populations of regulatory T cells has led to yet another therapeutic strategy. Several studies suggest an absence or a decrease in numbers of T suppressor cells in autoimmune individuals. Investigators are beginning to learn how to generate regulatory cells in autoimmune individuals. There are as yet no clinical trials that attempt to activate suppressor cells, but this strategy appears quite effective in mice.

In addition, the recent discovery of a subset of CD4+ T cells, T_H17 cells, which have been detected in several auto-inflammatory conditions, suggests that future strategies to treat autoimmune disease may try to regulate the balance between different sets of T cells.

SUMMARY

1. Tolerance is the state of lymphocyte unresponsiveness to antigen. There are several mechanisms for inducing B- and T-cell tolerance to self-antigen. These include anergy, deletion, receptor editing, and T-cell suppression.

2. Tolerance can be induced in both immature B and T lymphocytes (central tolerance) or mature B and T lymphocytes (peripheral tolerance). To be tolerized, a cell must express an antigen-specific receptor (BCR or TCR).

3. Central tolerance occurs in the bone marrow with respect to B cells and in the thymus with respect to T cells. Peripheral tolerance occurs in peripheral lymphoid organs.

4. Cell fate is influenced by the avidity of interaction of the BCR or the TCR for an autoantigen and the stage of development of the autoreactive lymphocyte when it encounters self-antigen.

5. Lack of costimulatory interactions can induce T- and/or B-cell anergy.

6. Anergy is a major mechanism of peripheral B- and/or T-cell tolerance.

7. T-cell suppression is mediated by $CD4^+$ $CD25^+$ T_{reg} cells. Foxp3 is a marker for T_{reg} cells.

8 Low-dose tolerance to food antigen induces T-cell suppression; high-dose tolerance induces T-cell anergy or deletion.

9. Immune privileged sites are protected from developing immune responses to pathogens, tumor cells, and histoincompatible tissue transplants. IL-10, TGF-β, and FasL play important roles in establishing immune privilege.

10. Autoimmunity is a condition in which the body mounts an immune response to one or more self-antigens.

11. Initiation of autoimmune diseases usually requires a combination of genetic and environmental events. Autoreactive clones of T and B cells exist normally but are held in check by homeostatic mechanisms. The breakdown of these controls by various mechanisms leads to the activation of autoreactive clones and autoimmune diseases.

12. A multiplicity of organs and tissues are involved in autoimmune disease, and the effector mechanisms of tissue damage may involve antibody, complement, T cells, and macrophages.

13. Alterations in the expression levels of genes involved in cell signaling, cell death and survival, cytokines, and immune clearance of apoptotic cells and immune complex may play a role in genetic susceptibility to autoimmune disease.

14. Autoimmunity may be triggered by environmental factors that can induce a release of sequestered self-antigens, molecular mimicry, or polyclonal activation.

15. Therapeutic strategies for the treatment of autoimmune diseases include cytotoxic or immunosuppressive drugs, anticytokine therapies, monoclonal antibodies that specifically block costimulatory interactions or that induce cell depletion, activation of suppressor T cells, and regulation of the balance between subsets of T cells.

REFERENCES

Bretscher PA, Cohn M (1968): Minimal model for the mechanism of antibody induction and paralysis by antigen. *Nature* 166:444–448.

Cambier JC, Gauld SB, Merrell KT, Vilen BJ (2007): B-cell anergy: From transgenic models to naturally occurring anergic B-cells? *Nature Rev Immunol* 7:633–643.

Davidson A, Diamond B (2001): Autoimmune diseases. *New Engl J Med* 345:340–350.

Frank MM, Austen KF, Claman HN, Unanue ER (eds) (1995): *Samter's Immunologic Diseases*, 5th ed. Boston: Little, Brown.

Fulcher DA, Lyons AB, Korn SL, Cook MC, Koleda C, Parish C, Fazekas de St. Groth B, Basten A (1996): The fate of self-reactive B-cells depends primarily on the degree of antigen receptor engagement and availability of T-cell help. *J Exp Med* 183:2313–2328.

Gay D, Saunders T, Camper S, Weigert M (1993): Receptor editing: An approach by autoreactive B-cells to escape tolerance. *J Exp Med* 177:999–1008.

Green DR, Ferguson TA (2001): The role of Fas ligand in immune privilege. *Nature Rev/Mol Cell Biol* 2:917–924.

Hahn BV (1998): Mechanisms of disease: Antibodies to DNA. *N Engl J Med* 338:1333.

Hartley SB, Crosbie J, Brink R, Kantor AB, Basten A, Goodnow C (1991): Elimination from peripheral lymphoid tissues of self-reactive B-lymphocytes recognizing membrane-bound antigens. *Nature* 353:765–769.

Kim JM, Rudensky A (2006): The role of the transcription factor Foxp3 in the development of regulatory T-cells. *Immunol Rev* 212:86–98.

Kishimoto H, Sprent J (2000): The thymus and negative selection. *Immunol Res* 21:315–323.

Leadbetter EA, Rifkin IR, Hohlbaum AM, Beaudette BC, Shlomchik MJ, Marshak-Rothstein A (2002): Chromatin–IgG complexes activate B-cells by dual engagement of IgM and toll-like receptors. *Nature* 416:603–607.

Mathis D, Benoist C (2007): A decade of AIRE. *Nature Rev Immunol* 7:645–650.

Miyara M, Sakaguchi (2007): Natural regulatory T-cells: Mechanisms of suppression. *Trends Mol Med* 13:108–116.

Nagler-Anderson C, Shi HN (2001): Peripheral nonresponsiveness to orally administered soluble protein antigens. *Crit Rev Immunol* 21:121–131.

Nemazee D (2006): Receptor editing in lymphocyte development and central tolerance. *Nature Rev Immunol* 6:728–740.

Nossal GJ, Pike BL (1980): Clonal anergy: Persistence in tolerant mice of antigen-binding B-lymphocytes incapable of responding to antigen or mitogen. *Proc Natl Acad Sci USA* 77:1602–1606.

O'Dell JR (1999): Anticytokine therapy—A new era in the treatment of rheumatoid arthritis? *New Engl J Med* 340:310.

Powell JD, Ragheb JA, Kitagawa-Sakakida S, Schwartz RH (1998): Molecular regulation of interleukin-2 expression by CD28 co-stimulation and anergy. *Immunol Rev* 165:287–300.

Rose NR (1998): The role of infection in the pathogenesis of autoimmune disease. *Semin Immunol* 10:5.

Sandel PC, Monroe JG (1999): Negative selection of immature B-cells by receptor editing or deletion is determined by site of antigen encounter. *Immunity* 10:289–299.

Shevach EM (2002): CD4$^+$CD25$^+$ suppressor T-cells: More questions than answers. *Nature Rev Immunol* 2:389–400.

Sorensen TL, Ransohogg RM (1998): Etiology and pathogenesis of multiple sclerosis. *Semin Neurol* 18:287.

Tiegs SL, Russell DM, Nemazee D (1993): Receptor editing in self-reactive bone marrow B-cells. *J Exp Med* 177:1009–1020.

Weiner H (2001): Oral tolerance: Immune mechanisms and the generation of T_H3-type TGF-beta-secreting regulatory cells. *Microb Infect* 3:947–954.

REVIEW QUESTIONS

For each question, choose the ONE BEST answer.

1. An individual normally does not make an immune response to a self-protein because:
   A) Self-proteins cannot be processed into peptides.
   B) Peptides from self-proteins cannot bind to MHC class I molecules.
   C) Peptides from self-proteins cannot bind to MHC class II molecules.
   D) Lymphocytes that express a receptor reactive to a self-protein are inactivated by deletion, anergy, or receptor editing.
   E) Developing lymphocytes cannot rearrange V genes required to produce a receptor for self-proteins.

2. Which of the following autoimmune diseases has been proven to be due to a single gene defect?
   A) systemic lupus erythematosus
   B) autoimmune lymphoproliferative syndrome
   C) multiple sclerosis
   D) rheumatoid arthritis
   E) Hashimoto thyroiditis

3. Rheumatoid factor, found in synovial fluid of patients with rheumatoid arthritis, is most frequently found to be:
   A) IgM reacting with L chains of IgG
   B) IgM reacting with H-chain determinants of IgG
   C) IgE reacting with bacterial antigens
   D) antibody to collagen
   E) antibody to DNA

4. In which of the following diseases do T_H1 CD4$^+$ cells, cytotoxic CD8$^+$ T cells, and autoantibody all contribute to the pathology?
   A) myasthenia gravis
   B) systemic lupus erythematosus
   C) Graves disease
   D) autoimmune hemolytic anemia
   E) type I diabetes mellitus

5. A 22-year-old woman has an erythematous rash on the malar eminences of her face that gets worse when she goes out in the sun. She has lost about 10 pounds, complains of generalized joint pain, and feels tired much of the time. Physical examination is normal except for the rash. Laboratory tests reveal a WBC count of 5500 (normal). Urinalysis shows elevated levels of protein in the urine but no RBCs, WBCs, or bacteria. Which one of the following is the most likely laboratory finding in this disease?
   A) decreased number of helper (CD4$^+$) T cells
   B) low level of C1 inhibitor
   C) high levels of antibodies to double-stranded DNA
   D) increased number of cytotoxic T cells
   E) low microbicidal activity of neutrophils

6. Blocking any of the following processes can result in peripheral tolerance in mature T cells except:
   A) the interaction of costimulatory molecules on T cells with their ligands on APC
   B) intracellular signal transduction mechanisms
   C) negative selection of thymocytes
   D) activation of the IL-2 gene
   E) the binding of antigen with MHC molecules

7. Which of the following is least likely to lead to autoimmunity?
   A) loss of suppressor T cells
   B) release of sequestered self-antigen
   C) genetic predisposition
   D) polyclonal activation
   E) increased clearance of immune complexes

8. A 30-year-old woman with a previous history of rheumatic fever has recently developed a heart murmur. The most likely cause is:
   A) circulating rheumatoid factor
   B) molecular mimicry of a streptococcal antigen and cardiac myosin
   C) a common variable immune deficiency
   D) a congenital abnormality

9. Curtis Jones, a retired sanitation worker, developed double vision. Upon neurologic examination he was observed to have weakness of his facial muscles and his tongue and abnormality in ocular movements. Several months later he developed difficulty in chewing, swallowing food, and breathing. Serologic tests revealed the presence of autoantibodies directed to receptors at the neuromuscular junction. The most likely diagnosis is:
   A) multiple sclerosis
   B) myasthenia gravis
   C) rheumatoid arthritis
   D) Hashimoto's thyroiditis
   E) Graves disease

ANSWERS TO REVIEW QUESTIONS

1. **D** Negative selection generally ensures that a lymphocyte expressing a receptor reactive to a self-protein is inactivated by deletion or anergy or receptor editing in the case of an autoreactive B cell.

2. **B** ALPS has been shown to arise as a direct consequence of a mutated Fas gene, which leads to impaired Fas-mediated apoptosis of lymphocytes. Most other autoimmune diseases (such as SLE, MS, RA, and Hashimoto's thyroiditis) are multigenic in origin; environmental triggers may play a role as well.

3. **B** Rheumatoid factor is generally an IgM antibody that reacts with determinants on the Fc portion of IgG.

4. **E** Autoantibody has been implicated in myasthenia gravis, Graves disease, SLE, and autoimmune hemolytic anemia. Type I insulin-dependent diabetes is mediated by effector T cells and autoantibodies.

5. **C** An erythematous rash that flares up upon sun exposure and generalized joint pains are common symptoms of systemic lupus erythematosus. The hallmark of this autoimmune disease is the production of antibodies to dsDNA. These antibodies may deposit in the skin, joints, and kidneys and result in the symptoms described by this patient. Deposition of antibodies in the kidneys can induce nephritis and lead to excretion of protein in the urine.

6. **C** Interfering with negative selection of thymocytes disrupts central rather than peripheral T-cell tolerance.

7. **E** A decrease (not an increase) in the clearance of immune complexes, as observed in certain complement deficiencies, would predispose the individual to autoimmune disease.

8. **B** Antibodies to the M protein of *Streptococcus pyogenes* have been found to cross-react with cardiac myosin and have been implicated in the heart valve damage characteristic of rheumatic fever.

9. **B** Antibodies to the acetylcholine receptor at the neuromuscular junction are believed to be the cause of myasthenia gravis. These autoantibodies block the binding of acetylcholine to the receptor, resulting in muscle weakness.

13

COMPLEMENT

 INTRODUCTION

The complement system plays a major role in defense against many infectious organisms as part of both the innate and antibody-mediated acquired immune responses. Named for some of the earliest observations of its activity—a heat-sensitive material in serum that "complemented" the ability of antibody to kill bacteria—we now know that complement comprises approximately 30 circulating and membrane-expressed proteins. Complement components are synthesized in the liver and by cells involved in the inflammatory response.

The biologic activities triggered by complement activation enhance pathways that remove microbial pathogens and they also directly attack the pathogen itself. Because these activities are so powerful, however, they may also damage the host. Thus, under normal conditions, complement activation is tightly regulated. In this chapter we describe the different pathways of complement activation, complement's key functions, and how complement activation is regulated. We will also describe the clinical conditions that result from either inappropriate complement activation or deficiency of complement components.

OVERVIEW OF COMPLEMENT ACTIVATION

There are three pathways of complement activation: the classical, lectin, and alternative pathways. The key features of each pathway are shown in Figure 13.1 and discussed in the paragraphs that follow. Each pathway is initiated when a complement component in serum binds to the surface of a pathogen. The **classical pathway** is activated when complement component C1 binds to an **antigen–antibody complex** (most often, antibody bound to the surface of a pathogen such as a bacterium); the **lectin pathway** is activated when **mannan-binding lectin** (**MBL**) binds to the terminal mannose residues on the surface of Gram-positive and Gram-negative bacteria, fungi, and yeast; and the **alternative pathway** is activated when complement component C3b deposits on the surface of a pathogen.

The early steps of each activation pathway involve sequential activation of successive complement components on the surface of the pathogen: The activation of one component induces an enzymatic function that acts on the next component in the cascade, splitting it into biologically active fragments, and so on. In addition, several activated complement components build up on the surface of the pathogen.

The three complement activation pathways converge with the cleavage of complement component C3 to form the critical intermediate, **C3b**, which covalently binds to the surface of the pathogen. In the alternative pathway, activation is triggered by the spontaneous deposition of C3b on the surface of the pathogen, so generation of further C3b molecules from C3 sets up an amplification loop that results in further triggering of the pathway.

C3b is an **opsonin**, which means that its deposition on the pathogen surface enhances pathogen uptake by

Immunology: A Short Course, Sixth Edition, By Richard Coico and Geoffrey Sunshine
Copyright © 2009 John Wiley & Sons, Inc.

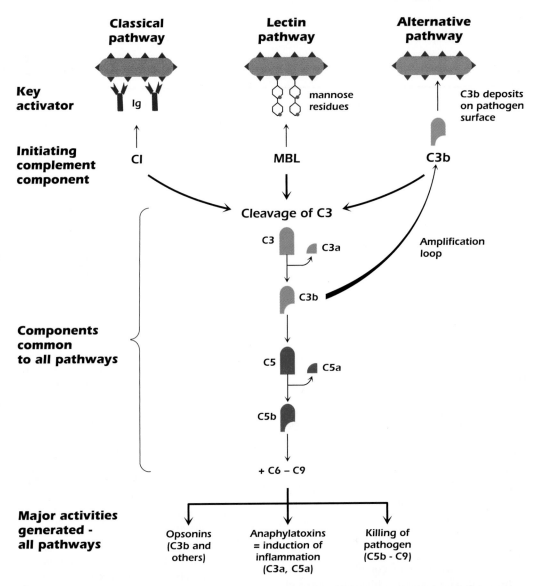

Figure 13.1. Summary of classical, lectin, and alternative complement activation pathways: key activators, initiating complement component, components common to all pathways, and major activities generated.

phagocytic cells (see also Chapter 4). The cleavage of C3 also produces a small fragment, *C3a*, which is released into the fluid phase. C3a is an *anaphylotoxin*, a molecule that induces potent inflammatory responses.

After C3b has bound to the pathogen surface, the next component in the sequence, C5, is cleaved to produce C5b and C5a. C5a, like C3a, is a small fluid-phase anaphylotoxin. C5b deposits on the surface of the pathogen, allowing the binding of components C6 through C9. These terminal components, C5b to C9, form a complex known as the membrane attack complex on the surface of the pathogen that leads to the death (lysis) of the pathogen.

Thus, all three pathways of complement activation result in three major biologic activities: the production

of opsonins on the pathogen surface, the synthesis of fluid-phase molecules that enhance inflammatory responses, and direct killing of the pathogen. All these activities lead to either rapid removal or direct destruction of the pathogen.

We now describe each of the pathways and biological activities in more detail.

Classical Pathway

The classical pathway was so named because it was the first complement pathway to be worked out. The component proteins are C1, C2, and so on, up to C9; the numbers designate the order in which the components were discovered, rather than their position in the activation sequence. Cleavage products are given lowercase letters, such as C3a or C4b. Large fragments such as C3b and C4b can be cleaved further to yield products such as C3c, C3d, and so on.

Activators. ***Antigen–antibody complexes*** are the major activators of the classical pathway, with antibody bound to the surface of a pathogen the predominant example. Antibody synthesis in response to pathogens is the key characteristic of the adaptive, humoral immune response. Thus, the classical complement pathway is a major effector mechanism of the adaptive immune response and leads to the elimination of pathogens.

Soluble antigen–antibody complexes also activate the classical pathway: Although they are normally removed by macrophages, they are found in autoimmune conditions such as SLE, which we discuss later in the chapter and in Chapter 17. Other activators of the classical pathway include some viruses (including HIV-1, discussed later in this chapter), necrotic cells and subcellular membranes (e.g., from mitochondria), aggregated immunoglobulins, and beta amyloid, found in Alzheimer's disease plaques. ***C-reactive protein***—a component of the inflammatory response (an "acute-phase reactant")—binds to the polysaccharide phosphocholine expressed on the surface of many bacteria (such as *Streptococcus pneumoniae*) and also activates the classical pathway.

Early Steps in the Classical Complement Pathway that Lead to C3 Cleavage. Figure 13.2 shows the predominant way in which the classical pathway is initiated: C1 binds to the Fc region of two closely spaced IgG molecules or one IgM molecule (IgM not shown in the figure) bound to an antigen expressed on the surface of a bacterium. Thus, IgM and IgG—and the IgG$_3$ subtype in particular—are effective activators of the classical complement pathway. Remember that in Chapters 7 and 10 we described how IgM is synthesized early in the immune response, in responses to both thymus-dependent and thymus-independent antigens; in addition, we noted that CD4$^+$ T cell responses to bacteria are skewed towards the development of T$_H$1 cells and secretion of interferon-γ, which favor the synthesis of IgG$_3$ in thymus-dependent antibody responses. Thus the synthesis of IgM or IgG$_3$ in the adaptive humoral immune response results in the binding of these antibodies to the pathogen that elicited them and ultimately leads to the elimination of the pathogen via complement activation.

Not all classes of immunoglobulins are equally effective at activating the classical complement pathway. Among human immunoglobulins, the ability to bind and activate C1 is, in decreasing order, IgM > IgG$_3$ > IgG$_1$ ≫ IgG$_2$. Other antibody subtypes—IgG$_4$, IgA, IgE, and IgD—do not bind or activate C1 and thus do not activate the classical complement pathway.

C1 is a complex of three different proteins: C1q (comprising six identical subunits) combined with two molecules each of C1r and C1s. As a consequence of C1q binding to the Fc region of the IgM or IgG bound to the antigen, C1s becomes enzymatically active. This enzymatically active form, known as ***C1s esterase***, cleaves the next component in the classical pathway, C4, into two pieces, C4a and C4b. C4a, the smaller piece, remains in the fluid phase, but C4b binds covalently to the surface of the pathogen. The C4b bound to the cell surface then binds C2, which is cleaved by C1s. Cleavage of C2 generates the fragments C2b, which remains in the fluid phase, and C2a. C2a binds to C4b on the surface of the cell to form a complex, C4b2a. The C4b2a complex is known as the ***classical pathway C3 convertase***; as we describe below, this enzyme cleaves the next component in the pathway, C3.

Lectin Pathway

Activators. Terminal mannose residues expressed by Gram-positive (*Staphylococcus aureus* and *Haemophilus influenzae* type b) and Gram-negative bacteria (*Klebsiella*, *Escherichia coli*), fungi (*Candida* and *Aspergillus fumigatus*), and yeast particles activate the lectin pathway. Because the lectin pathway is activated in the absence of antibody, it is part of the innate immune defenses.

The terminal mannose residues that activate the lectin pathway are not found on the surface of mammalian cells, so the lectin pathway of complement activation may be thought of as yet another way that the body discriminates between self and nonself. We referred to this critical concept earlier in the book, in both innate immunity (pattern recognition receptors for pathogens expressed on APC) and adaptive immunity (self-tolerance of T and B cells).

Early Steps in the Lectin Pathway That Lead to C3 Cleavage. Figure 13.2 shows that the lectin pathway is initiated when a pathogen, such as a bacterium, that expresses mannose on its surface binds to MBL (structurally homologous to C1q in the classical pathway). MBL is found in the circulation complexed with proteases, known as the ***mannose-associated serine proteases*** (***MASPs***). Once bound to the bacterium, one of the proteases, MASP-2, sequentially cleaves C4 and C2 to form C4b2a on the surface of the bacterium. As we discussed above, C4b2a is also formed in the classical pathway. Thus, the lectin and classical pathways converge at this point.

Alternative Pathway

Activators. The alternative pathway of complement activation is triggered by almost any foreign substance in the absence of specific antibody. Thus, the alternative pathway of complement activation is an effector arm of the

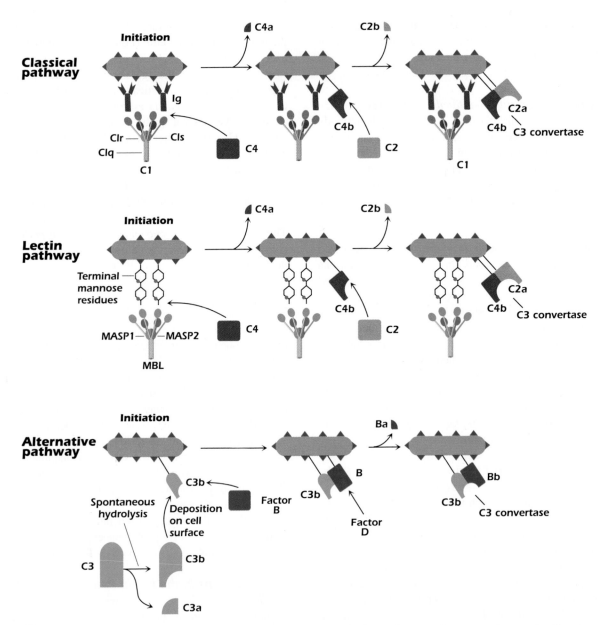

Figure 13.2. Early steps in activation of classical, lectin, and alternative complement pathways, leading to formation of C3 convertase, C4aC2b in both classical and lectin pathways, and C3bBb in alternative pathway.

innate immune defenses. The most widely studied activators include lipopolysaccharides from the cell walls of Gram-negative bacteria (which are *endotoxins*), the cell walls of some yeasts, and a protein present in cobra venom known as cobra venom factor. Some agents that activate the classical pathway—viruses, aggregated immunoglobulins, and necrotic cells—also trigger the alternative pathway.

Early Steps in Alternative Pathway That Lead to C3 Cleavage.
Deposition of C3b on the cell surface initiates the alternative pathway (see Fig. 13.2). C3b is generated in the circulation in small amounts by the spontaneous cleavage of a reactive thiol group in C3; this "preformed"

C3b can bind to proteins and carbohydrates expressed on cell surfaces, either of a pathogen or of a host (mammalian) cell. Thus, in a sense, the alternative pathway is always "on" and continual activation could damage cells of the host. However, as we describe in more detail below, mammalian cells regulate the progression of the alternative pathway. Microbial cells lack such regulators and cannot prevent the development of subsequent steps in the alternative pathway.

Following the deposition of C3b, the serum protein *factor B* combines with C3b on the cell surface to form a complex, C3bB. *Factor D* then cleaves factor B in the cell surface-associated C3bB, generating a fragment, Ba, that is released into the fluid phase and Bb, which remains attached to C3b. This C3bBb is the ***alternative pathway C3 convertase***, which cleaves C3 into C3a and C3b.

Steps Shared by All Pathways: Activation of C3 and C5

The left side of Figure 13.3 shows the first step that is common to all three complement pathways, C3 cleavage. The C3 convertase—C4b2a in the classical and lectin pathways and C3bBb in the alternative pathway—cleaves C3 into two fragments: The smaller, C3a, is released into the fluid phase and the larger, C3b, continues the complement activation cascade by binding covalently to the cell surface around the site of complement activation.

Note a unique feature of the alternative pathway: the amplification loop created by the generation of huge numbers of C3b molecules by the alternative pathway C3 convertase, C3bBb. Under normal conditions, C3bBb dissociates rapidly from the cell surface, but it can be stabilized by binding the serum protein ***properdin*** (also known as ***factor P***; Fig. 13.3). As a result, the properdin-stabilized C3bBb is able to bind and rapidly cleave high levels of C3 to C3b. As we described above, the deposition of C3b on a cell surface is the initiating step in the activation of the alternative pathway. Thus, the deposition on the cell surface of these rapidly produced and increased levels of C3b results in an almost explosive triggering of the alternative pathway. As we describe below, properdin's ability to activate this amplification loop is balanced by negative or regulatory molecules. Consequently, the alternative pathway is not continually activated.

C3b binding to either the classical/lectin or alternative pathway C3 convertases allows the next component in the sequence, C5, to bind and be cleaved (middle section of Fig. 13.3). For this reason, the C3 convertases with bound C3b are referred to as ***C5 convertases*** (C4b2a3b in the classical/lectin pathways, C3bBb3b in the alternative pathway.) The cleavage of C5 produces two fragments: C5a is released into the fluid phase and has potent anaphylatoxic properties. C5b binds to the cell surface and forms the nucleus for the binding of the terminal complement components, described in the next section.

Terminal Pathway

The terminal components of the complement cascades—C5b, C6, C7, C8, and C9—are common to the three complement activation pathways. Figure 13.4 shows that these

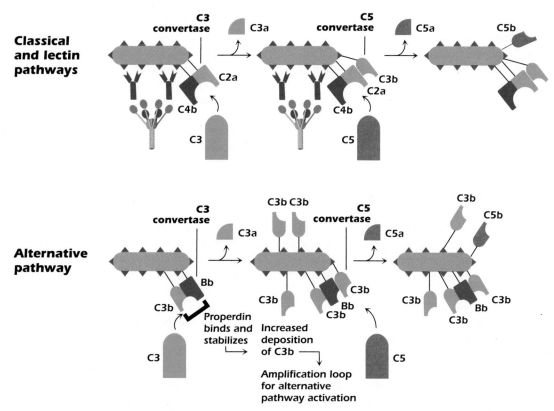

Figure 13.3. Cleavage of C3 by C3 convertase and C5 by C5 convertase in the classical and lectin pathways (top panel) and alternative pathway (bottom panel). In all the pathways, C3 is cleaved into C3b, which deposits on the cell surface, and C3a, released into the fluid phase. Similarly, C5 is cleaved into C5b, which deposits on the cell surface, and C5a, released into the fluid phase. In the alternative pathway, the stabilization of C3bBb by properdin increases C3b deposition on the cell surface and amplification of complement activation.

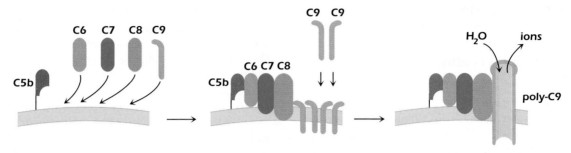

Figure 13.4. Formation of MAC. Late-stage complement components C5b-C9 bind sequentially to form a complex on the cell surface. Multiple C9 components bind to this complex and polymerize to form poly-C9, creating a channel that disrupts the cell membrane.

components bind to one another and form a membrane attack complex (MAC) that results in cell lysis.

The first step in MAC formation is C6 binding to C5b on the cell surface. C7 then binds to C5b and C6, C7 inserting into the outer membrane of the cell. The subsequent binding of C8 to C5b67 results in the complex penetrating deeper into the cell's membrane. C5b-C8 on the cell membrane acts as a receptor for C9, a perforin-like molecule (see Chapter 10) that binds to C8. Additional C9 molecules interact with the C9 molecule in the complex to form polymerized C9 (poly-C9). Poly-C9 forms a transmembrane channel that disturbs the cell's osmotic equilibrium: Ions pass through the channel and water enters the cell. The cell swells and the membrane becomes permeable to macromolecules, which then escape from the cell. The result is cell lysis.

REGULATION OF COMPLEMENT ACTIVITY

Uncontrolled complement activation can rapidly deplete complement components, leaving the host unable to defend against subsequent invasion by infectious agents. In addition, the fragments generated by complement activation (especially the cleavage products of C3, C4, and C5) induce potent inflammatory responses, which may damage the host. Indeed, complement activation is believed to play an adverse role in autoinflammatory conditions such as rheumatoid arthritis and in heart attacks when complement is activated by necrotic tissue (discussed later in the chapter). In addition, dysregulation of complement function in the eye has been suggested to play a role in age-related macular degeneration, the leading cause of visual impairment and blindness in the United States: A single amino acid change (attributable to a single-nucleotide polymorphism in the gene) in the complement regulator factor H, whose function we describe below, is associated with an almost threefold increased risk of developing the condition and may account for as many as 50% of all cases.

Normally, inappropriate activation of complement does not occur, because many steps in the complement pathways are negatively regulated by specific inhibitors. Some of these negative regulators are specific for one complement activation pathway, but many inhibit all the pathways. The importance of these complement regulators is underscored by the clinical conditions that arise when regulatory molecules are lacking: The individual may be either damaged by inflammatory responses or become susceptible to infectious diseases. Some of these conditions are described at the end of the chapter.

Many of the molecules that regulate complement activation are expressed on the surface of mammalian cells but not microbial cells. Consequently, damage to the host by complement activation is generally limited compared to damage to the pathogen.

C1 esterase inhibitor (C1INH) is a serum protein that inhibits the first step in the activation of the classical complement pathway. C1INH binds to C1r and C1s, causing them to dissociate from C1q and preventing complement activation. In addition, C1INH regulates the alternative pathway by inhibiting the function of C3bBb, and recent evidence indicates that it controls the lectin pathway by inhibiting MASP1 and MASP2. As described in the final section of the chapter, C1INH also inhibits the function of enzymes in other serum cascades, particularly those involved in clotting and in the formation of kinins, potent mediators of vascular effects. Other important regulators of complement activation are described below and shown in Figure 13.5.

C4b-binding protein (C4BP) is found in serum and *decay-accelerating factor (DAF, CD55), complement receptor (CR) 1 (CD35),* and *membrane cofactor protein (MCP, CD46)* are widely distributed cell surface molecules that regulate the classical and lectin pathway C3 convertase, C4b2a. Figure 13.5A shows that all these proteins can bind individually to C4b and displace the activated enzyme component, C2a.

Factor I, another serum protein, cleaves C4b on the cell surface after C2a has been displaced (Fig. 13.5A). Because factor I cleavage of C4b requires the presence of

A. **Classical pathway**

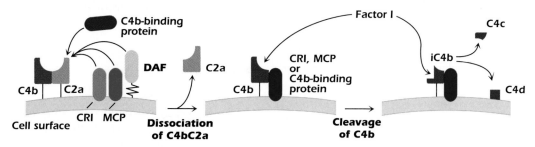

B. **Alternative pathway**

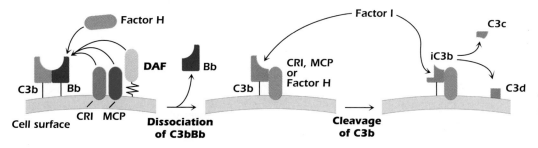

Figure 13.5. Regulators of C3 convertases in (A) classical pathway and (B) alternative pathway. Regulators may dissociate the convertase, cleave the complement component remaining on the cell surface, or act as a cofactor for this cleavage. C4 binding protein exclusively regulates the classical pathway and factor H regulates the alternative pathway. Factor I, DAF, CR1, and MCP regulate both pathways.

one or more of C4BP, MCP, and CR1, these molecules are referred to as **cofactors** for factor-I-mediated cleavage. Note that DAF dissociates the C4b2a complex but does not act as a cofactor for factor I. Factor I cleaves C4b into two fragments: C4c, released into the fluid phase, and C4d, which remains attached to the cell surface. C4c and C4d do not continue the complement cascade and have no known biologic activity.

Factor H, a serum protein, has two important regulatory functions in the alternative pathway. First, factor H competes with the previously described factor B for binding to C3b on a cell surface (shown in Fig. 13.2). Factor B binding to C3b continues the alternative pathway, but if factor H binds to C3b, the pathway stops. The nature of the surface to which the C3b is bound is important in determining which factor binds to C3b: The sialic acid coating of mammalian cells favors the binding of factor H, but bacterial cells lack sialic acid, so they favor the binding of factor B to C3b. As a result, mammalian cells are protected by the regulatory function of factor H, but bacterial cells are targeted for further activation of the complement pathway.

Figure 13.5B illustrates a second function of factor H: It binds to C3 convertase C3bBb in the alternative pathway and displaces Bb, preventing further activation of the complement cascade. Once factor H has bound to C3b, factor I cleaves C3b; thus, factor H is a cofactor for factor-I-mediated cleavage of C3b in the alternative pathway. C3b is cleaved stepwise, first to **iC3b** (indicating

an *inactive* C3b) and then to two additional fragments, **C3c**, which is released into the fluid phase and lacks biological function, and **C3d**, which remains attached to the cell surface. The breakdown products iC3b, C3c, and C3d do not continue the complement cascade, but as described above, iC3b and C3d have important biologic functions that we will describe in the next section.

Figure 13.5B also shows that the same cell surface molecules that inhibit the function of classical pathway C3 convertase C4b2a (DAF, MCP, and CR1) regulate the alternative pathway convertase, C3bBb. As we mentioned in the paragraphs above, factor I regulates both the classical and alternative pathways by cleaving C4b in the former and C3b in the latter.

The terminal pathway of complement activation and the formation of the MAC are also strictly regulated. Because the association of C5b with cell membranes is relatively nonspecific, the association of terminal pathway components C6–C9 with C5b on cell surfaces would form a MAC that could damage or lyse "innocent bystander" cells of the host. Both membrane-associated proteins and fluid-phase proteins prevent this from occurring. **CD59**, a widely distributed membrane protein, prevents lysis by binding to the C5b–C8 complex on the cell surface and preventing C9 polymerization. **S-protein (vitronectin)** and **SP-40,40 (clusterin)** are fluid-phase proteins that bind to C5b6, C5b67, C5b678, and C5b6789 and prevent interaction with membranes.

BIOLOGIC ACTIVITIES OF COMPLEMENT

The major functions of the complement system are summarized in the paragraphs below and shown in Figures 13.6 and 13.7. Complement components interact with a wide range of cells that express specific receptors. Table 13.1 lists the names, functions, and cellular pattern of expression of these receptors. The receptors fall into two broad categories: CR1 through CR4 and CRIg (a recently described receptor expressed on macrophages), which bind either to C3b and its further breakdown products or to C3b and C4b and their breakdown products; and receptors for C3a, C4a, and C5a, which bind the small soluble components generated by C3, C4, and C5 cleavage. (Distribution of the C4a receptor is not shown; it overlaps with the cellular distribution of the C3a receptor.)

Production of Opsonins

The most important function of complement in host defense is generally considered to be the generation of fragments with opsonic activity that deposit on the surface of pathogens (Fig. 13.6). C3b and C4b are the major opsonins generated, but iC3b, a fragment of C3b that does not activate complement, also has opsonic activity. Bacteria coated by opsonins are rapidly taken up and destroyed by phagocytic cells such as macrophages and

Opsonization

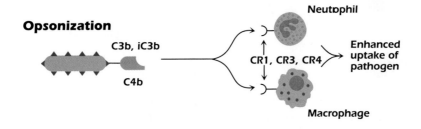

Anaphylatoxin production

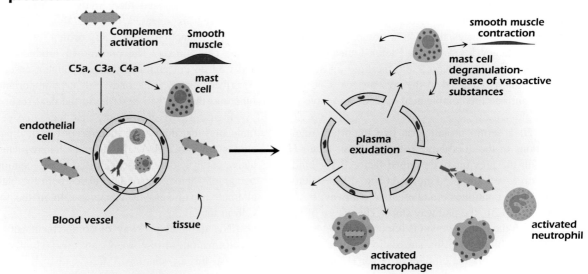

Cell lysis

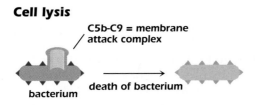

  Figure 13.6. Major functions of complement: production of opsonins, production of anaphylatoxins, and pathogen lysis.

Enhancement of B-cell responses

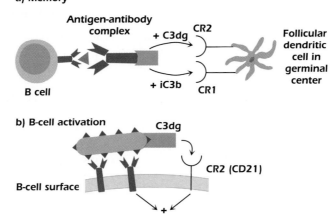

a) Memory

b) B-cell activation

Removal of immune complexes

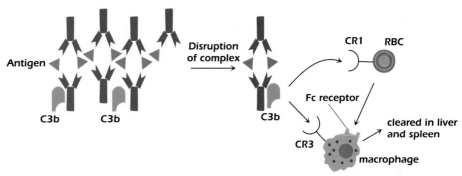

Removal of necrotic cells and subcellular membranes

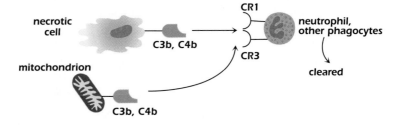

Responses to viruses

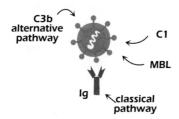

Figure 13.7. Other key functions of complement: enhancement of B-cell responses, removal of immune complexes, removal of necrotic cells and subcellular membranes, and responses to viruses.

neutrophils. These cells express the receptors CR1, CR3, and CR4, which have broad specificities for complement pathway-generated opsonins and for other complement components. The role of CR1 in regulating complement activation was described earlier in the chapter.

Production of Anaphylatoxins

The second major function associated with complement activation is the action of ***anaphylatoxins***. C5a is the most potent, followed by C3a; C4a is much less potent. The

TABLE 13.1. Complement Receptors

Complement Receptor	Cell Distribution	Complement Components Bound	Receptor Function
CR1 (CD35)	Erythrocytes, monocytes, macrophages, eosinophils, neutrophils, B cells, some T cells, follicular dendritic cells, mast cells	C3b, iC3b, C3c, C4b	Enhances phagocytosis; regulates complement activation pathways
CR2 (CD21)	Late precursor and mature B lymphocytes, some T cells (including thymocytes), follicular dendritic cells	C3b, iC3b, C3d/C3dg	Part of B-cell coreceptor: lowers threshold for B cell activation by antigen
CR3 (CD11b/CD18, also known as Mac-1)	Monocytes, macrophages, NK cells, granulocytes	iC3b (and many noncomplement components, including bacterial lipopolysaccharide and other surface molecules, and fibrinogen)	Enhances phagocytosis
CR4 (CD11c/CD18)	Myeloid cells, dendritic cells, activated B cells, NK cells, some cytotoxic lymphocytes, platelets	iC3b (and many noncomplement ligands, similar to those interacting with CR3)	Enhances phagocytosis
CRIg	Macrophages	C3b, iC3b	Enhances phagocytosis
C3a receptor	Smooth muscle cells, endothelial cells, epithelial cells, platelets, mast cells, macrophages, neutrophils, basophils, eosinophils	C3a	Mediates anaphylatoxic response
C5a receptor (CD88)	Smooth muscle cells, endothelial cells, epithelial cells, platelets, mast cells, macrophages, neutrophils, basophils, eosinophils.	C5a	Mediates anaphylatoxic response

name "anaphylatoxin" derives from the earliest recognition of their function: the ability to induce the shocklike characteristics of the systemic allergic or *anaphylactic* response (see Chapter 14). It is now understood that these small peptides play key roles in inducing an inflammatory response, which forms part of the body's defenses in removing an infectious agent that has penetrated the tissues.

The anaphylatoxins interact with receptors expressed on many different cell types (see Table 13.1). Figure 13.6 illustrates that they activate vascular endothelial cells (lining the walls of blood vessels), increasing the permeability of blood vessels and leading to local accumulation of fluid (edema) in the tissue. The influx into the tissue of fluid containing phagocytic cells (macrophages and neutrophils), antibodies, and complement components enhances the response to the pathogen. The anaphylatoxins are also **chemotactic** for neutrophils; that is, the cells migrate from an area of lesser concentration to an area of higher concentration. As a result, neutrophils circulating in the blood are activated, leave the circulation at the site of inflammation, and destroy the foreign material. The anaphylatoxins also induce smooth muscle contraction. Interaction of the anaphylatoxins with basophils or mast cells in tissues results in the release of many inflammatory mediators, including histamine. The effects of histamine and the anaphylatoxins on

vascular permeability and smooth muscle contraction are similar.

Lysis

The third major function of complement is the lysis of pathogens (Fig. 13.6). The terminal steps in the three complement activation pathways are the formation of a MAC on the surface of a cell. This results in the lysis of the cell, particularly a microbial pathogen.

Other Important Complement Functions

Enhancing B-Cell Responses to Antigens. The binding of complement component C3d or of the final breakdown product of C3, ***C3dg***, to CR2 (CD21) enhances antibody responses in several ways. Figure 13.7 shows two pathways that we have described previously: First, C3dg binds to antigen that is bound to Ig on the surface of a B cell. C3dg can bind simultaneously to CR2, which is part of the B-cell coreceptor (discussed in Chapters 7 and 10). Signaling through both the membrane Ig and the coreceptor augments activation of the B-cell. Thus, C3dg binding to antigen and the B-cell surface lowers the threshold for B-cell activation by as much as 1000-fold compared to binding in the absence of C3dg.

Second, in Chapter 7 we described how follicular dendritic cells in the germinal center bind antigen–antibody complexes and present antigen to proliferating B cells. This interaction is critical for the eventual development of memory cells. Follicular dendritic cells express the complement receptors CR2, which as we described above binds C3dg, and CR1, which binds iC3b. Thus follicular dendritic cells can present antigen–antibody complexes bound to one of these complement components to germinal center B cells. In this way, complement components also play a role in the induction of B-cell memory.

Third, B-cell processing of T-dependent antigens is more rapid when the antigen is bound to C3dg than when it is not; presumably the binding of C3dg to CR2 on the B-cell surface enhances uptake and processing of the antigen). This may be another way in which complement enhances B-cell responses to T-cell-dependent antigens.

Controlling Formation and Clearance of Immune Complexes.

When antibodies bind to multivalent antigens, cross-linking between the molecules tends to produce large antigen–antibody complexes that increase in size until they become insoluble. Although this precipitation of complexes has proved useful for identifying antigens and antibodies *in vitro* (see Chapter 5), the formation of large insoluble complexes *in vivo* can be detrimental to the host. As we describe in the final section of this chapter, people deficient in early components of the classical pathway components and in some autoimmune conditions such as SLE may show large insoluble immune complexes in tissues such as the skin and kidneys, inducing inflammation and damaging surrounding cells (see also Figure 12.9).

Deposition of C3b on a large antigen–antibody complex interferes with the bonds that keep the complex together. As a result, it breaks up into smaller pieces that can be cleared by macrophages (Fig. 13.7). Deposition of C3b on the antigen–antibody complex also allows binding to erythrocytes, which express the receptor CR1 on their surface. Erythrocytes clear the complexes from the circulation by transporting them through the circulation to the liver and spleen. In these organs, the complexes are transferred from the erythrocyte CR1 to macrophage CR3 and Fc receptors. Macrophages phagocytose the complexes and destroy them.

Removing Dead or Dying Cells.

Cells dying by necrosis can activate complement, leading to C4b and C3b deposition on the cell surface. The cell is then cleared by interacting with CR1 or CR3 on phagocytic cells (Fig. 13.7). Subcellular membranes, from organelles such as mitochondria and endoplasmic reticulum also directly activate both classical and alternative pathways and are cleared in a similar way. C-reactive protein, the acute-phase protein and component of the inflammatory response that we referred to earlier in the chapter, also binds to damaged and necrotic cells and activates the classical complement pathway. The same structure that C-reactive protein binds to on the surface of bacterial cells, the polysaccharide phosphocholine, is also exposed on damaged and necrotic mammalian cells. Recent evidence indicates that cells dying as a result of apoptosis may trigger complement activation.

In all these situations, complement removes dead or dying cells from the tissues and contributes to homeostasis. In some conditions, however, complement activation by dead or dying cells may have clinical consequences. Notable examples include complement activation by ischemia and reperfusion. In *ischemia*, an area of tissue dies after blood and oxygen supplies have been cut (important examples include cardiac tissue after a heart attack or brain tissue following a stroke). *Reperfusion* is the attempt to restore blood supply to the affected tissue. Complement activation is considered a major contributor to the inflammatory responses associated with both of these states, which damages healthy tissue. Complement-based therapies are currently being tested to reduce the deleterious effects of the inflammatory response.

Responses to Viruses.

Complement plays a role in defense against viral infection (Fig. 13.7). C1 can bind directly to and become activated by the surface of several viruses, including the type C retroviruses, lentiviruses, HIV-1, and HTLV-1. In addition, MBL of the lectin pathway binds and is activated by mannose residues on the surfaces of HIV-1, HIV-2, and influenza virus. Antibodies generated in the response against these viruses mediate further binding and activation of the classical pathway on the surface of the virus. Repeating subunits on the viral capsid or membrane surfaces activate the alternative pathway. Binding of complement proteins leads to opsonization and lysis of the virus by phagocytic cells. Complement binding also interferes with the ability of the virus to interact with the membrane of its target cells and thus blocks viral entry into the cell.

Many viruses use mechanisms that subvert the action of complement proteins. For example, some viruses produce proteins that mimic complement inhibitor function: the herpes viruses make proteins that have DAF- and/or MCP-like activities and others that block C5b-9 formation. In addition, vaccinia virus produces a protein that binds to C3b and C4b and inhibits complement activation: The protein has both decay-accelerating activity and acts as a cofactor for factor I. HIV-1, HTLV-1, simian immunodeficiency virus (SIV), and cytomegalovirus (CMV) capture the complement control proteins DAF, MCP, and CD59 when the virions bud from host cell membranes. As a consequence of these strategies, the viruses are protected from complement-mediated responses.

Some viruses also bind to complement receptors and thus gain entry into cells. One of the most studied interactions is the Epstein-Barr virus infection of human B lymphocytes: The virus's membrane glycoprotein, gp350/220, binds to CR2 (CD21) expressed on the B-cell surface, allowing the virus to be taken into the cell. Some viruses activate complement and use the C3b deposited on them to bind to host cell complement receptors; in this way, HIV-1 uses CR1, CR2, and CR3 to infect T cells, B cells, and monocytes. Other viruses bind to membrane-expressed complement regulators: Paramyxovirus (measles virus) uses MCP and viruses of the picornavirus family use DAF to infect epithelial cells.

 COMPLEMENT DEFICIENCIES

As we have described above, the complement system plays an important role in defending the host against microorganisms. It is particularly important in defending against what are known as *pyogenic* (pus-forming) bacteria, which include *Neisseria* species (the bacteria responsible for meningitis and some sexually transmitted diseases), *S. pneumoniae, H. influenzae*, and *S. aureus*. The major pathways of defense against these organisms appear to be the production of IgG antibody that binds to the bacteria accompanied by opsonization, complement activation, phagocytosis, and intracellular killing. Thus, genetic deficiencies or acquired conditions in which any one of these activities is diminished render a person particularly susceptible to these organisms. In addition, we have described the importance of complement in removing immune complexes from the circulation; we shall describe in this section how deficiencies of certain complement

components can result in immune complexes depositing in tissues, leading to inflammatory, autoimmune conditions.

Table 13.2 summarizes the clinical conditions that develop from deficiencies of either specific complement components or of regulators of complement function. Individuals genetically deficient in specific complement components are relatively rare (approximately 1 in 10,000 people), and deficiencies are not always associated with the development of a clinical condition. C3 deficiency is rare but can be severe and even life threatening because C3 is central to all the complement pathways. C3-deficient individuals are susceptible to recurrent pyogenic infections and may also develop inflammatory disorders associated with circulating immune complexes. One such disorder is ***membranoproliferative glomerulonephritis***, inflammation of the capillary loops in the glomeruli of the kidney, characterized by increased cell number and thickening of capillary walls.

Deficiencies in any of the classical pathway components C1, C4, or C2 are associated with increased susceptibility to autoimmune diseases such as SLE (see Chapter 12). The predisposition for SLE in these individuals appears to be the result of an impaired ability to process and clear immune complexes. Typically in SLE large insoluble immune complexes accumulate along the basement membrane in the kidney. Individuals deficient in C1, C4, or C2 also have an increased risk of infection with pyogenic bacteria. Individuals deficient in alternative pathway components or the later components common to all pathways, however, have an even higher risk of infection with pyogenic bacteria. This suggests that activation of the classical complement pathway may not be

⬤ TABLE 13.2. Complement Deficiencies

Deficient Complement Component	Effect on Complement Function	Clinical Condition
C3	C3b and other opsonic fragments not produced, terminal components not activated	Severe pyogenic infections and inflammatory conditions (glomerulonephritis)
C1, C4, or C2	No activation of classical pathway	Autoimmune conditions (SLE) and pyogenic infections
Properdin, factor B, or factor D	Inability to form MAC	Severe pyogenic infections
Mannose binding lectin	No activation of lectin pathway	Recurrent bacterial infections
C5, C6, C7, C8, or C9	Inability to form MAC	Recurrent neisserial infections
C1 inhibitor (C1INH)	Unregulated activation of all activation pathways	Angioedema
CD59, DAF	MAC damages host cells	Paroxysmal nocturnal hemoglobulinemia (hemolysis and thrombosis)
Factor H, factor I	Unregulated activation of C3	Glomerulonephritis, hemolytic-uremic syndrome
Complement receptor 3 (CR3)	Impaired adhesion and migration of leukocytes	Recurrent bacterial infections

as important as the alternative pathway in defense against these bacteria.

Deficiency of the alternative pathway component properdin, or of factors B or D, is associated with pyogenic, particularly neisserial, infections. Deficiency of mannose-binding lectin can be a major problem in early life, manifesting as severe recurrent infections. Individuals lacking components of the membrane attack complex C5b-C9 tend to get recurrent neisserial infections.

Deficiencies or disorders of complement receptors or complement regulatory proteins may also have serious consequences. Patients with a defect in CR3 may have a disorder known as leukocyte adhesion deficiency I (described in more detail in Chapter 17) in which adhesion and migration of all leukocytes is impaired. These patients suffer from recurrent pyogenic bacterial infections, but pus is not formed. Deficiency of factor H or factor I results in uncontrolled activation of the alternative pathway, leading to depletion of C3. The outcomes are similar to those seen in individuals with C3 deficiency described above: enhanced susceptibility to infection by pyogenic organisms and to immune complex diseases. Factor H deficiency is also associated with *hemolytic-uremic syndrome*, characterized by destruction of red blood cells, damage to endothelial cells, and in severe cases kidney failure.

The regulatory protein C1INH is the only control protein for classical pathway components C1r and C1s, and so deficiency results in uncontrolled cleavage of C2 and C4. (As we described above, C1INH also inhibits steps in both the lectin and alternative pathways.) Genetic deficiency of C1INH results in *hereditary angioedema (HAE)*.

Hereditary Angioedema

The condition is characterized by localized edemas in the skin and mucosa resulting from dilatation and increased permeability of the capillaries. The symptoms are recurrent attacks of swollen tissues, such as the face and limbs, pain in the abdomen, and swelling of the larynx, which can compromise breathing. The condition is thought to be the result of C1INH inhibiting the activity of enzymes in serum cascades other than the complement cascade; one of these serum pathways forms kinins, including bradykinin, which are potent vasodilators and inducers of vascular permeability and smooth muscle contraction. Deficiency of C1INH is thought to lead to increased production of these vascular mediators.

Paroxysmal nocturnal hemoglobinuria (PNH) is a rare acquired disorder that also involves complement regulatory proteins. The condition occurs primarily in young adults and is characterized by chronic destruction of red blood cells and thrombus formation (an aggregate of platelets and blood factors that causes vascular blockage), hemolytic anemia, and the presence of hemoglobin in urine, predominantly at night. The condition results from a somatic mutation in the gene that controls the production of the glycosylphosphatidylinositol (GPI) anchor that attaches many membrane proteins to the cell surface (see Chapter 6). In PNH, the anchor is not made properly and the proteins do not attach to the cell surface; they are secreted from the cell into the fluid phase. Several proteins are affected, including the complement regulatory proteins DAF and CD59. The absence of these molecules makes the red cell membrane particularly sensitive to complement-mediated lysis.

In other acquired conditions, C3 may become depleted to such an extent that immune complexes are not cleared or an individual becomes susceptible to infection. This can occur in some people who produce an autoantibody known as *C3 nephritic factor*: The antibody stabilizes the alternative pathway C3 convertase (C3bBb), generating a highly efficient and long-lived fluid-phase enzyme that cleaves C3. C3 nephritic factor has been described in some individuals with SLE and a rare disease known as partial lipodystrophy, involving the loss of fat from the upper part of the body. These conditions are also characterized by glomerulonephritis. Fat cells, particularly those in the upper part of the body, produce factor D, which cleaves C3bBb. The loss of fat cells in partial lipodystrophy may result from localized complement-mediated cell lysis.

SUMMARY

1 . The complement system—comprising approximately 30 serum- and membrane-expressed proteins—plays a key effector role in both innate immunity and antibody-mediated adaptive responses to microbial pathogens.

2 . Complement activation is a cascade that sequentially generates biologically active molecules. The major biologic activities generated by complement activation are opsonins (enhancing uptake of pathogens by phagocytic cells) and anaphylatoxins (inducing inflammatory responses). The biologically active complement components interact with specific receptors expressed on multiple cell types. Complement activation also results in the direct lysis of pathogens.

3. Complement can be initiated by three distinct pathways: (a) the classical pathway, predominantly by the binding of antigen–antibody complexes to complement component C1; (b) the lectin pathway, by terminal mannose residues on the surface of bacteria interacting with mannose-binding lectin; and (c) the alternative pathway, by the deposition of complement component C3b on the surface of the pathogen. The alternative pathway has an amplification loop that greatly enhances activation.

4. The three activation pathways converge with the cleavage of C3 to form C3b and C3a.

5. The final stages of all complement pathways are identical—the formation of a membrane attack complex, comprising components C5b through C9. Formation of the membrane attack complex leads to lysis of the cell.

6. The activity of complement and its components is tightly regulated by several proteins. These are found in the fluid phase (factors H and I, C1 inhibitor, C4b binding protein) and on the surface of many mammalian cells (DAF, MCP, and CR1). Complement regulator proteins are not expressed on the surface of microbial cells.

7. Complement has important functions in addition to the generation of opsonins, anaphylatoxins, and cell lysis. These include enhancing B-lymphocyte responses to antigen, controlling the formation and clearance of immune complexes, removal of dead and dying cells, and interactions with viruses.

8. Deficiencies of complement components, regulators of complement pathways, or receptors for complement components may result in increased susceptibility to infection or the development of inflammatory conditions.

REFERENCES

Atkinson JP, Goodship TH (2007): Complement factor H and the hemolytic uremic syndrome. *J Exp Med* 204:1245–1248.

Frank MM (2006): Hereditary angioedema: The clinical syndrome and its management in the United States. *Immunol Allergy Clin North Am* 26:653–668.

Haines JL, Hauser MA, et al (2005): Complement factor H variant increases the risk of age-related macular degeneration. *Science* 308:419

Riedemann NC, Ward PA (2003): Complement in ischemia reperfusion injury. *Am J Pathol* 162:363.

Roozendaal R, Carroll MC (2007): Complement receptors CD21 and CD35 in humoral immunity. *Immunol Rev* 219:157–166.

Rus H, Cudrici C, Niculescu F (2005): The role of the complement system in innate immunity. *Immunol Res* 33:103–112.

Takahashi K, Ip WE, Michelow IC, Ezekowitz RA (2006): The mannose-binding lectin: A prototypic pattern recognition molecule. *Curr Opin Immunol* 18:16–23.

Wallis R (2007): Interactions between mannose-binding lectin and MASPs during complement activation by the lectin pathway. *Immunobiology* 212:289.

Walport MJ (2001): Complement. *N Engl J Med* 344:1058–1066, 1140–1144.

 ## REVIEW QUESTIONS

For each question, choose the ONE BEST answer.

1. A patient is admitted with multiple bacterial infections and is found to have a complete absence of C3. Which complement-mediated function would remain intact in such a patient?
   A) lysis of bacteria
   B) opsonization of bacteria
   C) generation of anaphylatoxins
   D) generation of neutrophil chemotactic factors
   E) none of the above

2. Complement is required for:
   A) lysis of erythrocytes by the enzyme lecithinase
   B) NK-mediated lysis of tumor cells
   C) phagocytosis
   D) antibody-mediated lysis of bacteria
   E) all of the above

3. Which of the following is associated with the development of SLE?
   A) deficiencies in C1, C4, or C2
   B) deficiencies in C5, C6, or C7
   C) deficiencies in the late components of complement
   D) increases in the serum C3 level

E) increases in the levels of C1, C4, or C2

4. Activated fragments of C5 can lead to all of the following *except*:
A) contraction of smooth muscle
B) vasodilation
C) attraction of leukocytes to a site of infection
D) attachment of lymphocytes to macrophages
E) initiation of formation of membrane attack complex

5. The alternative pathway of complement activation is characterized by all of the following *except*:
A) activation of complement components beyond C3 in the cascade
B) participation of properdin
C) generation of anaphylatoxins
D) activation of C4
E) regulation by factor H

6. DAF regulates the complement system to prevent complement-mediated lysis of cells. This involves:
A) dissociation of the C3 convertase complex
B) blocking the binding of the C3 convertase to the surface of bacterial cells
C) inhibiting the membrane attack complex from binding to bacterial membranes
D) acting as a cofactor for the cleavage of C3b
E) causing dissociation of C5 convertase

7. The following activate(s) the alternative pathway of complement:
A) lipopolysaccharides
B) some viruses and virus-infected cells
C) fungal and yeast cell walls
D) many strains of Gram-positive bacteria
E) all of the above

ANSWERS TO REVIEW QUESTIONS

1. *E* All these functions are mediated by complement components that are generated later in the complement activation sequence than C3. Thus, all these functions are disrupted in the absence of C3.

2. *D* Complement is required for lysis of bacteria by IgM or IgG (classical pathway). Complement is not required for lysis of erythrocytes by lecithinase or for phagocytosis. However, opsonins such as C3b that are generated during complement activation can enhance phagocytosis. Although some tumor cells can initiate the alternate pathway of complement activation, complement plays no role in NK-mediated lysis of these cells.

3. *A* Inherited homozygous deficiency of one of the early proteins of the classical complement pathway (C1, C4, or C2) is strongly associated with the development of SLE. Such deficiencies probably result in abnormal processing of immune complexes in the absence of a functional classical pathway of complement fixation. Serum levels of C3 and C4 decrease in SLE due to the large number of immune complexes that bind to them. Deficiencies in the late components are associated with recurrent infections with pyogenic organisms.

4. *D* C5a is an anaphylatoxin, which induces degranulation of mast cells, resulting in the release of histamine, causing vasodilation and contraction of smooth muscles. C5a is also chemotactic, attracting leukocytes to the area of its release where an antigen is reacting with antibodies and activates the complement system; this is a part of the inflammatory response to an infection. C5b deposits on membranes and initiates the formation of the terminal

membrane attack complex. Neither C5a nor C5b promotes the attachment of lymphocytes to macrophages.

5. *D* The alternative pathway of complement activation connects with the classical pathway at the activation of C3. Thus, it does not require C1, C4, or C2. Properdin is essential for the activation through the alternative pathway, since it stabilizes the complex formed between C3b and activated serum factor B, C3bBb, which acts as a C3 convertase and activates C3. During the activation of the alternative pathway both C3a and C5a are generated; both are anaphylatoxins and cause degranulation of mast cells. Factor H is a key regulator of the alternative pathway.

6. *A* DAF is a cell surface regulator of complement activation that destabilizes the C3 convertases of the alternate and classical pathways (C3bBb and C4b2a, respectively). Like other regulators of complement activation—including CR1, factor H, and C4bBP—these proteins accelerate decay (dissociation) of the C3 convertase, releasing the component with enzymatic activity (Bb or C2a) from the component bound to the cell membrane (C3b or C4b).

7. *E* Each of these pathogens and particles of microbial origin can initiate the alternate pathway of complement activation. Teichoic acid from the cell walls of Gram-positive organisms, as well as parasites such as trypanosomes, can also activate complement via this pathway.

INTRODUCTION

Under some circumstances, immune responses produce damaging and sometimes fatal results. Such deleterious reactions are known collectively as *hypersensitivity*. The cellular and molecular mechanisms of such reactions are virtually identical to normal host defense responses. They cause immune-mediated damage to the host because they manifest as exaggerated reactions to foreign antigens or inappropriate reactions to self-antigens.

Coombs–Gell Hypersensitivity Designations

In the early 1960s, hypersensitivity reactions were divided into four types, designated I–IV by Coombs and Gell (1963) and summarized below. Although the lines of distinction used to separate these four types of hypersensitivity have blurred through the years as our knowledge of cellular and molecular immunology has grown, the Coombs–Gell designations are still relevant.

- **Type I.** IgE-mediated reactions (commonly called *allergic reactions* or *allergy*) are stimulated by the binding of IgE, via its Fc region, to high-affinity IgE-specific Fc receptors designated *FcεRI*. As we shall see later in this chapter, FcεRI are expressed on mast cells and basophils. Because of their high affinity for IgE, these receptors are usually bound to IgE even in the absence of antigen. When the IgE molecules do encounter antigens, a cascade of events is initiated that leads to destabilization and release of inflammatory mediators and cytokines from mast cells and basophils. This ultimately results in the clinical manifestations of type I hypersensitivity, which include rhinitis, asthma, and, in severe cases, anaphylaxis (from the Greek *ana*, which means "away from," and *phylaxis*, which means "protection"). Type I hypersensitivity reactions are rapid, occurring within minutes after challenge (reexposure to antigen). Consequently, allergic reactions are also called *immediate hypersensitivity*.

- **Type II.** Cytolytic or cytotoxic reactions occur when IgM or IgG antibodies bind inappropriately to antigen on the surface of self-cells and activate the complement cascade. This culminates in the destruction of the cells.

- **Type III.** Immune complex reactions occur when antigen–IgM or antigen–IgG complexes accumulate in the circulation or in tissue and activate the complement cascade. Granulocytes are attracted to the site of activation and damage results from the release of lytic enzymes from their granules. Reactions occur within hours of challenge with antigen.

- **Type IV.** Cell-mediated reactions—commonly called *delayed-type hypersensitivity (DTH)*—are mediated by T-cell-dependent effector mechanisms involving both CD4$^+$ T$_H$1 cells and CD8$^+$ cytotoxic T cells. Antibodies do not play a role in type IV hypersensitivity reactions. The activated T$_H$1 cells release cytokines that cause accumulation and activation of macrophages, which in turn cause local damage. This type of reaction has a delayed onset that may occur days or weeks after challenge with antigen.

This chapter deals with type I hypersensitivity. Hypersensitivity types II and III are discussed in Chapter 15; type IV hypersensitivity is discussed in Chapter 16.

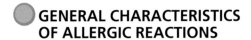

GENERAL CHARACTERISTICS OF ALLERGIC REACTIONS

The sequence of events involved in the development of allergic reactions can be divided into several phases: (1) the *sensitization phase*, during which IgE antibody is produced in response to an antigenic stimulus and binds to specific receptors on mast cells and basophils; (2) the ***activation phase***, during which reexposure (challenge) to antigen triggers the mast cells and basophils to respond by release of the contents of their granules; and (3) the ***effector phase***, during which a complex response occurs as a result of the effects of the many inflammatory mediators released by the mast cells and basophils. As noted above, the clinical manifestations of these effector mechanisms include rhinitis, asthma, and anaphylaxis.

Sensitization Phase

The immunoglobulin responsible for allergic reactions is ***IgE***. All normal individuals can make IgE antibody specific for a variety of antigens when antigen is introduced ***parenterally*** (entering the body via subcutaneous, intramuscular, or intravenous routes, not through the alimentary track) in the appropriate manner. However, as will be discussed below, some individuals are genetically predisposed to certain allergies. Note that allergic reactions can be elicited not only upon reexposure to the same antigen that initiated IgE synthesis but also to other antigens that have the same epitopes. Sensitization to ***allergens*** can occur through any means, including skin contact, ingestion, injection, and inhalation. Approximately 50% of the population generate an IgE response to airborne antigens that are encountered only on mucosal surfaces, such as the lining of the nose and lungs and the conjunctiva of the eyes. However, after repeated exposure to a large number of airborne allergens such as plant pollens, mold spores, house dust mites, and animal dander, approximately 20% of the general population develop clinical symptoms, resulting in seasonal or perennial allergic rhinitis. An outdated yet commonly used term used to describe the clinical symptoms induced by airborne allergens is ***hay fever***.

The term *atopy* (from the Greek word *atopos*, meaning "out of place") is frequently used to refer to IgE-mediated hypersensitivity and the adjective ***atopic*** to describe affected patients. Children of atopic individuals often suffer from allergies themselves, indicating that ***familial***

tendencies are common. Evidence suggests that IgE responses are genetically controlled by MHC-linked genes located on chromosome 6. Recently, other IgE regulatory genes have been implicated, including the high-affinity ***IgE Fc receptor (FcεRI) gene*** on chromosome 11 and the ***T_H2 IL-4 gene cluster*** on chromosome 5, which contains the genes for IL-3, IL-4, IL-5, IL-9, and IL-13.

T_H2 Cell Dependency of IgE Antibody Production. Several lines of evidence have demonstrated that IgE antibody production is T_H2-cell dependent. The mechanism by which these cells promote B-cell isotype switching has not been fully elucidated, although it is clear that certain cytokines produced by T_H2 cells, most notably IL-4 and IL-13, play a pivotal role. The administration of neutralizing antibodies to IL-4 in mice inhibits IgE production. In addition, IL-4 knockout mice cannot produce IgE following infection with *Nippostrongylus brasiliensis*—a nematode that induces high IgE responses in normal mice. A comparison of IL-4 levels in allergic versus nonallergic people has shown that IL-4 levels are significantly higher in the allergic population. Consistent with this observation, IgE levels are approximately 10-fold higher in allergic individuals. In normal individuals, the concentration of serum IgE is the lowest of all immunoglobulins. It has been suggested that the low levels of IgE antibody in nonallergic individuals are maintained by suppressor effects mediated by IFN-γ produced by T_H1 cells, which down-regulates IgE production. Thus, in normal individuals, a balance is maintained between T_H2-derived cytokines, which upregulate IgE responses, and T_H1-derived cytokines, which down-regulate IgE responses. Natural events such as infections with certain pathogens may disturb this balance and stimulate IgE-producing B cells. Therefore, allergic sensitization may result from failure of a control mechanism, leading to overproduction of IL-4 by T_H2 cells and, ultimately, increased IgE production by B cells. Once adequate exposure to the allergen has been achieved by repeated mucosal contact, ingestion, or parenteral injection, resulting in the production of IgE antibody, an individual is considered to be ***sensitized***. Once IgE antibody is made and secreted by allergen-stimulated B cells, it rapidly attaches to ***mast cells*** and ***basophils*** as it circulates past them.

Mast cells, the main effector cells responsible for allergic reactions, are a ubiquitous family of cells generally found around blood vessels in the connective tissue, in the lining of the gut, and in the lungs. They are large mononuclear cells that are heavily granulated and deeply stained by basic dyes (see Fig. 14.1). Mast cells are derived from progenitor cells that migrate to tissues (such as connective tissue and epithelium), where they differentiate into mature mast cells. In some species, including humans, circulating basophils also take part in allergic responses and function in

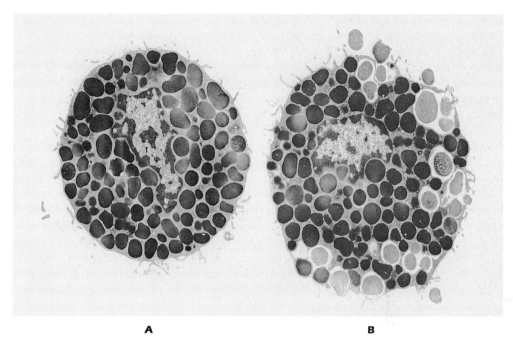

Figure 14.1. (A) Electron micrograph of normal mast cell illustrating large monocyte-like nucleus and electron-dense granules. (B) Mast cell that has been triggered and is beginning to release contents of granules, as seen by their decrease in opacity and formation of vacuoles connecting with exterior. (Photographs courtesy of Dr. T. Theoharides, Tufts Medical School.)

A   B

much the same way as tissue-based mast cells. Unlike mast cells, basophils mature in the bone marrow and are present in the circulation in their differentiated form. One of the most important features that mast cells and basophils share is receptors (FcεRI) on their cell membranes that bind with high affinity to the Fc portion of IgE. Once bound, the IgE molecules persist at the cell surface for weeks. The cell will remain sensitized as long as enough IgE antibody remains attached; the IgE molecules will trigger the activation of the cell when it comes into contact with antigen.

Sensitization may also be achieved passively, by transfer of serum that contains IgE antibody to a specific antigen. A procedure of historical interest only, known as the Prausnitz–Kustner (PK) test, was performed as a test for the antibodies responsible for anaphylactic reactions. Serum from an allergic individual was injected into the skin of a nonallergic person. After one to two days, during which the locally injected antibody diffused toward neighboring mast cells and became bound to them, the site of injection was said to be sensitized and would respond with an *urticarial reaction (hives)* when injected with the antigen to which the donor was allergic. Such a reaction in passively sensitized animals is called *passive cutaneous anaphylaxis (PCA)*.

Activation Phase

The activation phase of allergic reactions begins when the mast cell is triggered to release its granules and their inflammatory mediators. At least two of the receptors for the Fc portion of the IgE molecules must be bridged together in a stable configuration for the activation phase to occur. In the simplest and most immunologically relevant manner, this linkage is accomplished by a multivalent antigen that

can bind a different molecule of IgE to each of several epitopes on its surface, thus cross-linking them and effectively triggering the cell to respond by degranulating (see Fig. 14.2). The physiologic consequences of IgE-mediated mast cell degranulation depend on the dose of antigen and route of entry. Mast cells that degranulate within the *gastrointestinal tract* cause increased fluid secretion and peristalsis, which in turn can result in diarrhea and vomiting. In contrast, degranulation of mast cells in the *lung* causes a decrease in airway diameters and increased mucus

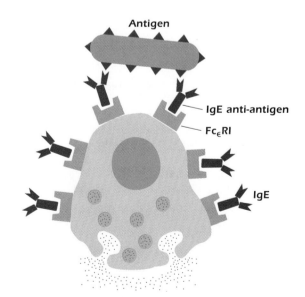

Antigen

IgE anti-antigen

FcεRI

IgE

Figure 14.2. Mast cell degranulation mediated by antigen cross-linking of IgE bound to IgE Fc receptors (FcεRI).

secretion. These events lead to congestion and blockage of the airways (coughing, wheezing, phlegm) and to swelling and mucus secretion in nasal passages. Finally, degranulation of mast cells present in the **blood vessels** causes increased blood flow and vascular permeability, resulting in increased fluid in tissues. This causes increased flow of lymph from the local lymph nodes, which in turn leads to increased numbers of cells and protein in tissue, all of which contribute to the inflammatory response.

Crosslinking of FcεRI receptors may also be accomplished in other experimentally useful ways, such as the addition of an antibody specific for IgE molecules or IgE receptor molecules on the surface of mast cells (Fig. 14.3A), exposure to sugar-binding lectins (Fig. 14.3B), or the use of chemical cross-linkers (Fig. 14.3C) or antibodies against FcεRI (Fig. 14.3D). As expected, dimers or aggregates of IgE will also cross-link these Fc receptors and activate mast cells to **degranulate**. Finally, activation of mast cells can also be achieved using calcium ionophores, which induce a rapid influx of calcium ions into the cell, triggering the signaling cascade leading to degranulation.

Mast cells may also be activated through mechanisms other than IgE Fc receptor cross-linking. Anaphylactoid reactions are produced by the **anaphylatoxins** C3a and C5a (products of complement activation; see Chapter 13)

as well as by various drugs such as codeine, morphine, and iodinated radiocontrast dyes. Physical factors such as heat, cold, or pressure can also activate mast cells; for example, **cold-induced urticaria** is an anaphylactic rash induced in certain individuals by chilling an area of skin. Finally, as noted above, certain lectins (sugar-binding molecules) can also cross-link IgE Fc receptors (see Fig. 14.3B). High concentrations of lectins are found in certain foods, such as strawberries. This might explain the urticaria induced in some individuals after eating these foods.

The triggering of a mast cell by the bridging of its receptors initiates a rapid and complex series of events culminating in the degranulation of the mast cell and the release of potent inflammatory mediators. Because of the ease with which its outcome can be measured, the mast cell has served as a model for the study of activation of cells in general. Among the events known to occur rapidly are receptor aggregation and changes in membrane fluidity; these result from methylation of phospholipids, which leads to a transient increase in intracellular levels of cyclic adenosine monophosphate (cAMP) followed by an influx of Ca^{2+} ions. The intracellular levels of cAMP and cyclic guanosine monophosphate (cGMP) are important in the regulation of subsequent events. In general, a sustained increase in intracellular cAMP at this stage will slow, or even stop, the process of degranulation. Thus, activation of adenylate cyclase, the enzyme that converts adenosine triphosphate (ATP) to cAMP, provides an important mechanism for controlling anaphylactic events.

As noted earlier, allergic reactions are often referred to as immediate hypersensitivity. This term is appropriate in light of the very rapid consequences of IgE Fc receptor cross-linking, beginning with microfilament transport of mast cell granules to the cell surface. Once at the cell surface, granule membranes fuse with the cell membrane and the contents are released to the exterior via exocytosis (see Fig. 14.1B). Depending on the extent of cross-linking on the cell surface, any cell can release some or all of its granules. This explosive release of granules is physiologic and does not imply lysis or death of the cell. In fact, the degranulated cells regenerate; once the contents of the granules have been synthesized, the cells are ready to resume their function.

Effector Phase

The symptoms of allergic reactions are entirely attributable to the inflammatory mediators released by the activated mast cells. It is helpful to place these mediators in two major categories (Fig. 14.4). The first category consists of basic **preformed mediators**, which are stored in the granules by electrostatic attraction to a matrix protein and are released as a result of the influx of ions, primarily Na^+ (Fig. 14.4A). Cytokines released from mast cells undergoing degranulation, including IL-3, IL-4, IL-5, IL-8, IL-9,

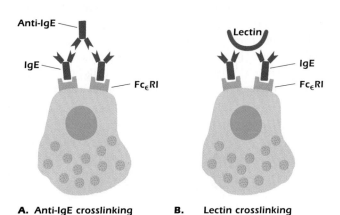

A. Anti-IgE crosslinking   **B.   Lectin crosslinking**

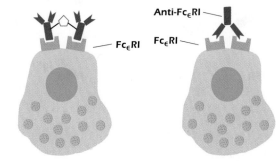

C. Chemical crosslinking   **D.   Anti FcεRI crosslinking**

Figure 14.3. **Induction of mast cell degranulation.**

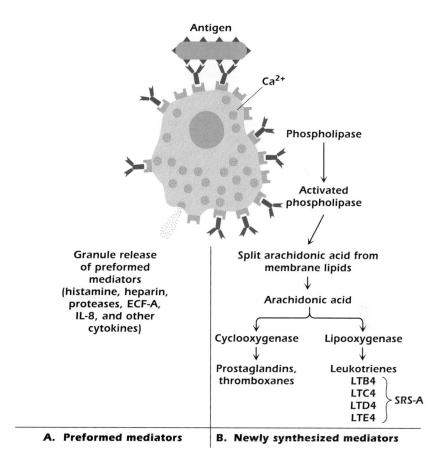

A. Preformed mediators

Granule release
of preformed
mediators
(histamine, heparin,
proteases, ECF-A,
IL-8, and other
cytokines)

B. Newly synthesized mediators

Antigen

Ca^{2+}

Phospholipase

↓

Activated
phospholipase

↓

Split arachidonic acid from
membrane lipids

↓

Arachidonic acid

Cyclooxygenase   Lipooxygenase

↓   ↓

Prostaglandins,   Leukotrienes
thromboxanes   LTB4
                               LTC4 } SRS-A
                               LTD4
                               LTE4

Figure 14.4. Mediators released during activation of mast cells.

TNF-α, and GM-CSF, also play a role in attracting and activating inflammatory cells to the site. Inflammatory cells participate in the so-called late-phase reactions of allergic responses (described later in this chapter) in concert with the second category of mast cell mediators—those synthesized *de novo*. The second category, newly formed mast cell mediators, consists of substances synthesized, in part, from membrane lipids (Fig. 14.4B). Many potent substances are released during degranulation; however, only the most important members of each category are considered here.

Preformed Mediators

Histamine. Histamine is formed in the cell by decarboxylation of the amino acid histidine; it is stored in the cell by binding via electrostatic interaction to an acid matrix protein called heparin. When released, histamine binds rapidly to a variety of cells via two major types of receptor, H1 and H2, which have different distribution in tissue and mediate different effects. When histamine binds to H1 receptors in smooth muscle, it causes constriction; when it binds to H1 receptors on endothelial cells, it causes separation at their junctions, resulting in vascular permeability. H2 receptors are involved in mucus secretion, increased vascular permeability, and the release of acid from stomach mucosa. All these effects are responsible for some of the major signs of systemic anaphylaxis: Difficulty

in breathing (asthma) or asphyxiation results from the constriction of smooth muscle around the bronchi in the lung, and the drop in blood pressure is a consequence of the extravasation of fluid into tissue spaces as the permeability of blood vessels increases. H1 receptors are blocked by antihistamines (e.g., Benadryl®), which compete directly for H1 receptor sites with histamine; when these drugs are given soon enough, they can counteract its effects. Blockage of H2 receptors requires other drugs, such as cimetidine. Some time following the introduction of antihistamines, it was noted that they were ineffective in controlling constriction of smooth muscle that was slower in onset and more persistent than that produced by histamine. This observation led to the discovery of the ***slow-reacting substance of anaphylaxis*** (SRS-A), now known to consist of a group of ***leukotrienes*** (see below).

Serotonin. Serotonin is present in the mast cells of a limited number of species, such as rodents. Its effects are similar to those of histamine; it causes constriction of smooth muscle and increases vascular permeability.

Chemotactic Factors. A variety chemotactic factors are released following degranulation of mast cells. Low-molecular-weight peptides called ***eosinophilic chemotactic factors*** (ECF) are also released upon degranulation. These produce a chemotactic gradient capable of attracting eosinophils to the site. The late-phase mediators—PAF and leukotrienes—also participate in the chemotaxis of inflammatory cells to the site; their roles will be covered below. Another important inflammatory cell attracted to the site is the *neutrophil*. Chemotaxis of these polymorphonuclear granulocytes occurs in response to IL-8 released by activated mast cells. As we shall see later, granulocytes are important in the late phase of IgE-mediated hypersensitivity. Other cells attracted to the site in response to mast-cell-derived chemotactic factors include basophils, macrophages, platelets, and lymphocytes.

In allergic reactions, eosinophils appear to serve as a late indicator of the presence of IgE-mediated reactions, especially the late-phase reaction discussed later in this chapter. Eosinophils may also release arylsulfatase and histaminase; these enzymes destroy several mediators of the hypersensitivity reaction, thus limiting it. Eosinophils have an additional function in parasitic worm infections, also discussed later in this chapter.

Heparin.   Heparin is an acidic proteoglycan that constitutes the matrix of the granule and to which basic mediators such as histamine and serotonin are bound. Its acidic nature accounts for the metachromatic (high-staining) properties of the mast cell when basic dyes, such as toluidine blue, are applied to it. Release of heparin causes inhibition of coagulation, which may be of some use in the subsequent recovery of the mast cell or further introduction of antigen into the reaction area; however, it is not directly involved in the symptoms of anaphylaxis.

Newly Synthesized Mediators
Leukotrienes.   When a preparation of smooth muscle, such as a guinea pig uterine horn, is treated with histamine, rapid contraction occurs. As noted above, this phenomenon was originally said to be due to the SRS-A. SRS-A is now known to consist of a set of peptides that are coupled to a metabolite of *arachidonic acid*. Collectively these coupled peptides are called *leukotrienes (LTs)*. The leukotrienes, which are named LTB4, LTC4, LTD4, and LTE4, cause prolonged constriction of smooth muscle when present in even minute amounts. They are considered to be the primary cause of antihistamine-resistant asthma in humans.

Thromboxanes and Prostaglandins.   Leukotrienes are only one of the complex products released from cell membrane lipids by phospholipases during mast cell triggering. Arachidonic acid is a polyunsaturated, long-chain hydrocarbon that can be oxygenated in two separate pathways (Fig. 14.4B): (1) by lipooxygenase to produce the above-mentioned leukotrienes and (2) by cyclooxygenase to produce *prostaglandins* and *thromboxanes*. Many of these latter compounds are vasoactive, cause bronchoconstriction, and are chemotactic for a variety of white cells, such as neutrophils, eosinophils, basophils, and monocytes.

Platelet-Activating Factor. Platelet-activating factor (PAF) induces platelets to aggregate and release their contents, which includes the mediators *histamine* and, in some species, *serotonin*. Activation of platelets may also induce release of metabolites of arachidonic acid, thus augmenting the effects of mast cell activation. PAF itself is one of the most potent causes of bronchoconstriction and vasodilation known; it rapidly produces shocklike symptoms, even when present in very small amounts.

Late-Phase Reaction

As mentioned above, many of the substances released during mast cell activation and degranulation are responsible for the initiation of a profound inflammatory response, which consists of infiltration and accumulation of eosinophils, neutrophils, basophils, lymphocytes, and macrophages. The most important of these elements, which constitute a large percentage of the cells activated during an inflammatory response, are eosinophils and neutrophils. This response, referred to as the *late-phase reaction*, often occurs within 48 h and may persist for several days (Fig. 14.5). The mast cell, degranulated by cross-linking of IgE by antigen on its surface, releases ECF-A, which recruits eosinophils to the reaction area. The passage of eosinophils and other leukocytes from the circulation to the tissue is facilitated by the increased vascular permeability caused by histamine and other mediators. Various cytokines, including GM-CSF, IL-3, IL-4, IL-5, and IL-13, play important roles in eosinophil growth and differentiation and in the cell adhesion of certain cell types. Together, these inflammatory mediators generate a second, milder wave of smooth muscle contraction than the immediate response, along with sustained edema. In the case of individuals suffering from allergic asthma, the late-phase reaction also promotes the development of one of the cardinal features of this form of asthma: airway hyperreactivity to nonspecific bronchoconstrictor stimuli such as histamine and methacholine.

Eosinophils can also bind to IgE through their expression of the low-affinity IgE Fc receptor (FcεRII or CD23). They also express Fc receptors to the Fc portion of IgG. Thus, both IgE- and IgG-bound antigen will bind to their respective Fc receptors, causing eosinophil activation. Like mast cells, once their receptors are triggered, they degranulate, releasing leukotrienes that cause muscle contraction. They also release PAF and *major basic protein*. Major basic protein has the ability to destroy various parasites (such as schistosomes) by

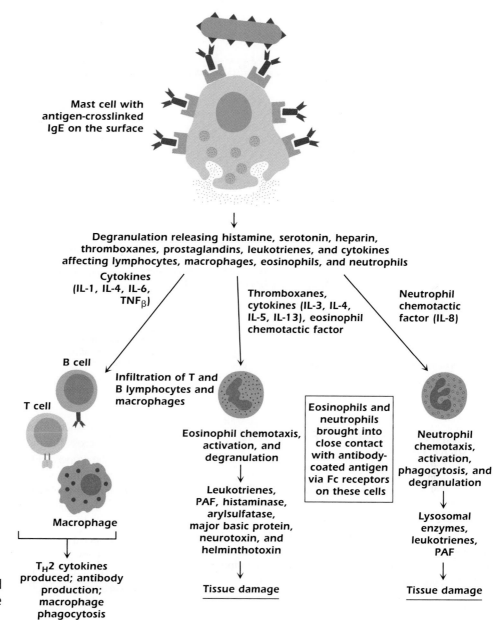

Figure 14.5. Late-phase reaction of type I IgE-mediated hypersensitivity showing some of mediators involved.

affecting their mobility and damaging their surfaces. Major basic protein is also toxic to mammalian respiratory tract epithelium. Finally, the eosinophilic degranulation releases *eosinophilic cationic protein (ECP)*, a potent neurotoxin and helminthotoxin. Although their activities are directed toward foreign invaders, all of these biologically active substances can cause damage to surrounding tissue.

Neutrophils recruited to the site in response to chemotactic factors come into close contact with antibody-coated antigen via the IgG Fc receptors that are normally expressed on these cells. Consequently, these cells become activated to phagocytose the antigen–antibody immune complexes. In addition, they release their powerful lysosomal enzymes,

which cause great tissue damage. Like degranulation products of eosinophils, degranulation products of neutrophils also include leukotrienes and PAF. T and B lymphocytes and macrophages also enter the area, further sensitizing or immunizing the host against the offending antigen or microorganism.

Figure 14.6 illustrates the general mechanism underlying allergic reactions. This dramatic series of events triggered and mediated by IgE is involved in the elimination of parasites, as described later in this chapter. Unfortunately, the same events take place in certain individuals when the antigen is a harmlesssubstance such as pollen, animal dander, or the common dust mite, resulting in tissue damage.

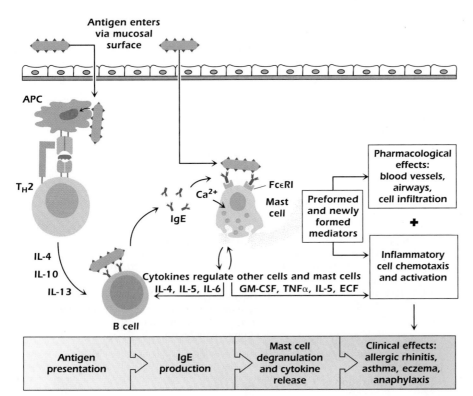

Figure 14.6. Overview of induction and effector mechanisms in type I hypersensitivity.

CLINICAL ASPECTS OF ALLERGIC REACTIONS

The clinical consequences of allergic reactions can range from localized reactions such as allergic rhinitis, asthma, atopic dermatitis, and food allergies to severe, life-threatening systemic reactions such as anaphylaxis. Although defined as localized anaphylaxis, asthmatic reactions can also be fatal. Mast cell degranulation is the central mechanism in each of these reactions.

Anaphylaxis

Allergic Rhinitis

Allergic rhinitis (commonly known as *hay fever*) is the most common atopic disorder worldwide. It is caused by airborne allergens that react with IgE-sensitized mast cells in the nasal passages and conjunctiva. Mediators released from mast cells increase capillary permeability and cause localized vasodilation, leading to the typical symptoms, which include sneezing and coughing.

Food Allergies

Another common atopic disorder, *food allergy*, is caused by the intake of certain foods (e.g., peanuts, rice, eggs).

Ingestion of such foods by susceptible individuals can trigger the cross-linking of allergen-specific IgE on mast cells of the upper and lower gastrointestinal tract. Mast cell degranulation and mediator release lead to localized smooth muscle contraction and vasodilation, often causing vomiting and diarrhea. In some cases, the allergen is absorbed into the bloodstream as a consequence of increased permeability of mucous membranes, allowing food allergens to be transported to mast cells present in skin. This causes *wheal and flare reactions* (*atopic urticaria*; see Fig. 14.7), commonly known as hives.

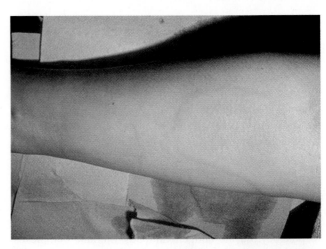

Figure 14.7. Wheal-and-flare reaction (atopic urticaria).

Atopic Dermatitis

A form of allergic reaction most frequently seen in young children, **allergic dermatitis** is caused by the development of inflammatory skin lesions induced by mast cell cytokines released following degranulation. These potent inflammatory cytokines released near the site of allergen contact stimulate chemotaxis of large numbers of inflammatory cells, especially eosinophils. The skin eruptions that develop are erythematous and pus (white cell) filled.

Asthma

Asthma is a common form of localized anaphylaxis. It is a chronic obstructive disease of the lower airways characterized by episodic exacerbations of at least partially reversible airflow limitation. The clinical manifestations of asthma are believed to be the result of three basic pathophysiologic events within the airways: (1) reversible obstruction, (2) augmented bronchial responsiveness to a variety of physical and chemical stimuli (airways hyperreactivity); and (3) inflammation. In recent years, the incidence and severity of asthma have increased dramatically in the United States. Mortality rates have been highest in children living in inner cities. Epidemiologic studies have suggested that the cockroach calyx is a major asthma-inducing allergen in these children. Many other allergens, including airborne pollens, dust, viral antigens, and various chemicals, can induce allergic asthma. Asthma may also be induced by phenomena ranging from exercise to exposure to cold temperatures independent of allergen exposure, a phenomenon known as intrinsic asthma.

Asthma

Airway inflammation is believed to play a major role in the pathogenesis of this disorder and is therefore a major target for pharmacologic intervention. Cytokine-induced recruitment of large numbers of inflammatory cells, particularly eosinophils, ultimately causes significant tissue injury. Tissue damage is mediated by the many toxic substances released by these inflammatory cells, including oxygen radicals, nitric oxide, and cytokines. These events lead to the development of mucus, buildup of proteins and fluids (edema), and sloughing off of epithelium, all of which combine to cause occlusion of the bronchial lumen. Adhesion molecules play a key role in the early events following inflammatory cell recruitment. Various cytokines released by T_H2 cells and by mast cells (such as IL-4, IL-13, and TNF-α) upregulate the expression of leukocyte and endothelial adhesion molecules, including ICAM-1, E-selectin, vascular cell adhesion molecule 1, and LFA-1. Once upregulated, eosinophil–endothelial cell adhesion increases, facilitating transendothelial migration

and prolonged survival within the lung tissue. Experimental adhesion molecule antagonists (e.g., anti-ICAM-1 monoclonal antibodies) are being investigated as candidate therapies for the treatment of asthma. Promising results using such immunotherapeutic reagents in animal models have stimulated interest in the development of antagonists that can be administered safely to humans.

 ## CLINICAL TESTS FOR ALLERGIES AND CLINICAL INTERVENTION

Detection

In a clinical setting, the degree of sensitivity to a particular allergen is usually determined by the patient's complaints and by the extent of skin test reactions. To avoid serious consequences from intradermal challenge in patients who may be extremely sensitive to certain allergens, a **skin-prick test** introducing minute amounts of antigen is administered first. A positive response to intradermal challenge, called wheal and flare, is characterized by **erythema** (redness due to dilation of blood vessels) and **edema** (swelling produced by release of serum into tissue) (Fig. 14.7). The reaction is the most rapid of all hypersensitivity reactions and reaches its peak within 10–15 min; it then fades, leaving no residual damage.

The size of the local skin reaction is roughly indicative of the degree of sensitivity to the allergen being administered. In addition, if the clinical history of symptoms correlates well with the time of contact with the antigen, the cutaneous anaphylactic response may be taken as evidence that those symptoms (e.g., sneezing, itchy eyes) are attributable to the allergen. Other, more quantitative, tests are used as well (see below).

More quantitative assays that correlate to some degree with clinical symptoms are available in the laboratory. One assay, known as the **radioallergosorbent test** (**RAST**), involves covalent coupling of the allergen to an insoluble matrix, such as paper disks or beads. The antigen-coated matrix is then dipped into a sample of the patient's serum and allowed to bind any antibody that is specific for the allergen. After the disk is washed, a radiolabeled antibody specific for IgE is added. The amount of radioactivity bound is a measure of the amount of specific IgE antibody in the serum sample. More commonly, fluorescent assays or ELISAs use enzyme-linked anti-IgE in lieu of radiolabeled antibody for the detection of allergen-specific IgE in patients' serum.

Intervention

Environmental Intervention. In some cases, the easiest way for individuals to control their allergies is to avoid exposure to known allergens, advice that is followed infrequently. If some pollens are the cause of the reaction, it may be possible for the patient to go to pollen-free areas during the season when the offending plant is pollinating.

TABLE 14.1. Pharmacologic Agents Used in Treatment of Allergies and Obstructive Pulmonary Diseases

Pharmacologic Category	Agent(s)	Pharmacologic Activity	Clinical Use
β Agonists (bronchodilators)	Albuterol	Relaxes contractions of the smooth muscle of the bronchioles; expands air passages of the lungs; short-acting (rescue therapy)	Asthma, bronchitis, and emphysema; prevention of exercise-induced bronchospasm
	Salmeterol	Similar to albuterol, except cannot be used for rescue therapy	Same as albuterol
	Epinephrine	Antagonist of histamine; relaxes smooth muscle and decreases vascular permeability	Acute attacks of bronchospasms associated with emphysema, bronchitis, or anaphylaxis
	Metaproterenol	Adrenergic agent that has primary β_2 activity; main effect is to relax the bronchioles	Same indications as epinephrine; may also be used for the prevention of bronchospasms associated with chronic obstructive pulmonary diseases
	Isoproterenol	Adrenergic agent has primary β_2 activity	Asthma, bronchitis, emphysema, and mild bronchospasms
Xanthine derivatives (bronchodilators)	Aminophylline	Directly relaxes smooth muscle of bronchi and pulmonary blood vessels	Prevents severe attacks of bronchial asthma; used in the treatment of apnea and bradycardia of prematurity in infants
	Theophylline	Directly relaxes smooth muscle of bronchi and pulmonary blood vessels; inhibits mast cell degranulation	Similar to aminophylline
Mast cell membrane stabilizers	Cromolyn sodium	Decreases or prevents mast cell degranulation; prevents Ca^{2+} influx	Used to treat or prevent mild bronchospasms associated with asthma; allergic rhinitis
Leukotriene modifiers	Zafirlukast	Binds to leukotriene receptors, thereby preventing airway edema, smooth muscle constriction, and altered inflammatory processes	Asthma
	Ziluton	Inhibits the formation of leukotrienes to prevent bronchoconstriction	Asthma
Antihistamines	Many are available, including fexofenadine (Allegra), loratidine (Claritin), and cetirizine (Zyrtec)	Primarily act by blocking the H1 receptors; inhibits smooth muscle (lung and gut) contraction, dilatation of small blood vessels, and mucus production	Allergic rhinitis, atopic dermatitis, hives, some rashes
Corticosteroids	Many are available, including hydrocortisone, methylprednisolone, prednisolone, prednisone, budesonide, flunisolide, and fluticasone propionate	Potent anti-inflammatory drugs with immunosuppressive activity when used in high doses; effects are numerous and widespread; immunomudulatory effects mainly act through inhibition of gene transcription (e.g., inhibition of COX-2 synthesis)	Asthma, allergic rhinitis, urticaria, eczema

Masks and *air filters* also have a useful role to play, but avoidance is usually difficult for the general allergic population.

Pharmacologic Intervention. Modern pharmaceutical chemistry has provided a host of drugs that are more or less effective at various stages in the evolution of allergic reactions. Many of these are bronchodilators developed to treat patients with obstructive pulmonary diseases such as asthma. Bronchodilators are agents that cause expansion of the air passages of the lungs. This allows the patient to breathe more easily and is of value in overcoming acute bronchospasms. Bronchodilators are also employed as adjuncts in prophylactic and symptomatic treatment of other obstructive pulmonary diseases, such bronchitis and emphysema. Table 14.1 provides a list of the major pharmacologic agents used to treat allergies and obstructive pulmonary diseases.

Immunologic Intervention. For many years, clinical immunologists have practiced a form of immunotherapy called *hyposensitization*. Over an extended period, patients are injected with increasing doses of the antigen to which they are sensitive. The improvement in symptoms noted in some patients has been ascribed to several different factors. The most popular rationale is based on the observation that such injections increase the synthesis of IgG antibody specific for the allergen. The circulating IgG presumably binds to and removes the allergen before it has a chance to reach and react with the IgE antibody on the surface of mast cells. Thus, the term *blocking antibody* has become associated with IgG antibody, and there is a rough correlation between titers of IgG antibody generated and clinical improvement.

Other findings during hyposensitization include an initial increase in levels of IgE antibody, followed by a prolonged decrease on continued therapy. This decrease has been linked to a decrease in intensity of symptoms and is attributed either to induction of tolerance or to a switch from T_H2 to T_H1 T cells. After repeated subclinical doses of the antigen, there is also a progressive decrease in the sensitivity of mast cells and basophils to triggering by antigen. It is likely that the apparent benefits of this immunologic therapy are due to more than one of these factors. Whatever the reason for improvement, this form of therapy is generally more successful in dealing with allergens that enter the circulation directly, such as bee-sting venom, than those allergens contacted via mucosal surfaces, such as pollen, against which IgG antibody therapy is unlikely to be effective.

Experimental immunotherapies for the treatment of IgE-mediated hypersensitivity are currently under investigation. A particularly promising therapy for the treatment of patients with asthma and allergic rhinitis employs the use of humanized anti-IgE monoclonal antibody (see Chapter 5) engineered so that it does not cross-link IgE

bound to mast cells and basophils. The use of plasmid DNAs encoding a specific antigen (used to induce hyporesponsiveness), cytokines such as IL-12 and IL-10 (used to cause a shift from T_H2 to T_H1 responses), anticytokines such as anti-IL-4 (used to inhibit IL-4 production), and cytokine receptor antagonists are also current areas of research.

Other immunologic intervention approaches have been attempted in experimental animals. For example, administration of a chemically altered allergen (e.g., ragweed pollen denatured by urea or coupled to polyethylene glycol) has been shown to suppress a primary or established IgE response. The mechanism may involve the induction of suppressor T_{reg} cells that are both antigen specific and isotype specific. The modified allergens do not combine with preexisting IgE antibodies and therefore do not trigger anaphylactic responses. Use of such modified allergens seems to offer another promising approach to treatment of allergy. Efforts have also been made to skew the T_H2 responses in the direction of T_H1 responses. The rationale for this approach is based on the key role that T_H2 cells play in allergic reactions by producing cytokines, such as IL4, that induce IgE class switching in B cells.

PROTECTIVE ROLE OF IgE

So far, we have focused on the properties of IgE associated with hypersensitivity reactions. What about the physiologic role of this immunoglobulin? Allergic reactions do have protective effects, which is evident when the sensitizing antigen is derived from one of many parasitic worms, such as helminths. The immune response to these worms favors the induction of IgE. Histamine and other mediators associated with the anaphylactic response are released in response to worm antigens cross-linking IgE on the surface of mast cells (and eosinophils). The effects of increased permeability due to histamine release bring serum components, including IgG antibody, to the site of worm infestation. The IgG antibody binds to the surface of the worm and attracts the eosinophils, which have migrated to the area as a result of the chemotactic effects of ECF-A. The eosinophils then bind to the IgG-coated worm via their membrane receptors for Fc and release the contents of their granules (Fig. 14.8 and 14.9). As noted earlier, eosinophils also express the low-affinity Fc receptor for IgE, which facilitates the binding of these cells to IgE-coated worms. The major basic protein released from the eosinophil granules coats the surface of the worm and leads, in some unknown way, to the death of the worm and its eventual expulsion from the body. As you can see, all components of the type I reaction combine to perform this protective function. This beneficial effect suggests that the wide range of responses involving IgE may have evolved from efforts to combat worm parasitism.

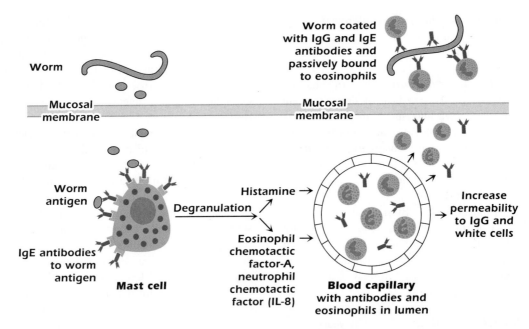

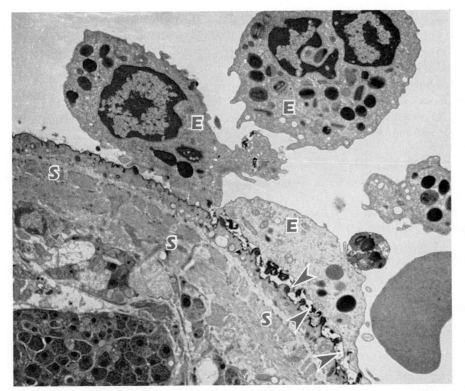

Figure 14.8. Destruction of worm by eosinophils that have migrated to area and been activated following IgE- and antigen-mediated mast cell degranulation.

Figure 14.9. Electron micrograph (×6000) of eosinophils (E) adhering to antibody-coated schistosomulum (S). The cell on the left has not yet degranulated, but the one on the right has discharged electron-dense material (arrows), which can be seen between the cell and the worm. (Photograph courtesy of Dr. J. Caulfield, Harvard Medical School.)

SUMMARY

1. Allergic reactions are mediated by IgE antibodies, which bind to high-affinity receptors specific for the Fc region of IgE (FcεRI) on the surface of mast cells and basophils. When these receptors are crosslinked following the binding of IgE to antigen, the cell responds by releasing its granules and their inflammatory mediators.

2. IgE responses are T-cell dependent. Allergens stimulate the induction of T_H2 cells, which release various cytokines (IL-4, IL-13) that stimulate B cells to undergo class switching to generate IgE responses.

3. Following antigen cross-linking of IgE on mast cells or basophils, the inflammatory mediators released by these cells have both early and late stage effects on the host; the latter may persist for several days.

4. The symptoms of allergic reactions can be attributed principally to the inflammatory mediators released by activated mast cells and basophils. Typical immediate symptoms of allergic reactions include increased vascular permeability, constriction of smooth muscles, and influx of eosinophils.

5. The early stage of allergic reactions is characterized by the release of preformed or rapidly synthesized short-lived mediators such as histamine and prostaglandins, which cause a rapid increase in vascular permeability and contraction of smooth muscle.

6. Late-stage allergic reactions are caused by induced synthesis and release of mediators including leukotrienes, cytokines, and chemokines released by activated mast cells. These recruit other leukocytes, including eosinophils and T_H2 cells, to the site of inflammation, causing sustained edema and a milder form of smooth muscle contraction than the immediate response. In an asthmatic reaction, airway hyperreactivity to nonspecific bronchoconstrictor stimuli such as histamine and methacholine also occurs.

7. Clinical manifestations of allergic reactions include localized reactions such as allergic rhinitis, atopic dermatitis, food allergies, and obstructive pulmonary diseases such as asthma, bronchitis, and emphysema.

8. Systemic reactions can lead to life-threatening anaphylaxis.

9. Despite the dangerous systematic reactions produced by type I hypersensitivity reactions mediated by IgE, the value of this immunoglobulin probably lies in its ability to combat parasitic infections.

10. Common therapeutic agents used to treat allergic reactions include bronchodilators (beta agonists and xanthine derivatives), corticosteroids, cromolyn sodium, antihistamines, and leukotriene modifiers.

REFERENCES

Bacharier LB, Geha RS (2000): Molecular mechanisms of IgE regulation. *J Allergy Clin Immunol* 105:S547.

Bevan MA, Metzger H (1993): Signal transduction by Fc receptors: The FcεRI case. *Immunol Today* 14:222.

Coombs RRA, Gell PGH (1963): The classification of allergic reactions underlying disease. In Gell PGH, Coombs RRA (eds): *Clinical Aspects of Immunology*. Oxford, UK: Blackwell.

Finkelman, FD (2007): Anaphylaxis: Lessons from mouse models. *J Allergy Clin Immunol* 120(3):506.

Golden DB (2007): What is anaphylaxis? *Curr Opin Allergy Clin Immunol* 7(4):331.

Heusser C, Jardieu P (1997): Therapeutic potential of anti-IgE antibodies. *Curr Opin. Immunol.* 9:805.

Kuhn R (2007): Immunoglobulin E blockade in the treatment of asthma. *Pharmacotherapy* 27(10):1412.

Naclerio R, Solomon W (1997): Rhinitis and inhalant allergins. *JAMA* 278:1842.

Peters-Golden M, Henderson WR Jr (2007): Leukotrienes. *N Engl J Med* 357(18):1841.

Ray A, Cohen L (1999): T_H2 cells and GATA-3 in asthma: New insights into the regulation of airway inflammation. *J Clin Invest* 104:985.

Townley RG (2007): Interleukin 13 and the beta-adrenergic blockade theory of asthma revisited 40 years later. *Ann Allergy Asthma Immunol* 99(3):215.

Umetsu DT, Dekruyff RH (2006): Immune dysregulation in anthma. *Curr Opin Immunol* 18(6):727.

Umetsu DT, Dekruyff RH (2006): The regulation of allergy and asthma. *Immunol Rev* 212:238.

REVIEW QUESTIONS

For each question, choose the ONE BEST answer.

1. A 22-year-old male with significant cat allergies visits a home with multiple cats. Two hours later, he arrives at an urgent care center with a severe exacerbation of asthma. He is treated with a short-acting bronchodilator and epinephrine. Initially, his symptoms resolved after treatment; however, 8 h later he is forced to go to the emergency room with another exacerbation. What is the most likely cause of his symptoms?
   A) additional IgE cross-linking on mast cells leading to lipid mediator and cytokine release
   B) CD4$^+$ T$_H$1 cell production of IFN-γ
   C) complement activation leading to mast cell degranulation by C5a and C3a
   D) eosinophil and basophil infiltration leading to release of proinflammatory mediators
   E) neutrophil recruitment and release of cytoplasmic granule components

2. A 21-year-old male who is allergic to cat dander is exposed to a friend's cat while wearing a facial mask to reduce his contact with the allergen. Nevertheless, several hours later, he is wheezing and coughing. Which of the following best explains this individual's allergic reaction?
   A) Mast cells in his gastrointestinal tract degranulated following the cross-linking of allergen-specific IgE on their surface and the inflammatory mediators traveled to his lung.
   B) Mast cells in his blood vessels degranulated following the cross-linking of allergen-specific IgE on their surface, causing a systemic inflammatory response.
   C) Mast cells in his lung degranulated following the cross-linking of allergen-specific IgE on their surface.
   D) Mast cells in his skin degranulated following the cross-linking of allergen-specific IgE on their surface, causing a systemic inflammatory response.

3. The usual sequence of events in an allergic reaction is as follows:
   A) The allergen combines with circulating IgE; then the IgE–allergen complex binds to mast cells.
   B) The allergen binds to IgE fixed to mast cells.
   C) The allergen is processed by APC and then binds to histamine receptors.
   D) The allergen is processed by APC and then binds to mast cells.
   E) The allergen combines with IgG.

4. Epinephrine:
   A) causes bronchodilation
   B) is effective even after anaphylactic symptoms commence
   C) relaxes smooth muscle
   D) decreases vascular permeability
   E) all of the above

5. A human volunteer agrees to be passively sensitized with IgE specific for a ragweed antigen (allergen). When challenged with the allergen intradermally, he displays a typical skin reaction due to an immediate hypersensitivity reaction. If the injection with sensitizing IgE was preceded by an injection (at the same site) of Fc fragments of human IgE followed by intradermal injection with allergen, which of the following outcomes would you predict?
   A) No reaction would occur because the Fc fragments would interact with the allergen and prevent it from gaining access to the sensitized mast cells.
   B) No reaction would occur because the Fc fragments would interact with the IgE antibodies, making their antigen-binding sites unavailable for binding to antigen.
   C) No reaction would occur because the Fc fragments would interact with FcεR receptors on mast cells.
   D) The reaction would be exacerbated due to the increased local concentration of IgE Fc fragments.
   E) The reaction would be exacerbated due to the activation of complement.

6. The following mechanism(s) may be involved in the clinical efficacy of desensitization therapy to treat patients with allergies to known allergens:
   A) enhanced production of IgG, which binds allergen before it reaches mast cells
   B) skewing of T-cell responses from T$_H$2 to T$_H$1
   C) decreased sensitivity of mast cells and basophils to degranulation by allergen
   D) decreased production of IgE antibody
   E) all of the above

7. Antihistamines:
   A) block H1 receptors and inhibit smooth muscle contraction, dilatation of small blood vessels, and mucus production
   B) directly bind to histamine, blocking its inflammatory effect
   C) influence the activity of leukotrienes
   D) inhibit binding of IgE to mast cells
   E) are adrenergic agents that mainly relax the bronchioles

8. In the RAST assay for ragweed pollen:
   A) The patient's serum is first mixed with a radiolabeled anti-IgE.
   B) Only IgE anti-ragweed antibodies are detected.
   C) The patient's serum competitively inhibits binding of the anti-IgE.
   D) Monovalent IgE is used.
   E) Complement is utilized.

9. Anaphylactic reactions:
   A) evolve in minutes and abate within 30 min
   B) may be followed by inflammatory reactions hours later
   C) are the consequences of released pharmacologic agents
   D) may involve components of mast cell granule matrix
   E) all of the above

ANSWERS TO REVIEW QUESTIONS

1. *D* The timing of the symptoms exhibited in this individual are characteristic of late-phase allergic reactions in which eosinophil infiltration occurs. This recruitment of eosinophils as well as the passage of other leukocytes from the circulation to the tissue is facilitated by the increased vascular permeability caused by proinflammatory cytokines and histamine.

2. *C* Despite the use of protective barriers such as facial masks to prevent an individual's inhalation of allergens, small amounts of airborne antigens such as cat dander can enter by this route and cause degranulation of IgE-sensitized mast cells in the lung.

3. *B* Allergic individuals have already made IgE responses to specific allergens. IgE binds passively to cells expressing high-affinity Fc receptors for IgE (e.g., mast cells) and interacts with the allergen when present. This results in cross-linking of the high-affinity FcεR, resulting in mast cell degranulation. The allergen does not need to be processed by APC in order to bind to IgE.

4. *E* All are effects of epinephrine and make it useful for treatment of acute anaphylactic symptoms.

5. *C* Since the IgE Fc fragments would bind to the high-affinity FcεR expressed on the surface of mast cells, the allergen-specific

IgE would not have access to these receptors and therefore would not bind to these cells. When the allergen is introduced intradermally, it would bind to the allergen-specific IgE at the site, but this would not result in cross-linking of FcεR, which are saturated with soluble IgE Fc fragments. Hence no immediate hypersensitivity reaction would take place.

6. *E* All are considered to be involved to varying degrees in injection therapy.

7. *A*. Antihistamines act by blocking H1 histamine receptors, NOT histamine itself. They do not act by influencing the activity of leukotrienes or by binding to IgE on mast cells and are not adrenergic agents.

8. *B* The RAST assay measures IgE antibody that is allowed to bind to allergen coupled to an insoluble matrix. It detects IgE anti-ragweed antibodies. It does not utilize monovalent IgE, and complement is not utilized in the test.

9. *E* All are true. A and C are true of the classic wheal-and-flare response, while B and D describe features of the late-phase response, which is a complication of some anaphylactic reactions.

15

HYPERSENSITIVITY: TYPES II AND III

INTRODUCTION

Hypersensitivity reactions characterized as type II and type III reactions are mediated by antibodies belonging to the IgG, IgM, and in some cases IgA or IgE isotypes. The distinction between these two forms of hypersensitivity lies in the type and location of antigen involved and the way in which antigen is brought together with antibody. *Type II hypersensitivity reactions* are stimulated by the binding of antibody directly to an antigen on the surface of a cell. *Type III hypersensitivity reactions* are stimulated by antigen–antibody immune complexes. The target antigens involved in type II and type III hypersensitivity reactions are often self-antigens.

TYPE II HYPERSENSITIVITY

Three different antibody-mediated mechanisms are involved in type II hypersensitivity reactions. The targeted cell is either damaged or destroyed through a variety of mechanisms associated with (1) complement-mediated reactions, (2) antibody-dependent cell-mediated cytotoxicity, and (3) antibody-mediated cellular dysfunction. As illustrated by the examples presented below, many of these reactions are manifestations of antibody-mediated autoimmunity. The mechanisms of generation of autoantibodies were discussed in Chapter 12. The antibodies involved in these hypersensitivity reactions are either directed against normal self-antigens (e.g., cross-reactive antibodies elicited following an infection) or modified self-antigens (e.g., drug-induced autoantibodies elicited after the binding of drugs to certain cell membranes).

Complement-Mediated Reactions

In complement-mediated hypersensitivity reactions, antibodies react with cell membrane self-antigens, leading to complement fixation. This activates the complement cascade, as discussed in Chapter 13, and leads to *lysis* of the cell. Alternatively, binding of antibody to the cell surface and subsequent activation of complement (to yield C3b) effectively opsonize the target cell (Fig. 15.1A). *Opsonization* culminates in the phagocytosis and destruction of the cell by macrophages and neutrophils expressing surface Fc receptors or receptors that bind C3b. Blood cells are most commonly affected by this mechanism. Interestingly, IgG Fc receptor knockout mice fail to mount type II (and type III) hypersensitivity reactions—a finding that underscores the pivotal role played by IgG Fc receptors in initiating these reaction cascades.

Antibody-Dependent, Cell-Mediated Cytotoxicity

Antibody-dependent cell-mediated cytotoxicity (ADCC) utilizes Fc receptors expressed on many cell types (such as NK cells, macrophages, neutrophils, and eosinophils) to bring these cells into contact with antibody-coated target

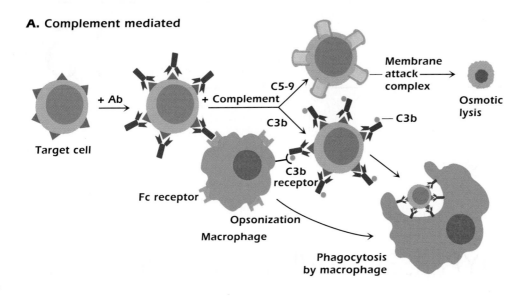

A. Complement mediated

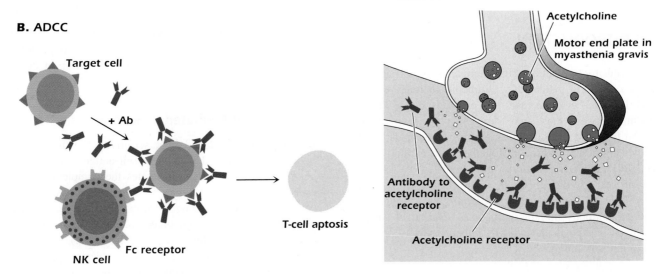

B. ADCC

C. Antireceptor antibodies

Figure 15.1. Three mechanisms of antibody-mediated injury in type II hypersensitivity. (A) Complement-mediated reactions lead to lysis of cells or render them susceptible to phagocytosis. (B) In ADCC, IgG-coated target cells are killed by cells that bear Fc receptors for IgG (such as NK cells and macrophages). (C) Antireceptor antibodies disturb the normal function of receptors. In this example, acetylcholine receptor antibodies impair neuromuscular transmission in myasthenia gravis.

cells (Fig. 15.1B). Lysis of these target cells requires contact but does not involve phagocytosis or complement fixation. Instead, ADCC-mediated lysis of target cells is analogous to that of cytotoxic T cells and involves the release of cytoplasmic granules (modified lysosomes) containing **perforin** and **granzymes**. Once released from the lytic granules, perforins insert into the target cell membrane and polymerize to form pores. Granzymes, which consist of at least three serine proteases, enter the cytoplasm of the target cell and activate events leading to apoptosis.

ADCC reactions are typically triggered by IgG binding to IgG-specific Fc receptors (FcϵIII, also known as CD16). However, IgE antibodies can also be involved in ADCC. In this situation, the low-affinity IgE Fc receptor (FcϵRII) expressed on certain cells, including eosinophils (see Chapter 14), binds to the Fc portion of IgE antibodies bound to target antigens such as parasites (see Fig. 14.8).

Antibody-Mediated Cellular Dysfunction

In some type II hypersensitivity reactions, antibodies bind to **cell surface receptors** that are critical for the functional integrity of the cell (Fig. 15.1C). When autoantibodies bind to such receptors, they impair or dysregulate cell function without causing cell injury or inflammation.

In the following section, we provide several examples of clinically important type-II-antibody-mediated hypersensitivity reactions.

 EXAMPLES OF TYPE II HYPERSENSITIVITY REACTIONS

Transfusion Reactions

Transfusion of ABO-incompatible blood results in complement-mediated cytotoxic reactions. For example, for reasons that are still not completely clear, people with type O blood have IgM anti-A and anti-B antibodies (*isohemagglutinins*) in their circulation, which react with the A and B blood group substances, respectively. If such a person were to be transfused with RBCs expressing the type A blood group antigen, the consequences could be disastrous. Since there is a considerable amount of IgM anti-A antibody in this person's circulation, all the transfused type A RBCs cells will bind to some antibody. There would be similar consequences if this person were transfused with RBCs expressing the type B blood group antigen. As you learned in Chapter 13, a single IgM molecule is sufficient to activate many complement molecules. Because of the efficiency of IgM antibody in activating complement and the absence of repair mechanisms, RBCs will be lysed intravascularly by the destructive action of complement on their membranes. Not only does this nullify the desirable effects of the transfusion, but also the individual is faced with the risk of kidney damage from blockage by large quantities of RBC membrane plus the possible toxic effects of the release of the heme complex.

Drug-Induced Reactions

In some people, certain drugs act as *haptens,* combining with cells or with other circulating blood constituents and inducing antibody formation. When antibody combines with cells coated with the drug, cytotoxic damage results. The type of pathologic injury depends on the type of cell that binds the drug. For example, some drugs can bind to platelets and cause them to become immunogenic. The antibody responses cause lysis of the platelets and resulting thrombocytopenia (low blood platelet count). This disorder, in turn, can give rise to *purpura* (hemorrhage into the skin, mucous membranes, and internal organs), the main problem in drug-induced thrombocytopenia. Withdrawal of the offending drug leads to a cessation of symptoms. Other drugs, such as chloramphenicol (an antibiotic), may bind to WBCs; phenacetin (an analgesic) and chlorpromazine

(a tranquilizer) may bind to RBCs. An immune response to these drugs can lead to *agranulocytosis* (decrease in granulocytes) of WBCs and hemolytic anemia in the case of RBCs. Damage to the target cell in these examples may be mediated by either of the two mechanisms described above: cytolysis via the complement pathway or phagocytosis mediated by receptors for Fc or C3b.

Although the preceding discussion emphasizes type II reactions induced by drugs, hypersensitivity to drugs may also induce IgE-mediated immediate type I hypersensitivity reactions (see Chapter 14), type IV delayed-type hypersensitivity reactions (discussed in Chapter 16), and the immune-complex-mediated reactions (type III) discussed below.

Rh Incompatibility Reactions

A somewhat similar mechanism occurs in the rhesus (Rh) incompatibility reaction seen in infants born of parents with Rh-incompatible blood groups. Rh antigens are so named because rabbit antisera raised against rhesus monkey RBCs agglutinate the erythrocytes from approximately 85% of humans tested. RBCs from such individuals are therefore said to be Rh$^+$; cells from the remaining 15% of the population are considered Rh$^-$. Rh$^-$ mothers can become sensitized to Rh antigens during their first pregnancy if the child has Rh$^+$ RBCs. This occurs as a result of the release of some of the baby's RBCs into the mother's circulation during birth. If the mother is sufficiently immunized to produce anti-Rh antibody of the IgG isotype, subsequent Rh$^+$ fetuses will be at risk because IgG antibody is capable of crossing the placenta, as you learned in Chaper 4. In second or subsequent pregnancies, when the anti-Rh IgG antibodies have crossed the placenta, they bind to the Rh antigen on the RBCs of the fetus. Because the density of Rh antigen on the surface of RBCs is low, these antibodies usually fail to agglutinate or lyse the cells directly. However, the antibody-coated cells are readily destroyed by the opsonic effect of the Fc portions of the IgG, which interact with the receptors for Fc on the phagocytic cells of the reticuloendothelial system. The result is progressive destruction of fetal or newborn RBCs. The pathologic consequences of decreased transport of oxygen include jaundice associated with the breakdown of hemoglobin, a condition known as hemolytic disease of the newborn (*erythroblastosis fetalis*). Prevention of this Rh incompatibility reaction can be achieved by the administration of anti-Rh antibodies to the mother within 72 h of parturition to effectively block the sensitization phase. This also causes a rapid clearance of Rh$^+$ cells from the mother's circulation. One widely used preparation of anti-Rh antibodies involves the use of antibodies (*Rhogam*) against the D antigen, now known to be the strongest immunogen and the most important of all the Rh antigens.

Reactions Involving Cell Membrane Receptors

An example of antibody-mediated cellular dysfunction due to reactivity with a cell receptor is seen in the autoimmune disease *myasthenia gravis*.

Myasthenia Gravis

Antagonistic autoantibodies reactive with *acetylcholine receptors* in the motor end plates of skeletal muscles impair neuromuscular transmission, causing muscle weakness (see Fig. 15.1C). Conversely, autoantibodies can serve as agonists in some cases, causing stimulation of the target cells. For example, in Graves disease antibodies directed against thyroid-stimulating hormone receptor on thyroid epithelial cells stimulate the cells, resulting in hyperthyroidism. Myasthenia gravis and Graves disease are discussed in more detail in Chapter 12, which deals with the subject of autoimmunity.

Reactions Involving Other Cell Membrane Determinants

As a consequence of certain infectious diseases or for other reasons, some individuals produce autoantibodies reactive against their own blood cells. When RBCs are the target, binding of anti-RBC autoantibody shortens RBC life span or destroys them altogether. Destruction can be complement mediated, resulting in RBC hemolysis. It can also be mediated by phagocytosis following the binding of phagocytes to (1) the Fc regions of autoantibodies or (2) C3b bound to autoantibodies. This may lead to progressive anemia if the production of new RBCs cannot keep pace with RBC destruction. Occasionally, the antibody only binds effectively at lower temperatures (so-called *cold agglutinins*), in which case lowering of body temperature, particularly in the arms and legs, leads to effective antibody binding and destruction of the RBCs.

Another example of cell destruction by autoantibodies is *idiopathic thrombocytopenia purpura*. In this condition, antibodies directed to platelets result in platelet destruction by complement or by phagocytic cells with Fc or C3b receptors. A decrease in platelet numbers may lead to bleeding (purpura). Similarly, autoantibodies directed against granulocytes can induce agranulocytosis, predisposing individuals to various infections. Finally, autoantibodies may form against other tissue components; antibodies formed against basement membrane collagen cause *Goodpasture's syndrome* (see Chapter 12), and those directed against desmosomes result in *pemphigus vulgaris*.

TYPE III HYPERSENSITIVITY

Under normal conditions, circulating *immune complexes* comprised of antibodies bound to foreign antigens are removed by phagocytic cells. Phagocytosis is facilitated by the binding of the Fc regions of the antibodies present in such complexes to IgG Fc receptors expressed on these cells. In addition, RBCs that have C3b receptors may bind immune complexes that have fixed complement and transport them to the liver, where the complexes are removed by phagocytic Kupffer cells. A recently discovered innate immune mechanism for the disposal of immune complexes was identified. It involves a *histidine-rich glycoprotein (HRG)* which is abundantly synthesized by the liver and released into the bloodstream. In contrast to the other known immune complex clearing mechanisms, such as the complement system, HRG does not require preactivation. HRG is therefore more readily available to remove immune complexes from circulation. Interestingly, HRG also has the ability to clear apoptotic cells by binding naked DNA. Through its interactions with naked DNA and immune complexes, HRG may mask epitopes recognized by autoantibody-producing B cells (such as rheumatoid factors and anti-DNA antibodies). The latter property may regulate adaptive immune system activation and indicates that HRG may play an important role in ameliorating autoimmune reactions.

What happens when physiologic mechanisms for clearing immune complexes are overwhelmed by large quantities of such complexes? When this happens, immune complexes of a certain size can inappropriately deposit in the tissues and trigger a variety of systemic pathogenic events known as *type III hypersensitivity reactions*. If such a reaction is systemic, it is also referred to as *systemic immune complex disease*. Localized reactions are also known as *localized immune complex disease*. Both of these can be associated with immune complex deposition in the joints, kidneys, skin, choroid plexus, and ciliary artery of the eye. The tissue damage caused by these immune complexes varies, depending on the site of localization. For example, if the site of immune complex deposition is joint meniscus, this may lead to destruction of synovial membranes and cartilage.

The generation of immune complexes can be stimulated by *exogenous antigens* such as bacteria and viruses or, as in the case of the Arthus reaction described below, by intradermal or intrapulmonary exposure to large amounts of foreign protein. Alternatively, *endogenous antigens* can serve as a target for autoantibodies, in which case the clinical outcome is considered an autoimmune phenomenon (see Chapter 12). DNA is the endogenous antigen in SLE.

Systemic Lupus Erythematosus

Patients with SLE often have both systemic (multiorgan) and localized manifestations of immune complex disease. Localized tissue injury occurs as a result of the formation of antigen–antibody complexes (*in situ* immune complexes) at extravascular sites such as the glomeruli of the kidneys. Immune complexes are also formed *in situ* on the glomerular basement membrane in a variety of glomerular diseases.

The mechanism of injury in immune-complex-mediated disease is the same regardless of whether immune complex deposition is systemic or local. Central to the pathogenesis of tissue injury is the fixation of complement by the immune complexes, activation of the complement cascade, and release of biologically active fragments (such as anaphylotoxins C3a and C5a; see Chapter 13). Complement activation results in increased vascular permeability and stimulates the recruitment of polymorphonuclear phagocytes that release lysosomal enzymes (such as neutral proteases), which can damage the glomerular basement membrane.

IgG is the immunoglobulin isotype usually involved in type III hypersensitivity reactions, but IgM can also be involved. As with type II hypersensitivity reactions, IgG Fc receptors (CD16) expressed on leukocytes play a pivotal role in initiating type III reaction cascades. The antibody–antigen complexes may fix complement and/or activate effector cells (primarily neutrophils) that cause tissue damage. C3a and C5a generated by complement activation induce mast cells and basophils to release arachidonic acid metabolites and chemokines that attract additional basophils, eosinophils, macrophages, and neutrophils to the area. The polymorphs release their lysosomal enzymes at the surface of the affected tissues. Macrophages are stimulated to release TNF-α and IL-1, while platelets form microthrombi and contribute to cellular proliferation by releasing platelet-derived growth factor (PDGF).

Systemic Immune Complex Disease

The pathogenesis of systemic immune complex disease can be divided into three phases. In the first phase, antigen–antibody immune complexes form in the circulation (Fig. 15.2A). This is followed by deposition of immune complexes in various tissues (Fig. 15.2B), which initiates the third phase—inflammatory reactions in various tissues (Fig. 15.2C). Several factors help to determine whether immune complex formation will lead to tissue deposition and disease. The size of the complexes appears to be important. Very large complexes formed under conditions of antibody excess are rapidly removed from the circulation by phagocytic cells and are rendered harmless. Because small or intermediate complexes circulate for longer periods of time and bind less avidly to IgG Fc receptors expressed on phagocytic cells, they tend to be more pathogenic than large complexes. A second factor that can influence the development of systemic immune complex disease is the integrity of the mononuclear phagocytic system. An intrinsic dysfunction of this system increases the probability of persistence of immune complexes in the circulation. Overloading the phagocytic system with large quantities of immune complexes also compromises its ability to mediate their clearance from the circulation. For reasons that are not well understood, the favored sites of immune complex deposition are the kidneys, joints, skin, heart, and small vessels. Localization in the kidney can be explained, in part, by the filtration function of the glomeruli.

Serum Sickness. The prototype of systemic immune complex disease is ***serum sickness***. This term derives from observations made at the turn of the twentieth century by von Pirquet and Schick regarding the consequences of the treatment of certain infectious diseases, such as diphtheria and tetanus, with antisera made in horses. It was well known that the pathologic consequences of infection by both the *Corynebacterium* and the *Clostridium* organisms were due to the secretion of exotoxins that are extremely damaging to host cells (Chapter 20). The bacteria themselves are relatively noninvasive and of little consequence. Hence the strategy that evolved to treat these diseases was to neutralize the toxins rapidly, before quantities large enough to kill the host became fixed in tissues. Since active immunization required several weeks to produce useful levels of antibody, it was necessary to protect the individual through passive immunization. Large amounts of a preformed antitoxin antibody were injected as soon as the disease was diagnosed in order to prevent death by toxin. Horses, which were readily available, easily immunized, and capable of yielding large quantities of useful antisera, were the animals of choice for the production of antitoxin. Today, we know that the administration of large quantities of ***heterologous serum*** (serum from another species) causes the recipient to synthesize antibodies to the foreign immunoglobulin. This leads to the formation of antigen–antibody complexes, which results in the clinical symptoms associated with serum sickness. Serum sickness can also occur in patients as a secondary reaction to the administration of nonprotein drugs. The classic clinical manifestations consist of fever, arthralgia, lymphadenopathy, and skin eruption. In addition, the potential development of serum sickness is becoming an important consideration in administration of monoclonal antibodies made in rodents for treatment of malignancy, graft rejection, or autoimmune disease.

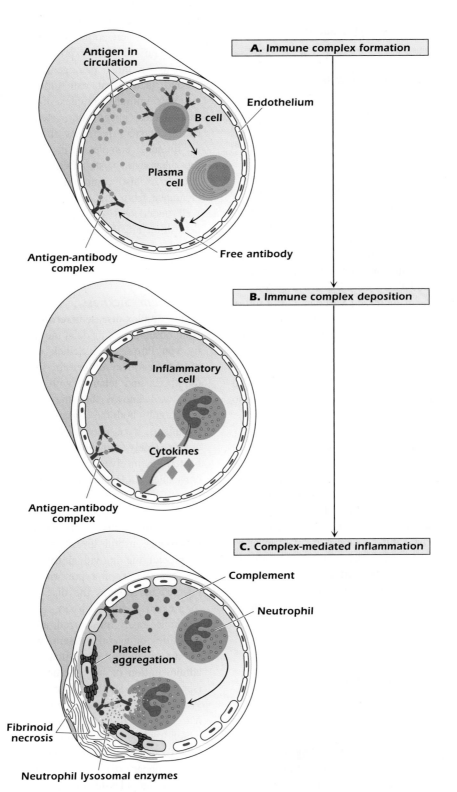

Figure 15.2. Three sequential phases in induction of systemic type III (immune complex) hypersensitivity: (A) immune complex formation; (B) immune complex deposition; (C) complex-mediated inflammation.

Infection-Associated Immune Complex Disease.
Perhaps the best example of infection-associated immune complex diseases is ***rheumatic fever***. In susceptible individuals, this disease is associated with infections (such as those of the throat) caused by ***group A streptococci*** and involves inflammation and damage to the heart, joints, and kidneys. A variety of antigens in the cell walls and membranes of streptococci have been shown to be cross-reactive with antigens present in human heart muscle, cartilage, and glomerular basement membrane. It is presumed that antibody to the streptococcal antigens binds to these components of normal tissue and induces inflammatory reactions via a pathway similar to that described above. The ensuing immune complexes participate in both the inflammation of joints and the damage characteristic of this disease.

In a variety of other infections, some individuals produce antibodies that cross-react with some constituent of normal tissue. For example, individuals predisposed to ***Goodpasture's syndrome*** (see Chapter 12) sometimes develop the disease following viral respiratory infections. The pulmonary hemorrhage and glomerulonephritis of Goodpasture's patients are caused by antibodies that bind directly to basement membrane in the lung and kidney, activate complement, and cause membrane damage through the accumulation of neutrophils and release of degradative enzymes. Goodpasture's syndrome is sometimes considered to be a type II hypersensitivity reaction, since it also involves an antibody-mediated cytotoxic effect on normal cells. The distinction between this infection-associated antibody-mediated disease and the immune complex disease of serum sickness is that microscopic examination of Goodpasture's lesions reveals a linear, ribbonlike deposit along the basement membrane (Fig. 15.3), as would be expected if an even carpet of antibody were bound to surface antigens. By contrast, in serum sickness the pileup of

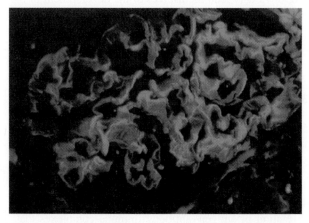

Figure 15.3. Ribbonlike deposit of antibody along basement membrane (associated with Goodpasture's syndrome) revealed by fluorescent antibodies to human Ig. (Courtesy of Dr. Angelo Ucci, Tufts University Medical School.)

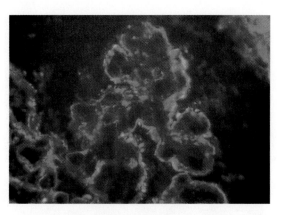

Figure 15.4. "Lumpy-bumpy" staining pattern of fluorescent antibody specific for human immunoglobulin: immune complex deposits in glomerular basement membrane associated with serum sickness. (Courtesy of Dr. Angelo Ucci, Tufts University School of Medicine.)

preformed immune complexes on the basement membrane leads to so-called lumpy-bumpy deposits (Fig. 15.4).

There may be times during the course of a number of other infectious diseases (such as malaria, leprosy, and dengue) when large amounts of antigen and antibody exist simultaneously and cause the formation and deposition of immune aggregates. Thus, the complex of symptoms in any of these diseases may include a component attributable to a type III hypersensitivity reaction.

Complement Deficiency. As noted above, most immune complexes do not cause damage because they are removed from circulation before they become lodged in the tissues. Complexes that contain C3b bind to erythrocytes bearing CR1. The erythrocytes deliver the complexes to mononuclear phagocytes within the liver and spleen for removal by phagocytosis. The components of the classical complement pathway reduce the number of antigen epitopes that antibodies can bind by intercalating into the lattice of the complex, resulting in smaller, soluble complexes. It is these smaller complexes that bind most readily to the erythrocytes. In patients with complement deficiencies affecting C1, C2, and C4 (see Chapter 13), the complexes remain large and bind poorly to the erythrocytes. These non-erythrocyte-bound complexes are taken up rapidly by the liver and then released to be deposited in tissues such as skin, kidney, and muscle, where they can cause inflammatory reactions.

Localized Immune Complex Disease

In 1903, a French scientist named Maurice Arthus immunized rabbits with horse serum by repeated intradermal injection. After several weeks, he noted that each succeeding injection produced an increasingly severe reaction at

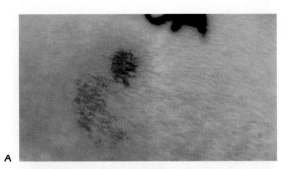

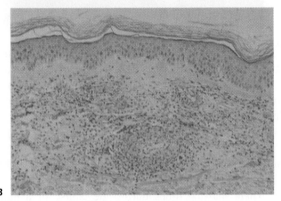

Figure 15.5. Type III hypersensitivity Arthus reaction: (A) gross appearance, showing hemorrhagic appearance (purpura); (B) histologic features of Arthus reaction showing neutrophil infiltrate. (Courtesy of Dr. M. Stadecker, Tufts University Medical School.)

the site of inoculation. At first, a mild erythema (redness) and edema (accumulation of fluid) were noticed within 24 h of injection. These reactions subsided without consequence by the following day, but subsequent injections produced larger edematous responses, and by the fifth or sixth inoculations the lesions became hemorrhagic with necrosis and were slow to heal. This phenomenon, known as the **Arthus reaction**, is the prototype of localized immune complex

reactions. As with systemic immune complex hypersensitivity reactions, localized reactions involve soluble antigens. The local inflammatory responses occur following reactivity of antigen with already formed, antigen-specific IgG antibody. When preformed antibodies come in contact with antigen at the appropriate concentrations (antibody excess) in or near vessel walls, insoluble immune complexes form and accumulate as they would on a gel diffusion plate (see Chapter 5). The subsequent pathophysiologic events are very similar to those described in the systemic pattern (see Fig. 15.2). The end result is rupture of the vessel wall and hemorrhage, accompanied by necrosis of local tissue (Figs. 15.5A,B).

A clinical example of Arthus-type hypersensitivity reactions is seen in a disease called *farmer's lung*. This is an intrapulmonary type III hypersensitivity reaction that occurs in patients with *extrinsic allergic alveolitis* (allergen-induced inflammation of the alveoli). As its name implies, farmer's lung sometimes occurs in individuals involved in farming; thus it is classified as an occupational disease. In sensitive individuals, exposure to moldy hay leads, within 6–8 h, to severe respiratory distress (pneumonitis). Affected individuals make large amounts of IgG antibody specific for the spores of thermophilic actinomycetes that grow on spoiled hay. Inhalation of the bacterial spores leads to a reaction in the lungs that resembles the Arthus reaction seen in skin, namely, the formation of antigen–antibody aggregates and consequent inflammation.

There are many similar pulmonary type III reactions that bear names related to the occupation or causative agent, such as pigeon breeder's disease, cheese washer's disease, bagassosis (bagasse is sugarcane fiber), maple bark stripper's disease, paprika worker's disease, and the increasingly rare thatched roof worker's lung. Dirty work environments, involving massive exposure to potentially antigenic material, obviously lend themselves to the development of these forms of occupational disease.

SUMMARY

1. Type II hypersensitivity reactions involve damage to target cells and are mediated by antibody through three major pathways. In the first pathway, antibody (usually IgM, but also IgG) activates the entire complement sequence and causes cell lysis.

2. In the second type II hypersensitivity pathway, antibody (usually IgG) engages receptors for Fc on phagocytic cells, and C3b engages receptors on phagocytic cells with C3b receptors, causing destruction of the antibody and/or C3b-coated target through ADCC. These reactions usually involve circulating blood cells, such as RBCs, WBCs, and platelets, and the consequences are those that would be expected from destruction of the particular type of cell.

3. The third type II hypersensitivity pathway leads to dysfunctional cellular consequences caused by the binding of disease-causing antagonistic or agonistic autoantibodies to cell surface receptors (such as occurs in myasthenia gravis or Graves disease, respectively).

4. Type III hypersensitivity reactions involve the formation of antigen–antibody immune complexes that can activate the complement cascade and induce acute inflammatory responses. Release of certain products of complement (C3a and C5a) causes a local increase in vessel permeability and permits the release of serum (edema) and the chemotactic attraction of neutrophils. In the process of ingesting

the immune complexes, the neutrophils release degradative lysosomal enzymes that produce the tissue damage characteristic of these reactions.

5. If the site of a type III reaction is a blood vessel wall, the outcome is hemorrhage and necrosis; if the site is a glomerular basement membrane, loss of integrity and release of protein and RBCs into the urine results; and if the site is a joint meniscus, destruction of synovial membranes and cartilage occurs.

6. Multiple forms of type III hypersensitivity reactions exist ranging from localized to systemic reactions. The reactions manifested depend on the type and location of antigen and the way in which it is brought together with antibody. In all cases, however, the outcome depends on complement and granulocytes as mediators of tissue injury.

REFERENCES

Carlson JA, Chen KR (2006): Cutaneous vasculitis update: Small vessel neutrophilic vasculitis syndromes. *Am J Dermatopathol* 28:486.

Chang S, Carr W (2007): Urticarial vasculitis. *Allergy Asthma Proc* 28(1):97.

Cuellar ML (2002): Drug-induced vasculitis. *Curr Rheumatol Rep* 4:55.

Dixon FJ, Cochrane CC, Theofilopoulus AN (1988): Immune complex injury. In Samter M, Talmage DW, Frank MM, Austen KF, Claman HN (eds): *Immunological Diseases*, 4th ed. Boston: Little, Brown.

Gorgani NN, Theofilopoulos AN (2007): Contribution of histidine-rich glycoprotein in clearance of immune complexes and apoptotic cells: Implications for ameliorating autoimmune diseases. *Autoimmunity* 40:260.

Nimmerjahn F, Ravetch JV (2006): Fc gamma receptors: Old friends and new family members. *Immunity* 24:19.

REVIEW QUESTIONS

For each question, choose the ONE BEST answer.

1. Which of the following most likely involves a reaction to a hapten as its etiologic cause?
   A) Goodpasture's syndrome following a viral respiratory infection
   B) hemolytic anemia following treatment with penicillin
   C) rheumatoid arthritis following a parasitic infection
   D) farmer's lung following exposure to moldy hay

2. In an experimental mouse model for the study of autoimmune hemolytic anemia, intravenous administration of a monoclonal IgA antibody specific for a RBC antigen did not cause anemia to occur. The best explanation for this observation is:
   A) The IgA would localize in the gastrointestinal tract.
   B) The Fc region of the IgA antibody does not bind receptors for Fc receptors on phagocytic cells.
   C) IgA cannot activate complement beyond the splitting of C2.
   D) The IgA used has a low affinity for the RBC antigen.
   E) The IgA used requires a secretory component to exert an effect.

3. The glomerular lesions in immune complex disease can be visualized microscopically with a fluorescent antibody against:
   A) IgG heavy chains
   B) κ light chains
   C) C1
   D) C3
   E) all of the above

4. Immune complexes are involved in the pathogenesis of which of the following rheumatic-fever-associated diseases?
   A) poststreptococcal glomerulonephritis
   B) pigeon breeder's disease
   C) serum sickness
   D) autoimmune hemolytic anemia
   E) pemphigus vulgaris

5. The final damage to vessels in immune-complex-mediated arthritis is due to:
   A) cytokines produced by T cells
   B) histamine and SRS-A
   C) the C5, C6, C7, C8, C9 membrane attack complex
   D) lysosomal enzymes of polymorphonuclear leukocytes
   E) cytotoxic T cells

6. Serum sickness is characterized by:
   A) deposition of immune complexes in blood vessel walls when there is a moderate excess of antigen
   B) phagocytosis of complexes by granulocytes
   C) consumption of complement

D) appearance of symptoms before free antibody can be detected in the circulation

E) all of the above

7. Type II hypersensitivity:
A) is antibody-independent
B) is complement-independent
C) is mediated by CD8$^+$ T cells
D) requires immune complex formation
E) involves antibody-mediated destruction of cells

8. A patient is suspected of having farmer's lung. A provocation test involving the inhalation of an extract of moldy hay is performed. A sharp drop in respiratory function is noted within 10 min and returns to normal in 2 h only to fall again in another 2 h. The most likely explanation is:

A) The patient has existing T-cell-mediated hypersensitivity.
B) This is a normal pattern for farmer's lung.
C) The patient developed a secondary response after the inhalation of antigen.
D) The symptoms of farmer's lung are complicated by an IgE-mediated reactivity to the same antigen.
E) All of the above.

ANSWERS TO REVIEW QUESTIONS

1. *B* Penicillin can function as a hapten, binding to red blood cells and inducing a hemolytic anemia. A, C, and D are examples of immune aggregate (type III) reactions requiring complement and neutrophils for pathologic effects.

2. *B* Since phagocytic cells have Fc receptors for IgG, bound IgA would not cause engulfment and damage. Thus, A, C, D, and E are false.

3. *E* The lesions in immune complex disease are dependent on the presence of antigen, antibody, and complement. Hence all can be demonstrated by immunofluorescence at a lesion: A and B, because they are parts of IgG; C and D, because they are the early components of complement activated by the immune aggregates.

4. *A* Rheumatic fever is a disease associated with infections caused by group A streptococci. It involves the development of antistreptococci antibodies that are cross-reactive with antigens present in human heart muscle, cartilage, and glomerular basement membrane.

5. *D* Neither T cells nor mast cells are responsible for the final tissue damage in immune complex disease. Therefore A, B, and E can be eliminated. The final lytic complex of complement is similarly not involved, since complement activation up to C5 is sufficient to bring in the polymorphonuclear leukocytes, whose lysosomal enzymes cause the tissue damage.

6. *E* All are characteristics of serum sickness.

7. *E* Type II hypersensitivity reactions occur following development of antibodies against target antigens expressed on normal cells or cells with altered membrane determinants. Antibodies bind to the surface of these cells and mediate damage or destruction by one or more mechanisms, including complement-mediated reactions. CD8$^+$ cytotoxic T cells and immune complexes are not involved in these reactions.

8. *D* The onset of symptoms in type III hypersensitivity reactions in farmer's lung and similar occupational diseases usually occurs several hours after exposure to the causal antigen. The appearance of breathing difficulties within minutes would create a strong suspicion that a type I anaphylactic response is also present. Presumably the patient made both IgE and IgG antibodies to the actinomycete antigens. A positive wheal-and-flare reaction on skin testing would provide further confirmation.

16

HYPERSENSITIVITY: TYPE IV

INTRODUCTION

In contrast to the antibody-mediated hypersensitivity reactions discussed in the previous two chapters, *type IV hypersensitivity* is cell mediated. In marked contrast with type I hypersensitivity (mediated by IgE), which is immediately available to react with allergens, type IV responses involve the activation, proliferation, and mobilization of antigen-specific T cells. Because of the delay in the immune response compared to antibody-mediated hypersensitivity reactions, type IV hypersensitivity is often referred to as *delayed-type hypersensitivity (DTH)*. Like antibody-mediated hypersensitivity, DTH reactions can result in damage to host cells and tissues. The harmful effects of DTH are caused by the release of inappropriately large amounts of cytokines (including chemokines) by activated T cells. Chemokines attract and activate other mononuclear cells that are not antigen specific, including monocytes and macrophages. It is the recruitment and activation of these antigen-nonspecific cells that bears primary responsibility for the deleterious outcome of type IV hypersensitivity reactions.

Depending on the antigen involved, DTH reactions mediate aspects of immune function that can be either beneficial (resistance to viruses, bacteria, fungi, and tumors) or harmful (allergic dermatitis, autoimmunity). Other antigens capable of eliciting DTH reactions include those expressed by foreign cells in transplantation settings or one of many chemicals (serving as haptens) capable of penetrating skin and coupling to body protein carriers.

Cutaneous DTH reactions are initiated when CD4 memory T cells are activated by Langerhans cells and other APC in the skin. Upon activation, CD4 T cells release inflammatory mediators, which recruit effector cells to the site of antigen administration. While the monocyte/macrophage is thought to be the major effector cell in this model, $CD8^+$ cytolytic T cells and NK cells are also thought to serve this function. Activated effector cells mount an inflammatory response that results in the elimination of antigen and the extravasation of plasma accompanied by swelling at the site of challenge. The magnitude of the response to the antigen is measured as an increase in swelling at the site of challenge (such as that seen during the development of a tuberculin skin reaction).

GENERAL CHARACTERISTICS AND PATHOPHYSIOLOGY OF DTH

The clinical features of type IV hypersensitivity reactions vary, depending on the sensitizing antigen and the route of antigen exposure. These variations include contact hypersensitivity, tuberculin-type hypersensitivity, and granulomatous hypersensitivity (see next section). In general, however, a common pathophysiologic mechanism accounts for each of these variations. The major events involve three steps: (1) activation of antigen-specific inflammatory T_H1 and T_H17 cells in a previously sensitized individual; (2) elaboration of proinflammatory cytokines by antigen-specific T_H1 and T_H17 cells; and (3) recruitment

Immunology: A Short Course, Sixth Edition, By Richard Coico and Geoffrey Sunshine
Copyright © 2009 John Wiley & Sons, Inc.

and activation of antigen-nonspecific inflammatory leuko-cytes. These events typically occur over a period of several days (48–72 h).

Mechanisms Involved in DTH

The mechanisms involved in the sensitization to DTH and the elucidation of the reaction following antigenic challenge are now quite well understood. As in antibody-mediated hypersensitivity reactions, previous exposure to the antigen is required to generate DTH. Such exposure (the *sensitization stage*; Fig. 16.1A) activates and expands the number of antigen-specific T_H1 and T_H17 cells; when subsequently challenged with the same antigen, this increased population of cells responds by producing cytokines that promote DTH reactions (the *elicitation stage*; Fig. 16.1B). During the elicitation phase, activated T_H1 and T_H17 T cells mediate the activation and recruit-ment of antigen-nonspecific inflammatory cells to the area of the reaction, including macrophages, NK cells, cytotoxic $CD8^+$ T cells, neutrophils, and B cells. The sensitization stage typically occurs over one to two weeks, during which normal mechanisms of T cell activation occur (see Chapter 10). In contrast, the elicitation stage requires approximately

18–48 h from the time of antigenic challenge to recruit and activate these cells—a period that culminates in the histologic and clinical features of DTH. The clinical manifestations of DTH can last for several weeks or, in some cases, can be chronic (e.g., DTH occurring in certain autoimmune diseases such as myasthenia gravis).

The antigen-challenged T cells produce several cytokines during the elicitation stage, most notably chemokines and IFN-γ, which cause chemotaxis and activation of macrophages (Fig. 16.2). The recruitment and activation of antigen-nonspecific cells by antigen-specific T_H1 and T_H17 cells demonstrate the interaction between acquired and innate immunity discussed in Chapter 2. Another cytokine produced by these cells is IL-12. IL-12 suppresses the T_H2 subpopulation and promotes the expansion of the T_H1 and T_H17 subpopulations, thereby driving the production of more and cytokines that in turn activate more macrophages. Thus, IL-12 plays an important role in DTH. Table 16.1 summarizes the important cytokines involved in DTH reactions.

DTH reactions also involve $CD8^+$ T cells, which are first activated and expanded during the sensitization stage of the response. These cells can damage tissues by cell-mediated cytotoxicity (see Chapter 10). Activation

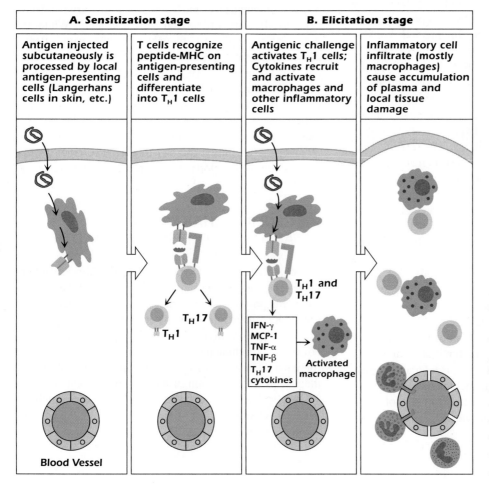

Figure 16.1. DTH reaction. (A) Stage of sensitization by antigen involves presentation of antigen to T cells by APC, leading to the release of cytokines and differentiation of T_H0 T cells to T_H1 and T_H17 cells. (B) Challenge with antigen (the elicita-tion stage) involves antigen presen-tation to T_H1 cells by APC, leading to T_H1 and T_H17 activation, release of cytokines, and recruitment and activation of macrophages.

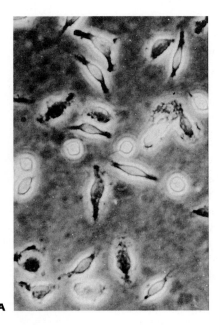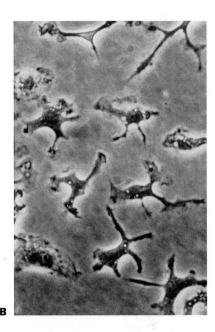

 Figure 16.2. Effect of IFN-γ on peritoneal macrophages. (A) Normal macrophages in culture as they are just beginning to adhere. (B) Macrophages that after activation with IFN-γ have adhered, spread out with development of numerous pseudopodia, and grow larger. More lysosomal granules are also visible. (Courtesy of Dr. M. Stadecker, Tufts University Medical School.)

A   **B**

TABLE 16.1. Cytokines Involved in DTH Reactions

Cytokine[a]	Functional Effects[b]
IFN-γ	Activates macrophages to release inflammatory mediators
Chemokines MCP-1 RANTES MIP-1α MIP-1β	Recruit macrophages and monocytes to the site
TNFα	Causes local tissue damage
TNFβ	Increases expression of adhesion molecules on blood vessels

[a]MCP, membrane cofactor protein; MIP, macrophage inflammatory protein; TNF, tumor necrosis factor.
[b]Additional functional effects are described in Chapter 11.

of CD8$^+$ T cells occurs as a consequence of the ability of many chemicals capable of inducing DTH reactions to cross the cell membrane (such as pentadecacatechol, the chemical that induces *poison ivy*). Within the cell, these chemicals react with cytosolic proteins to generate modified peptides; these peptides are translocated to the endoplasmic reticulum and delivered to the cell surface in the context of class I MHC molecules. Cells presenting such modified self-proteins are subsequently damaged or killed by CD8$^+$ T cells.

It should be obvious from the preceding discussion that many of the effector functions in DTH are performed by activated macrophages. In the most favorable circumstances, DTH results in destruction of an infectious organism (see below) that may have elicited the response in the first place. This destruction is believed to result predominantly from ingestion of the organism by macrophages. Given the involvement of T_H1 and T_H17 cells, the cellular reactions occur within a cytokine milieu containing IFN-γ, which further activates the phagocytes. The phagocytized infectious agent is then degraded by lysosomal enzymes and by-products of the burst of respiratory activity such as peroxide and superoxide radicals. Foreign tissues, tumor tissue, and soluble or conjugated antigens are dealt with in a similar manner.

EXAMPLES OF DTH

Contact Sensitivity

Contact sensitivity (sometimes called *contact dermatitis*) is a form of DTH in which the target organ is the skin and the inflammatory response is produced as the result of contact with sensitizing substances on its surface. Thus, it is primarily an epidermal reaction characterized by eczema at the site of contact with the allergen, which typically peaks 48–72 h after contact. The prototype for this form of DTH is *poison ivy dermatitis* (Fig. 16.3A). The offending substance is contained in an oil secreted by the leaves of the poison ivy vine and other related plants. These oils contain a mixture of catechols (dihydroxyphenols) with long hydrocarbon side chains. These features allow it to penetrate the skin by virtue of its lipophilicity (allowing it to dissolve in skin oils) and its ability to couple covalently (by formation of quinones) to some carrier molecules on cell surfaces. Other contact sensitizers are generally also lipid-soluble haptens. They have a variety of chemical forms, but all have in common the ability to penetrate skin and form hapten carrier conjugates. Chemicals such as 2,4-dinitrochlorobenzene (DNCB) are used to induce contact sensitivity. Since virtually every normal individual is capable of developing contact hypersensitivity to a test dose of this compound, it is frequently used to assess a patient's potential for T cell reactivity (cell-mediated immunity). Metals such as nickel and chromium, which are present in some jewelry and clasps of undergarments, are also capable of inducing contact sensitivity, presumably by way of chelation (ionic interaction) by skin proteins.

Contact sensitivity is initiated by presentation of the offending allergen by APC in the skin (*Langerhans cells*) to T cells expressing antigen-specific TCRs. It is not yet known whether the sensitizer couples directly to components on the cell surface of the Langerhans cell or couples first to proteins in serum or tissue that are then taken up by the Langerhans cells. The initial contact results in expansion of antigen-specific clones of T_H1 cells. Subsequent contact (challenge) with the sensitizing antigen triggers the elicitation stage of DTH discussed earlier. The histologic appearance of this variant of DTH shows mononuclear infiltrates in the dermis (Fig. 16.3B) that manifest as the separation of epidermal cells, *spongiosis* (an inflammatory intercellular edema of the epidermis), and blister formation (Fig. 16.3A).

In many cases, enough of the sensitizing antigen remains at the site of the initial contact so that in approximately one week, when sufficient T cell expansion has taken place, the remaining antigen serves as the challenging antigen, causing the elicitation phase to occur without new contact with the sensitizing antigen.

The commonly performed procedure for testing for the presence of contact sensitivity is the *patch test*. A solution of the suspected antigen is spread on the skin and covered by an occlusive dressing. The appearance, within three days, of an area of *induration* (raised thickening) and *erythema* (redness) indicates sensitivity.

Granulomatous Hypersensitivity

Unlike DTH associated with most contact dermatitis reactions, in which the antigen is readily eliminated, lesions resulting from *granulomatous hypersensitivity* resolve slowly and result in little tissue damage. In some circumstances, the antigen may persistent as a chronic source of immune stimulation. For example, schistosomal eggs and lipid-encapsulated mycobacteria are resistant to enzymatic degradation and therefore can be present for prolonged periods of time (lifelong, in some cases). Under these circumstances, continuous accumulation of macrophages leads to clusters of epithelioid cells, which fuse to form giant cells in *granulomas*. The maximal reaction time for the development of a granuloma is 21–28 days. The pathological changes result from the inability of macrophages to destroy phagocytized pathogens (e.g., *Mycobacterium leprae*) or to degrade large inert antigens. Granulomas can be destructive because of their displacement of normal tissue and can

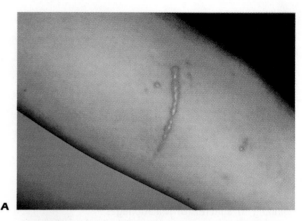

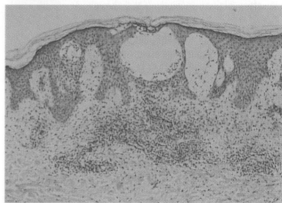

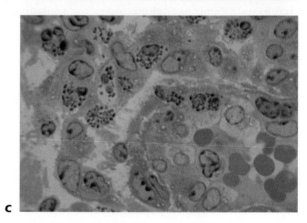

Figure 16.3. (A) Type IV contact sensitivity reaction gross appearance of reaction to poison ivy. (B) Type IV contact hypersensitivity reaction histologic appearance showing intraepithelial blister formation and mononuclear infiltrate in dermis. (C) Cutaneous basophil reaction showing basophils and some mononuclear cells 24 h after skin test. (Courtesy of Dr. M. Stadecker, Tufts University Medical School.)

result in caseous (cheesy) necrosis. This is typical in such diseases as tuberculosis caused by infection with *Mycobacterium tuberculosis*, in which a cuff of lymphocytes surrounds the core and may cause considerable fibrosis.

Granulomatous hypersensitivity may thus be attributable more to the persistent attempts of the host to isolate and contain the pathogen than to the effects of the invading organisms. In diseases such as smallpox, measles, and herpes, the characteristic *exanthems* (skin rashes) are partly attributable to DTH responses to the virus, with additional destruction attributable to the attack by cytotoxic $CD8^+$ T cells against the virally infected epithelial cells.

Tuberculin-Type Hypersensitivity

Tuberculin-type reactions are *cutaneous inflammatory reactions* characterized by an area of firm red swelling of the skin that is maximal at 48–72 h after challenge. The term tuberculin-type is derived from the prototype DTH reaction in which a lipoprotein antigen called tuberculin, isolated from *M. tuberculosis*, was used to test for evidence of exposure to the causative agent of tuberculosis (TB). However, note that soluble antigens from other organisms, including *M. leprae* and *Leishmania tropica*, may also induce tuberculin-type DTH reactions. Today, TB tests are performed by intradermally injecting a more purified lipoprotein extract isolated from *M. tuberculosis* called *purified protein derivative* (*PPD*). The PPD test (also called the Mantoux test) is extremely useful for public health surveillance of TB. If an individual has been previously sensitized to antigens expressed by *M. tuberculosis* as a consequence of infection with this organism, the characteristic tuberculin-type lesion will appear at the site of injection within 48–72 h. Evidence of erythema and induration appears, reaching maximal levels 72 h after the challenge (see Fig. 16.4A). The induration can easily be distinguished from *edema* (fluid accumulation) by absence of pitting when pressure is applied. Even when they are severe, these reactions rarely lead to necrotic damage and resolve slowly. A biopsy taken early in the reaction reveals primarily mononuclear cells of the monocyte/macrophage series with a few scattered lymphocytes. Characteristically, the mononuclear infiltrates appear as a perivascular cuff before extensively invading the site of deposition of antigen (see Fig. 16.4B). Neutrophils are not a prominent feature of the initial reaction. In more severe cases, tuberculin-type hypersensitivity reactions may progress toward granulomatous hypersensitivity (discussed above). Biopsies of tissue in which this occurs show a more complex pattern, with the arrival of B cells and the formation of granulomas in persistent lesions. The hardness or induration is attributable to the deposition of fibrin in the lesion.

While the PPD test is usually very reliable, false-negative or false-positive reactions may be seen in some situations. Immunosuppressed individuals (such as those infected with human immunodeficiency virus and some individuals on high-dose chemotherapy) may have false-negative PPD reactions due to the inability of antigen-specific T cells to respond (anergy; see Chapter 12).

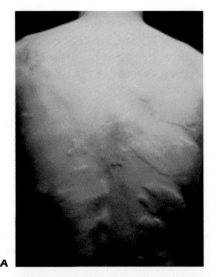

A

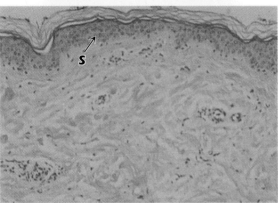

B

Figure 16.4. (A) Type IV DTH reaction (tuberculin reaction)—gross appearance showing induration and erythema 48 h after tuberculin test. (Courtesy of A. Gottlieb, Tulane University Medical School.) (B) Type IV DTH reaction—histologic picture showing dermal mononuclear cell infiltrate (*arrow*). (Courtesy of M. Stadecker, Tufts University Medical School.)

When PPD is used to test individuals for exposure to *M. tuberculosis*, those who have been vaccinated with a nonpathogenic attenuated strain of the organism that causes TB in cattle (the *Mycobacterium bovis* or BCG) may also generate false-positive reactions. The efficacy of the BCG vaccine against human pulmonary TB varies enormously in different populations. The prevailing hypothesis attributes this variation to interactions between the vaccine and the mycobacteria common in the environment, but the precise mechanism has not yet been elucidated. Routine BCG vaccination is not performed in many countries, including the United States, because of its questionable efficacy and the impact such a practice would have on our ability to confirm whether individuals have been exposed to *M. tuberculosis*.

Allograft Rejection

As you will learn in more detail in Chapter 18, if an individual receives a graft of cells, tissues, or organs taken from an *allogeneic donor* (a genetically different individual of the same species), it will usually become vascularized and be accepted initially. However, if the genetic differences are within the MHC, T cell-mediated rejection of the graft ensues, with a duration and intensity related to the degree of incompatibility between donor and recipient. After vascularization, there is an initial invasion of the graft by a mixed population of antigen-specific T cells and antigen-nonspecific monocytes through the blood vessel walls. This inflammatory reaction soon leads to destruction of the vessels; this deprivation of nutrients is quickly followed by necrosis and breakdown of the grafted tissue.

Additional Examples of DTH

An unusual form of DTH has been observed in humans following repeated intradermal injections of antigen. The response is delayed in onset (usually by about 24 h) but consists entirely of erythema, without the induration typical of classic delayed-hypersensitivity reactions. When this condition was studied experimentally, it was found that the erythema was attended by a cellular infiltrate but that the predominant cell type was the basophil (Fig. 16.3C). Studies in guinea pigs showed that the response was primarily mediated by T cells and was subject to the same MHC restrictions as classic T cell-mediated responses. When classic delayed hypersensitivity was present, however, infiltrates of basophils were not seen. Thus, cutaneous basophil hypersensitivity seemed to be a variant of T cell-mediated responses, but its exact mechanism was unknown. The picture was complicated still further when it was shown that passive transfer of serum could, under some circumstances, evoke a basophil response.

The physiologic significance of cutaneous basophil hypersensitivity remained a mystery until it was shown that guinea pigs bitten by certain ticks had severe cutaneous basophil hypersensitivity reactions at the site of attachment of the tick. The infiltration of basophils and, presumably, the release of inflammatory mediators from their granules resulted in death of the tick and its eventual detachment. Thus, cutaneous basophil hypersensitivity may have an important role in certain forms of immunity to parasites. More recently, basophil infiltrates have also been found in contact dermatitis with allergens such as poison ivy, rejection of renal grafts, and some forms of conjunctivitis. All of these observations indicate that basophils may play a role in some types of delayed hypersensitivity disease.

Other examples of DTH include reactions to self-antigens in certain autoimmune diseases, such as myasthenia gravis, rheumatoid arthritis, type I diabetes, and multiple sclerosis (see Chapter 12). Like the persistent infections that can cause chronic DTH reactions, these reactions are often chronic as a result of the continuous clonal activation of autoreactive T_H1 cells.

● TREATMENT OF DTH

Therapies to treat T cell-mediated hypersensitivity vary in accordance with the variant of DTH involved. In most cases, DTH reactions such as contact dermatitis and tuberculin-type reactions resolve after a period of days to weeks following removal of the antigen. Corticosteroids, applied either topically or systemically, constitute a very effective treatment for these forms of DTH. In more severe variants of DTH, such as pathogen-induced granulomatous hypersensitivity, allograft rejection, and those seen in certain autoimmune diseases, more aggressive forms of immunosuppressive therapy are commonly used, including drug treatment with cyclosporine or topical calcineurin inhibitors (such as tacrolimus; see Chapter 18 for additional discussion of immunosuppressive therapies).

SUMMARY

1. The normal events associated with cell-mediated immunity that are crucial for protection against intracellular parasites such as viruses, many bacteria, and fungi can also cause DTH reactions.

2. The major events leading to DTH reactions involve three steps: (a) activation of antigen-specific inflammatory T_H1 and T_H17 cells in a previously sensitized individual; (b) elaboration of proinflammatory cytokines (e.g., IFN-γ) and T_H17 family cytokines by the antigen-specific T_H1 and T_H17 cells, respectively; and (c) recruitment and activation of antigen-nonspecific inflammatory leukocytes.

3. There are several varieties of DTH, including (a) contact hypersensitivity characterized by eczema which peaks 48–72 h after allergen contact; (b) granulomatous hypersensitivity characterized by a granuloma, which is maximal 21–28 days after antigen is introduced; and (c) tuberculin-type hypersensitivity characterized by an area of firm red erythema (redness) and induration (raised thickening) that is maximal 48–72 h after challenge.

4. Other variants include reactions occurring in certain T-cell-mediated autoimmune diseases (e.g., myasthenia gravis, rheumatoid arthritis, type I diabetes,

5. Cytotoxic CD8$^+$ T cells can also participate in the damage associated with DTH reactions.

6. Phagocytic macrophages are the major histologic feature of DTH and account for the protective outcome of this form of hypersensitivity when pathogens are involved.

and multiple sclerosis) and in some individuals who have received allografts.

7. When macrophages are unable to destroy a pathogen, a granuloma is induced (granulomatous hypersensitivity). Granulomas can also develop following phagocytosis of inert substances. Granulomas are characterized histologically by the presence of macrophages, epithelioid cells, giant cells, and CD4 and CD8 lymphocytes.

REFERENCES

Brandt L, Feino CJ, Weinreich OA, Chilima B, Hirsch P, Appelberg R, Andersen P (2002): Failure of the *Mycobacterium bovis* BCG vaccine: Some species of environmental mycobacteria block multiplication of BCG and induction of protective immunity to tuberculosis. *Infect Immun* 70:672.

Burger D, Dayer JM (2002): Cytokines, acute-phase proteins, and hormones: IL-1 and TNF-alpha production in contact-mediated activation of monocytes by T lymphocytes. *Ann NY Acad Sci* 966:464.

Fyhrquist-Vanni N, Alenius H, Lauerma A (2007): Contact dermatitis. *Dermatol Clin* 25:613.

Posadas SJ, Pichler WJ (2007): Delayed drug hypersensitivity reactions—New concepts. *Clin Exp Allergy* 37:989.

Romano A, Demoly P (2007): Recent advances in the diagnosis of drug allergy. *Curr Opin Allergy Clin Immunol* 7:299.

Sicherer SH, Leung DY (2007): Advances in allergic skin disease, anaphylaxis, and hypersensitivity reactions to foods, drugs, and insects. *J Allergy Clin Immunol* 119:1462.

Vukmanovic-Stejic M, Reed JR, Lacy KE, Rustin MH, Akbar AN (2006): Mantoux Test as a model for a secondary immune response in humans. *Immunol Lett* 107:93.

Wollina U (2007): The role of topical calcineurin inhibitors for skin diseases other than atopic dermatitis. *Am J Clin Dermatol* 8:157.

REVIEW QUESTIONS

For each question, choose the ONE BEST answer.

1. Which of the following does not involve cell-mediated immunity?
   A) contact sensitivity to lipstick
   B) rejection of an allograft
   C) serum sickness
   D) the Mantoux test
   E) immunity to chicken pox

2. A positive delayed-type hypersensitivity skin reaction involves the interaction of:
   A) antigen, complement, and cytokines
   B) antigen, antigen-sensitive T cells, and macrophages
   C) antigen–antibody complexes, complement, and neutrophils
   D) IgE antibody, antigen, and mast cells
   E) antigen, macrophages, and complement

3. Delayed skin reactions to an intradermal injection of antigen may be markedly decreased by:
   A) exposure to a high dose of X irradiation
   B) treatment with antihistamines
   C) treatment with an antineutrophil serum
   D) removal of the spleen
   E) decreasing levels of complement

4. Which of the following statements is characteristic of contact sensitivity?
   A) The best therapy is oral administration of the antigen.
   B) Patch testing with the allergen is useless for diagnosis.
   C) Sensitization can be passively transferred with serum from an allergic individual.
   D) Some chemicals acting as haptens induce sensitivity by covalently binding to host proteins acting as carriers.
   E) Antihistamines constitute the treatment of choice.

5. Positive skin tests for delayed-type hypersensitivity to intradermally injected antigens indicate:
   A) A humoral immune response has occurred.
   B) A cell-mediated immune response has occurred.
   C) Both T- and B-cell systems are functional.
   D) The individual has previously made IgE responses to the antigen.
   E) Immune complexes have been formed at the injection site.

6. T-cell-mediated immune responses can result in:
   A) formation of granulomas
   B) induration at the reaction site
   C) rejection of a heart transplant

D) eczema of the skin in the area of prolonged contact with a rubberized undergarment

E) all of the above

7. Which one of the following statements about the PPD skin test is true?

A) It is specific for *Mycobacterium tuberculosis*.

B) It can be positive in an individual who was previously immunized with BCG.

C) It does not distinguish between present and past tuberculosis infections.

D) Induration can vary, so a positive test depends upon the underlying immune status of the patient tested.

E) B, C and D are all true.

ANSWERS TO REVIEW QUESTIONS

1. *C* Serum sickness is mediated by an antibody–antigen complex that involves components of the complement system and neutrophils. All other answers involve cell-mediated immunity to a significant extent.

2. *B* Cell-mediated reactions result from the triggering of T cells by antigen with recruitment of macrophages. Antibody, complement, and mast cells do not play roles in this process, although they do play a role in immediate hypersensitivity responses.

3. *A* High doses of X irradiation will destroy T cells, which are responsible for initiating the response. Histamine, neutrophils, the spleen, and complement do not play a role, and any treatment that affects them would not affect a DTH response.

4. *D* The allergens involved are those capable of penetrating skin and binding to host carrier proteins; thus D is correct. In certain experimental situations, oral ingestion of antigen was shown to induce suppression after subsequent induction of contact sensitivity, but it has not yet been shown to be an effective therapeutic maneuver in humans; thus A is wrong. B is wrong because patch testing consists of application of the offending allergen under an occlusive dressing, and a positive DTH response after 24–48 h is considered evidence of sensitivity. Passive transfer of

cell-mediated immune responses is accomplished with T cells, not serum; thus C is wrong. Corticosteroids, not antihistamines, constitute the treatment of choice for contact sensitivity, so E is also incorrect.

5. *B* A delayed-type hypersensitivity reaction, evidenced by erythema and induration within 24–72 h of antigen injection, indicates that a cell-mediated reaction has occurred. Such reactions do not involve antibody produced by B cells, so A, C, D, and E are all incorrect.

6. *E* All of these effects are manifestations of cell-mediated immunity. Formation of granulomas is characteristic of a chronic DTH reaction. Induration usually takes place at the reaction site. Rejection of the heart is an example of an allograft response. Some of the chemicals used to cure rubber can induce contact sensitivity reactions such as eczema after prolonged skin exposure.

7. *E* Each of the statements except for statement A are true. Positive PPD tests occur in immunocompetent individuals who have been infected with *M. tuberculosis*. However, positive reactions to PPD tests will also occur in individuals previously vaccinated with *Mycobacterium bovis*, also known as BCG.

17

IMMUNODEFICIENCY DISORDERS AND NEOPLASIAS OF THE LYMPHOID SYSTEM

Contributed by SUSAN R.S. GOTTESMAN

INTRODUCTION

At first glance, the connection between immunodeficiency syndromes and neoplasias of the lymphoid system is not apparent: Immunodeficiency syndromes are characterized by *absences* or deficiencies, whereas neoplasias reflect *excesses* or uncontrolled proliferations. So why are they discussed in the same chapter? The relationship between these two types of immune system disorders demonstrates the fine tuning and integration of the elements of the immune system. Deficiencies, particularly in a single arm of the immune system, affect the ability of the remaining elements to control their growth. For this reason, immunodeficiencies are fertile ground for the development of neoplasia. Because autoimmune phenomena are further manifestations of the loss of immune regulation that frequently accompany immunodeficiency, three seemingly disparate disease states—immunodeficiency, autoimmunity, and lymphoid neoplasia—often coexist in a single individual. Primary autoimmune diseases were discussed in Chapter 12; autoimmune reactions resulting from immunodeficiency or leading to lymphoid malignancy will be highlighted throughout this chapter.

As you have learned in previous chapters, the immune response is mediated by T and B lymphocytes, NK cells, myeloid/monocytic lineage cells, dendritic cells, and complement. The interactions among these cells, their soluble mediators (antibodies and cytokines), and complement are tightly controlled. Disorders in the development and differentiation of the cells, synthesis of their products, or interactions among them may lead to immune deficiencies with clinical severities ranging from mild to fatal. However, clinical consequences of deficiencies in which the immune system shows **redundancy** (overlap in the functions of one component with another) are noticeably absent. For example, parts of the cytokine network normally exhibit redundancy and rarely come to medical attention.

Although inborn immunodeficiency diseases (conditions present at birth) are generally rare, early descriptions of these "experiments of nature" shed light on the functioning of the immune system. Animal models that mimicked different types of human immunodeficiencies illuminated the cellular subdivisions of specific immunity into T and B lymphocytes—that is, cell-mediated versus humoral immunity. Today, information gained from analyzing these rare immunodeficiency syndromes and lymphoid neoplasms at the molecular level is applied to their treatment and to the development of immunotherapies for autoimmune diseases and lymphoid and nonlymphoid malignancies. The chapter begins with descriptions of inborn and acquired immunodeficiency syndromes and concludes with neoplasias of the immune system.

IMMUNODEFICIENCY SYNDROMES

Immunodeficiencies are divided into two major categories: in *primary immunodeficiencies*, which may be hereditary or acquired, the deficiency is the cause of disease; in *secondary immunodeficiencies* the immune deficiency is a result of other diseases or conditions.

Primary immunodeficiencies can be categorized on the basis of clinical presentation. These categories correspond roughly to the arm of the immune system that is malfunctioning: (1) T- or cell-mediated immunity; (2) B- or antibody-mediated immunity; (3) both B- and T-cell immunity; (4) nonspecific immunity mediated by phagocytic cells and/or NK cells; and (5) complement activation. Abnormalities of cytokine, chemokines, and their receptors do not form a separate category but are incorporated into groups 1–4 since they are the means used by cells to communicate and function.

An expressed immune response is often the result of interactions among several cell types; for example, a deficiency of antibody production and B-cell function may actually be caused by an underlying problem in T cells or in T–B-cell interaction. Classification based on the apparent *expressed* defect, rather than its underlying cause (which may be unknown), is a useful framework for diagnosing new patients. This method of classification also allows correlation with animal models in which the fundamental immune defect may be more readily identified.

Immunodeficiency should always be suspected in a patient with recurrent infections. As shown in Table 17.1, the types of infection can often facilitate diagnosis of the underlying problem. For example, recurrent bacterial otitis media (ear infection) and bacterial pneumonia are common in individuals with B-cell and antibody deficiency. Increased susceptibility to fungal, protozoan, and viral infections is seen with T-cell and cell-mediated immunodeficiencies. Systemic infections with bacteria that are normally of low virulence, superficial skin infections, or infections with *pyogenic* (pus-producing) organisms suggest deficiencies in phagocytic cells. Recurrent infections with pyogenic microorganisms are associated with complement deficiencies. Of particular significance is the occurrence of *opportunistic infections*, diseases caused by microorganisms present in the environment that are nonpathogenic in immunocompetent individuals. *Pneumocystis jiroveci*, cytomegalovirus (CMV), *Toxoplasma gondii, Mycobacterium avium*, and *Candida* are among the most common culprits in opportunistic infections associated with deficiencies in cell-mediated immunity.

Primary Immunodeficiency Syndromes

With the exception of IgA deficiency (discussed later in this chapter), the frequency of primary immunodeficiency syndromes is very low—about 1 in 10,000. Approximately 50% of all cases are antibody deficiencies, 20% are combined deficiencies in antibody- and cell-mediated immunity, 18% are phagocytic disorders, 10% are disorders of cell-mediated immunity alone, and 2% are complement deficiencies. Figure 17.1 shows that, in general, the earlier the genetic defect or block occurs in development, the more arms of the immune system are affected and the more severe the disease.

 TABLE 17.1. Major Clinical Manifestations of Immune Disorders

Disorder	Associated Diseases
Deficiency	
B-lymphocyte deficiency—deficiency in antibody-mediated immunity	Recurrent bacterial infections such as otitis media and recurrent pneumonia
T-lymphocyte deficiency—deficiency in cell-mediated immunity	Increased susceptibility to viral, fungal, and protozoal infections
T- and B-lymphocyte deficiency—combined deficiency of antibody and cell-mediated immunity	Acute and chronic infections with viral, bacterial, fungal, and protozoal organisms
Phagocytic cell deficiency	Systemic infections with bacteria of usually low virulence; infections with pyogenic bacteria; impaired pus formation and wound healing
NK cell deficiency	Viral infections, associated with several T-cell disorders and X-linked lymphoproliferative syndromes
Complement component deficiency	Bacterial infections; autoimmunity
Unregulated Excess	
B lymphocytes	Monoclonal gammopathies; other B-cell malignancies; lymphoproliferative syndromes
T lymphocytes	T-cell malignancies; autoimmune lymphoproliferations
Complement components	Angioedema due to defect in Cl esterase inhibitor

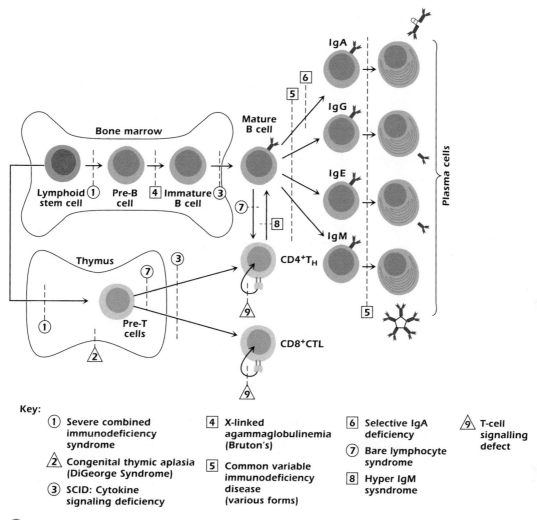

Key:
- ① Severe combined immunodeficiency syndrome
- ⚠2 Congenital thymic aplasia (DiGeorge Syndrome)
- ③ SCID: Cytokine signaling deficiency
- 4 X-linked agammaglobulinemia (Bruton's)
- 5 Common variable immunodeficiency disease (various forms)
- 6 Selective IgA deficiency
- 7 Bare lymphocyte syndrome
- 8 Hyper IgM sysndrome
- ⚠9 T-cell signalling defect

⬤ Figure 17.1. Sites of defective lymphopoietic development associated with primary immunodeficiency syndromes. (*Circles*) Lesions presenting as combined immunodeficiencies; (*triangles*) lesions presenting as T-cell disorders; (*squares*) lesions presenting as predominantly B-cell or humoral immune deficiencies.

Severe Combined Immunodeficiency Diseases.
Originally called Swiss-type agammaglobulinemia, SCID comprises a heterogeneous group of diseases in which both cell-mediated immunity and antibody production are defective (see Figure 17.1). Individuals with SCID are susceptible to virtually every type of microbial infection (viral, bacterial, fungal, and protozoal), most notably CMV, *P. jiroveci*, and *Candida*. Vaccination with attenuated live virus could prove fatal in infants with SCID.

Severe Combined Immunodeficiency Disease

Patients can be subclassified at initial evaluation according to the lymphocyte subsets present in their blood (Table 17.2). One group, designated as T⁻B⁺, has essentially absent T cells and normal or increased numbers of nonfunctioning B cells. This group of patients may also lack NK cells. A second group, T⁻B⁻, has severe lymphopenia due to the absence of both T and B cells. A few patients are T⁺B⁺, and rare patients are T⁺B⁻. The preferred treatment for all SCID patients is a T-cell-depleted bone marrow transplant from an HLA-matched sibling donor.

T⁻B⁺ Subgroup
X-LINKED SCID. Patients with X-linked SCID constitute 40–50% of SCID cases, with the majority of those showing T⁻B⁺ lymphopenia and lacking NK cells. Mutations have been found in the gene located on the X chromosome that codes for the γ chain, which is common to the receptors for IL-2, IL-4, IL-7, IL-9, and IL-15 (see Chapter 11). Thus, the mutation impairs responses to a multitude of cytokines (Fig. 17.2A).

TABLE 17.2.   Severe Combined Immunodeficiency Diseases

Specific Disorder	Underlying Deficiency	Mode of Inheritance[a]
T^-B^+ *subgroup*		
X-linked SCID	Mutated γ chain of cytokine receptors	X linked
Autosomal recessive SCID	Mutated JAK3 tyrosine kinase	AR
T^-B^- *subgroup*		
Adenosine deaminase deficiency	ADA enzyme	AR
Purine nucleoside phosphorylase deficiency	PNP enzyme	AR
Recombinase deficiency	Rag 1 or Rag 2 enzyme	AR
T^+B^- *Subgroup*		
Omenn's syndrome	Partial Rag deficiency	AR
T^+B^+ *Subgroup*		
Bare lymphocyte syndrome	MHC class II transcription activator (4 proteins)	AR
	MHC class I TAP defect	AR
ZAP-70 deficiency	Kinase domain of TCR-associated PTK, ZAP-70	AR
Multisystem Disorders		
Wiskott–Aldrich syndrome	WAS protein	X linked
Ataxia telangectasia	ATM protein for DNA repair	AR

[a] AR: autosomal recessive.

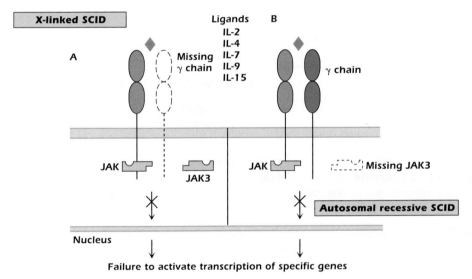

Figure 17.2. T^-B^+ subgroup. (A) Cytokine receptors that share the common γ chain fail to generate intracellular signals following ligand binding when this chain is missing. (B) Cytokine receptor signaling mediated by the common γ chain is defective when JAK3 tyrosine kinase is missing. Both result in SCID.

AUTOSOMAL RECESSIVE SCID.   A small subgroup of patients characterized by $T^-B^+NK^-$ lymphopenia show an autosomal recessive (rather than X-linked) pattern of inheritance. These individuals have a phenotype identical to the X-linked SCID group and cannot be distinguished clinically. Mutations are localized in the gene for JAK3 tyrosine kinase (Fig. 17.2B), the intracellular molecule responsible for transmitting signals from the γ hain of the receptors (see Chapter 11). Expression of JAK3 is normally restricted to hematopoietic cells.

An even smaller group of patients with autosomal recessive SCID present with $T^-B^+NK^+$ lymphopenia.

These individuals have mutations in the IL-7Rα chain or in a chain of CD3.

Animal models with targeted defects have proven very instructive in delineating these human deficiencies. In mouse gene knockout models (see Chapter 5), γ-chain knockouts, like SCID patients, have defective development of both T- and B-cell lineages. IL-7 and IL-7R knockouts bear a greater resemblance to SCID patients, suggesting that in the mouse IL-7 is crucial for T-cell/B-cell development and/or function and that the absence of IL-7 is not compensated for by other cytokines. In contrast, IL-2 knockouts show only some immune dysfunction, with normal T- and B-cell development and without a SCID phenotype.

T⁺B⁻ Subgroup

ADENOSINE DEAMINASE DEFICIENCY. Adenosine deaminase (ADA), an enzyme in the purine salvage pathway, is a ubiquitously expressed *housekeeping enzyme* (an enzyme used in the everyday function of all or most cells). Individuals lacking this enzyme account for approximately 20% of SCID patients and show an autosomal recessive pattern of inheritance. The deficiency results in buildup of toxic wastes, causing symptom progression over time and making early detection and treatment particularly critical in this group of patients.

ADA deficiency has its greatest impact on the immune system, resulting in failure of both T- and B-lymphocyte development. Many patients have an associated characteristic skeletal abnormality. The reason these patients do not exhibit even more multisystem problems is not completely understood. Investigation of this rare genetic disease has shown the particular importance of the salvage pathway in lymphocyte development and differentiation and has led to the development of antileukemic drugs to stop the growth of malignant lymphocyte precursors. ADA-deficient patients lacking a matched sibling marrow donor were the first group to be treated with gene therapy by transfecting a functional gene for ADA. However, even after years of development, this experimental approach remains fraught with great difficulties. Continuous enzyme supplementation is an alternative treatment.

PURINE NUCLEOSIDE PHOSPHORYLASE DEFICIENCY. A mutation in another enzyme in the purine salvage pathway, purine nucleoside phosphorylase (PNP), also leads to a buildup of toxic products that are particularly damaging to the neurologic system and to T cells. Eventually, all lymphoid tissues—thymus, tonsils, lymph nodes, and spleen—are depleted. Paradoxically, even though children with this condition are markedly immunodeficient, autoimmune disease is common in these patients.

RECOMBINASE DEFICIENCIES AND RADIOSENSITIVITY SCID. Recombination-activating genes (*RAG*) 1 and 2 code for enzymes involved in the rearrangement of the Ig genes in pre-B cells and the TCR genes in pre-T cells (see Chapters 6 and 9). Both enzymes are absolutely required for gene rearrangement, so mutations in either result in complete absence of T cells, B cells, and Ig. Maturation stops at the pre-T- and pre-B-cell stages. Typically, NK-cell function is intact. Mutations in genes for other proteins (such as Artemis), which are involved in Ig and TCR recombination and DNA repair, will generate a similar clinical picture. The relationship with DNA repair accounts for the radiosensitivity.

T⁺B⁻ Subgroup

OMENN SYNDROME. Omenn syndrome is a "leaky" SCID with reduced but partial Rag protein activity. A complete understanding of this disease is still lacking. The clinical presentations of patients with Omenn syndrome are similar to those with severe graft-versus-host (GVH) disease (discussed in Chapter 19) rather than to those lacking Rag protein activity. Although they are severely immunodeficient (cannot mount an effective immune response to any pathogen), Omenn syndrome patients demonstrate dysregulation of the immune system resulting in an attack against self. These patients are T⁺B⁻ by peripheral blood analysis and have massive skin and gastrointestinal infiltration by eosinophils and activated T cells, which produce T$_H$2-type cytokines (see Chapters 10 and 11). This results in a hyper-IgE syndrome and malnutrition due to protein loss. The success rate of bone marrow transplants in individuals with Omenn syndrome is low compared with other types of SCID patients; failures are due to graft rejection. Thus, although Omenn syndrome patients are immunodeficient, they still require pretreatment with immunosuppressive therapy.

T⁺B⁺ Subgroup

BARE LYMPHOCYTE SYNDROME. Bare lymphocyte syndrome (BLS) results from the failure to express HLA (the human MHC) molecules and is thus a defect in antigen presentation rather than an intrinsic lymphocyte cellular abnormality. BLS is divided into three groups, depending on which class of HLA molecules is missing: class I, class II, or both classes I and II. Only those individuals lacking expression of HLA class II molecules consistently show immunodeficiencies. Circulating T- and B-cell numbers may be normal; however, in the absence of HLA class II molecules, protein antigens cannot be presented to CD4⁺ T cells (Fig. 17.3). Therefore, collaboration does not occur between APC (B cells, macrophages/monocytes, dendritic cells) and CD4⁺ T cells. As a result, help is not provided to B cells for antibody production or to T cells for cytotoxic T-cell generation (see Chapter 10). This results in a clinical presentation of combined immunodeficiency. Since MHC class II expression is required on thymic epithelial cells for positive selection of CD4⁺ T cells, proportionately fewer CD4⁺ T cells are produced in the thymus (see Fig. 17.1, defect 7). Therefore, most patients have a decreased proportion of CD4⁺ to CD8⁺ T cells, resulting in a reversed CD4:CD8 T-cell ratio. The CD4⁺ T cells present are functional, as demonstrated by their ability to respond when stimulated *in vitro*. Since GVH disease can still occur in these patients, HLA matched bone marrow donors are required for treatment.

The mutation responsible for BLS affecting class II molecules is not in the HLA class II genes themselves but in one of the four genes that code for regulatory factors

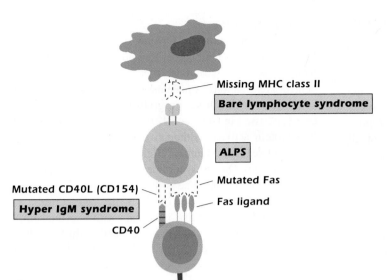

Figure 17.3. Missing cell membrane determinants required for normal T-cell–APC interactions result in several primary immunodeficiency syndromes, including bare lymphocyte syndrome, hyper-IgM syndrome, and Fas deficiency.

required to transcribe the class II genes. A better understanding of this transcription failure in BLS could result in the development of methods to turn off HLA class II expression. Theoretically these could then be applied to prevent graft rejection of transplanted organs (such as the kidney and liver) in immunocompetent individuals.

Few patients deficient in HLA class I expression have been identified; some were discovered serendipitously. This is undoubtedly due to the fact that not all individuals with deficient HLA class I expression show clinically significant immunodeficiency. Those who do usually present with chronic inflammatory lung disease late in childhood. As in BLS patients with defective HLA class II expression, patients with HLA class I deficiency do not have a mutation in the HLA class I gene, but rather have a mutated gene for the **transporter protein** (*Tap*). As described in Chapter 9, Tap transports peptides generated in the cytosol into the endoplasmic reticulum, where they interact with and stabilize the structure of MHC class I molecules. In the absence of the *Tap* gene product, expression of MHC class I molecules on the cell surface is very low. In the case of HLA class I deficiencies, positive selection of CD8$^+$ T cells in the thymus is defective, and their peripheral blood levels are decreased. For reasons that are unclear, when patients with this defect are symptomatic, they have recurrent bacterial pneumonias rather than the expected viral infections.

ZAP-70 MUTATION.   Patients with a mutation in the T-cell tyrosine kinase ZAP-70, which transduces the signal transmitted through the TCR, also present with a SCID-like phenotype. This will be described in more detail later in this chapter.

Other Multisystem Disorders. In addition to the combined immunodeficiency diseases we have just

discussed, several multisystem inherited disorders result in a SCID-like clinical picture.

WISKOTT–ALDRICH SYNDROME.   Wiskott–Aldrich syndrome is an X-linked disease showing a classic triad of symptoms: (1) bleeding diathesis (tendency to bleed) due to thrombocytopenia (low platelet level in blood) and small platelet size, (2) recurrent bacterial infections, and (3) paradoxically, allergic reactions (including eczema, elevated IgE levels, and food allergies). Over the longer term, patients have an increased risk of developing malignancies, particularly of the lymphoid system. The genetic basis of the disease is a mutation in the X-linked gene coding for the Wiskott–Aldrich syndrome protein (WASP), which is expressed in all hematopoietic stem cells. WASP interacts with the cytoskeleton; it allows remodeling after receptor engagement, contributes to the immune synapse between interacting cells, and affects maturation and migration of cells of both the adaptive and innate immune systems. In cells of patients with this syndrome, the cytoskeleton cannot effectively reorganize in response to stimuli.

The immune defects are variable, but both T and B cells are functionally abnormal, with T-cell numbers particularly decreased. Characteristically, patients are unable to respond to polysaccharide antigens. Treatment consists of antibiotics and antiviral agents given promptly with each infection. Reconstitution of T and B cells has been reported following bone marrow transplantation. Without treatment, the average life expectancy is approximately three years. With extension of survival, the incidence of malignancies would be expected to increase.

ATAXIA TELANGIECTASIA.   Ataxia telangiectasia (AT) is another multisystem genetic disorder in which neurologic symptoms (staggering gait or ataxia) and abnormal vascular dilatation (telangiectasia) accompany increased susceptibility to infections; lymphopenia (low lymphocyte numbers in peripheral blood); thymic hypoplasia; and depressed levels of IgA, IgE, and sometimes IgG. The immune defect involves both cellular and humoral (T-cell-dependent and T-cell-independent) immune responses; T-dependent regions of lymphoid tissues are affected most severely. The genetic basis of this syndrome is a mutation in the gene coding for a protein known as ATM, part of a pathway activated when the cell suffers DNA breaks from ionizing radiation and oxidative damage. AT patients have impaired development of T and B cells. The normal generation of both lineages involves critical phases of extensive cell proliferation, apoptosis, and DNA recombination events; all of these may be dysregulated with a mutated, nonfunctional ATM protein. AT children also have a greatly increased risk of developing malignancies, particularly lymphoid neoplasms. This may be the result of an ATM-dependent defect in DNA repair or cell cycle arrest following chromosomal damage. AT has been grouped with **Bloom syndrome** and **Fanconi's anemia;** all three disorders show similar variable immunodeficiencies and susceptibility to DNA damage.

In summary, the causes underlying severe defects in both cell-mediated and humoral immunity are varied. They range from mutations in enzymes found in all cells, which should have global effects in the body (such as deficiencies in ADA and PNP), to mutations involving signaling proteins specifically expressed in T cells (such as the ZAP-70 mutation).

Animal models have been informative, both in understanding the defects observed in human syndromes and in helping delineate steps in normal T- and B-cell development. The SCID mutant mouse strain, which has a genetic defect in a protein repairing double-stranded DNA breaks, was the first mouse model used for the study of this group of diseases. Since then, knockout mouse models for the majority of these spontaneous human genetic diseases have been produced as a means to study these diseases (see Chapter 5). In addition, SCID mice and nude mice (discussed later in this chapter), with diminished ability to reject foreign tissues, can be used as "living test tubes" to study the growth of human hematopoietic stem cells and human tumors.

Immunodeficiency Disorders Associated with T Cells and Cell-Mediated Immunity.

As noted in Table 17.1, patients with T-cell-associated deficiency diseases are susceptible to viral, fungal, and protozoal infections. In addition, because T cells are required to help B cells produce antibodies to T-dependent antigens (see Chapter 10), patients with T-cell-associated deficiencies also exhibit selective defects in antibody production. Consequently, T-cell-deficient patients may be difficult to distinguish clinically from SCID patients.

Congenital Thymic Aplasia (DiGeorge Syndrome).

DiGeorge syndrome is a T-cell deficiency in which the thymus, as well as other nonlymphoid organs, develops abnormally. The syndrome is caused by defective migration of fetal neural crest cells into the third and fourth pharyngeal pouches. This usually takes place during week 12 of gestation. In DiGeorge syndrome, the heart and face develop abnormally and the thymus and parathyroids fail to form, resulting in **thymic aplasia** and **hypoparathyroidism** along with cardiac disease. Due to the lack of the thymic structure, there is an absence of mature T cells, and immunodeficiency occurs. The athymic nude mouse is an animal model of DiGeorge syndrome; in these animals, the thymus and hair follicles do not develop.

DiGeorge Syndrome

DiGeorge syndrome is not hereditary; it occurs sporadically and is generally the result of a deletion in chromosome 22q11. Newborns present with hypocalcemia (low serum calcium levels), resulting from absence of the parathyroid glands, and have symptoms of congenital cardiac disease. Affected children suffer from recurrent or chronic infections with viruses, bacteria, fungi, and protozoa. They have either no or very few mature T cells in the periphery (blood, lymph nodes, or spleen) (see Fig. 17.1, defect 2). Although B cells, plasma cells, and serum Ig levels may be normal, many patients fail to mount an antibody response after immunization with T-dependent antigens. The lack of helper T cells, which are required for Ig isotype switching, results in the absence of IgG and other switched isotypes following immunization. The IgM response to T-independent antigens is intact. Since individuals with DiGeorge syndrome lack T cells and fail to generate normal antibody responses, they should *never* be immunized with live attenuated viral vaccines.

Children with DiGeorge syndrome used to be treated with a fetal thymus graft, which resulted in the appearance of host-derived T cells within a week. The fetal thymus used for transplantation needed to be <14 weeks gestation to avoid GVH reactions, which would occur if mature donor thymocytes were transferred into the immunoincompetent recipient. This donor fetal thymus provided the environment (the thymic epithelial cells) for development of recipient T cells from the patient's normal lymphoid precursors. Although the T cells produced were normal, cell-mediated immunity and help for antibody production were not fully restored. The recipient's T cells learned the MHC of the transplanted thymus as "self" and sometimes collaborated poorly with the body's own APC in the periphery (see Chapters 8 and 9). Because this treatment strategy was not entirely successful, therapy now mostly occurs in response to symptoms. Some patients have small remnants of thymic tissue, allowing delayed (though still diminished) T-cell maturation. The other medical problems associated with the syndrome, such as congenital heart disease, add to the overall poor prognosis.

T-Cell Deficiencies with Normal Peripheral T-Cell Numbers.

A number of patients have been identified with functional rather than numerical defects in their T cells. Clinically, they may present with opportunistic infections and a strikingly high incidence of autoimmune disease. Family studies show autosomal recessive patterns of inheritance. Molecular analysis demonstrates that the underlying causes are heterogeneous, with deficient expression of ZAP-70 tyrosine kinase, CD3ϵ, or CD3γ (Fig. 17.4).

As described in Chapter 10, ZAP-70 is required for intracellular transduction of signal after binding of the TCR. For reasons that are not clear, patients defective in ZAP-70 expression present with a SCID-type clinical picture (defective cell-mediated and humoral immunity). The absence of T-cell activity suggests that ZAP-70 plays a critical role in the function of mature T cells (see Fig. 17.1, defect 3); however, the reason for the effect on B-cell function is unclear and raises the possibility of a similar role in B cells. In addition, although the peripheral blood counts, lymph nodes, and thymus are essentially normal, CD8$^+$ T cells are missing in patients defective in ZAP-70 expression. This indicates that ZAP-70 is also required for CD8$^+$ T-cell differentiation in the thymus.

Mutations in CD3 chains are quite rare; only a handful of patients with such defects have been described. Mouse models confirm that all the CD3 peptide chains are required for normal signaling through the TCR. It is not clear, however, that these mouse models accurately mimic the few patients reported.

Autoimmune Lymphoproliferative Syndrome.

Autoimmune lymphoproliferative syndrome (ALPS) is an autosomal dominant disease characterized by massive proliferation of lymphoid tissue with early lymphoma development. This genetic defect results in systemic autoimmune phenomenon (hence its name) and increased susceptibility to chronic viral infections only. Patients have an increased number of double-negative (CD4$^-$CD8$^-$) T cells but may eventually develop B-cell lymphomas. Most ALPS patients have a mutation in the gene coding for the Fas protein (CD95) (see Fig. 17.3). Signaling through this protein normally activates *apoptosis*, or programmed cell death (see Chapters 10 and 12). Without activation of apoptosis, cells that should have died, such as autoimmune cells, continue to live, and immune responses that should have been turned off persevere. The unchecked proliferation of B cells then provides fertile ground for transforming mutations that lead to B-cell lymphomas. Most ALPS patients have one normal and one mutated Fas molecule, which suggests that the mutated Fas molecule interferes with the function of the normal molecule when they are cross-linked. Some ALPS patients have defects in other components of the apoptosis pathway, such as Fas ligand or caspase 10.

Autoimmune Lymphoproliferative Syndrome

Two mouse strains—*lpr* and *gld*—have phenotypes similar to those of ALPS patients. The *lpr* mice have a mutation in their Fas gene and *gld* mice have a mutation in their Fas ligand gene. For many years, *lpr* mice were studied as a model for autoimmune disease, specifically SLE, before their Fas gene defect was discovered.

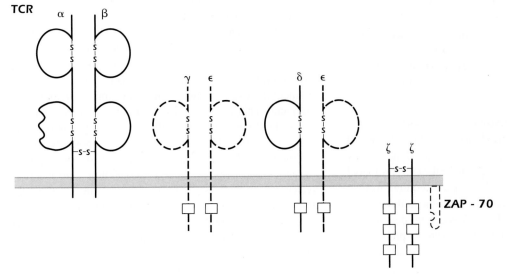

Figure 17.4. Deficiencies of molecules (shown with dashed lines) involved in T-cell signaling through the antigen-specific TCR.

Chronic Mucocutaneous Candidiasis. Chronic mucocutaneous candidiasisis is a poorly defined collection of syndromes characterized by *Candida* infections of skin and mucous membranes. This ubiquitous fungal organism is normally nonpathogenic. These patients usually have normal T-cell-mediated immunity to microorganisms other than *Candida* and normal B-cell-mediated immunity (antibody production) to all microorganisms including *Candida*. Thus, they have only a selective defect in the functioning of T cells. This disorder affects both males and females, is particularly prevalent in children, and may be inherited.

B-Cell- or Immunoglobulin-Associated Immunodeficiency Disorders.

B-cell- or immunoglobulin-associated immune diseases range from defective B-cell development with complete absence of all Ig classes to deficiencies in a single class or subclass of Ig. Patients suffer from recurrent or chronic infections that may start in infancy (Bruton's or X-linked agammaglobulinemia) or in young adulthood. Evaluation includes analysis of B-cell number and function and immunoelectrophoretic and quantitative determinations of Ig class and subclass.

X-Linked Agammaglobulinemia. First described in 1952 by Bruton, X-linked agammaglobulinemia (XLA) is also called ***Bruton's agammaglobulinemia***. The disorder, which is relatively rare (1 in 100,000), is first noticed at five to six months of age, when the infant has lost the maternally derived IgG that had passed through the placenta. At that age, the infant presents with serious and repeated bacterial infections as a result of severe depression or virtual absence of all Ig classes.

X-Linked Agammaglobulinemia

The major defect lies in the inability of pre-B cells, which are present at normal levels, to develop into mature B cells. The *BTK* gene, which is mutated in XLA, normally codes for a tyrosine kinase enzyme residing in the cytosol. *BTK* is essential for signal transduction from the pre-BCR on developing B cells. Without this signal, the cell develops no further (see Fig. 17.1, defect 4). Only the nonmutated X chromosome is active in all mature B cells from female carriers of the mutant gene. XLA is therefore one of several inherited immunodeficiency diseases in which a mutation in a cytoplasmic tyrosine kinase is responsible for the disorder (see above descriptions of the JAK3 form of SCID and the ZAP-70 form of T-cell deficiency).

Analysis of the blood, bone marrow, spleen, and lymph nodes of XLA patients reveals near absence of mature B cells and plasma cells, explaining the depressed Ig levels. Characteristically, affected children have markedly underdeveloped tonsils. The limited numbers of B cells appear normal in their ability to become plasma cells. Infants with XLA have recurrent bacterial otitis media, bronchitis, septicemia, pneumonia, arthritis, meningitis, and dermatitis. The most common microorganisms found to cause infections in these patients are *Haemophilus influenzae* and *Streptococcus pneumoniae*. Frequently, patients suffer from malabsorption due to infestation of the gastrointestinal tract with *Giardia lamblia*. Unexpectedly, XLA patients are also susceptible to infections by viruses that enter through the gastrointestinal tract, such as echovirus and polio. The infections do not respond well to antibiotics alone; treatment consists of periodic injections of **intravenous γ-globulin (IVGG)** containing large amounts of IgG (discussed further in Chapter 20). Although such passive immunization has maintained some patients for 20–30 years, the prognosis is guarded, as chronic lung disease due to repeated infections often supervenes.

Two other rare mutations, μ heavy-chain deficiency and λ5 chain deficiency, result in an identical clinical picture as a result of the same underlying pathophysiology. The λ5 chain is part of the surrogate light chain on pro-B cells and, along with the μ heavy chain and a third chain, form the pre-B cell. These pro-B or pre-B cells do not have functional receptors (pre-BCR) to receive the signals necessary to allow their survival and continued maturation. Both of these mutations have autosomal recessive patterns of inheritance.

Transient Hypogammaglobulinemia. At five to six months of age, passively transferred maternal IgG disappears, and IgG production by the infant begins to rise. Premature infants may have transient IgG deficiency if they are not yet able to synthesize Ig. Occasionally, a full-term infant may also fail to produce appropriate amounts of IgG, even when levels of IgM and IgA are normal. The cause appears to be a deficiency in number and function of helper T cells. Transient hypogammaglobulinemia may persist from a few months to as long as two years. It is not sex-linked and can be distinguished from the non-X-linked inherited agammaglobulinemias by the presence of normal numbers of B cells in the blood. Although treatment is usually not necessary, affected infants need to be identified, since they should not be given immunizations during this period.

Common Variable Immunodeficiency Disease. Patients with common variable immunodeficiency disease (CVID) have markedly decreased serum IgG and IgA levels, with normal or low IgM and normal or low peripheral B-cell numbers. The cause of the disease, which affects both males and females, is not entirely clear and is probably not uniform. Onset may occur at any age, with peaks at 1–5 years and 15–20 years. Affected individuals suffer from recurrent respiratory and gastrointestinal infections with pyogenic bacteria and, paradoxically, from autoimmune diseases associated with autoantibodies such as hemolytic anemia, autoimmune thrombocytopenia, and SLE. Many also have disorders of cell-mediated immunity. Long term, these patients have a high incidence of cancers, particularly lymphomas and gastric cancers.

Common Variable Immunodeficiency Syndrome

CVID is characterized by a failure in maturation of B cells into antibody-secreting cells (see Fig. 17.1, defect 5). This defect may be due to an inability of the B cells to proliferate in response to antigen, normal proliferation of B cells without secretion of IgM, secretion of IgM without class switching to IgG or IgA (due to an intrinsic B-cell or T-cell abnormality), or failure of glycosylation of IgG heavy chains. In most cases, the disorder appears to be the result of diminished synthesis and secretion of Ig. The disease is familial or sporadic, with unknown environmental influences triggering onset. In the peripheral blood, patients will have normal or near-normal numbers of B cells but usually a marked reduction of memory B cells (CD27$^+$/IgD$^-$ B cells). Memory B cells are those which have been exposed to antigen in the germinal center, where they have hypermutated and isotype switched their immunoglobulin genes and now are ready to respond rapidly with high-affinity antibody on reexposure to antigen.

Treatment depends on severity. For severe disease with many recurrent or chronic infections, IVGG therapy is indicated. Treated patients can have a normal life span. Women with CVID have normal pregnancies but, of course, do not transfer maternal IgG to the fetus.

Selective Immunoglobulin Deficiencies. Several syndromes are associated with selective deficiency of a single class or subclass of Ig. Some of these are accompanied by compensatory elevated levels of other isotypes, such as the increased IgM levels in cases of IgG or IgA deficiency.

IgA deficiency is the most common immunodeficiency disorder in the Western world, with an incidence of approximately 1 in 800 (see Fig. 17.1, defect 6). The cause is unknown but appears to be associated with decreased release of IgA by B lymphocytes. IgA deficiency can also occur transiently as an adverse reaction to drugs. Patients may suffer from recurrent sinopulmonary viral or bacterial infections and/or celiac disease (defective absorption in the bowel); alternatively, they may be entirely asymptomatic. Isolated IgA deficiency may also precede full-blown expression of CVID; the two disorders are often found in the same families.

Treatment of symptomatic patients with IgA deficiency consists of broad-spectrum antibiotics. Therapy

with immune serum globulin is not useful because commercial preparations contain only low levels of IgA and because *injected* IgA does not reach the areas of the secretory immune system, where IgA is normally the protective antibody. Furthermore, patients may mount antibody responses (usually IgG or IgE) to the IgA in the transferred immune serum, causing hypersensitivity reactions. The prognosis for selective IgA deficiency is generally good, with many patients surviving normally.

Selective deficiencies in other Ig isotypes include *IgM deficiency*, a rare disorder in which patients suffer from recurrent and severe infections with polysaccharide-encapsulated organisms such as pneumococci and *H. influenzae*. Selective deficiencies in subclasses of IgG have been described but are even rarer.

Disorders of T–B Interactions. There are at least two diseases in which the T- and B-cell lineages appear to mature normally but demonstrate abnormal interactions between them. Although both disorders described below are due to underlying T-cell abnormalities, the predominant clinical symptoms are in the B-cell or humoral immune response.

Hyper-IgM Syndrome. Patients with hyper-IgM syndrome (HIGM) present with recurrent respiratory infections at one to two years of age; very low serum IgG, IgA, and IgE; and normal to elevated IgM (see Fig. 17.1, defect 8). The B cells, which are normal in number, are functional *in vitro* and will isotype switch when appropriately stimulated. The T cells are also normal in number, subset distribution, and proliferative responses to mitogens. The most common form, X-HIGM, is caused by a mutation in the *CD40L* gene on the X chromosome, which results in the absence of CD40 ligand (CD154) on T$_H$ cells (see Fig. 17.3). CD40L binds to CD40 expressed on B cells (see Chapter 10). This interaction is necessary for B-cell proliferation, class switching, and even germinal center formation. CD40–CD40L interaction also plays a role in macrophage–T$_H$1 cell interaction; this aspect may explain the propensity of these patients to develop opportunistic infections, particularly *Pneumocystis carinii* pneumonia (PCP), and their poorer prognosis compared to XLA patients. For the same reason, DTH reactions are absent.

Hyper-IgM Syndrome

A second group of patients with presentations similar to X-HIGM have a defect in the CD40 molecule and thus an autosomal recessive pattern of inheritance. A third group, with a defect downstream in the interaction between CD40 and a modulator of the transcription factor NF-κB (see Chapter 10), has an X-linked mode of inheritance.

As is common in genetic disorders involving intracellular regulatory molecules, these children show abnormalities in nonimmune system cells as well, reflecting the ubiquitous use of these molecules in many types of cells.

Recently, two more groups of patients with HIGM have been described. One has a mutation in activation-induced cytidine deaminase (AID), the molecule essential for somatic hypermutation and isotype switching, and a second has a mutation in uracil-DNA glycosylase, an enzyme also active in isotype class switching.

X-Linked Lymphoproliferative Syndrome (Duncan Syndrome).

X-linked lymphoproliferative syndrome (XLPS) was originally observed in six maternally related males of the Duncan family, hence its common name. This rare disease is usually due to a mutation in the gene coding for the SLAM (signaling lymphocyte activation molecule)–associated protein (SAP), located on the X chromosome. SAP is an intracytoplasmic molecule that links several surface receptors with downstream molecules in T cells, B cells, NK cells, eosinophils, and platelets. In spite of the wide distribution of the molecule among numerous hematopoietic cell lineages, any abnormalities are usually subtle and undetected until patient exposure to EBV. EBV exposure results in a severe course of infectious mononucleosis, which may be fatal. Presumably this is the result of impaired killing of infected cells by T and NK cells. Development of malignant lymphoma or dysgammaglobulinemia frequently follows survival from infection or may occur without prior EBV exposure. The lymphomas are predominantly aggressive B-cell lymphomas at extranodal sites, particularly the gastrointestinal tract. Burkitt's lymphoma (described later in the chapter) is the most common type. Although the pattern of lymphomas is similar to those in other patients with poorly controlled EBV-induced B-cell proliferations due to T-cell defects (such as in AIDS or immunosuppressed transplant patients), the incidence is much greater in XLPs. An inability of T cells to regulate B-cell growth once it has been initiated is considered to be a major part of the underlying defect. Prognosis is extremely poor.

X-Linked Lymphoproliferative Syndrome

Phagocytic Dysfunctions.

Phagocytic cells—polymorphonuclear leukocytes and macrophages/monocytes—play a critical role in both innate and acquired immunity to pathogens, acting either alone or in concert with lymphocytes. Inherited deficiencies affecting phagocytic cell function have helped identify many of the molecules required at each step of the phagocyte's elimination of pathogens. These steps and the associated deficiencies include the following: migration and adhesion of phagocytic cells (leukocyte adhesion deficiency), phagocytosis and lysosomal fusion (Chédiak–Higashi syndrome), and respiratory burst for killing (chronic granulomatous disease) (Fig. 17.5). Phagocytic dysfunction may also be secondary; causes include extrinsic factors, such as drugs and systemic diseases (e.g., diabetes mellitus), or defects in other arms of the immune system.

Leukocyte Adhesion Deficiency.

As discussed in Chapter 11, for leukocytes to arrive at sites of infection

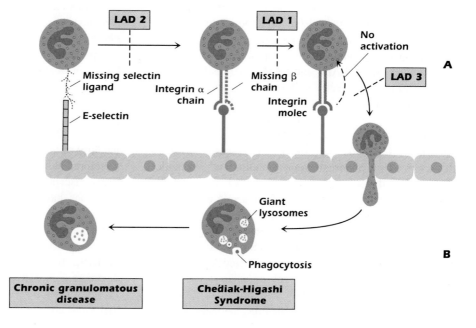

Figure 17.5. (A) Defects in cell adhesion disrupt the ability of leukocytes to interact with vascular endothelium, causing impairment of migration of these cells from the blood to sites of infection. (B) Impairments in mechanisms required for phagocytosis result in defective intracellular killing of microorganisms.

in tissues, they must first leave the bloodstream. This is accomplished in a series of steps. The first one consists of the cell's slow rolling along the endothelium through the interaction of selectins on endothelium and selectin ligands on leukocytes (see Figure 11.3). Chemoattractants then cause the cell to stop rolling. The cell adheres more firmly, followed by transendothelial migration. These latter steps involve the interaction of leukocyte integrins with their ligands on endothelial cells.

Leukocyte adhesion deficiency (LAD) is a group of disorders in which the interaction between the leukocyte and the vascular endothelium is disrupted (Fig. 17.5A). *LAD1* is an autosomal recessive disease mapping to chromosome 21. Patients have a defect in the β subunit of integrin molecules preventing their expression. The β subunit is common to three integrins found on granulocytes, monocytes, and lymphocytes: LFA-1(CD11a/CD18), Mac-1 (CD11b/CD18), and p150,95 (CD11c/CD18). As a result, adhesion and migration of all white blood cells are impaired. LAD1 individuals suffer from recurrent soft tissue bacterial infections and have increased WBC counts but without pus formation or effective wound healing. As expected, lymphocyte function is also affected due to the lack of LFA-1 expression. Newborns with LAD1 characteristically have delayed separation of their umbilical cord.

LAD3, a disorder clinically identical to LAD1, has recently been identified. Individuals with LAD3 express both integrin chains, but the molecule does not become activated in response to stimuli. The leukocytes are therefore able to roll but do not arrest in response to endothelial cell signals, similar to LAD1 (Fig. 17.5A).

LAD2 individuals have a defect in selectin ligands; therefore, cells from these patients cannot roll along the endothelial surface (Fig. 17.5A). The underlying defect in LAD2 is in fucose metabolism, which results in the absence of fucosylated ligands available for binding to selectins. Although the immunodeficiency symptoms are milder, the defect in fucose metabolism results in other developmental abnormalities. As in LAD1 and LAD3, there is little or no pus formation, and affected children do not show classical clinical signs of severe infection.

Chédiak–Higashi Syndrome. Chédiak–Higashi syndrome (CHS) is an autosomal recessive disease characterized by abnormal giant granules and organelles (Fig. 17.5B) due to a mutation of the *LYST* gene; this gene codes for a protein that may have a role in organelle protein trafficking. Lysosomes and melanosomes are particularly affected, resulting in defects in pigmentation; abnormalities in neutrophil, NK-cell, and platelet function; and neurologic abnormalities. Neutrophils show diminished intracellular killing of organisms, the result of both defective degranulation and impaired fusion of lysosomes with phagosomes. With time, patients develop massive infiltrates of lymphocytes and macrophages in the liver, spleen, and lymph nodes. Pyogenic organisms such as *Streptococcus* and *Staphylococcus* cause recurrent, sometimes fatal infection. Prognosis is poor.

Chronic Granulomatous Disease. In chronic granulomatous disease (CGD), the final step in killing of ingested organisms is defective (Fig. 17.5B) and the continued intracellular survival of the organisms results in granuloma formation. In normal individuals, activated neutrophils and mononuclear phagocytes kill organisms via the *respiratory burst*, which consumes oxygen and generates hydrogen peroxide and free superoxide radicals. Mutations in any of the four subunits of the enzyme that catalyzes the burst (NADPH oxidase) can result in CGD. The most common form of CGD is due to a mutation in one of the membrane-bound subunits of NADPH oxidase, gp91^{phox}, which is coded for by the *CYBB* gene located on the X chromosome. Thus, the majority of patients show an X-linked recessive pattern of inheritance. The other subunits of NADPH oxidase are coded for by autosomal genes. CGD patients with mutations in these other subunits show autosomal recessive inheritance. Mutations in these patients occur mostly in one of the two cytosolic subunits of the enzyme, p47^{phox} or p67^{phox}.

Symptoms appear during the first two years of life. Patients have enhanced susceptibility to infection with organisms that are normally of low virulence, such as *Staphylococcus aureus, Serratia marcescens*, and *Aspergillus*. Associated abnormalities include lymphadenopathy (increase in lymph node size) and hepatosplenomegaly (increase in liver and spleen size) due to the chronic and acute infections. Treatment consists of aggressive immunization and therapy with wide-spectrum antibiotics, antifungal agents, and interferon-γ.

Other disorders with reduced or absent levels of phagocyte-associated enzymes include *glucose-6-phosphate dehydrogenase, myeloperoxidase*, and *alkaline phosphatase*; all of these result in decreased intracellular killing of organisms.

IL-12/23-Interferon-γ Deficiency. A mutation in any of the molecules operative in the interactions among IL-12, IL-23, IFN-γ, and their receptors results in an inability of monocytes to respond with secretion of TNF-α; therefore, individuals carrying these mutations are selectively susceptible to weakly pathogenic mycobacteria. Five mutations have been identified: IFN-γR1 (ligand-binding chain) and IFN-γR2 (signal-transducing chain), both on APC; STAT1 (transducing signal from IFN-γR); IL−12β (p40 subunit) produced by APC; and IL-12Rβ$_1$ (β subunit of IL-12 receptor) on T and NK cells. This group of disorders demonstrates the importance of IFN-γ and IL-12 in controlling mycobacterial infections but also suggests that there are compensation mechanisms for other effects of these cytokines. Immunization with live BCG, common in some parts of the world, is dangerous for patients with this defect.

Natural Killer Cell Deficiency.

Very little is known about NK-cell deficiency in humans; only a few such cases have been reported. Animal studies suggest that NK-cell deficiency impairs allograft rejection and is linked to higher susceptibility to viral diseases and increased metastases from tumors. NK-cell defects are seen in SCID, in some T-cell and phagocytic cell disorders, and in X-linked lymphoproliferative syndrome.

Diseases Caused by Abnormalities in Complement System.

As described in Chapter 13, complement is important in the opsonization and killing of bacteria and altered cells, in chemotaxis, and in B-cell activation. Complement components also participate in the elimination of antigen–antibody complexes, preventing immune complex deposition and subsequent disease. Deficiencies in complement are inherited as autosomal traits; heterozygous individuals have half the normal level of a given component. For most components, this is sufficient to prevent clinical disease. Normally, the half-life of activated complement components is carefully controlled by inhibitors, which break down the products or dissociate the immune complexes.

Deficiencies of Early Complement Components.

The early components of complement are particularly important in generating the opsonin, C3b (Fig. 17.6). Patients with deficiencies of C1, 4, or 2 from the classical pathway or with deficiency in C3 itself have increased infections with encapsulated organisms (*S. pneumoniae*, *Streptococcus pyogenes*, *H. influenza*) and increased rheumatic diseases. The reason for the latter is the improper clearance of immune complexes as a consequence of low C3b generation, and often the autoimmune disease is most striking. In fact, SLE is the most common presenting symptom of some complement deficiencies. SLE in these individuals is of earlier onset and more severe than without this association and can occur in the absence of autoantibodies that are frequently found in other cases of SLE (see Chapter 12). Deficiencies of mannose-binding lectin, which binds to the surface of microbes without antibody and activates the classical pathway, also result

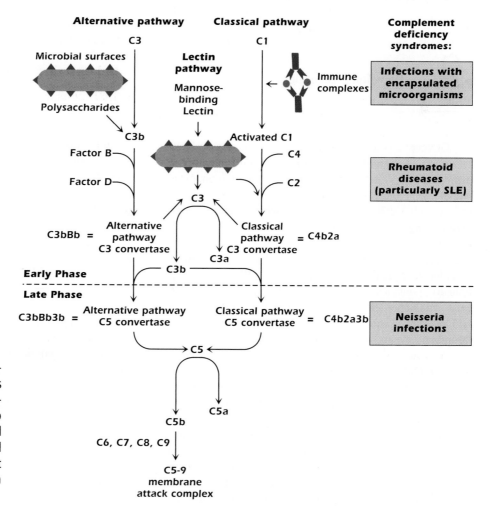

Figure 17.6. Complement cascade showing that deficiencies in early-phase complement components predispose individuals to infections caused by encapsulated microorganisms and rheumatoid syndromes. Late-phase complement deficiencies are associated with *Neisseria* infections.

in risk of bacterial infections and lupuslike symptoms. Since all the complement activation pathways—classical, mannose-binding lectin, and alternative—activate C3, deficiencies of C3 itself are associated with the most severe symptoms, particularly infectious complications.

Deficiencies of Late Complement Components.
Deficiencies of the late complement components (C5–C9) interfere with the generation of the MAC. The MAC is directly lytic and responsible for the primary defense against Gram-negative bacteria, particularly *Neisseria meningitidis* (Fig. 17.6).

Defective Control of Complement Components
HEREDITARY ANGIOEDEMA. In hereditary angioedema, patients lack a functional *C1 esterase inhibitor*. (The disorder is also referred to as C1 esterase inhibitor deficiency.) Without this inhibitor, the action of C1 on C4, C2, and the kallikrein system is uncontrolled, generating large amounts of vasoactive peptides. These peptides cause increased blood vessel permeability. Patients suffer from localized edema, which is life threatening when it occurs in the larynx and obstructs the airway passage. Treatment includes avoidance of precipitating factors (usually trauma) and infusion of C1 esterase inhibitor, if available.

Hereditary Angioedema

GLYCOSYL PHOSPHATIDYL INOSITOL PROTEIN DEFICIENCIES. A family of proteins with GPI anchors is expressed on the membranes of RBCs, lymphocytes, granulocytes, endothelial cells (blood vessel lining cells), and epithelial cells. These proteins, which include *decay-accelerating factor* (DAF or CD55) and *CD59*, protect the cells against spontaneous lysis by complement (see Fig. 13.4). In the absence of these cell surface inhibitors, granulocytes, platelets, and particularly RBCs are susceptible to spontaneous lysis by complement. Rare families exist with inherited mutations in DAF, CD59, or all the GPI proteins. Patients show symptoms of severe anemia, thrombotic events, and chronic infections.

An acquired form of the disease, called *paroxysmal nocturnal hemoglobinuria (PNH)*, is more common. In PNH, patients have a deficiency in an enzyme required for the production of all the GPI-anchored proteins due to an acquired somatic mutation in an early myeloid stem cell. The three nonlymphoid lineages (granulocytes, platelets, and erythrocytes) are affected. In many patients, the stem cells with this mutation eventually acquire additional mutations, dominate the normal cells in the bone marrow, and stop maturing, resulting in acute myelogenous leukemia.

During the chronic course of PNH, intravascular hemolysis occurs, more prominently in the kidneys at night where the acidic environment activates the alternative complement pathway. This clinical presentation is reflected in its name, paroxysmal nocturnal hemoglobinuria.

Secondary Immunodeficiency Diseases

As noted at the beginning of this chapter, secondary immunodeficiency diseases are the consequence of other diseases. By far, the most common cause of immunodeficiency disorders worldwide is malnutrition. In developed countries, immunodeficiency is more often *iatrogenic*, inadvertently caused by medical treatment, particularly from the use of chemotherapeutic agents in cancer therapy or deliberate immunosuppression for organ transplantation or autoimmune disease. Secondary immunodeficiencies can be seen in untreated autoimmunity or overwhelming infections by bacteria. Malignancies of the immune system also frequently suppress the nonmalignant components, resulting in increased susceptibility of these patients to infection.

ACQUIRED IMMUNODEFICIENCY SYNDROME

Initial Description and Epidemiology

In 1981, several cases of an unusual pneumonia caused by PCP were reported in homosexual males in the San Francisco area of California. This was followed by the recognition of an aggressive form of Kaposi's sarcoma in a similar population in New York City. Since those first cases of AIDS were recognized until today, over 20 million people have died worldwide and over 30 million are currently infected.

Acquired Immunodeficiency Syndrome

AIDS is caused by infection with HIV. The virus is transferred through blood and body fluids. Blood, semen, vaginal secretions, breast milk, and (to a small extent) saliva of an infected individual all contain free virus or cells harboring virus. Thus, HIV can be transmitted through sexual contact, sharing of needles, transfusion of blood or blood products, placental transfer, passage through the birth canal, and breast feeding.

Although first recognized in sexually active homosexual males in large U.S. cities, AIDS has no sexual preference. Worldwide, heterosexual transmission is most common. In the United States, although homosexual males and intravenous drug abusers still constitute the major infected groups, the greatest increase in incidence rate is among heterosexual women and minorities (African-Americans and Hispanics). Transmission of the virus through transfusion of blood and blood products has been virtually eliminated in the United States through screening of donors, testing of collected blood units, and heat-inactivation of clotting factor concentrates. For reasons that will become clear later in the discussion, a dangerous "window period" still exists during which infection of blood units or organs cannot be detected. Transmission from mother to infant, which accounts for >80% of the pediatric cases, can be greatly diminished by antiviral therapy of the expectant mother and avoidance of vaginal childbirth and breast feeding. However, these positive statements are almost as a footnote to an epidemic that continues to spread worldwide without signs of abating, particularly in Africa and Southeast Asia.

Human Immunodeficiency Virus

HIV is an enveloped human retrovirus of the lentivirus family. Two strains of HIV have been described, HIV-1 and HIV-2. HIV-2, the less virulent strain, is found mostly in Western Africa. The viral particle contains two identical single strands of genomic RNA and three enzymes; *integrase, protease*, and *reverse transcriptase* (Fig. 17.7). These are packaged in the *p24* core antigen with *p7*, a nucleoprotein, and *p9*; all of these are surrounded by the *p17* matrix protein. The viral envelope, which is derived from the host cell membrane, displays viral glycoproteins, including *gp120* and *gp41*, which are critical for infection. The gp120, which is noncovalently bound to the transmembrane protein gp41, has high affinity for CD4; therefore, all cells expressing CD4 are potential targets for the virus.

These include macrophages/monocytes and dendritic cells as well as CD4$^+$ T cells.

After binding to CD4, gp120 undergoes a conformational change and must then also bind a second molecule (a coreceptor) on the surface of the target cell for HIV to enter the cell. Several *chemokine receptors* (see Chapter 11) are coreceptors for HIV. The particular coreceptor used by the virus depends on the variant of the gp120 molecule expressed on its surface. Variation in gp120 therefore determines what is referred to as the *tropism* of the virus, dictating which CD4$^+$ target cell can be infected by that viral particle. *Macrophage tropic HIV* uses the chemokine receptor CCR5 and requires only a low level of CD4 on the host cell. CCR5 is expressed by macrophages and dendritic cells, both of which express low levels of surface CD4. *Lymphotropic HIV* uses the chemokine receptor CXCR4 expressed on T cells and requires a high density of CD4 on the cell surface. HIV variants using CCR5 are called R5, and those using CXCR4 are termed X4; variants able to bind both chemokine coreceptors are referred to as R5X4. Both coreceptors are G-coupled proteins with seven transmembrane spanning domains. CCR5 normally binds the chemokines, RANTES, monocyte chemotactic protein 1α (MIP−1γ), and MIP−1ε. CXCR4 binds stromal derived factor 1.

CCR5 is thought to be the major coreceptor for the establishment of primary infection, since individuals with mutations in CCR5 appear to be at least partially protected. If an individual is first infected with a macrophage tropic variant via sexual contact, viral infection can be established in the macrophages and dendritic cells of MALT. These infected cells will then provide a *reservoir* of virus both

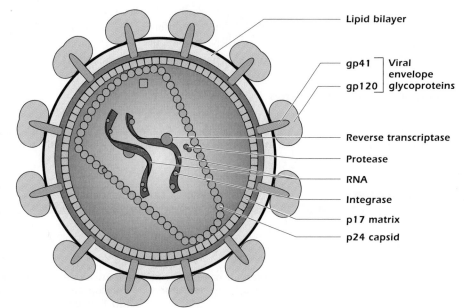

Figure 17.7. Structure of HIV-1 showing two identical RNA strands (viral genome) and associated enzymes. The enzymes include reverse transcriptase, integrase, and protease packaged in a cone-shaped core composed of p24 capsid protein with surrounding p17 protein matrix, all of which are surrounded by a phospholipid membrane envelope derived from the host cell. Virally encoded membrane proteins (gp41 and gp120) are bound to the envelope.

Lipid bilayer

gp41 } Viral envelope
gp120 } glycoproteins

Reverse transcriptase

Protease

RNA

Integrase

p17 matrix

p24 capsid

locally and distally, since they are not killed by the infection and are capable of migrating throughout the body. Exposure of HIV-infected cells to antigen promotes viral replication (particularly in the macrophages), a switch to the lymphotropic form, and further, rapid dissemination in the body. Thus, the tropism of the virus produced within the infected individual changes over time. This evolution is due to mutations in the gp120 gene that result in alterations in its amino acid sequence.

Following the binding of gp120 to CD4 and its coreceptor, gp41 penetrates the cell membrane, allowing fusion of the viral envelope with the cell membrane and subsequent viral entry. In the host cell, viral RNA is replicated to a cDNA copy by the viral enzyme reverse transcriptase. The cDNA may remain in the cytoplasm or may enter the nucleus and be integrated into the host genome as a provirus with the help of the viral enzyme integrase. Viral replication continues at a low level, sometimes for several years, so that HIV infection remains in a relatively, but not truly, "latent" phase.

The HIV genome has a long terminal repeat (LTR) region at each end (Fig. 17.8). The LTR is required for viral integration and has binding sites for regulatory proteins. When the T cell is activated by antigen, a cascade of reactions leads to activation of the transcription factor NF-κB. NF-κB binds to a promoter region in LTR, activating transcription of the provirus by host RNA polymerase.

Transcription of the provirus produces a long mRNA transcript that is spliced at alternative sites for the synthesis of different proteins. The first two proteins made are *tat* and *rev*. Tat enters the nucleus, where it acts as a transcription factor. It binds to the LTR region and increases the rate of viral transcription. Rev also acts in the nucleus, binding to the Rev-responsive element in the viral mRNA transcript. Rev binding increases the RNA transport rate to the cytoplasm. When the mRNA is transported more rapidly into the cytoplasm, less splicing occurs in the nucleus and different proteins can then be made from these mRNA forms. In this second wave of viral protein synthesis, the structural

components of the viral core and envelope are produced in precursor form. In the third wave, unspliced RNA is transported to the cytoplasm and serves as the RNA for the new viral particles and for the translation of *gag* and *pol*: *gag* codes for p24, p17, and p7/p9; *pol* codes for the viral protease, reverse transcriptase, and integrase. The protease cleaves these products of *gag* and *pol*, which are first synthesized as a single polyprotein.

Release of virus from CD4$^+$ T cells frequently results in lysis of the cell. Macrophages and dendritic cells are generally not killed by HIV; therefore they can serve as reservoirs, transporting virus to other parts of the body (lymphoid tissue and central nervous system) and producing a small number of particles without cytopathic consequences. Dendritic cells carry the virus mostly on their surface, whereas the macrophages allow a constant low level of viral production. The stimulation of infected macrophages and T cells by cytokines or antigen results in increased viral replication and the productive phase.

Clinical Course

The clinical course of HIV infection can be divided into three phases: acute infection, chronic latent phase, and crisis phase.

Acute Infection. Upon initial infection with HIV, many patients are asymptomatic. Others will show a flu-like illness characterized by fever, sore throat, and general malaise starting two to four weeks after infection and lasting one to two weeks. During this time, there is a viremia (virus in peripheral blood) and a precipitous drop in the number of circulating CD4$^+$ T cells. The immune system responds by generating CTLs and antibodies specific for the virus. The CTLs, which kill virally infected cells, are partially responsible for the drop in CD4$^+$ T cells. At this point the patient will **seroconvert**, express detectable antibody specific for HIV proteins. The number of CD4$^+$ T cells in the peripheral blood then partially recovers. Infected macrophages

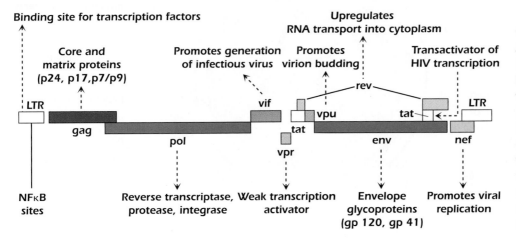

Figure 17.8. The genes and proteins of HIV-1. The HIV-1 RNA genome is flanked by LTR regions required for viral integrations and regulation of the viral genome. Several viral genes overlap, resulting in different reading frames; this allows the virus to encode many proteins in a small genome. The functions of the gene products are also shown.

and dendritic cells disseminate the virus to lymphoid tissue throughout the body.

Chronic Latent Phase. Although the immune response seems standard for a viral infection, it merely contains rather than eradicates the virus. The extremely high rate of mutation of the virus may explain the ineffectiveness of the immune response. A "latent" phase is established which may last as long as 15 years. During this relatively asymptomatic period, a low level of viral replication continues, associated with a gradual decline in CD4$^+$ T-cell number. HIV is therefore never truly latent.

In contrast to what might be expected, the number of viral-infected T cells in the peripheral blood is extremely low. The lymph nodes are the predominant location of infected cells. As described above, macrophages act as a reservoir. Follicular dendritic cells of the germinal center (see Chapter 7) not only function as a reservoir but also present virus on their surface. This results in continuous presentation of virus to T and B cells, culminating in the intense follicular (germinal center) hyperplasia and lymphadenopathy typical of this phase.

The T cells undergo a slow rate of lysis, which eventually results in involution of the lymph node. This T-cell death seems to be the result of a combination of factors. First, production of virus in the cells causes lysis. Second, the infected cell seems to be more susceptible to apoptosis. Third, CTLs kill some of the infected cells. Finally, uninfected CD4$^+$ T cells may be killed in a bystander antibody-dependent cell-mediated cytotoxicity-like mechanism as a result of binding of soluble gp120 and anti-gp120 antibody to their surface CD4 molecules.

During this phase, patients' peripheral CD4$^+$ T-cell counts, CD4:CD8 T-cell ratios, and viral loads are monitored. In healthy individuals, the CD4:CD8 T-cell ratio is approximately 2, but in this phase of HIV infection the ratio is reversed, with CD8 T cells outnumbering CD4 T cells. A reversed CD4:CD8 T-cell ratio can be seen in other viral infections but is usually due to an increase in CD8$^+$ T cells rather than a decrease in CD4$^+$ T cells as seen in HIV. As the number of CD4$^+$ T cells reaches progressively lower values, the patient becomes symptomatic, entering the final crisis phase, AIDS.

Crisis Phase. AIDS was originally recognized by the clinical appearance of unusual infections and malignancies; these continue to be the hallmarks of the full-blown disease. The Centers for Disease Control and Prevention (CDC) has identified illnesses that are considered AIDS-associated (Table 17.3). Diagnosis of any of these (or a defined threshold CD4 T-cell level of <200 cells/µL or <14% of T cells) labels the patient as having AIDS rather than merely being HIV-infected. The illnesses fall into three categories—unusual malignancies, opportunistic infections, and general debilitating

 TABLE 17.3. AIDS-Associated Diseases Defined by CDC[a]

Infections—frequently disseminated
  Fungal
    Candidiasis
    Cryptococcosis
    Histoplasmosis
    Coccidioidomycosis
    Cryptosporidiosis
  Parasitic
    Toxoplasmosis
    Pneumocystis
    Cryptosporidiosis
    Isosporiasis
  Bacterial
    Mycobacteriosis (including atypical)
    Salmonella
  Viral
    Cytomegalovirus (CMV)
    Herpes simplex virus
    Progressive mutifocal leukoencephalopathy

Neoplasms
  Sarcoma
    Kaposi's sarcoma
  Lymphoma
    Burkitt's lymphoma
    Diffuse large B-cell lymphoma
    Primary effusion lymphoma
    Primary CNS lymphoma
  Carcinoma
    Invasive cancer of uterine cervix

General conditions
  HIV encephalopathy and dementia
  Wasting syndrome
  CD4$^+$ T-cell count < 200/µL is AIDS defining

[a]Selected illnesses are discussed in the text.

syndromes—reflecting the primary effects of HIV on the immune system and CNS.

Several concurrent factors appear to initiate this symptomatic or crisis phase. The gradual drop in CD4$^+$ T cells eventually results in an ***immunodeficient state*** that leaves the individual susceptible to opportunistic infections, similar to patients with primary immunodeficiency syndromes and immunosuppressed transplant patients. ***Activation of virally-infected T cells*** by antigen results in stimulation of viral transcription and progeny formation. This leads to accelerated T-cell death, exacerbating the immunodeficient state. Rapid viral replication also increases the *viral mutation* rate, allowing the virus to escape from any remaining immune controls.

The patterns of AIDS-associated illnesses in an individual may partially reflect the mode of HIV transmission (sexual transmission vs. intravenous drug use). This is suggested by differences in the infections and malignancies seen among AIDS patients with different HIV exposures as well as the contrast between AIDS patients and other immunosuppressed individuals. Some individuals infected with HIV may be coinfected with other sexually transmitted organisms, some of which may lead to aggressive forms of cancer in the immunodeficient state of the patient. In fact, all of the malignancies seen in AIDS patients are believed to be caused by oncogenic DNA viruses. For instance, *human papillomavirus (HPV)* is associated with the development of cervical cancer in women. Exposure to HPV, combined with the individual's immunodeficient state, may be responsible for a markedly increased incidence and aggressiveness of *invasive cervical cancer* in HIV$^+$ women. The CDC includes invasive cervical cancer in the AIDS-associated malignancies.

The aggressive form of *Kaposi sarcoma (KS)* is virtually unique to AIDS patients, particularly male homosexuals, and may occur early in the course of the disease. KS is an abnormal proliferation of small blood vessels; in its usual form, it presents as a slow-growing tumor on the skin of the lower extremities of elderly men. *Human herpes virus 8 (HHV-8)* has been identified in KS from AIDS patients. This virus is also associated with an unusual form of aggressive lymphoma seen in AIDS patients called *primary effusion lymphoma*. Again, this malignancy is more common in male homosexual AIDS patients; some of them have the lymphoma and KS concurrently.

Aggressive *B-cell lymphomas*, mostly *EBV- associated lymphomas*, are seen at an incidence similar to that observed in immunosuppressed transplant patients. These lymphomas are usually *Burkitt* or *diffuse large B-cell lymphomas* (see below) and often involve sites outside the lymph nodes (extranodal). In AIDS patients, the CNS is a frequent site of primary lymphoma. Two other malignancies are not AIDS defining but have a more aggressive course in AIDS patients: squamous cell carcinoma of the head and neck region (also possibly associated with HPV) and atypical Hodgkin lymphoma.

The infectious diseases associated with AIDS reflect the inability of the patient's markedly depressed cell-mediated immune system to handle organisms that are normally nonpathogenic (opportunistic infections). As in any T-cell immunodeficient patient, *PCP* is a major infectious complication. *Candidiasis* is also frequently seen. Granuloma formation—a T-helper-cell-dependent function—is poor in these patients, leading to uncontrolled *mycobacterial infections*. *Mycobacterium avium*, not normally a human pathogen, can cause overwhelming infection. Cryptosporidia, *M. avium*, and CMV, among the most common organisms infecting the gastrointestinal tract in AIDS patients, can cause severe diarrhea. The CNS is susceptible to infection by *Cryptococcus, Toxoplasma*, and CMV.

The multiple infections cause continuous cell necrosis (death), a major feature of AIDS. The organisms and cell debris provide chronic antigenic stimulation to a deficient immune system. The B cells show evidence of responding to that stimulation; patients have polyclonal hypergammaglobulinemia (elevated serum Ig), circulating immune complexes, and markedly increased plasma cell production. In spite of this B-cell activity, patients are unable to mount an effective antibody response to newly encountered antigens, perhaps due to the T-cell defect; however, they also have particular difficulty with T-cell-independent responses to encapsulated organisms. In addition, B cells infected with EBV (normally eliminated by T cells) are susceptible to additional transforming events, resulting in the B-cell malignancies discussed above.

The CNS is infected with HIV, presumably via macrophage transport. The virus infects microglia cells (bone-marrow-derived cells in the same lineage as the macrophage), oligodendrocytes, and astrocytes. This may start the process, resulting in AIDS-related *dementia* and progressive *encephalopathy*. In total, up to 50% of AIDS patients show CNS symptoms and more than 70% have CNS changes at autopsy.

Finally, these patients suffer from *cachexia*, or wasting syndrome, to a degree much more severe than can be attributed to their concurrent illnesses. It is thought that HIV alters the cytokine profile of the macrophages to increase TNF production, leading to the development of extreme weight loss and fatigue.

The clinical course of AIDS has changed, at least for individuals in developed countries with access to medication. The first improvement was seen in the early, prophylactic, and aggressive treatment of infections, particularly PCP. Initially, most patients died early from infection. With the aggressive treatments, more began surviving long enough to develop the malignancies, which took prominence among AIDS patients in the 1990s. A second, more recent improvement was the introduction of multiple antiviral therapies, which prolong the chronic phase of HIV infection, thus delaying entry of the individual to full-blown AIDS (see below).

Prevention, Control, Diagnosis, and Therapy of HIV Infection

Prevention and control of HIV are best accomplished by avoiding unprotected contact with blood and body fluids from infected individuals. Education and public awareness of both what to avoid and what is safe (casual contact) are required to control the disease and to prevent possible panic.

All blood donations in the United States have been tested for antibodies to HIV since 1985. Because the development of an antibody response after exposure to HIV can take up to five weeks, this testing still leaves a long window of time period in which a recently infected individual might not be detected. Consequently, each blood donor is screened by an interview process and asked direct questions orally and in writing about high-risk behavior. Viremia following infection precedes the immune response; testing for viral RNA, which requires an amplification step, is very sensitive and has significantly decreased but not eliminated the window period. The HIV NAT (nucleic acid testing) can be set up to detect either proviral cDNA in WBCs or viral RNA in plasma. The latter also forms the basis for the quantitative viral load test (see below).

HIV$^+$ women who are pregnant are placed on antiviral therapy to decrease viral load and thereby diminish risk of transplacental transfer of virus. Cesarean sections are performed to eliminate infection during passage through the birth canal. Finally, exposure through breast milk is avoided.

For individuals accidentally exposed to infected products, therapy is administered as soon as possible after exposure to prevent establishment of infection.

Diagnosis of HIV infection is generally made by detection of antibodies to the viral particles by ELISA and confirmed by Western blot analysis, which detects antibodies to individual viral proteins (see Chapter 5). Patients are monitored by following their absolute CD4$^+$ T-cell count in the peripheral blood and monitoring viral titers by quantitative analysis of viral RNA (viral load). CD4 counts above 500/µL are not associated with opportunistic infections. The CDC has designated CD4 counts below 200/µL as an indicator of full-blown AIDS, making it one of the AIDS-defining criteria.

Therapy using azidothymidine (AZT), a nucleoside inhibitor of reverse transcriptase, was the first promising treatment for HIV infection. Protease inhibitors form a second class of therapeutic agents, and nonnucleoside reverse transcriptase inhibitors a third. Drug resistance to single agents develops rapidly, however, because HIV is capable of an amazing rate of spontaneous mutation during the course of infection in a single individual. The mutations arise from the lack of fidelity of the reverse transcriptase and RNA polymerase.

Individuals who are HIV-positive but asymptomatic are placed on **triple-agent antiviral therapy**, referred to as **highly active antiretroviral therapy (HAART)**. HAART combines three drugs from at least two of the inhibitor classes directed against HIV's reverse transcriptase and protease. It is hoped that the triple-agent therapy will delay the appearance of mutant strains. This therapy prevents infection of new cells; however, previously infected cells remain until they are lysed. After initiating therapy, the fall in viral titers is rapid and dramatic, but a small baseline titer almost always remains. As you might expect, discontinuation of the drugs for a prolonged period results in a resurgence of virus. Mutations may allow escape from control by these agents, so there is still a great need to develop an extensive arsenal of drugs to treat the disease. However, HAART, especially when initiated early, has changed the landscape of the AIDS epidemic in developed nations. HIV infection in individuals from those countries with access to the medications has gone from being a virtual death sentence to being a chronic disease. However, this glimmer of hope should not in any way minimize the seriousness of this infection. In addition, the therapy is not without side effects, including suppression of hematopoietic cells, nausea, and malaise. Long-term survivors are beginning to struggle with age-related diseases at younger ages and additional time is needed to evaluate how successful this approach truly is.

As discussed earlier, infections and other AIDS-associated diseases must also be treated; it was the successful institution of prophylactic treatment for infection that first led to extension of life span and improved quality of life.

Many infectious diseases have been controlled by vaccines, the most effective way of preventing the spread of infection through a population. Vaccines induce a long-lasting immune response prior to exposure to the infectious agent (Chapter 20). The development of a vaccine for HIV presents serious challenges, however. First, we do not yet know which effector arm of the immune system—antibody, CTL, and so on—needs to be boosted to mount a response that will eliminate the virus on entry into the organism. HIV escapes eradication despite both antibody and cytotoxic T-cell responses in recently infected individuals. Second, the ability of the virus to "hide out" in reservoir cells and its high mutation rate are major problems that need to be overcome for vaccination to be effective. Third, the availability of animal models, in which candidate vaccines for other infectious diseases are tested extensively, is limited due to their lack of susceptibility to infection by HIV. The best model is the simian monkey, which develops a disease similar to AIDS after infection with simian immunodeficiency virus (SIV). Lastly, testing of vaccines in humans presents a host of ethical problems. An understanding of the molecular biology and structure of all components of HIV throughout its life cycle will be essential to development of a safe vaccine.

NEOPLASMS OF LYMPHOID SYSTEM

A common theme throughout this chapter has been the idea that dysregulation of the immune system can result in the emergence of neoplasms, particularly neoplasms of lymphoid cells. This is true for patients with primary immunodeficiency diseases and AIDS as well as immunosuppressed transplant patients (see also Chapter 19). In these circumstances, the malignancies are most often aggressive B-cell lymphomas, frequently associated with EBV infection. Although malignant transformation of any element of the immune system can occur in the absence of clinically apparent immunodeficiency, when tumors are analyzed at the molecular level, dysregulation intrinsic to the malignant cells or imposed upon them by the environment becomes obvious. In this section, we first describe general concepts of lymphoid neoplasms followed by specific examples of important types.

Referring to a malignancy as a *leukemia* implies that the malignant cells are predominantly present in the circulation and/or bone marrow. A *lymphoma* presents as a solid mass in the lymph nodes, spleen, thymus, or extranodal organs. Sometimes the same malignant cell type can show either presentation (*leukemia/lymphoma*).

In 1996, the World Health Organization (WHO) recommended a classification system based on cell of origin (B vs. T/NK cell) and stage of differentiation [immature (precursor) vs. mature (peripheral)] (Table 17.4). These tumors are considered outgrowths of a transformed lymphoid cell that appears frozen in development. They have the same surface markers and many of the same properties as the corresponding normal cells at that developmental stage. However, the malignant cells may not continue to mature, may accumulate in large numbers, and all originate from a single clone (in other words, they are *monoclonal*). They will occupy the same sites or traffic in the same pattern as their normal counterparts—for example, bone marrow for immature B cells, thymus for immature T cells—until they spill over into additional locations.

Southern blot analysis of DNA extracted from B- or T-cell neoplasms shows a single band for the Ig genes and TCR genes, respectively. This demonstrates that all the tumor cells have the same rearrangement of these genes and establishes the monoclonality of that lymphoid growth. For some lymphoid neoplasms, a unique molecular abnormality has been identified, which may contribute to the transformation of that cell. These molecular changes are also incorporated into the classification scheme. Since the WHO classification is based on cell of origin rather than clinical presentation, leukemias are no longer designated separately from lymphomas if they are derived from the same malignant cell type. The WHO grouping makes practical sense, because the treatment is often based on the malignant cell type.

B-Cell Neoplasms

***Precursor B-Cell Lymphoblastic Leukemia/
Lymphoma.*** B-cell acute lymphoblastic leukemias

TABLE 17.4. World Health Organization Classification for Lymphoid Neoplasms[a]

B-Cell Neoplasms

**Precursor B-cell lymphoblastic
    leukemia/lymphoma**

Mature B-cell neoplasms

Chronic lymphocytic leukemia/small
    lymphocytic lymphoma/prolymphocytic leukemia

Follicular lymphoma

Mantle cell lymphoma

Marginal-zone lymphoma of mucosa-associated lymphoid tissue (MALT) type

    mucosa-associated lymphoid tissue (MALT) type

Nodal marginal-zone lymphoma

Splenic marginal-zone lymphoma

Hairy cell leukemia

Diffuse large B-cell lymphoma (including subtypes:
    mediastinal, primary effusion, intravascular)

Burkitt's lymphoma

Plasma cell myeloma

Lymphoplasmacytic lymphoma

**B-cell proliferations of uncertain malignant
    potential**

Lymphomatoid granulomatosis

Post-transplant lymphoproliferative disorders

T/NK cell neoplasms

**Precursor T-cell lymphoblastic
    leukemia/lymphoma**

Mature T-cell/NK-cell neoplasms (selected)

T-cell large granular lymphocytic leukemia

NK-cell leukemia

Peripheral T-cell lymphoma (unspecified)

Mycosis fungoides

Sezary syndrome

Primary cutaneous anaplastic large-cell lymphoma

Systemic anaplastic large-cell lymphoma

Extranodal NK/T-cell lymphoma, nasal type

Intestinal T-cell lymphoma

Hepatosplenic γδ T-cell lymphoma

Adult T-cell leukemia/lymphoma

Hodgkin lymphoma

Nodular lymphocyte predominant Hodgkin lymphoma

Classical Hodgkin lymphoma

Nodular sclerosis

Mixed cellularity

Classical, lymphocyte rich

Lymphocyte depleted

[a]Selected neoplasms are discussed in the text.

(B-ALLs) correspond to the pro-B-, pre-B-, or immature B-cell stages of development as demonstrated by the expression of surface CD markers along with the extent of Ig gene rearrangement and protein expression in the individual patient's leukemia cells (Fig. 17.9). The malignant cells may express the blast or stem cell marker CD34 (particularly pro-B cells) and will express CD10 and CD19, which are early B-cell markers. Similar to the normal pro-B or pre-pre-B cell and pre-B cell, corresponding B-ALLs express terminal deoxynucleotidyl transferase (TdT) in the nucleus. The expression of this enzyme, normally required to rearrange the Ig genes (and TCR genes), reflects the fact that B-ALL cells are in the process of gene rearrangement. These cells do not yet express a complete Ig molecule on their surfaces and

have only cytoplasmic μ chains if at the pre-B-cell stage. Chemotherapy has been successful in treating children with these leukemias.

Mature B-Cell Neoplasms.

Burkitt's Lymphoma/Leukemia. Burkitt's may present as a leukemia or lymphoma; both forms are characterized by a translocation that places the ***c-myc oncogene*** next to either the Ig H-chain gene or one of the two L-chain genes [t(8;14), t(8;22), or t(2,8)] (Fig. 17.10). The c-*myc* protein is normally involved in activating genes for cell proliferation when a resting cell receives a signal to divide. Translocation to the Ig genes leads to increased expression of c-*myc* and increased cell proliferation. Antigenic stimulation of the B cell may possibly initiate

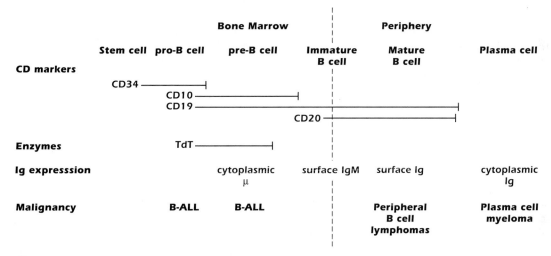

Figure 17.9. Correlation of B-cell development with B-cell malignancies.

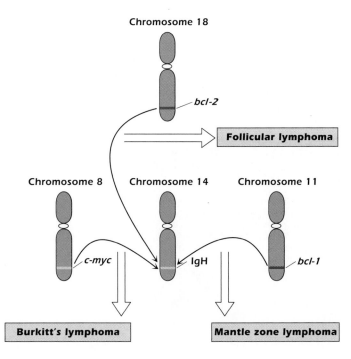

Figure 17.10. Some B-cell neoplasms associated with translocations of genes to chromosomal locus encoding Ig H-chain gene on chromosome 14.

overexpression of c-*myc*, now under the control of the Ig gene.

In equatorial Africa, this lymphoma is endemic in children and is associated with EBV infection of the B cells. Burkitt's lymphoma is one of the malignancies seen in patients immunosuppressed medically or with AIDS. In these patients, the EBV genome is sometimes but not always found in the lymphoma cells.

Follicular Lymphoma.   The normal cell counterpart of follicular lymphomas is the B cell of the germinal center (Fig. 17.11). As described in Chapter 7, B cells stimulated by antigen enter a primary follicle, generating a germinal center. The B cells may respond by proliferating and undergoing affinity maturation, by Ig isotype switching, and by differentiating into memory or plasma cells. If their antibody is a poor match for that antigen or of low affinity, the cell undergoes *apoptosis* or cell death. In follicular lymphomas, the *bcl-2 gene*, which produces a protein that interferes with apoptosis, is translocated to the Ig H-chain gene [t(14;18)] (see Fig. 17.10). This results in continuous expression of bcl-2 protein, preventing death of the cells. In fact, these B-cell neoplasms have a low rate of proliferation and a long chronic clinical course. They display the phenotype (surface CD markers) of normal follicular center B cells: CD19$^+$, CD20$^+$, CD10$^+$, and surface Ig.

Follicular Lymphoma

Mantle Cell Lymphoma.   The normal germinal center is surrounded by a collar of small, quiescent B cells that have not responded to antigen (see Fig. 17.11). A neoplasm of these mantle zone cells has the same B-cell phenotype as its normal counterpart: CD19$^+$, CD20$^+$, CD5$^+$, and sIgM. The majority of mantle cell lymphomas demonstrate overexpression of *cyclin D1* protein, usually, but not always

the result of the translocation of the *bcl-1 gene* to the Ig H-chain gene [t(11;14)] (see Fig. 17.10). Cyclin D1 is normally responsible for promoting cell cycle progression from G$_1$ to S phase, leading to cell division. Mantle cell lymphoma has a higher proliferative rate and a more aggressive course than follicular lymphomas.

Marginal-Zone Lymphoma.   Marginal-zone lymphomas commonly arise in MALT and are often associated with chronic antigenic stimulation or autoimmune disease. For example, chronic *Helicobacter pylori* infection of the stomach may lead to the development of gastric lymphoma, which is thus preventable by antibiotic treatment. Patients with autoimmune thyroiditis (*Hashimoto thyroiditis*) and autoimmune disease of the salivary glands (*Sjögren's syndrome*) have a high incidence of B-cell lymphoma development in the affected organ.

The association between autoimmune disease or infection and lymphoma suggests two interesting hypotheses which are not mutually exclusive. First, chronic antigenic stimulation, particularly in response to a limited number of epitopes, provides fertile ground for the development of a B-cell lymphoma. B cells may be particularly vulnerable to developing transforming mutations as they continue to undergo somatic mutation of their Ig genes in response to stimulation. The second hypothesis is that a defect in the regulation of the B cells, whether intrinsic or due to lack of T-cell down-regulation, leads to both autoimmune disease and, eventually, lymphoma.

As described earlier in this section, the malignant cells of the immune system follow the trafficking patterns of their normal counterparts. Marginal-zone lymphomas of MALT remain localized for a prolonged period and then follow the circulatory pattern for normal MALT cells, traveling to other MALT sites in the body.

Chronic Lymphocytic Leukemia/Small Lymphocytic Lymphoma.   Chronic lymphocytic leukemia (CLL) or small lymphocytic lymphoma (SLL) was originally thought to be a malignant transformation of a subset of B

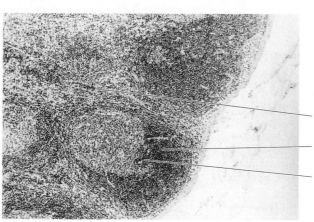

Sites of:

T-cell lymphomas (CLL/SLL)

Mantle cell lymphomas

Follicular lymphomas

Figure 17.11. Section through normal lymph node showing sites that become involved by T- and B-cell lymphomas. CLL/SLL, mantle cell lymphoma, and follicular lymphoma are all B cell derived.

cells known as B-1 cells (see Chapter 7). In some patients, it presents first with a leukemic picture, with blood and bone marrow involvement (CLL); in others it presents first in the lymph nodes (SLL) (see Fig. 17.11). Similar to B-1 cells, CLL/SLL cells express the mature B-cell markers sIgM, CD19, and CD20, as well as CD5. A subgroup has hypermutated Ig genes, suggesting post-germinal center origin and therefore the transformation of a different B-cell subset than B-1.

Chronic Lymphocytic Leukemia/Small Lymphocytic Lymphoma

Most CLL cases (>65%) have a deletion in chromosome 13 at q14.3. This region codes, not for a protein, but for microRNA (miRNA 15 and 16), which has the normal function of down-regulating the mRNA for *bcl-2*. Therefore, CLL cells often have overexpression of *bcl-2* as the result of posttranscriptional control.

CLL is the most common leukemia in North America and Western Europe and is seen mostly in older individuals. These patients are extremely susceptible to infection, suggesting that their nonmalignant cells are not functioning properly. Autoimmune antibodies are common, particularly against RBCs, resulting in autoimmune hemolytic anemia. The antibodies may be produced by the malignant clone or, more often, by nontransformed B cells. The association of this autoimmune condition with a leukemia/lymphoma again suggests that a lymphoid neoplasm arises in the setting of immune dysregulation or causes it. CLL has a long clinical course, but eventually there is massive involvement of every organ, peripheral blood, and bone marrow.

Diffuse Large B-Cell Lymphoma. The diffuse large B-cell lymphomas are a heterogeneous group of lymphomas that may arise *de novo* at a single site, may progress from one of the above-described slow-growing lymphomas (such as follicular lymphoma), or may be a consequence of a poorly controlled transforming viral infection (EBV or HHSV8) in immunosuppressed individuals. In all cases, the cells generally express the B-cell markers CD19 and CD20 and surface Ig.

Historically, the behavior of the *de novo* diffuse large B-cell lymphomas has been unpredictable. Gene expression microarray analysis (see Chapter 5) has divided the lymphomas into two major groups based on their gene activation patterns and has demonstrated a correlation between these two groups and response to therapy. Those lymphomas with gene expression profiles similar to germinal center B cells had a much better response and prognosis than those with gene expression profiles resembling that of activated or immunoblastic B cells. Similarly, two subgroups could be delineated based on having a translocation or mutation of the *bcl-6* gene.

These genetic alterations result in this protein's continued expression. The *bcl-6* gene codes for a transcriptional regulator that normally represses the set of genes required for plasma cell differentiation and maintains the transcription of genes that allow the B cell to continue as a B cell in the germinal center (i.e., undergo further affinity maturation and isotype switching). Lymphoma patients showing mutations or translocations of *bcl-6*, have a better prognosis as compared with those with other B-cell lymphomas.

The association of EBV infection with diffuse large B-cell lymphomas and Burkitt's lymphoma in immuno-suppressed patients illustrates the consequences of a breakdown in the immune system's ability to regulate aberrant cell growth. EBV infection of B cells (via the EBV receptor CD21) leads to polyclonal B-cell proliferation. In healthy individuals, these expanded EBV-infected B cells are removed by the body's CTLs (see Chapter 10). In situations in which T cells are lacking, the infected B cells continue to expand; some may acquire even more mutations, such as *c-myc* translocation, that lead to transformation, independent growth, and the accumulation of additional mutations. For patients on immunosuppressive therapy with an atypical B-cell proliferation, it is still possible to prevent the development of lymphoma by withdrawing the immunosuppressive treatment and allowing the body's immune system to handle the abnormal proliferation. Of course, this option is not possible in AIDS patients.

Plasma Cell Neoplasms. Neoplastic growths of plasma cells may occur at a single site, resulting in a ***plasmacytoma***. If they occur at multiple sites, predominantly throughout the bone, they are called ***multiple myeloma*** or ***plasma cell myeloma***. Similar to normal plasma cells, IL-6 functions as an autocrine growth factor for myeloma cells.

Plasma Cell Neoplasms

The neoplastic plasma cells may continue to synthesize and secrete their Ig product. In many cases, this secreted monoclonal protein causes more difficulties for the patient than the malignant cells themselves. Light-chain deposits called ***amyloid*** can cause organ failure, especially in the kidneys. As described in Chapter 4, excretion in the urine of free light chains derived from multiple myeloma patients—***Bence Jones proteins***—led to an early understanding of Ig light-chain structure.

The monoclonal product of myeloma cells is detected in the serum and sometimes in the urine as a spike, known as an M spike in the γ region of an electrophoretic evaluation (see Fig. 4.1). A spike, rather than a broad band, forms because all the immunoglobulins are identical and migrate to the same place by size and charge (see Chapter 5). Most cases produce monoclonal IgG; IgA is the next most frequent Ig isotype found. The levels of all other normal immunoglobulins are severely decreased in these patients, who are immunosuppressed with respect to antibody production and therefore susceptible to infection. Before the appearance of full-blown myeloma, patients may have a small amount of monoclonal Ig in their serum for many years. Many individuals remain at this stage, never progressing to disease. Small M spikes may also be found in association with other lymphoid neoplasms, such as CLL, or even with nonmalignant conditions.

Lymphoplasmacytic Lymphoma (Waldenström's macroglobulinemia). Lymphoplasmacytic lymphoma/ Waldenström's macroglobulinemia is a neoplasm of a single clone of B cells; the microscopic appearance of the clone is a mixture of lymphocytes, plasma cells, and something in between—lymphoplasmacytoid cells. The neoplastic cells involve the lymph nodes, bone marrow, and spleen. Although uncommon, these lymphomas are of interest to immunologists because they overproduce and secrete monoclonal IgM, thus making it accessible for study. The large size and high concentration of the IgM in the blood may combine to slow blood flow and clog vessels (hyperviscosity syndrome). In some patients, the IgM has an abnormal structure, causing it to precipitate in the cold (cryoglobulin); this results in circulatory problems in the patient's extremities (fingers and toes).

T-Cell Neoplasms

Precursor T-Cell Acute Lymphoblastic Leukemia/ Lymphoma. Precursor T-cell acute lymphoblastic

leukemia/lymphoma (T-ALL) is a neoplasm of immature T cells with characteristics identical to those of thymocytes frozen in their immature state. As Figure 17.12 shows, T-ALLs express the pan-T markers CD2, CD5, and CD7, which appear early in T-cell development in the thymus. Some T-ALLs have the characteristics of immature or early thymocytes and do not express CD4 or CD8 (they are double negative). Most T-ALLs are slightly more mature, expressing both CD4 and CD8 (double positive) but little or no CD3 on their surface, similar to common thymocytes. These cells have not yet completed rearrangement of their TCR genes and still express TdT. T-ALL presents as a leukemia or as a thymic mass. Treatment has not been as successful as for B-ALL.

Mature T-Cell Neoplasms. Peripheral T-cell lymphomas have varied presentations. They are found wherever T cells normally migrate—namely, skin, lung, vessel wall, gastrointestinal tract, and lymph nodes. They also retain some of the functions of normal mature T cells; consequently, cytokine production by the neoplastic cells results in a background of inflammatory cells, including eosinophils, plasma cells, and macrophages. Peripheral T-cell lymphomas usually have a more aggressive course than B-cell lymphomas. Two will be highlighted here: cutaneous T-cell lymphoma and adult T-cell leukemia/lymphoma.

Cutaneous T-Cell Lymphoma. When confined to the skin, this cutaneous T-cell lymphoma is still known by its historical name, ***mycosis fungoides***, because patients were originally believed to have a chronic fungal infection of the skin that waxed and waned over many years. We now understand that the skin disease is due to infiltration of the

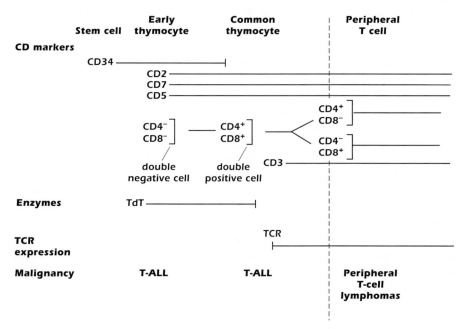

Figure 17.12. Correlation of T-cell development with T-cell malignancies.

epidermis by malignant CD4$^+$ T cells. Eventually, the cells may spread to the lymph nodes and even into the blood. These malignant T cells in the circulation are called Sezary cells, and the patient is said to have **Sezary syndrome**.

Adult T-Cell Leukemia/Lymphoma. Adult T-cell leukemia/lymphoma (ATLL) is an aggressive T-cell neoplasm that was described in the 1970s in a region of Japan, where it is endemic. It is also found in the Caribbean, parts of central Africa, and a small region of the southeast United States. ATLL is a neoplasm of mature, usually CD4$^+$ T cells. IL-2 is an autocrine growth factor for these cells. In early attempts at treatment, the neoplasm was found to respond temporarily—for a few months—to administration of an antibody (known as anti-Tac) specific for the α chain of the IL-2 receptor (CD25).

ATLL is caused by the retrovirus HTLV-1, which was described and isolated before recognition of AIDS and HIV. The proviral genomic structure is similar to HIV, containing an LTR and coding for structural and regulatory proteins as well as viral enzymes, reverse transcriptase, integrase, and protease. Tax, the viral protein that transactivates HTLV-1 transcription by binding to the LTR region, also activates host genes, including those coding for IL-2, IL-2R α chain, and a parathyroid-like hormone (not normally expressed by T cells). Therefore, activation of proviral transcription is associated with activation and proliferation of host T cells. Patients with ATLL frequently have extreme elevations in serum calcium levels as a result of the increased synthesis of the parathyroid-like hormone.

Transmission of HTLV-1 is similar to that of HIV; it is acquired through contact with blood and body fluids, with more efficient transfer through breast milk. Thus, many patients are infected with HTLV-1 during infancy. The incubation period of this virus is long, typically 20–40 years. The virus primarily infects the CD4$^+$ T-cell subset and also infects the nervous system. A subset of patients presents with neurologic disease.

Fortunately, only a very low proportion (approximately 1%) of infected patients develop ATLL. The trigger for the development of disease after so many years is unknown. The CD4$^+$ T cells harbor the virus in a quiescent state. Unlike HIV, the virus is not cytolytic for these cells once activated. To the contrary, HTLV-1 leads to transformation and continuous proliferation of the T cells. Once a patient is diagnosed with ATLL, survival is generally 6–12 months. Blood supplies in the United States and the United Kingdom are screened for this virus.

Hodgkin Lymphoma

Hodgkin lymphoma is characterized by the presence of relatively small numbers of large, binucleate malignant cells called Reed–Sternberg cells (described below) in a reactive background of small T cells, eosinophils, plasma cells, macrophages, and fibroblasts. This reactive milieu is the result of abundant cytokine production, particularly IL-5, by the tumor cells and/or background cells. Patients show clinical signs of increased cytokine production: fever, night sweats, and weight loss. Characteristically, these patients demonstrated evidence of depressed cell-mediated immune responses with no DTH reaction to common test antigens and increased susceptibility to viral and parasitic infections.

The lineage origin of the Reed–Sternberg cell, which expresses no lineage-specific markers and is characterized by the expression of only CD15 and CD30, was the subject of much debate. Recent studies applying molecular techniques to analysis of single malignant cells have shown rearrangements in the Ig genes, supporting a B-cell origin. The finding of hypermutation in those Ig genes suggests that the Reed–Sternberg cell derives from a post-germinal center B cell. Although the malignant cell has been identified as a B cell (and is large), this lymphoma behaves differently from large B-cell lymphomas and is therefore classified separately. Lymphomas overall are grouped as Hodgkin versus non-Hodgkin lymphomas.

Immunotherapy

The expanding knowledge of lymphoma biology combined with the technical advances in monoclonal antibody and protein production has led to the development of a new generation of treatment options. Currently, chimeric and humanized monoclonal antibodies directed against CD20, in particular, are widely used for the treatment of B-cell lymphomas. These antibodies are generally used alone ("cold"), causing tumor cell elimination by opsonization of antibody-coated cells. Additional agents to block cytokines or cytokine receptors, which stimulate the proliferation of malignant cells, are being combined with conventional chemotherapy. Conventional chemotherapies, which are largely nonspecific agents, kill all dividing cells. The technology used in developing these new specific therapies is also widely applicable to drug development for the treatment of autoimmune diseases and nonlymphoid cancers, such as breast cancer.

The immune system normally works as a finely tuned network, responding to foreign invaders, causing no harm to itself, and returning to a more quiescent state (but with memory) once the threat is over. Eliminating, chronically stimulating, or allowing uncontrolled growth of any single component perturbs the remaining elements. Thus, without proper regulation of the network, the occurrence of any one of the major categories of disorders—immunodeficiency, autoimmune disease, or lymphoid neoplasm—allows the emergence of one or both of the other two disease types.

SUMMARY

1. Immunodeficiency disorders are referred to as primary when the deficiency is the cause of disease and secondary when the deficiency is a result of other diseases or the effects of treatment regimens.

2. Immunodeficiency diseases may be due to disorders in the development or function of B cells, T cells, phagocytic cells, or components of complement.

3. Immunodeficiency disorders predispose patients to recurrent infections. The type of infection that develops is sometimes characteristic of the particular arm of the immune system that is deficient. Defects in humoral immunity lead to increased susceptibility to bacterial infections; in cell-mediated immunity, to viral and fungal infections; in phagocytic cells, to pyogenic organisms; and in complement components, to bacterial infections and autoimmunity.

4. Immune deficiencies constitute one type of defect or disorder of the immune system. Other aspects of such disorders are the unregulated proliferation of B or T lymphocytes, the overproduction of lymphocyte or phagocytic cell products, and the unregulated activation of complement components. This may account for the association of immune deficiencies with autoimmune disease and malignancies.

5. HIV causes a massive immunosuppressive illness known as AIDS by infecting and killing CD4$^+$ T lymphocytes.

6. Lymphoid neoplasms are uncontrolled monoclonal proliferations that can be related to their normal cell counterparts by surface markers and stage of differentiation. Many lymphoid neoplasms have specific chromosomal translocations, causing dysregulation of cell proliferation and death. Some are associated with viral infections such as EBV and HTLV-1, acting as either growth promoters or oncogenic viruses.

REFERENCES

Ammann AJ (1994): Mechanisms of immunodeficiency. In Stites DP, Terr Al, Parslow TG (eds): *Basic and Clinical Immunology*, 8th ed. East Norwalk, CT: Appleton & Lange.

Anderson DC, Springer TA (1987): Leukocyte adhesion deficiency: An inherited defect in Mac-1, LFA-1, and p150, 95 glycoproteins. *Annu Rev Med* 38:175.

Bacchelli C, Buckridge S, Thrasher A, Gaspar HB (2007): Translational minireview series on immunodeficiency: Molecular defects in common variable immunodeficiency. *Clin Exp Immun* 149:401–409.

Baltimore D, Feinberg MB (1989): HIV revealed: Towards a natural history of the infection. *N Engl J Med* 132:1673.

Berger EA, Murphy PM, Farber JM (1999): Chemokine receptors as HIV-1 coreceptors: Roles in viral entry, tropism and disease. *Annu Rev Immunol* 17:657.

Buckley RH (2004): Molecular defects in human severe combined immunodeficiency and approaches to immune reconstitution. *Ann Rev Immunol* 22:625–655.

Cavazzana-Calvo M, Hacein-Bay S, de Saint Basile G, De Coene F, Selz F, Le Deist F, Fischer A (1996): Role of interleukin-2 (IL-2), IL-7, and IL-15 in natural killer cell differentiation from cord blood hematopoietic progenitor cells and from γc transduced severe combined immunodeficiency X1 bone marrow cells. *Blood* 88:3901–3909.

Chiorazzi N, Ferrarini M (2003): B cell chronic lymphocytic leukemia: Lessons learned from studies of the B cell antigen receptor. *Annu Rev Immunol* 21:841–894.

Cicardi M, Zingale L, Zanichelli A, Deliliers DL (2007): Established and new treatments for hereditary angioedema: An update. *Mol Immunol* 44:3858–3861.

Cimmino A, Calin GA, Fabbri M, Iorio MV, Ferracin M, Shimizu M, Wojcik SE, Aqeilan RI, Zupo S, Dono M, Rassenti L, Alder H, Volinia S, Liu CG, Kipps TJ, Negrini M, Croce CM (2005): MiR-15 and miR-16 induce apoptosis by targeting BCL2. *Proc Natl Acad Sci USA* 102:13944–13949.

Clerici M, Shearer GM (1994): The T_H1-T_H2 hypothesis of HIV infection: New insights. *Immunol Today* 14:107.

Cunningham-Rundles C, Ponda PP (2005): Molecular defects in T- and B-cell primary immunodeficiency diseases. *Nature Rev Immunol* 5:880–892.

Espeli M, Rossi B, Mancini SJC, Roche P, Gaunthier L, Schiff C (2006): Initiation of pre-B cell receptor signaling: Common and distinctive features in human and mouse. *Sem Immunol* 18:56–66.

Fahey JL (1993): Update on AIDS. *Immunologist* 1:131.

Fauci AS (1993): Multifactorial nature of human immunodeficiency virus disease: Implications for therapy. *Science* 262:1011.

Geier JK, Schlissel MS (2006): Pre-BCR signals and the control of Ig gene rearrangements. *Sem Immunol* 18:31–39.

Green WC (1993): AIDS and the immune system. *Sci Am* (Sept):99.

Hazenberg MD, Hamann D, Schuitemaker H, Miedema F (2000): T-cell depletion in HIV-1 infection: How CD4$^+$ T cells go out of stock. *Nature Immunol* 1:285.

Helbert MR, Lage-Stehr J, Mitchison NA (1993): Antigen presentation, loss of immunologic memory and AIDS. *Immunol Today* 14:340.

Jaffe ES, Harris NL, Stein H, Vardiman JW (eds) (2001): *World Health Organization Classification of Tumours. Pathology and Genetics of Tumours of Haematopoietic and Lymphoid Tissues.* Lyon, France: IARC Press.

Jain A, Ma CA, Liu S, Brown M, Cohen J, Strober W (2001): Specific missense mutations in NEMO result in hyper-IgM syndrome with hypohydrotic ectodermal dysplasia. *Nature Immunol* 2:223–228.

Kawakami Y, Kitaura J, Hata D, Yao L, Kawakami, T (1999): Functions of Bruton's tyrosine kinase in mast and B cells. *J Leukocyte Biol* 65:286–290.

Kohler H, Muller S, Nara P (1994): Deceptive imprinting in the immune response against HIV-1. *Immunol Today* 15:475.

Lusso P, Gallo RC (1995): Human herpes virus 6 in AIDS. *Immunol Today* 16:67.

McLean-Tooke A, Spickett GP, Gennery AR (2007): Immunodeficiency and autoimmunity in 22q11.2 deletion syndrome. *Scand J Immunol* 66:1–7.

Nomura K, Kanegane H, Karasuyama H, Tsukada S, Agematsu K, Murakami G, Sakazume S, Sako M, Tanaka R, Kuniya Y, Komeno T, Ishihara S, Hayashi K, Kishimoto T, Miyawaki T (2000): Genetic defect in human X-linked agammaglobulinemia impedes a maturational evolution of pro-B cells into a later stage of pre-B cells in the B-cell differentiation pathway. *Blood* 96:610–617.

Ochs HD, Smith CIE, Puck JM (2007): *Primary Immunodeficiency Diseases.* New York: Oxford University Press.

Orkin SH (1989): Molecular genetics of chronic granulomatous disease. *Annu Rev Immunol* 7:277.

Quartier P, Bustamamente J, Sanai O, Plebani A, Debre M, Deville A, Litzman J, Levy J, Fermand JP, Lane P, Horneff G, Aksu G, Yakin I, Davies G, Texcan I, Ersoy F, Catalan N, Imai K, Fischer A, Durandy A (2004): Clinical immunologic and genetic analysis of 29 patients with autosomal recessive hyper-IgM syndrome due to activation-induced cytidine deaminase deficiency. *Clin Immunol* 110:22–29.

Rosenberg ZF, Fauci AS (1990): Immunopathogenic mechanisms of HIV infection: Cytokine induction of HIV expression. *Immunol Today* 11:176.

Snapper SB, Rosen FS (1999): The Wiskott-Aldrich Syndrome Protein (WASP): Roles in signalling and cytoskeletal organization. *Annu Rev Immunol* 17:905.

Straus SE, Sneller M, Lenardo MJ, Puck JM, Strober W (1999): An inherited disorder of lymphocyte apoptosis: The autoimmune lymphoproliferative syndrome. *Ann Intern Med* 130:591–601.

Wamatz K, Denz A, Dräger R, Braun M, Groth C, Wolff-Vorbeck G, Eibel H, Schlesier M, Peter HH (2002): Severe deficiency of switched memory B cells (CD27^{+1}IgM$^-$IgD$^-$) in subgroups of patients with common variable immunodeficiency: A new approach to classify a heterogeneous disease. *Blood* 99:1544–1551.

Zhu Y, Nonoyama S, Morio T, Muramatsu M, Honjo T, Mizutani S (2003): Type two hyper-IgM syndrome caused by mutation in activation-induced cytidine deaminase. *J Med Dent Sci* 50:41–46.

REVIEW QUESTIONS

For each question, choose the ONE BEST answer.

1. An eight-month-old baby has a history of repeated Gram-positive bacterial infections. The most probable cause for this condition is:
   A) The mother did not confer sufficient immunity to the baby *in utero*.
   B) The baby suffers from erythroblastosis fetalis (hemolytic disease of the newborn).
   C) The baby has a defect in the alternative complement pathway.
   D) The baby is allergic to the mother's milk.
   E) None of the above.

2. A 50-year-old worker at an atomic plant who previously had a sample of his own bone marrow cryopreserved was accidentally exposed to a minimal lethal dose of radiation. He was subsequently transplanted with his own bone marrow. This individual can expect to:
   A) have recurrent bacterial infections
   B) have serious fungal infections due to deficiency in cell-mediated immunity
   C) make antibody responses to thymus-independent antigens only
   D) all of the above
   E) none of the above

3. Which of the following immune deficiency disorders is associated exclusively with an abnormality of the humoral immune response?
   A) X-linked agammaglobulinemia (Bruton's agammaglobulinemia)
   B) DiGeorge syndrome
   C) Wiskott–Aldrich syndrome
   D) chronic mucocutaneous candidiasis
   E) ataxia telangiectasia

4. A sharp increase in levels of IgG with a spike in the IgG region seen in the electrophoretic pattern of serum proteins is an indication of:
   A) IgA or IgM deficiency
   B) plasma cell myeloma
   C) macroglobulinemia
   D) hypogammaglobulinemia
   E) severe fungal infections

5. Patients with DiGeorge syndrome may fail to produce IgG in response to immunization with T-dependent antigens because:
   A) They have a decreased number of B cells that produce IgG.
   B) They have increased numbers of suppressor T cells.
   C) They have a decreased number of T helper cells.
   D) They have abnormal antigen-presenting cells.
   E) They cannot produce IgM during primary responses.

6. A two-year-old child has had three episodes of pneumonia and two episodes of otitis media. All the infections were demonstrated to be pneumococcal. Which of the following disorders is most likely to be the cause?
   A) an isolated transient T-cell deficiency
   B) a combined T- and B-cell deficiency
   C) a B-cell deficiency
   D) transient anemia
   E) AIDS

7. A healthy woman gave birth to a baby. The newborn infant was found to be HIV-seropositive. This finding is most likely the result of:
   A) the virus being transferred across the placenta to the baby
   B) the baby's making anti-HIV antibodies
   C) the baby's erythrocyte antigens cross-reacting with the virus
   D) the mother's erythrocyte antigens cross-reacting with the virus

   E) maternal HIV-specific IgG being transferred across the placenta to the baby

8. Immunodeficiency disease can result from a:
   A) developmental defect of T lymphocytes
   B) developmental defect of bone marrow stem cells
   C) defect in phagocyte function
   D) defect in complement function
   E) all of the above

9. A nine-month-old baby was vaccinated against smallpox with attenuated smallpox virus. He developed a progressive necrotic lesion of the skin, muscles, and subcutaneous tissue at the site of inoculation. The vaccination reaction probably resulted from:
   A) B-lymphocyte deficiency
   B) reaction to the adjuvant
   C) complement deficiency
   D) T-cell deficiency
   E) B- and T-lymphocyte deficiency

10. The most common clinical consequence(s) of C3 deficiency is (are):
    A) increased incidence of tumors
    B) increased susceptibility to viral infections
    C) increased susceptibility to fungal infections
    D) increased susceptibility to bacterial infections
    E) all of the above

ANSWERS TO REVIEW QUESTIONS

1. *E* None of these is likely to be the underlying cause for the history. The baby is probably hypogammaglobulinemic. Hypogammaglobulinemia leads to recurrent bacterial infections. Viral and fungal infections are controlled by cell-mediated immunity, which is normal in hypogammaglobulinemic individuals. Answer A is incorrect because the mother's IgG, which passed through the placenta, would have a half-life of 23 days, and would therefore not be expected to remain in the baby's circulation for 8 months. At this age, any Ig present in the baby's circulation is synthesized by the baby. Answer B is irrelevant, since erythroblastosis fetalis is caused by the destruction of the newborn's Rh+ erythrocytes by the Rh− mother's antibodies to Rh antigen. Answer C is unlikely since the classical complement pathway would still be protective; a defect in the alternative pathway would not result in the selective inability to protect from only Gram-positive bacterial infections. Answer D is incorrect because, even if allergic to the mother's milk, the baby should not suffer from increased frequency of bacterial infections.

2. *E* The autologous bone marrow cells, which contain stem cells, will replicate, differentiate, and repopulate the hematopoietic-reticuloendothelial system, rendering the individual immunologically normal. Thus the individual is not expected to have bacterial, viral, or fungal infections or to respond to antigens differently from a normal individual.

3. *A* The only immunodeficiency disorder that is associated with an abnormality exclusively of the humoral response is X-linked (Bruton's) agammaglobulinemia. DiGeorge syndrome results from thymic aplasia, in which there is a deficiency in T cells that influence IgG responses, which require T helper cells. Wiskott–Aldrich syndrome is associated with several abnormalities. Ataxia telangiectasia is a disease with defects in both cellular and humoral immune responses, with T-cell-dependent areas of lymphoid tissues the most severely affected. Chronic mucocutaneous candidiasis is a poorly defined collection of syndromes associated with a selective defect in the functioning of T cells.

4. *B* This pattern is characteristic of plasma cell myeloma (IgG myeloma). Plasma cell myeloma may be recognized by the synthesis of large amounts of homogeneous antibody of any one isotype. Although patients with plasma cell myeloma may suffer from a decreased synthesis of other Ig isotypes, the electrophoretic pattern is not necessarily an indication of IgA or IgM deficiency.

5. *C* Patients with DiGeorge syndrome have a decreased number of T cells, in particular, T helper cells, which are essential for the IgG response to T-dependent antigens. These patients have normally functioning B cells and are capable of responding to T-independent antigens or with only IgM responses (primary responses) to T-dependent antigens.

6. *C* The cause of the two-year-old's infections is very likely B-cell deficiency, which is characterized by recurrent bacterial infections leading to otitis media and pneumonia. T-cell deficiency would usually result in viral, fungal, and protozoal infections. The same is true for combined T- and B-cell deficiency. Answer D (transient anemia) is irrelevant in this case; anemia is not generally associated with increased infections. It is unlikely that with a history of only pneumococcal infections the child would have AIDS. The latter syndrome is associated more with characteristic infections such as *Pneumocystis carinii* and various viral infections.

7. *E* The most likely explanation is that the "healthy" mother has been infected with HIV-1 and is making anti-HIV IgG, which is transferred to the fetus and newborn transplacentally. While it is possible that the HIV was transferred to the infant across the placenta, this would not cause the newborn to make antibodies to the virus at this young age. Thus answers A and B are incorrect. Answers C and D are false because this unlikely situation would result in the recognition of the viral antigen as "self" and the individual would not make antiself antibodies.

8. *E* All are correct. Immunodeficiency disorders may result from defects in the development of bone marrow stem cells into lymphocytes and other cells that participate in the immune response. They can also result from defects in phagocyte functions, which are important in phagocytosis and presentation of antigen. Immunodeficiency disorders may also result from defects in complement function and absence or malfunction of one or more of the complement components, activators, or regulators.

9. *D* T-cell deficiency would result in the absence of the crucial immunologic defenses against viral infection—that is, cell-mediated immunity. Cell-mediated immunity plays the major role in immunity to viral infections, much greater than the role of either antibody or complement. In fact, individuals with impaired T-cell-mediated immunity should not be vaccinated with live virus, which, even if attenuated, may cause a serious infection.

10. *D* Deficiency in C3 is associated with increased susceptibility to bacterial infections, because C3 plays an important role in the opsonization and destruction of bacteria. C3 is a component of all the complement activation pathways: alternative, classical, and mannose-binding lectin pathways. Cell-mediated immunity is generally more important in the resistance of the host to viral and fungal infections. In general, cell-mediated immunity is also considered to be more important than complement in the resistance of the host to tumors.

18

TRANSPLANTATION

 INTRODUCTION

As you have already learned, the immune system has evolved as a way of discriminating between self and non-self. Once foreignness has been established, the immune system proceeds toward its ultimate goal of destroying the foreign material, whether it is a microorganism, the product of a microorganism, a substance present in the environment, or a tumor cell. Chapter 19 will describe the immune mechanisms that occur in response to a tumor.

The same self/nonself discriminating power of the immune system is undesirable in certain therapeutic settings, such as the transplantation of cells, tissues, or organs from one individual to another. Prior to the advent of effective immunosuppressive therapies, organ transplants uniformly culminated in the phenomenon of graft rejection with one notable exception—blood transfusions. *Graft rejection* is a phenomenon in which transplanted tissue or cells expressing donor-derived MHC determinants that are disparate from those of the host are destroyed by immune-mediated mechanisms. Blood transfusions represent the earliest and most successful cell-based "transplants" and continue to be the most common. The reason for this success is due to the fact that RBCs do not express MHC antigens. In addition, they express only a limited number of different types of RBC antigens; these include four ABO blood group antigens and two Rh blood group antigens. Therefore, it is relatively easy to match donor and recipient RBCs. Matching prevents rapid antibody-mediated destruction of

donor RBCs. By contrast, the MHC antigens expressed on other cells, tissues, and organs are genetically polymorphic in the population, so matching donor and recipient is extremely difficult.

Our current understanding of the cellular and molecular mechanisms associated with graft rejection and effective immunosuppressive therapies has made transplantation of various cells, tissues, and organs for therapeutic purposes very commonplace (Table 18.1). For example, over 10,000 kidneys are transplanted each year with a high success rate. Transplantations of heart, lungs, cornea, liver, and bone marrow that were considered groundbreaking and newsworthy as recently as 25 years ago have now become commonplace. Although its incidence has been reduced significantly with advances in immunosuppressive therapies, rejection remains a significant factor. Thus, transplantation immunology continues to be a major area of research.

RELATIONSHIP BETWEEN DONOR AND RECIPIENT

Before we discuss the immunologic mechanisms associated with graft rejection, it is important to understand the various types of transplantation. These are shown in Figure 18.1 and are described below:

1. An *autograft* is a graft or transplant from one area to another on the same individual, such as the transplantation of normal skin from one area

Immunology: A Short Course, Sixth Edition, By Richard Coico and Geoffrey Sunshine
Copyright © 2009 John Wiley & Sons, Inc.

TABLE 18.1. Transplantation of Specific Organs and Tissues

Organ/Tissue	Clinical Uses	Comments
Skin	Burns, chronic wounds, diabetic ulcers, venous ulcers	Commonly autologous grafts; increasing use of artificial skin consisting of stromal elements and cultured cells of allogeneic or xenogeneic origin
Kidney	End-stage renal failure	Graft survival now exceeds 85% at one year even with organs from unrelated donors
Liver	Hepatoma and biliary atresia	Successful in about two-thirds of recipients at 1 year
Heart	Cardiac failure	Survial rates in excess of 80% at 1 year
Lung	Advanced pulmonary or cardiopulmonary diseases	Sometimes performed together with heart transplantation
Bone marrow	Incurable leukemias and lymphomas, congenital immunodeficiency diseases	Risk of GVH disease a unique feature of bone marrow transplantation; increasingly, transplantation of hematopoietic stem cells being used
Cornea	Blindness	HLA matching not advantageous since this is a "privileged" site that normally lacks lymphatic drainage
Pancreas	Diabetes mellitus	Pancreas and kidney transplantation sometimes performed together; success rates approaching that seen with kidney transplants

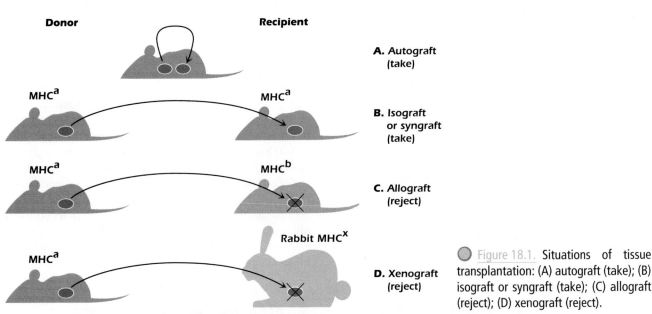

Figure 18.1. Situations of tissue transplantation: (A) autograft (take); (B) isograft or syngraft (take); (C) allograft (reject); (D) xenograft (reject).

of an individual to a burned area of the same individual (Fig. 18.1A). The graft is recognized as autochthonous or *autologous* (self), and no immune response is induced against it. Barring technical difficulties in the transplantation process, the graft will survive or "take" in its new location.

2. An *isograft* or *syngraft* is a graft or transplant of cells, tissue, or organ from one individual to another individual who is *syngeneic* (genetically identical) to the donor (Fig. 18.1B). An example of an isograft is the transplantation of a kidney from one identical

(homozygotic) twin to the other. As in the case of an autograft, the recipient, who is genetically identical with regard to the donor MHC and all other loci, recognizes the donor's tissue as "self" and does not mount an immune response against it. The donor and recipient are described as *histocompatible*.

3. An *allograft* is a graft, or transplant, from one individual to an MHC-disparate individual of the same species (Fig. 18.1C). Because of the high degree of MHC polymorphism within a given outbred species, this *allogeneic* transplant will result in rejection of

the grafted foreign tissue. The donor and recipient, in this case, are considered *nonhistocompatible* or *histoincompatible*.

4. A *xenograft* is a graft between a donor and a recipient from different species (Fig. 18.1D). The transplant is recognized as foreign, and the immune response mounted against it will destroy or reject the graft. Donor and recipient are described as histoincompatible.

IMMUNE MECHANISMS RESPONSIBLE FOR ALLOGRAFT REJECTION

The most direct evidence that the immune response is involved in graft rejection is provided by experiments in which skin is transplanted from one individual to a genetically different individual of the same species (the allogeneic transplant described above). Skin from a mouse with black hair transplanted onto the back of an MHC-disparate white-haired mouse appears normal for one or two weeks. However, after approximately two weeks, the skin allograft begins to be rejected and is completely sloughed off within a few days. This process is called *first-set rejection*. Following this rejection, if the recipient is transplanted with another piece of skin from the same initial donor, the graft is rejected within six to eight days. This accelerated rejection is termed a *second-set rejection*. By contrast, if the first-set rejection is followed by a skin graft from a different MHC-disparate mouse strain, rejection occurs at a rate similar to that of the initial graft—with so-called *first-set kinetics*. Thus, second-set rejection is an expression of specific immunologic memory for antigens expressed by the graft. The participation of CD4$^+$ and CD8$^+$ T cells in second-set rejection can be shown by transferring these cells from an allograft-sensitized individual into a normal syngeneic recipient. If the normal syngeneic recipient is transplanted with the same allograft that was used on the original T-cell donor, a second-set rejection ensues. This establishes that T cells primed in the initial grafting mediate the accelerated rejection in the second host. However, antibodies can also contribute to the destruction of grafted tissue in second-set rejection.

Many other lines of evidence establish the immunologic nature of graft rejection:

1. Histologic examination of the site of the rejection reveals lymphocytic and monocytic cellular infiltration reminiscent of the DTH reaction (see Chapter 16); both CD4$^+$ and CD8$^+$ cells are present at the site (and, as we shall see later, both play a crucial role in graft rejection).

2. Animals that lack T lymphocytes (such as athymic mice or humans with DiGeorge syndrome; see Chapter 17) do not reject allografts.

3. The process of rejection slows down considerably or does not occur at all in individuals treated with immunosuppressive drugs.

Direct evidence for the immunologic basis of graft rejection comes from the observation that in the absence of immunosuppressive therapy animals transplanted with foreign tissues or cells generate alloreactive T cells and alloantigen-specific antibodies that ultimately destroy the graft.

CATEGORIES OF ALLOGRAFT REJECTION

Clinically, allograft rejections fall into three major categories: (1) hyperacute rejection, (2) acute rejection, and (3) chronic rejection. The following are descriptions of the rejection reactions that might be observed after transplantation of a kidney; they also apply to rejection of other tissues.

Hyperacute Rejection

Hyperacute rejection occurs within a few minutes to a few hours of transplantation. It is a result of destruction of the transplant by so-called *preformed antibodies* to incompatible MHC antigens and, in some cases, to carbohydrates expressed on transplanted tissues (e.g., on endothelial cells). Preformed antibodies are those that have been produced in the recipient prior to transplant. In some cases, these preformed antibodies are generated as a result of previous transplantations, blood transfusions, or pregnancies. These cytotoxic antibodies activate the complement system followed by platelet activation and deposition; this causes swelling and interstitial hemorrhage in the transplanted tissue which decrease the flow of blood. Thrombosis with endothelial injury and fibrinoid necrosis are often seen in cases of hyperacute rejection. The recipient may have fever and leukocytosis and may produce little or no urine. The urine the recipient does produce may contain various cellular elements, such as erythrocytes. Cell-mediated immunity is not a factor in hyperacute rejection.

Acute Rejection

Acute rejection occurs in a recipient who has not previously been sensitized to the transplant. This form of rejection is mediated by T cells and is believed to result from their direct recognition of alloantigens expressed by the donor cells (as discussed in more detail later in this chapter). Acute rejection is commonly experienced by individuals who receive mismatched tissue or by allograft recipients who are given immunosuppressive treatment insufficient to prevent rejection. For example, an acute rejection reaction may begin a few days after transplantation of a kidney, with a complete loss of kidney function within 10–14 days. Acute rejection of a kidney is accompanied by a rapid decrease in renal function. Enlargement and tenderness of the grafted kidney, a rise in serum creatinine level, a fall in urine output, decreased renal blood flow, and presence of blood cells and proteins in the urine are characteristic of acute rejection. Histologically, cell-mediated immunity, manifested by intense infiltration of lymphocytes and macrophages, takes place at the rejection site. The acute rejection reaction may be reduced by immunosuppressive therapy with corticosteroids, cyclosporine, and other drugs, as we shall see later in this chapter.

Chronic Rejection

Chronic rejection, which is caused by both antibody- and cell-mediated immunity, occurs in allograft transplantation months or years after the transplanted tissue has assumed its normal function. In cases of kidney transplantation, chronic rejection is characterized by slow, progressive renal failure. Histologically, the chronic reaction is accompanied by proliferative inflammatory lesions of the small arteries, thickening of the glomerular basement membrane, and interstitial fibrosis. Because the damage caused by immune injury has already taken place, immunosuppressive therapy at this point is useless, and little can be done to save the graft.

It is important to understand that the rate, extent, and underlying mechanisms of rejection may vary from those presented above for kidney transplantation; these factors depend on the transplanted tissue and site of the transplanted graft. The recipient's circulation, lymphatic drainage, and expression of MHC antigens on the graft, along with several other factors, determine the rejection rate. For example, bone marrow and skin grafts are very sensitive to rejection compared to heart, kidney, and liver grafts.

ROLE OF MHC MOLECULES IN ALLOGRAFT REJECTION

Antigens that evoke an immune response associated with graft rejection are referred to as *transplantation antigens* or *histocompatibility antigens*. Indeed, the major histocompatibility complex was so named because of its central role in graft rejection. Why do these molecules serve as the major antigenic targets for the T cells ultimately responsible for graft rejection? There are at least two reasons. First, as discussed in Chapter 8, gene products of the MHC are cell surface proteins. All nucleated cells express class I MHC

molecules, but class II molecules are normally expressed only on a subset of hematopoietic cells and by thymic stromal cells. Other cell types may also be induced to express class II MHC following their exposure to the proinflammatory cytokine IFN-γ (see Chapter 11). In an organ transplantation scenario, when a donor and recipient are MHC disparate (allogeneic), the immune response will be directed predominantly against foreign MHC class I antigens expressed on the cells in the grafted tissue. Second, foreign MHC molecules activate an enormous number of T-cell clones in the recipient. It is estimated that up to 5% of all T-cell clones in the body may be activated in response to alloantigen activation, orders of magnitude higher than the response to other antigens. The nonself-MHC molecules with their bound peptides cross-react with T-cell receptors expressed on many different T-cell clones. Other mechanisms that also contribute to the presentation of transplant alloantigens to the recipient's T cells are discussed below.

Mechanisms of Alloantigen Recognition by T Cells

As we discussed in Chapters 8 and 9, the T cells are educated within the thymus to recognize foreign antigens within the context of self-MHC, specifically, the allelic phenotype encountered in the thymus during T-cell differentiation. Thus, the exposure of an individual to nonself-MHC molecules expressed on the graft represents an artificial but clinically relevant situation.

There are two mechanisms of alloantigen recognition by T cells: direct and indirect. When T cells are exposed to foreign cells expressing nonself-MHC (either class I or class II), many clones are "tricked" into activation because their TCRs bind to (ligate) the foreign MHC–peptide complex being presented. This *direct recognition* mechanism (Fig. 18.2A) is presumably due to the recognition of foreign MHC bound to donor-derived peptides. It is important to recall that MHC molecules can, and do, bind physiologically to self-peptides. Self-proteins are routinely digested within cytosolic organelles called proteosomes, and peptides are delivered to the endoplasmic reticulum where they can bind to MHC class I molecules. Such MHC–self-peptide complexes are believed to stabilize the structure of the MHC molecules and are of no consequence when expressed on the surface of cells in a normal individual because there is tolerance to self-peptides. When foreign peptides are bound to donor MHC molecules expressed by grafted cells, the donor MHC–peptide complex has functional cross-reactivity with the self-MHC–peptide combination and thus activates peptide-specific T cells. Hence, when donor-derived peptides are presented to T cells by APC that are "passengers" in the transplanted tissue (donor dendritic cells, in particular), they are recognized as foreign. Activation of these passenger APC occurs in response to "danger

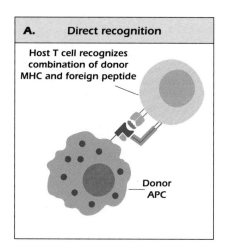

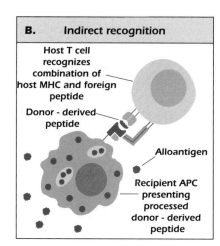

Figure 18.2. (A) Direct and (B) indirect recognition of alloantigens in grafted organs and tissues.

signals" they encounter because of the unavoidable injurious consequences of organ transplantation. Donor APC activation is evidenced by their increased expression of MHC class II molecules, increased expression of T-cell costimulatory molecules, and use of chemokine receptors to facilitate their trafficking to host secondary organs. In short, these activated APC become potent stimulators of host T cells.

The *indirect recognition* of T-cell alloantigens involves the APC of the recipient (Fig. 18.2B). Host APC process alloantigenic proteins and present the resulting peptides on self-MHC molecules to T cells expressing TCRs for these foreign epitopes. This is essentially the same process by which epitopes derived from any other foreign protein activate peptide-specific T cells. It is now known that a major source of the donor-derived peptides presented in this direct fashion are the *minor H antigens* encoded by genes outside the MHC. Responses to minor H antigens are generally mediated by CD8$^+$ T cells because they are presented by class I MHC molecules. As we will discuss later in this chapter, minor H antigens appear to be important in bone marrow transplantation and have been implicated in GVH disease (discussed later in this chapter) in cases of HLA-matched bone marrow transplantations.

In short, direct activation of T cells by alloantigens is due to recognition of donor-derived MHC antigens expressed by donor cells serving as APC (see Fig. 18.2A). Indirect activation of T cells occurs via recognition of donor-derived cellular peptides (mostly minor H antigens) bound to MHC antigens expressed by host APC (see Fig. 18.2B). The relative contribution of these two mechanisms to graft rejection is not known. The direct mechanism of alloantigen recognition is believed to be of importance in acute rejection of grafts. The destruction of donor cells in such cases is directly mediated by T cells. In contrast, indirect alloantigen recognition by T cells also involves activation of host macrophages, which cause tissue damage and fibrosis. Indirect activation leads to the development of cytotoxic alloantibody responses, which may also play a role in the destruction of the graft.

Role of T-Cell Lineages and Cytokines in Allograft Rejection

Alloactivation of T cells generates both allospecific CD4$^+$ and CD8$^+$ cells. The cytokines produced are synthesized mainly by activated CD4$^+$ T-cell clones. The most important cytokines generated during these responses are IL-2, IFN-α, IFN-β, IFN-γ, TNF-α, and TNF-β. IL-2 is important for T-cell proliferation and for differentiation of CTL and T$_H$1 cells participating in the DTH reactions associated with allograft rejection. IFN-γ is important for the activation of macrophages, which migrate to the graft area and cause tissue damage; TNF-β is cytotoxic to the cells present in the graft. IFN-α, IFN-β, TNF-β, and TNF-α increase the expression of class I molecules, while IFN-γ increases the expression of class II molecules on both host and allograft cells, thus increasing the effectiveness of antigen recognition and enhancing graft rejection.

It is now clear that, in addition to the roles played by the T$_H$1 cells, other CD4$^+$ T-cell lineages also participate in graft rejection (Fig. 18.3). As we have discussed in preceding chapters, depending on the microenvironment in peripheral lymphoid organs, helper CD4$^+$ T cells differentiate in different types of effector cells that mediate different types of responses. In the presence of IL-12, T$_H$1 cells dominate and mediate IFN-γ-dependent macrophage activation and DTH (see Chapter 16). In the presence of IL-4, T$_H$2 cells mediate IL-5-dependent eosinophilic rejection. In the presence of TGF-β, IL-6, and IL-23, T$_H$17 cells emerge and are thought to mediate neutrophilic rejection. In the presence of TGF-β alone, T$_{reg}$ cells dominate and promote allograft acceptance by multiple mechanisms, including IL-9-dependent mast cell recruitment.

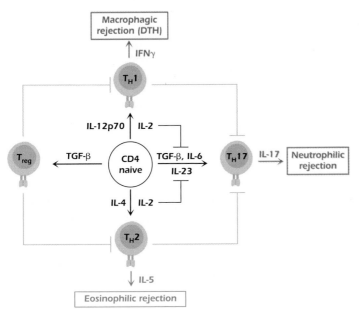

Figure 18.3. Allograft activation of multiple CD4$^+$ T cells, leading to graft rejection.

LABORATORY TESTS USED IN TISSUE TYPING

In order to minimize the risks of graft rejection, laboratory tests are performed prior to transplantation to determine the MHC phenotypes of both the donor and recipient. These tests are often referred to as *tissue typing*. Tissue typing in humans involves assays that determine HLA allele expression on donor and host cells (usually peripheral blood lymphocytes for convenience). This information is then used to assess the magnitude of MHC parity/disparity between the two individuals. It also predicts the potential outcome of a transplant procedure. With the advent of highly effective immunosuppressive drugs, attempts to match donor and recipient by the similarity of their HLA antigens is becoming less essential in certain organ transplant settings (such as the kidney). Nevertheless, HLA analyses are critical in order to minimize the occurrence of graft-versus-host disease in some transplants, including bone marrow transplantation (see below).

Historically, HLA typing was conducted using serologic methods. Panels of HLA-specific monoclonal antibodies were used to phenotype the MHC antigens expressed on cells using immunofluorescence methods (Chapter 5). With the advent of the PCR in the 1980s, molecular typing became possible. Genetic variations in the PCR-amplified DNA can then be detected in a number of ways, including restriction fragment length polymorphism (RFLP), PCR fingerprinting, sequence analysis, allele-specific oligonucleotide typing, and PCR sequence-specific primer typing. These highly sensitive methods are far more accurate than serologic typing because they can detect differences at the level of a single amino acid.

Molecular genotyping of donor and recipient HLA antigens has also eliminated the need to carry out functional assays for tissue typing. The classic approach to functional assessment of HLA compatibility between donor and host cells is the *mixed-leukocyte reaction* (MLR). This method, still used in some experimental settings, involves the coculturing of leukocytes from donor and recipient leukocytes for several days. Donor T cells respond to allogeneic MHC (allo-MHC) antigens expressed on the recipient cells and are stimulated to produce cytokines and proliferate in the presence of these antigens (see Table 18.2). The same is true for recipient leukocytes, which will proliferate in the presence of alloantigens on the donor cells. The proliferation is usually measured by introducing a radioactively labeled precursor to DNA (such as radiolabeled thymidine) into the culture. The greater the extent of proliferation, the more DNA is synthesized by the proliferating cells, and the more radioactivity is incorporated into the cells' DNA.

In most cases, it is essential to ascertain whether the recipient lymphocytes will react against the donor histocompatibility antigen; it is not as important to determine whether the donor lymphocytes will react against the recipient alloantigens. For this reason, the MLR is set up as a "one-way MLR," in which the donor cells have been treated with mitomycin C or X irradiation to prevent their proliferation. In this way, the only cells with the ability to proliferate are the recipient T cells. Under these conditions, recipient CD4$^+$ T cells will proliferate when stimulated with foreign MHC class II molecules. This response will lead to the production of cytokines, which help activate alloreactive cytotoxic CD8$^+$ T cells. The functional activity of such cells can subsequently be measured in assays of CTL cells (see Chapters 5 and 10).

TABLE 18.2. Cases of Mixed-Lymphocyte Reaction Associated with Different Transplantation Situations

Transplantation Situation	HLA Relationship	Treatment of Reacting Leukocytes	MLR
Tissue between identical twins	HLA identical (syngeneic)	No treatment	(−) No reaction
Tissue between nonrelated donor and recipient	HLA different (allogeneic)	No treatment	(+) Reaction intensity depends on the degree of HLA difference between donor and recipient
Tissue between nonrelated donor and recipient	HLA different (allogeneic)	Donor's cells are treated with a mitotic inhibitor, thus testing reactivity of only recipient cells (performed to test for donor–recipient match)	(+) This is a one-way MLR; reaction intensity depends on the degree of HLA difference between donor and recipient
Bone marrow transplantation, or tissue grafting to an immunoincompetent recipient	HLA different (allogeneic)	Recipient's cells are treated with a mitotic inhibitor, thus testing reactivity of only donor's cells (performed to avoid GVH reaction)	(+) This is a one-way MLR; reaction intensity depends on the degree of HLA difference between donor and recipient

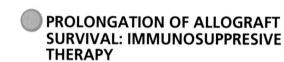 PROLONGATION OF ALLOGRAFT SURVIVAL: IMMUNOSUPPRESIVE THERAPY

A major clinical issue in transplantation immunology is to determine how the components and regulatory interactions involved in graft rejection might be manipulated to allow acceptance of an allograft or xenograft. Nonspecific approaches using immunosuppressive drugs that reduce the overall immunocompence of the recipient to all foreign antigens have been used with success to achieve this goal. However, because patients must be treated chronically with these drugs to maintain the immunosuppressed state, they are predisposed to opportunistic infections and malignancies. Chemoprophylaxis using antimicrobial drugs is utilized in patients undergoing nonspecific, generalized immune suppression to help reduce the incidence of infections, but the potential for malignancy cannot be addressed prophylactically.

More recently, experimental strategies that target responses to the antigens of a particular donor have been investigated. The ultimate goal of this approach is to achieve lasting tolerance to the donor tissue. As discussed in Chapter 12, there are several mechanisms by which T- and B-cell tolerance to self-antigens is achieved. These include clonal deletion, anergy, and suppression. Although tolerance-inducing strategies have been combined with conventional immunosuppressive therapies (discussed below) in clinical trials, none of these strategies have been used to replace such chronic therapy in clinical transplantation.

Currently, immunosuppressive drugs are used for three purposes:

Induction Therapy. Induction therapy is used to suppress the immune system approximately two weeks pretransplantation to reduce the incidence of immediate rejection of the graft.

Maintenance Therapy. In order to ensure that the immune system is kept at bay to facilitate graft survival over time, combinations of synergistic immunosuppressive drugs are used to interfere with specific immune mechanisms (such as T-cell activation). Typically, doses of immunosuppressive drugs used in maintenance therapy are lower than in induction therapy to allow the immune system to function (albeit suboptimally) and to minimize the incidence of opportunistic infections.

Specific Treatments. In some cases, episodes of acute rejection may occur months or years after transplantation. Immunosuppressive drugs are used in these situations, typically at dose levels similar to those used in induction therapy regimens.

Several of the standard and experimental immunosuppressive agents used in transplantation are listed in Table 18.3 and discussed below. They are commonly used in various combinations to prevent graft rejection in transplantation of heart, kidney, lungs, pancreatic islet cells, liver, and other organs and tissues.

Anti-Inflammatory Agents

Corticosteroids, such as *prednisone, prednisolone*, and *methylprednisolone*, are powerful anti-inflammatory agents. As pharmacologic derivatives of the glucocorticoid family of steroid hormones, their physiologic effects result from binding to intracellular steroid receptors expressed

⬤ TABLE 18.3. Immunosuppressive Drugs Used in Transplantation

Inhibitors of lymphocyte gene expression	Corticosteroids
	Cyclosporine (Neoral)
	FK-506
Inhibitors of cytokine signal transduction	Anti-CD25
	Rapamycin
	Leflunomide
Inhibitors of nucleotide synthesis	Azathioprine (Imuran)
	Mercaptopurine
	Chlorambucil
	Cyclophosphamide

in almost every cell of the body. The immunosuppressive action of corticosteroids is due to several effects, most of which are a consequence of corticosteroid-induced regulation of gene transcription. Corticosteroids down-regulate the expression of several genes that code for inflammatory cytokines. These include IL-1, IL-2, IL-3, IL-4, IL-5, IL-8, TNF-α, and GM-CSF. Corticosteroids also inhibit expression of adhesion molecules, which in turn inhibits leukocyte migration to sites of inflammation. Corticosteroids therefore inhibit the activity of inflammatory cells. In addition, they promote the release of cellular endonucleases, leading to the induction of apoptosis in lymphocytes and eosinophils. In addition, they reduce phagocytosis and killing by neutrophils and macrophages and reduce expression of MHC class II molecules. In this way, corticosteroids inhibit T-cell activation and T-cell function.

Despite these beneficial anti-inflammatory effects, it is important to acknowledge that corticosteroids also have potent toxic effects, including fluid retention, weight gain, diabetes, thinning of the skin, and bone loss. Therefore, the efficacy of corticosteroids in the control of disease involves the judicious use of these agents to strike a careful balance between their beneficial and toxic effects. As will be discussed below, given the growing arsenal of immunosuppressive therapies, corticosteroids are often used in combination with other pan-immunosuppressive agents in an effort to keep the dose and toxic side effects to a minimum.

Cytotoxic Drugs

Antimetabolites that suppress the immune response include the purine antagonists azathioprine, mercaptopurine, and mycophenolate mofetil, all of which interfere with the synthesis of RNA and DNA by inhibiting inosinic acid, the precursor for the purines, adenylic and guandylic acids. Chlorambucil and cyclophosphamide, compounds that alkylate DNA, also interfere with the metabolism of DNA.

These agents were originally developed to treat cancer. The observation that they are also cytotoxic to lymphocytes led to their use as immunosuppressive therapeutic agents. However, because they interfere with DNA synthesis in many tissues in the body, they have a range of toxic effects, including anemia, leukopenia, thrombocytopenia, intestinal damage, and hair loss. Fatal reactions to these cytotoxic drugs have also been reported. As noted above, the availability of other immunosuppressive agents allows cytotoxic drugs to be used in combination therapies at lower, less toxic doses.

Agents that Interfere with Cytokine Production and Signaling

A highly effective immunosuppressive therapy involves the use of drugs that interfere with calcineurin—a phosphatase crucial for intracellular events leading to cytokine gene transcription—IL-2 in particular (see Chapter 10). These drugs, which are commonly used as supplements to immunosuppressive antimetabolite and cytotoxic drugs, include cyclosporine and FK-506 (tacrolimus). They exert their pharmacologic effects by binding to immunophilins B, a family of intracellular proteins involved with lymphocyte signaling pathways. Upon binding to immunophilins, these agents interfere with the signal transduction pathways needed for clonal expansion of lymphocytes.

Cyclosporine is a cyclic peptide derived from a soil fungus (*Tolypocladium inflatum*). When it forms a complex with **cyclophilin**—a cytoplasmic immunophililn—the complex binds to and blocks the phosphatase activity of calcineurin. Ultimately, this inhibits TCR signal transduction and suppresses synthesis of IL-2 receptors and production of IL-4 and IFN-γ. In addition, cyclosporine is known to induce the synthesis of TGF-β, a cytokine with immunosuppressive capability. Cyclosporine is effective when administered before transplantation but is ineffective in suppressing ongoing rejection. Evidence indicates that cyclosporine is nephrotoxic and associated with an increased risk of cancer when administered longterm. It has been suggested that these and other side effects are largely due to the TGF-β-inducing property of cyclosporine.

FK506 (tacrolimus) is a macrolide compound obtained from the filamentous bacterium *Streptomyces tsukabaenis*. Macrolides have a multimembered lactone ring attached to one or more deoxy sugars. Although its structure is considerably different from that of cyclosporine, its biologic and immunosuppressive activities are similar. FK506 binds to a different cytoplasmic immunophilin (FK506-binding protein). Like cyclosporine, it interferes with T-cell activation by blocking calcineurin activity and the production of cytokines.

Another drug that interferes with cytokine production by T cells is rapamycin (Sirolimus). Like FK506, rapamycin is a macrolide compound; it is derived from the bacterium *Streptomyces hygroscopicus*. Like cyclosporine and FK506, rapamycin inhibits T-cell activation, but it does so using a different pharmacologic mechanism. Unlike cyclosporine and FK506, which block calcineurin activity, rapamycin inhibits T-cell activation by blocking signal transduction mediated by IL-2 and other cytokines, not by inhibiting IL-2 production.

Immunosuppressive Antibody Therapy

Antilymphocyte antibody preparations, such as horse antilymphocyte and rabbit antithymocyte globulin (ATG), have been used as adjuncts to standard immunosuppressive therapy for many years. While this therapeutic approach can effectively remove unwanted lymphocytes, treatment of humans with large amounts of foreign protein has the disadvantage of inducing a serum sickness caused by the formation of immune complexes (see Chapter 15). Nevertheless, ATG is still used today to treat acute graft rejection. Clearly, the challenge for those attempting to develop new antibody-based therapies for transplant patients is to develop antibodies that are less immunogenic but maintain their targeted effects. Monoclonal antibodies and engineered mouse–human chimeric antibodies or humanized antibodies are being used to this end (see Chapter 5). The first mouse monoclonal antibody to be used as an immunosuppressive agent in humans was OKT3, which is directed against CD3 expressed on T cells. More recently, two chimeric antibodies (Daclizamab and Basiliximab) with specificity for the IL-2 receptor α-chain (CD25) have been used. They down-regulate expression of the IL-2 receptor on activated T cells—a phenomenon that interferes with the ability of T cells to proliferate in response to IL-2. The advent of engineered antibodies holds great promise in reducing the limitations of alloantibody therapy by minimizing the antigenicity of these proteins.

New Immunosuppressive Strategies and Frontiers

The use of antibodies to several other molecules important for T-cell adhesion (such as anti-ICAM-1) and T-cell activation is currently under investigation. In the latter category, a humanized mouse antibody against human CD154 (also known as CD40 ligand) has recently been shown to prevent acute renal allograft rejection in nonhuman primates. Other target antigens include the costimulatory molecules CD80 (B7.1) and CD86 (B7.2). As discussed in Chapter 10, binding of CD80 and CD86 to CD28 initiates a cascade of T-cell activation events. Conversely, binding of CD152 (CTLA-4), an alternate ligand for these costimulatory molecules, delivers inhibitory signals to the responding T cells. As predicted, blocking CD28 ligation interferes with the transmission of signals needed for gene

expression and T-cell activation. Thus, antibodies that interfere with costimulatory molecule-mediated T-cell activation may have efficacy in transplant patients. A related experimental approach uses the inhibitory ligand CTLA-4 to suppress the function of these costimulatory molecules. In animal studies, injection of soluble CTLA-4 has been found to allow the long-term survival of certain grafted tissues. Evidence suggests that the mechanism responsible for the beneficial effect of CTLA-4 involves the blocking of costimulation of the T cells that recognize donor antigens, thus inducing a state of unresponsiveness (anergy).

Our knowledge of CD4$^+$ T-cell lineages and the cytokines they produce has grown considerably in recent years. The discovery of T_H17 T cells that produce a family of IL-17 cytokines (Chapter 11) and the resurgence of interest in and investigation of T cells with suppressive activity (T_{reg} cells) have given rise to new hypotheses regarding immune mechanisms for transplant rejections and, by extension, new approaches to prevent rejection (see Fig. 18.2). For example, it has been suggested that skewing of responses toward T_H17 or T_H1 and away from T_{reg} cells may be responsible for acute rejection of organ transplants. Blocking key cytokines *in vivo*, most notably IL-6, may result in a shift from T_H17 toward a regulatory phenotype (T_{reg}) to help prevent transplant rejection.

It is clear from the above discussion that several experimental approaches are currently under investigation with the hope of finding immunosuppressive agents that will be less toxic and will not leave the recipient helpless to opportunistic infections. However, with all the experimental approaches mentioned above, the main agents that are most commonly used today for clinical immunosuppression are corticosteroids, cyclosporin, FK506, and azathioprine.

HEMATOPOIETIC STEM CELL TRANSPLANTATION

Transplantation of hematopoietic stem cells constitutes a special transplantation situation because it is performed mostly between an immunocompetent donor and an immunocompromised recipient. Historically, the procedure involved the use of bone marrow as a source; today, peripheral blood is more commonly used.

Hematopoietic stem cell transplantation (HCT) is used to treat a variety of conditions, including SCID, Wiskott–Aldrich syndrome (see Chapter 17), and advanced leukemia. HCT is also used to treat blood cell diseases such as thalassemia and sickle cell diseases, in which a mutant gene is inherited. The mutant gene expresses itself only in the blood-forming hematopoietic cells. In these patients, transplantation of hematopoietic stem cells is a form of gene therapy: the genetically abnormal blood-forming stem cells are replaced with normally functioning cells.

The ultimate goal of HCT is to restore or reconstitute normal hematopoiesis of the recipient. Hematopoietic stem cells give rise to all blood cell lineages (see Chapter 2). Small numbers of these pluripotent cells also circulate in the blood. This finding, along with our knowledge about the cytokines that control the proliferation and differentiation of hematopoietic stem cells (known as granulocyte colony-stimulating factors, or G-CSFs), has given rise to the clinical use of G-CSF to increase the numbers of hematopoietic stem cells in both the marrow and the blood. The quantitation of these cells is facilitated by their unique expression of CD34. The administration of G-CSF induces myeloid precursor cells to differentiate into mature neutrophils. Neutrophils produce proteases that are able to cleave the proteins that anchor CD34$^+$ cells to the bone marrow microenvironment. Thus, CD34$^+$ hematopoietic stem cells are mobilized to enter the periphery, where sufficiently large quantities of cells can be recovered for use in HCT. Because of the efficacy and convenience of this procedure, peripheral blood from G-CSF-treated individuals is being used increasingly as a source of hematopoietic stem cells.

The two most common types of HCT are *allogeneic HCT* and *autologous HCT*. In rare cases, HCT is used when transplantation is performed between identical twins (syngeneic transplantation). Syngeneic stem cell transplantation is associated with a relatively low immunologic risk because of the genetic similarity between donor and recipient. Autologous HCT is an important therapy but, strictly speaking, it is not transplantation; it is a technique of obtaining stem cells from blood or marrow and returning them to the same individual. Therefore, immunologic transplantation barriers do not exist. This procedure is commonly used to treat patients with hematologic malignancies such as leukemia, lymphoma, or myeloma. The stem cells are recovered from the bone marrow or blood and stored frozen (cryopreserved) while the patient is treated intensively with chemotherapy and/or irradiation to control the malignancy and to markedly decrease the number of malignant cells in marrow and blood. Finally, the autologous stem cells are infused into the patient so that blood cell production can be restored.

Allogeneic HCT involves the use of donor cells obtained from blood, bone marrow, or umbilical cord sources and placental blood in which the concentration and growth of blood cell-forming stem cells is even greater than in the blood of adults. Unlike autologous HCT, where there is no risk of immune reactivity to the infused cells, in allogeneic HCT, two potential immune rejection outcomes may result: (1) The donor stem cells and the hematopoietic cells to which they give rise may be rejected by the recipient (host-versus-graft effect) or (2) an immune reaction to host MHC antigens may occur (graft-versus-host disease, see below). When the recipient is immunocompetent, immune rejection by host T cells is usually prevented by

intensive immunosuppressive therapy of the recipient prior to the transplant (induction therapy). This approach is also used in patients with malignancies; the rapidly dividing cancer cells are destroyed via induction therapy prior to HCT. Patients with immunodeficiency diseases (such as SCID) do not require such induction therapy since there is no risk of rejection by the host. To reduce the risk of graft-versus-host disease, T cells are rigorously eliminated from the donor cell population. This removal, which can be achieved by a number of methods (such as treatment with monoclonal anti-T-cell antibodies and complement), widens the choice of bone marrow donors.

GRAFT-VERSUS-HOST DISEASE

As noted above, HCT from a donor to an HLA-disparate recipient results in a reaction mounted by the grafted T cells against the recipient's MHC (and/or minor H) antigens. This response manifests as *graft-versus-host disease* (*GVHD*). GVHD occurs when immunocompetent lymphoid cells are transplanted into individuals who are immunologically compromised (such as those who have undergone high-dose radiation therapy or chemotherapy). GVHD can be either acute or chronic. Acute GVHD is responsible for 15–40% of HCT transplant mortality and is the major cause of morbidity after allogeneic HCT; chronic GVHD occurs in up to 50% of patients who survive three months after HCT.

Two important principles help to explain the pathophysiology of acute GVHD. First, it represents an exaggerated but "normal" inflammatory response against foreign antigens (the ubiquitous host alloantigens in this case). Second, donor lymphocytes encounter tissues in the recipient that have often been profoundly damaged due to an underlying disease of the host or pre-HCT therapy regimens such as radiation or chemotherapy.

In humans, GVHD may produce splenomegaly (enlarged spleen), hepatomegaly (enlarged liver), lymphadenopathy (enlarged lymph nodes), diarrhea, anemia, weight loss, and other disorders in which the underlying causes are inflammation and destruction of tissue. GVHD is initiated by donor-derived T cells that recognize the recipient's MHC antigens (and minor H antigens) as foreign. Standard procedures are used to eliminate virtually all mature T cells from the donor hematopoietic stem sell source, but the pluripotent stem cells will give rise to donor-derived T cells over time. Interestingly, most of the innate inflammatory cells that participate in the destruction of host cells in GVHD are host cells recruited to the site of the reaction by cytokines (mainly TNFα and IL-1) released by activated donor participating in the GVH reaction. Unless the reaction is controlled, GVHD activates destructive immune defense mechanisms carried out by donor- and host-derived cells that may lead to death of the recipient. GVHD can be modulated and controlled using a variety of immunosuppressive agents. Administration of calcineurin inhibitors such as cyclosporine or tacrolimus, along with short-course methotrexate, has become the standard immunosuppressive regimen for allogeneic HCT.

 XENOGENEIC TRANSPLANTATION

It is estimated that more than 50,000 people who need organ transplants die each year while waiting for a compatible donor. Studies are underway regarding the use of nonhuman organs to address the critical shortage of human organs available for transplantation. For ethical and practical reasons, species closely related to the human, such as the chimpanzee, have not been widely used. Attention has focused on the pig, which has some organs that are anatomically similar to ours. Interestingly, the human T-cell response to xenogeneic MHC antigens is not as strong as the response to allogeneic MHC molecules.

The major problem with using organs from other species in human recipients is the existence of natural or preformed antibodies to carbohydrate moieties expressed on the graft's endothelial cells. As a consequence, the activation of the complement cascade occurs rapidly and hyperacute rejection ensues. Another concern is the possibility that animal organs and tissues may harbor viruses that might infect humans. This fear is underscored by the possibility that the HIV pandemic may have been caused by the transmission of a virus from monkeys to humans. In the United States, the CDC and other public health agencies have drafted guidelines to monitor patients who receive xenografts using sensitive assays to detect imported viruses.

 THE FETUS: A TOLERATED ALLOGRAFT

A puzzling phenomenon associated with allograft rejection is that the fetus, which expresses paternal histocompatibility antigens that are not expressed by the mother, is not rejected by the mother as an allograft. It is known that the mother can mount an antibody response against fetal antigen, as exemplified by anti-Rh antibodies produced by Rh$^-$ mothers. More importantly, women who have experienced multiple births have antibodies to the father's MHC antigens. It appears that in most cases the antibodies are harmless to the fetus, and it is the mother's ability (or, rather, inability) to respond with the production of cytotoxic T cells against the fetus that is important. There is evidence that fetal trophoblast cells, which constitute the outer layer of the placenta and come in contact with maternal tissue, do not express polymorphic MHC class I or class II molecules; they appear to express only the nonpolymorphic class Ib MHC molecule, HLA-G. Thus, the fetal trophoblast does not prime for a cellular immune response associated with allograft rejection.

It has been suggested that the major function of HLA-G is to provide a ligand for the KIRs on maternal NK cells, thus preventing them from killing the fetal cells (see Chapter 2). HLA-G is also expressed in thymic medullary epithelium, where it might ensure T-cell tolerance to this molecule. Finally, no cells expressing large amounts of MHC class II molecules (e.g., dendritic cells) have been found in the placenta.

Other factors that affect the immune response and may be involved in the fetal–maternal relationship include cytokines, complement inhibitory proteins, and other as-yet-unknown factors. α-Fetoprotein, a protein synthesized in the yolk sac and fetal liver, also appears to be important to the survival of the fetus and has been demonstrated to have immunosuppressive properties. The fetus is only the most spectacular of several tissues in the body that do not initiate an immune response or are not affected by immune components; these are referred to as *immunologically privileged sites*. Increased knowledge of the immunologic mechanisms responsible for the mother's tolerance of the fetus may provide new insights for the purposeful induction of tolerance in grafted cells, tissues, and organs.

SUMMARY

1. Alloreactive T cells are principally responsible for allograft rejection. Alloantigen-specific antibodies are responsible for hyperacute rejection and can also participate in other types of rejection.

2. The most important transplantation antigens, which cause rapid rejection of the allograft, are derived from the donor MHC, called HLA in humans and H-2 in mice. Genetic differences between donor and host can also result in allogeneic cellular peptides (minor H antigens) being presented by host MHC molecules to T cells. Reactions to these allogeneic proteins can also lead to graft rejection.

3. Two mechanisms for host T-cell alloantigen recognition are known to exist: (a) Direct activation of T cells by alloantigens is due to recognition of donor-derived MHC antigens expressed by donor cells serving as APC and (b) indirect activation of T cells occurs via recognition of donor-derived cellular peptides (mostly minor H antigens) bound to MHC antigens expressed by host APC.

4. The degree of histocompatibility between donor and recipient can be determined by serologic or, more commonly, molecular tissue typing.

5. Survival of allografts is prolonged using a cocktail of immunosuppressive agents, including anti-inflammatory agents, cytotoxic agents, antimetabolites, and agents that interfere with IL-2 production and cytokine-mediated signaling. Newer modalities include the use of biologic agents that target costimulatory molecules associated with T-cell activation.

6. The fetus is a natural allograft that is tolerated. Multiple factors appear to be involved in this form of tolerance, including the absence of MHC class I and II molecules on fetal trophoblast cells and the "absence" of MHC class II expression on placental cells.

REFERENCES

Afzali B, Lombardi G, Lechter RI, Lord GM (2007): The role of T helper 17 (Th17) and regulatory T cells (Treg) in human organ transplantation and autoimmune disease. *Clin Exp Immunol* 148:32.

Alegre ML, Florquin S, Goldman M (2007): Cellular mechanisms underlying acute graft rejection: Time for reassessment. *Curr Opin Immunol* 19:563.

Auchincloss H Jr, Sachs D (1998): Xenogeneic transplantation. *Annu Rev Immunol* 16:433.

Auchincloss H Jr, Sykes M, Sachs D (1998): Transplantation immunology. In Paul WE (ed): *Fundamental Immunology*, 4th ed. New York: Lippincott-Raven.

Beniaminovitz A, Itescu S, Lietz K, Donovan M, Burk EM, Groff BD, Edward N, Mancini DM (2000): Prevention of rejection in cardiac transplantation by blockade of the interleukin-2 receptor with a monoclonal antibody. *N Engl J Med* 342:613.

Charlton B, Auchincloss H Jr, Fathman CG (1994): Mechanisms of transplantation tolerance. *Annu Rev Immunol* 12:707.

Devetten M, Armitage JO (2007): Hematopoietic cell transplantation: Progress and obstacles. *Ann Oncol* 18:1450.

Ferrara JLM, Deeq HJ (1991): Graft versus host disease. *N Engl J Med* 324:667.

Hunt JS (1992): Immunobiology of pregnancy. *Curr Opin Immunol* 4:591.

Kirk, AD (1999): Treatment with humanized monoclonal antibody against CD154 prevents acute renal allograft rejection in nonhuman primates. *Nat Med* 5:686.

LaRosa DF, Rahman AH, Turka L (2007): The innate immune system in allograft rejection and tolerance. *J Immunol.* 178: 7503.

Nash RA, Antin JH, Karanes C (2000): Phase 3 study comparing methotrexate and tacrolimus with methotrexate and cyclosporine for prophylaxis of acute graft-versus-host disease after marrow transplantation from unrelated donors. *Blood* 96:2062.

Schreiber SL, Crabtree GR (1992): The mechanism of action of cyclosporin A and FK-506. *Immunol Today* 13:136.

Sun Y, Tawara, I, Toubai, T (2007): Pathophysiology of acute graft-versus-host disease: Recent advances. *Translat Res* 150:197.

⬤ REVIEW QUESTIONS

For each question, choose the ONE BEST answer.

1. In clinical transplantation, preformed cytotoxic antibodies reactive against MHC antigens expressed on the grafted tissue cause:
   A) chronic rejection
   B) hyperacute rejection
   C) acute rejection
   D) delayed-type hypersensitivity
   E) no serious problems

2. Following transplantation of a solid organ, skewing an immune response in a direction that promotes activation of T_H1 and T_H17 T cells would be expected to:
   A) help prevent rejection of allografts
   B) minimize progression of autoimmune diseases
   C) promote allograft rejection
   D) promote antibody responses
   E) induce regulatory T cells

3. Which of the following is a pathophysiologic mechanism for activation of donor APC in individuals who have received organ transplants?
   A) their exposure to damaged cells in the recipient
   B) generation of antibodies against donor MHC antigens by host B cells
   C) failure of regulatory T cells in the recipient to suppress APC activation
   D) polyclonal activation of recipient T cells
   E) production of IL-4 by T_H2 cells

4. Transplant rejection may involve:
   A) cell-mediated immunity
   B) activation of T_H17 cells
   C) complement-dependent cytotoxicity
   D) release of IFN-γ by alloreactive T_H1 cells
   E) all of the above

5. Molecular HLA genotyping of peripheral blood lymphocytes from an individual in need of a kidney transplant donor confirms the expression of the following alleles: HLA-A1, -A3; HLA-B7, -B8; HLA-DR3, -DR4. What would be the most likely outcome of a renal transplant performed in this individual using a donor with the following HLA genotype: HLA-A1, A1; HLA-B8, -B22; HLA-DR3, -DR4?
   A) The graft would be accepted with no need for immuno-suppressive therapy.
   B) The graft would undergo hyperacute rejection.
   C) The graft would be rejected even if immunosuppressive therapy were used.
   D) The graft would be accepted if maintenance immunosuppressive therapy were used.

6. A clinical trial investigating the efficacy of a humanized anti-CD28 monoclonal antibody in prolonging kidney allograft survival shows that patients treated with this biologic reagent have significantly fewer episodes of chronic rejection. The probable mechanism responsible for this effect is best explained by:
   A) binding of anti-CD28 to B cells, which blocks their interaction with B7.1 and B7.2 expressed on T cells
   B) formation of circulating CD28-anti-CD28 immune complexes
   C) binding of anti-CD28 to T cells, which interferes with signal transduction needed for T-cell activation
   D) binding of anti-CD28 to suppressor T-cells, which then become activated
   E) binding of anti-CD28 to B and T cells, which interferes with signal transduction and activation of both populations

ANSWERS TO REVIEW QUESTIONS

1. B Hyperacute rejection is caused by preformed cytotoxic, complement-fixing antibodies that cause platelet activation and deposition, which in turn causes swelling and hemorrhage in the transplanted tissue. This occurs minutes to hours following transplantation and quickly leads to a decrease in the flow of blood through the tissue and ultimate rejection of the graft. Because choices A, C, and D are T-cell mediated, they are incorrect. Choice E is wrong for obvious reasons.

2. C Because T_H1 and T_H17 cells produce proinflammatory cytokines, skewing immune responses to activate these cells would promote allograft rejection. Skewing the response in the T_{reg} direction would be expected to promote allograft survival.

3. A Activation of donor APC present in the allograft tissue as "passenger APC" is mediated, in large part, by their exposure to disease-related or radiation/chemotherapy-induced damaged host cells.

4. E All are correct. The important process in the rejection of an allotransplant is cell-mediated immunity. Here, T cells, which recognize the alloantigens, become activated; the T cells release cytokines, one of which is IFN-γ, which recruits and activates phagocytic cells that, together with cytotoxic T cells, destroy the graft. However, the reaction to the allotransplant may also involve antibodies (IgM and IgG), which can cause damage to tissue via activation of complement and the recruitment of polymorphonuclear cells to the site of the reaction. The polymorphonuclear cells would damage the graft by the release of their lysosomal enzymes.

5. B The only mismatched HLA allele between the donor and recipient is the HLA-B22 expressed by the donor; all other HLA alleles are matched. Thus, with appropriate maintenance immunosuppressive therapy, the engrafted kidney would most likely survive long term.

6. C Experimental models have demonstrated that injection of allografted mice with anti-CD28 monoclonal antibody prolongs survival of the allograft. Blocking CD28 ligation interferes with the transmission of signals needed for gene expression (such as IL-2 synthesis) and T-cell activation. B7.1 and B7.2 are costimulatory molecules that ligate CD28 expressed on antigen-presenting cells, leading to T-cell activation.

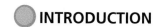

19

TUMOR IMMUNOLOGY

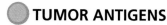

INTRODUCTION

Immune responses against tumor cells occur, in large part, due to expression of surface components on malignant cells that give rise to antigenic structures. Experimental evidence for this phenomenon was provided by mouse studies; when tumor cells were injected subcutaneously into syngeneic (MHC-matched) mice, the cells formed nodules that grew for a few days and then regressed. When identical tumor cells were reinjected into the mice, the tumor cells did not produce nodules or grow. The mice that rejected the tumor had generated an immune response to the tumor. Subsequently, it has been demonstrated that *tumor-specific transplantation antigens (TSTAs)*, known more commonly as *tumor antigens*, are present on many tumors in a variety of animal species, including humans.

The major focus of this chapter concerns the role of the immune system in tumor cell destruction. It is believed that tumor cells are generated in normal individuals and then destroyed by normal immune effector mechanisms, without notice or consequence, throughout life. Obviously, these immunologic mechanisms are not always successful. The hope is that our growing knowledge of host defense mechanisms and the phenomenon of immunosurveillance will provide new insights into prevention and better treatment of cancer. *Immunosurveillance* is the ability of innate and adaptive immune mechanisms to seek and destroy tumor cells. Understanding the cellular and molecular mechanisms responsible for immunosurveillance

is a major goal of tumor immunology. Two other goals of tumor immunology are (1) to elucidate the immunologic relationship between the host and the tumor and (2) to utilize the immune response to tumors for the purpose of diagnosis, prophylaxis, and therapy. Various approaches to meeting these goals will be discussed in this chapter.

TUMOR ANTIGENS

Advances in immunologic and molecular biologic methodology have greatly facilitated the identification of tumor antigens capable of eliciting immune reactions. Before defining the different categories of tumor antigens, it is important to underscore the principal biologic mechanisms that may lead to the appearance of immunogenic tumor antigens; these include mutation, gene activation, and clonal amplification. Like normal immune responses to foreign antigens, the immunogenic potential of tumor antigens is manifested when their expression stimulates immune effector mechanisms. The antigenic prerequisites that apply to foreign immunogens also apply to tumor antigens. As discussed in Chapter 3, a substance must possess the following characteristics in order to be immunogenic: (a) foreignness, (b) high molecular weight, (c) chemical complexity, and (d) degradability with the ability to interact with host MHC antigens. Immunogenic tumor antigens fulfill these criteria and thus have the potential to induce immune responses. Nonimmunogenic

Immunology: A Short Course, Sixth Edition, By Richard Coico and Geoffrey Sunshine
Copyright © 2009 John Wiley & Sons, Inc.

tumor antigens are, in many cases, self-antigens to which some degree of tolerance exists. This poses major barriers to both *de novo* and vaccine-induced tumor immunity. As we shall see later in this chapter, efforts to overcome these barriers include the use of peptides derived from self-antigens expressed on tumor cells; these peptides are engineered to contain altered amino acids in order to increase the immunogenicity of the tumor antigen.

Some tumor antigens consist of structures that are unique to the cancerous cells and are not present on their normal counterparts. Other tumor antigens may be common to both malignant and normal cells but are only unmasked on malignant cells. Still other tumor antigens represent structures that are present on fetal or embryonic cells but disappear from normal adult cells. These latter antigens are referred to as *oncofetal antigens*. Some tumor antigens are qualitatively not different from those found on normal cells but are overexpressed (present at significantly higher levels) on the cancer cell. These overexpressed structures are typically products of *oncogenes*. For example, the level of *human epidermal growth factor receptor* (*HER*) in certain breast and ovarian cancers is high due to overexpression of the *HER-2/neu-1* oncogene. Another example is the elevated products of the *ras* oncogene present on some human prostate cancer cells. The structural features of the tumor antigens arising by these various mechanisms are often similar from individual to individual. This similarity has sometimes translated to therapeutic advances in the treatment of cancer, because commonly expressed tumor antigens can serve as targets for immune-based therapy (such as monoclonal antibodies against HER to treat breast and ovarian cancer). Finally, oncogenic retroviruses (such as the human T-cell leukemia virus) that can transform normal cells into cancer cells also induce tumor cell antigens with extensive structural similarity.

Normal genes that were previously silent may also be activated by *carcinogens*. It is generally assumed that unique tumor antigens on carcinogen-induced tumors are products of mutated genes that are often predisposed to such mutations due to the presence of so-called hot spots. There is little or no cross-reactivity between carcinogen-induced tumors. This absence of cross-reactivity is probably due to the random mutations induced by the chemical or physical carcinogens, which lead to a wide array of different antigens. For example, if the chemical carcinogen methylcholanthrene is applied in an identical manner to the skin of two genetically identical animals or to two similar sites on the same individual, the cells of the developing tumors (sarcomas in this case) will exhibit antigens unique to each tumor, with no immunologic cross-reactivity. Similarly, there is little or no cross-reactivity between tumors induced by physical means, such as ultraviolet light or by X-irradiation.

Carcinogens can also cause clonal amplification of single cells expressing a particular normal antigen and can convert an otherwise nonimmunogenic molecule to an immunogenic antigen. The carcinogen-induced transformation event(s) that cause the emergence of such expanded clones most likely affect genes with mutation-sensitive hot spots while sparing the genes responsible for the production of other, normal proteins. When these normal proteins are *clonotypic* (only expressed by single clones of cells), their expression is amplified dramatically, making them immunogenic if tolerance can be broken. For example, the idiotypes of antigen-specific receptors expressed by B or T cells may not be sufficient to elicit a response in the normal host but may serve as target antigens for tumor cells bearing the same idiotype.

The following sections provide overviews of the various categories of tumor antigens and the immune effector mechanisms that play a role in preventing tumor cell development. Our expanding knowledge of these areas of tumor immunology continues to facilitate the development of clinically useful tumor-specific immunotherapies.

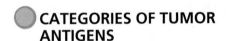

CATEGORIES OF TUMOR ANTIGENS

Tumor antigens may be classified into several major categories (Table 19.1). The categories differ in both the factors that induce the malignancy and the immunochemical properties of the tumor antigens.

Normal Cellular Gene Products

Some tumor antigens are derived from normal genes that, under normal circumstances, are programmed to be expressed only during embryogenesis; these are the aforementioned oncofetal antigens. Examples include the *melanoma-associated antigen (MAGE)* family of proteins, none of which are expressed in any normal adult tissues except for the testes (an immunologically privileged site). MAGE antigens are candidate tumor vaccine antigens because their expression is shared by many melanomas. Another category of oncofetal antigens, the *cancer testes (CT) antigens*, are encoded by genes that are normally expressed only in the human germline. The CT antigens are expressed in various tumor types, including melanoma and carcinomas of the bladder, lung, and liver. Like many other tumor-associated antigens, the MHC restriction elements of the antigenic epitopes have been identified for both MAGE-1 and CT antigens. This information is being exploited in experiments aimed at developing immunogenic tumor peptide vaccines. The goal is to identify peptides that can be presented by class I MHC antigens on APC to activate cytotoxic (CD8[+]) T-cell responses.

TABLE 19.1. Categories of Tumor Antigens

Category		Type of Antigen	Name of Antigen	Types of Cancer
Normal cellular gene products	Embryonic	Oncofetal antigens	MAGE-1	Several
			MAGE-2	Several
			CEA	Lung, pancreas, breast, colon, stomach
			AFP	Liver, Melanoma; carcinoma of bladder, lung, and liver testis
	Differentiation	Normal intracellular enzymes	Prostate-specific antigen CT antigen	Prostate
			Tyrosinase	Melanoma
		Oncoprotein	HER-2/neu	Breast, ovary
		Carbohydrate	Lewis	Lymphoma
	Clonal amplification	Immunoglobulin idiotype	Specific antibody of B-cell clone	Lymphoma
Mutant cellular gene products	Point mutations	Oncogene product	Mutant RAS proteins	Several
		Suppressor gene product	Mutant p53	Several
		CDK	Mutant CDK-4	Melanoma
Viral gene products	Transforming viral gene	Nuclear proteins	E6 and E7 proteins of HPV	Cervical

Other examples of oncofetal antigens include the *carcinoembryonic antigen (CEA)* and α-*fetoprotein (AFP)*. CEA is found primarily in serum of patients with cancers of the gastrointestinal tract, especially cancer of the colon. Elevated levels of CEA have been detected in the circulation of patients with some types of lung cancer, pancreatic cancer, and some types of breast and stomach cancer. However, elevated levels of CEA have also been detected in the circulation of patients with nonneoplastic diseases such as emphysema, ulcerative colitis, and pancreatitis as well as in the sera of alcoholics and heavy smokers. AFP is normally present at high concentrations in fetal and maternal serum but absent from the serum of normal individuals. AFP is secreted rapidly by cells of a variety of cancers, particularly in patients with hepatomas and testicular teratocarcinomas.

Finally, amplified clones of malignant B or T cells expressing antigen-specific receptors represent yet another example of how normal cellular gene products can be characterized as tumor antigens. The idiotype of the particular immunoglobulin or TCR expressed by the transformed B or T cell, respectively, effectively identifies that clone as a unique population of malignant cells.

Mutant Cellular Gene Products

Several tumor antigens are products of mutated genes. In every case, these antigens were the result of a *somatic mutation* (a genetic change absent from autologous normal DNA). Often, these mutations occur in genes that encode functionally important parts of the expressed protein. There are several well-characterized examples of tumor antigens that are derived from mutant cellular gene products. *Chronic myelogenous leukemia (CML)* is characterized by the *Philadelphia chromosome*, a shortened chromosome 22 resulting from a reciprocal translocation between the *bcr* gene on chromosome 22 and the *abl* gene on chromosome 9 [t(9;22)]. The molecular equivalent of t(9;22) can be detected in virtually all cases of CML. It manifests with the expression of a *bcr/abl* fusion gene that encodes chimeric RNAs, which produce copious amounts of tyrosine kinase encoded by the *abl* gene This chimeric gene product appears, at least in part, to be responsible for uncontrolled cell proliferation. Targeted therapy with a potent inhibitor of the *bcr/abl*-derived tyrosine kinase (Imatinib) has been shown to be highly efficacious in the treatment of CML and a number of other malignancies including gastrointestinal stromal tumors.

Another example of a mutant cellular gene product is seen in many cases of familial melanoma. This disease is associated with a mutation in *cycline-dependent kinase-4 (CDK-4)* that reduces binding to its inhibitor (p16INK-4), which happens to be a tumor suppressor protein. Yet another example of a tumor antigen generated by a mutant cellular gene is the mutant *p53 protein*. The p53 mutation generates

TABLE 19.2. Activation of Cellular Protooncogenes in Human Cancers

Protooncogene	Activation Mechanism	Chromosomal Change	Associated Cancer
c-*myc*	Genetic rearrangement	Translocation: 8-14. 8-2, or 8-22	Burkitt's lymphoma
c-*abl*	Genetic rearrangement	Translocation, 9-22	CML
c-*H-ras*	Point mutation		Bladder carcinoma
c-*K-ras*	Point mutation		Lung and colon carcinoma
N-*myc*	Gene amplification		Neuroblastoma

common conformational changes in p53a, a protein that normally acts as a suppressor of cellular growth. Mutations in p53 are among the most common seen in tumors of human and experimental animals. They typically occur in evolutionarily conserved regions of the *p53* gene and result in overproduction of the protein, which then serves as an immunogenic antigen for autologous B and T cells. Antibody and T-cell responses are also seen when mutations occur in *ras* oncogene-encoded proteins. Mutant *ras* proteins, resulting from a glycine substitution at position 12 of *ras*, represent one of the most common mutations in human cancers.

Experimental evidence shows that tumor immunity *in vivo* can be induced against normal p53 by mutant p53 peptides if the mutant peptides are administered to animals with IL-12 to promote T-cell responses toward a proinflammatory T_H1 phenotype. Because p53 is commonly overexpressed in cancer cells, the emerging cytotoxic T-cell responses can destroy tumor cells. Furthermore, p53 knockout mice can be induced to generate cytotoxic T cells specific for normal p53 that, on adoptive transfer into p53 wild-type mice, can eradicate tumors overexpressing p53 without causing autoimmunity in the host.

Tumor Antigens Encoded by Oncogenes

Although a full discussion of carcinogenesis is beyond the scope of this chapter, it is important to summarize the *oncogene theory* in order to better understand the properties of those oncogene-derived proteins that can become tumor antigens. All retroviral oncogenes are known to have close relatives in the genomes of virtually all normal vertebrate cells called c-*onc* genes or *protooncogenes*. The gene products of protooncogenes have been identified as proteins with known functions in normal cells, such as growth factor receptors and signal transducers. The oncogene theory postulates that, when such protooncogenes are mutated or activated by other aberrant mechanisms, they overexpress or inappropriately express the mutated forms of their gene products, thereby contributing to neoplastic transformation and the development of cancer. Oncogenes are aberrantly activated in somatic cells in many forms of human cancer, including carcinoma, sarcoma, leukemia, and lymphoma. The chief mechanisms of activation are chromosomal translocation, point mutation, and gene amplification.

Table 19.2 gives a partial list of the known protooncogenes and their associated cancers.

Animal studies have shown that tumors induced by oncogenic viruses exhibit extensive immunologic cross-reactivity. This is because any particular oncogenic virus induces the expression of the same antigens in a tumor, regardless of the tissue of origin or the animal species. For example, animal DNA viruses such as polyoma, SV40, and Shope papilloma virus induce tumors that exhibit extensive cross-reactivity within each virus group. Many leukemogenic viruses, such as Rauscher leukemia virus, induce the formation of tumors that exhibit cross-reactivity not only within each virus group but also between some groups. There is considerable evidence to suggest that several human cancers, such as Burkitt's lymphoma, nasopharyngeal carcinoma, T-cell leukemia, and hepatocellular carcinoma, are caused by viruses.

As you might expect, the viral proteins, which ultimately serve as tumor antigens, are expressed intracellularly as predominantly nuclear proteins. In order for CTLs to recognize these antigens, they must be processed and presented as class I MHC-associated peptides. Studies using SV40-specific CTLs have confirmed that these cells can recognize processed fragments of proteins that are primarily located intracellularly. The unique tumor antigens of cells transformed by SV40 and several other viruses, including polyoma virus, adenovirus, and HPV, have been studied extensively; in many cases, they are clearly related to the transformed phenotype and the establishment of malignancy. Such viruses have so-called *early-region genes*, designated *E1A/E1B* and *E6/E7*, that are transcribed during early stages of viral replication and in transformed cells by adenovirus and human papilloma virus, respectively. Like other categories of tumor antigens, these proteins are candidate targets for therapy.

Immunologic Factors Influencing the Incidence of Cancer

In the late 1950s, a hypothesis emerged to help explain the primary reason for development of T-cell-mediated immunity during the evolution of vertebrates. It was proposed that the main function of this arm of the immune system was to provide specific defense against altered self or neoplastic cells. The term ***immunosurveillance*** was coined to describe the concept of immunologic resistance against the development of cancer. However, there is growing recognition that immunosurveillance represents only one dimension of the complex relationship between the immune system and cancer. The concept of immunosurveillance is well supported by studies of immunocompromised animals and epidemiologic studies of patients with various immunodeficiencies (primary, secondary, or acquired); an increased incidence of cancer is correlated with these states, but only cancers associated with viruses or, in some cases, UV exposure. By contrast, most common forms of cancer are not increased in immunocompromised individuals. However, patients with immunodeficiency diseases are usually susceptible to viral infections and certain malignant neoplasms (Table 19.3).

The absence of immunosurveillance in spontaneous cancers or those induced by carcinogens does not imply that such tumors do not express immunogenic tumor antigens. These tumor cells, like those induced by viruses, are sensitive to immunologic destruction. Nevertheless, the natural development of tumor-specific immune responses sometimes fails to prevent cancer from developing. Indeed, recent work has shown that the immune system may also promote the emergence of primary tumors with reduced immunogenicity that are capable of escaping immune recognition and destruction. This finding prompted the development of the cancer ***immunoediting hypothesis*** to more broadly encompass the potential host-protective and tumor-sculpting functions of the immune system throughout tumor development. Cancer immunoediting is a dynamic process composed of three phases: ***elimination, equilibrium***, and ***escape*** (Fig. 19.1). Elimination represents the classical concept of cancer immunosurveillance, equilibrium is the period of immune-mediated latency after incomplete tumor destruction in the elimination phase, and escape refers

to the final outgrowth of tumors that have outstripped all immunologic restraints. In the elimination phase, cells and molecules of the innate and adaptive immune systems, which comprise the cancer immunosurveillance network, may eradicate the developing tumor and protect the host from tumor formation. If this process is not successful, the tumor cells may enter the equilibrium phase, where they may be maintained chronically or immunologically sculpted by immune "editors" to produce new populations of tumor cell variants. These variants may eventually evade the immune system by a variety of mechanisms and become clinically detectable in the escape phase. Even at early stages of tumorigenesis, these cells may express distinct tumor-specific markers and generate proinflammatory "danger" signals that initiate the cancer immunoediting process (Fig. 19.1B).

EFFECTOR MECHANISMS IN TUMOR IMMUNITY

Until recently, most of the information concerning tumor antigen-specific immune effector mechanisms and their capacity to destroy tumor cells has been derived from experiments with transplantable tumors in animals or from *in vitro* experiments. There is now ample evidence to suggest that adaptive and innate immune responses play important roles in the relationship between the host and the tumor in humans as well.

Immune effector mechanisms that are potentially capable of destroying tumors *in vitro* are summarized in Table 19.4. In general, destruction of tumor cells by these mechanisms is more efficient in the case of dispersed tumors (i.e., when the target tumor cells are in a single-cell suspension) than in the case of solid tumors, probably because dispersed cells are more accessible to immune action.

TABLE 19.3. Malignant Neoplasms with an Increased Incidence In Immunodeficiency Patients

Type of Immunodeficiency	Cancer	Associated Virus[a]
Primary (congenital)	Hepatocellular carcinoma	HBV
	B-cell lymphoma	EBV
Secondary (e.g., drug-induced)	B-cell lymphoma	EBV
	Squamous cell carcinoma (skin)	HPV
	Hepatocellular carcinoma	HBV
	Cervical carcinoma	HPV
AIDS	Cellular carcinoma	HBV
	Cloagenic or oral carcinoma	HPV
	B-cell lymphoma	EBV

[a]HBV, hepatitis B virus; EBV, Epstein-Barr virus; HPV, human papilloma virus.

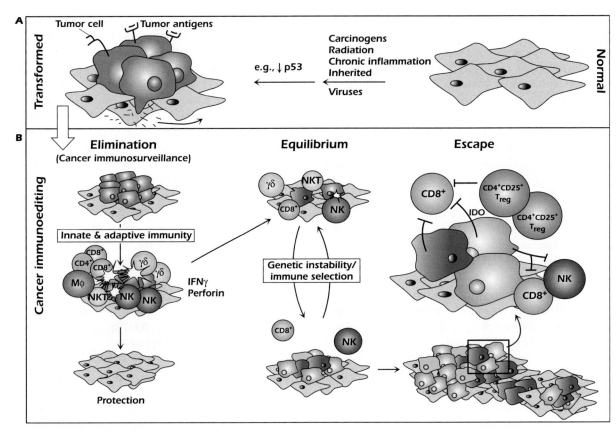

Figure 19.1. Three phases of cancer immunoediting: elimination, equilibrium, and escape. (Adapted from GP Dunn, LJ Old, and RD Schreiber (2007): *Immunity* 21:137.)

TABLE 19.4. Effector Mechanisms in Cancer Immunity

Effector Mechanism	Comments
Antibodies and B cells (complement-mediated lysis, opsonization)	Role in tumor immunity poorly understood
T cells (cytolysis, apoptosis)	Critical for rejection of virally and chemically induced tumors
NK cells (cytolysis, ADCC, apoptosis)	Tumor cells not expressing one of the MHC class I alleles are effectively rejected by NK cells
LAK cells (cytolysis, apoptosis)	Antitumor responses seen in certain human cancers following cancers following adoptive transfer of LAK cells
Macrophages and neutrophils (cytostasis, cytolysis, phagocytosis)	Can be activated by bacterial products to destroy or inhibit tumor cell growth
Cytokines (apoptosis, recruitment of inflammatory cells)	Growth inhibition can occur using adoptively transferred tumor cells transfected with certain cytokines (e.g., GM-CSF)

The character and magnitude of an immune response to tumor antigens depend on the context of antigen presentation. In normal immune responses, when dendritic cells (DCs) acting as APC encounter certain danger signals resulting from cellular damage or invasion by a pathogen (e.g., double-stranded RNA), they are activated and mature to produce cytokines that promote differentiation of $CD4^+$ T_H0 cells to T_H1 cells (Chapter 11). Such

DC activation therefore promotes cell-mediated immune responses. Alternatively, when activated DCs polarize T_H0 cells toward a T_H2 phenotype, antibody responses are facilitated. Both types of immune responses can theoretically participate in the destruction of tumor cells. However, many therapeutic immune-based strategies are aimed at promoting cell-mediated responses since tumor cell destruction by CTLs is the major goal.

B-Cell Responses to Tumors

Both IgM and IgG antibodies have been shown to destroy tumor cells *in vitro* in the presence of complement. Several studies conducted with mice indicate that antitumor antibodies are effective *in vivo* in destroying some leukemia and lymphoma cells and in reducing metastases in several other tumor systems. However, other studies *in vivo* and *in vitro* show that the same antibodies in the presence of complement are ineffective in destroying the cells of the same tumor in a solid form.

Destruction of Tumor Cells by Opsonization and Phagocytosis.

Destruction of tumor cells by phagocytic cells has been demonstrated *in vitro*, but only in the presence of antitumor immune serum and complement. The relevance of this finding *in vivo* is unknown.

Antibody-Mediated Loss of Adhesive Properties of Tumor Cells.

Metastatic activity of certain types of tumors requires the adhesion of the tumor cells to each other and to the surrounding tissue. Antibodies directed against tumor cell surfaces may interfere with the adhesive properties of the tumor cells. Like destruction by opsonization and phagocytosis, the relevance of this mechanism *in vivo* is unknown.

Cell-Mediated Responses to Tumor Cells

Destruction of Tumor Cells by T Lymphocytes.

Destruction of tumor cells *in vitro* by tumor antigen-specific T cells has been demonstrated numerous times for a variety of tumors, both dispersed and solid. Moreover, from many studies with experimental animals (primarily but not exclusively mice), there is good evidence that tumor-specific, cytotoxic T cells are responsible for destruction of virally induced tumors *in vivo*. As discussed below, certain cytokines are essential players in antitumor responses mediated by CTLs, including IFN-α and TNF. CD4$^+$ helper T cells also play a major role in the induction, regulation, and maintenance of such CTLs.

Antibody-Dependent Cell-Mediated Cytotoxicity.

Antibody-dependent cell-mediated cytotoxicity (ADCC) involves (1) the binding of tumor-specific antibodies to the surface of the tumor cells; (2) the interaction of various cells, such as granulocytes and macrophages, which possess surface receptors for the Fc portion of the antibody attached to the tumor cell; and (3) the destruction of the tumor cells by substances released from these cells that carry receptors for the Fc portion of the antibody. The importance of this mechanism in the destruction of tumor cells *in vivo* is still unclear.

Destruction of Tumor Cells by NK Cells, NK/T Cells, and Cytokine-Activated Killer Cells.

As discussed in earlier chapters, NK cells are a lymphoid population representing the 10–20% of peripheral blood mononuclear cells able to lyse MHC class I-negative tumor and virus-infected cells (see Fig. 2.5). Most NK cells are localized in peripheral blood, lymph nodes, spleen, and bone marrow, but they can be induced to migrate toward sites of inflammation by different chemoattractants, including chemokines.

NK cells have receptors for the Fc region of IgG (CD16) and can participate in ADCC (see Chapter 4). Like activated macrophages, NK cells secrete TNF-α, which induces hemorrhage and tumor necrosis; however, the exact mechanism by which NK cells recognize and kill the tumor cells is still not clear. More recently, evidence has been obtained indicating that NK/T cells is another innate immune cell population that is essential for tumor elimination *in vivo* (see Chapter 2).

Cytokine-activated killer cells [historically and currently called lymphokine-activated killer (LAK) cells] are tumor-specific killer cells obtained from the patient. They have been used with minimal success to treat patients with solid tumors; newer strategies using T cells isolated from the tumor called tumor-infiltrating lymphocytes (TILs) and adoptively transferred to patients are showing some therapeutic promise.

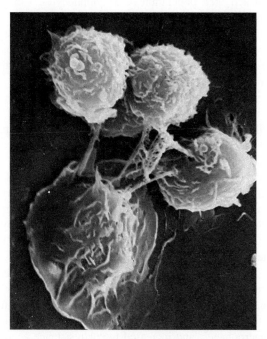

Figure 19.2. Scanning electron micrograph showing activated macrophage with filopodia extending to surface of three melanoma cells (× 4500). (Photograph courtesy of Dr. K.L. Erickson, School of Medicine, University of California, Davis. Reproduced with permission of Lippincott/Harper and Row.)

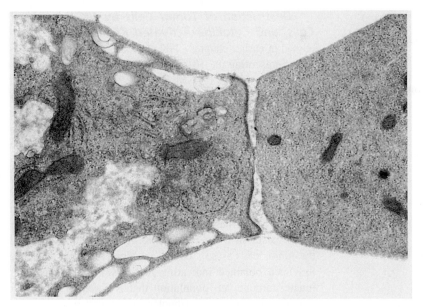

Figure 19.3. **The kiss of death.** An electron micrograph showing a contact point between an activated macrophage (left) and a melanoma cell after 18 h of coculture, leading to cytolysis of the melanoma target cell. Flocculent material is found between the cells; a dense plate is associated with the cell membranes of the macrophage process; microtubules also appear in these projections ($\times$ 26, 000). (Photograph courtesy of Dr. K. L. Erickson, School of Medicine, University of California, Davis. Reproduced with permission of Lippincott/Harper and Row.)

Destruction of Tumor Cells by Activated Macrophages and Neutrophils. Macrophages and neutrophils are generally not cytotoxic to tumor cells *in vitro*. They can be activated by bacterial products *in vitro* to cause selective cytostasis or cytolysis of malignant cells. Macrophages may also become highly cytotoxic (Figs. 19.2 and 19.3) when they are activated by cytokines; most notable among these is IFN-γ produced by an activated population of T lymphocytes, which, by themselves, are not cytotoxic.

These CD4$^+$ T cells are tumor specific: They release IFN-γ after activation by tumor antigen. Other cytokines released by these antigen-activated T lymphocytes attract macrophages to the area of the antigen. IFN-γ also prevents migration of macrophages away from the antigen. The mechanism of activation of macrophages by T cells specific for tumor antigen is similar to mechanisms involved in DTH reactions in allograft rejection or in the killing of microorganisms: Antigen-specific T cells become activated by antigen, and they release cytokines, which attract and activate macrophages. These activated macrophages are cytotoxic to the microorganism, to tumor cells, and even to "self"-cells in the vicinity of the activated macrophages. The damaging and killing activity of activated macrophages is due to several products that they release, notably lysosomal enzymes and TNF-α. Mounting evidence indicates that destruction of tumor cells by activated macrophages occurs *in vivo*. For example, resistance to a tumor can be abolished by specific depletion of macrophages, and increased tumor resistance accompanies an increase in the number of activated macrophages. Finally, activated macrophages are frequently found at the site of regression of a tumor. However, the relationship between the tumor and the tumor-associated macrophages is quite complex. On the one hand, macrophages can

and do kill tumor cells. On the other, macrophages and tumor cells have been shown to produce reciprocal growth factors, leading to an almost symbiotic relationship. Thus, changes in the delicate balance between macrophages and tumor cells may drastically affect the fate of the tumor.

Cytokines

As discussed above, and in Chapter 11, cytokines have a variety of ancillary functions that can facilitate immune effector mechanisms in cancer immunity. Depending on the cytokines produced, immune effector mechanisms may be stimulated or inhibited. Consequently, acquired and/or innate immunity may either stimulate or inhibit the growth of premalignant or malignant cells. The growth-promoting effects of cytokines can be seen in certain tumor cells that produce and respond to cytokines in an autocrine fashion. Similarly, production of TGF-β by some tumor cells promotes tumor growth due to the angiogenic and immunosuppressive properties of this cytokine.

Cytokines such as TNF-α and IFN-γ have antitumor effects because, among other functions, they upregulate MHC class I and class II antigens on some tumor cells. Decreased expression of these antigens allows tumor cells to evade the actions of cytotoxic T cells and NK cells. Cytokine upregulation of MHC antigens thereby facilitates important cell-mediated effector mechanisms. The effects of sustained high levels of certain cytokines have been studied using tumor cells transfected with cytokine genes. Transfection with genes coding for cytokines IL-1, IL-7, IL-12, GM-CSF, or IFN-γ followed by adoptive transfer of such cells into tumor-bearing mice has been shown to inhibit tumor growth significantly. GM-CSF and IL-12 are commonly used in preclinical and clinical tumor vaccines.

LIMITATIONS OF THE EFFECTIVENESS OF IMMUNE RESPONSES AGAINST TUMORS

There is no question that an immune response can be induced against tumors. Why, then, in spite of the immune response, does the tumor continue to grow in the host? Several possible mechanisms may be operational, either alone or in combination with one another. As shown in Table 19.5, tumor-related and host-related factors may influence the escape of tumor cells from destruction by the immune system.

Tumor-related factors that relate to defective immunosensitivity range from the lack of an antigenic epitope to resistance of tumor cells to tumoricidal effector pathways.

TABLE 19.5. Mechanisms of Tumor Escape from Immunologic Destruction

Tumor-related	*Failure of tumor to provide a suitable antigenic target*
	• Lack of antigenic epitope (tumor antigen)
	• Lack of MHC class I molecule
	• Deficient antigen processing by tumor cell
	• Antigenic modulation
	• Antigenic masking of tumor
	• Resistance of tumor cell to tumoricidal effector pathway
	Failure of tumor to induce an effective immune response
	• Lack of antigenic epitope
	• Decreased MHC or tumor antigen expression by tumor
	• Lack of costimulatory signal
	• Production of inhibitory substances (e.g., cytokines) by tumor
	• Shedding of tumor antigen and tolerance induction
	• Induction of T-cell signaling defects by tumor burden
Host-related	*Failure of host to respond to antigenic tumor cells*
	• Immune suppression or deficiency of host, including apoptosis and signaling defects of T-cells due to carcinogen (physical, chemical), infections, or age
	• Deficient presentation of tumor antigens by host APC
	• Failure of host effectors to reach the tumor (e.g., stromal barrier)
	• Failure of host to kill variant tumor cells because of immunodominant antigens on parental tumor cells
	• T_{reg} hindrance of tumor immunity

Defective immunogenicity of the tumor may also account for a tumor's escape from immunologic destruction. Here, again, the lack of an antigenic epitope heads the list of possible mechanisms. Several other mechanisms, including lack of expression of costimulatory molecules by tumor cells, shedding of tumor antigens, and subsequent tolerance induction, may also contribute to the failure of such cells to induce immune responses. Finally, the stromal environment is critical for preventing or permitting the immunologic destruction of tumor cells. Under certain circumstances, the stroma is the site for paracrine stimulatory loops that cause rapid malignant growth and thereby impede immunologic destruction.

Host-related mechanisms that promote the evasion of tumors from immunologic destruction are also summarized in Table 19.5. Mechanisms include immune suppression, T_{reg} hindrance of tumor immunity, deficient presentation of tumor antigens by APC, and failure of host effectors to reach the tumor due to stromal barriers. Alternatively, the possible privileged-site setting of the tumor may facilitate immune evasion. Finally, studies have shown that expression of an immunodominant tumor antigen tends to prevent sensitization to other tumor antigens, thus warding off immune attack on variants.

Nonspecific immune suppression mediated by tumor cells can also allow tumors to escape from immunologic destruction. Certain types of tumors synthesize various compounds, such as prostaglandins, that reduce many aspects of immune responsiveness. However, the role of this mechanism in the escape from destruction by the immune response is still unclear.

Finally, the immune response and its various components have a finite capacity for the effective destruction of tumors (or, for that matter, of invading microorganisms). Thus, while immunization may result in effective protection against an otherwise lethal dose of tumor cells, it is ineffective if the dose of tumor cells is sufficiently large. In the face of an immune response, the progression of the growth of a tumor in an immunocompetent host may be due to a rapid increase in the mass of the tumor, which outstrips the increase in immune responsiveness; the large mass of the tumor eventually overwhelms any effects of the immune response.

IMMUNODIAGNOSIS

Immunodiagnosis of tumors may be performed to achieve two separate goals: (1) the immunologic detection of antigens specific to tumor cells and (2) the assessment of the host's immune response to the tumor. Immunodiagnosis is predicated on immunologic cross-reactivity, and immunologic methods may be used to detect tumor antigens and other "markers" in cases where tumor antigens exhibit similarities from individual to individual. In the presence of such immunologic cross-reactivity, antibody or lympho-cytes from individuals with the same type of tumor would be expected to react with the cross-reactive tumor antigens, regardless of the individual from whom they have been derived. Although this approach is useful in monitoring patients for tumor recurrence after therapy, no tumor marker has undisputed specificity or sensitivity for application in early diagnosis or mass cancer screening.

As discussed earlier in this chapter, tumor cells may express cytoplasmic, cell surface, or secreted products that are different in nature and/or quantity from those produced by their normal counterparts. Because of the generally weak antigenicity of the tumor-specific markers, such qualitative or quantitative differences have generally been demonstrated by the use of antibodies produced in xenogeneic animals. The use of mouse monoclonal antibodies has greatly enhanced the specificity of immun-odiagnosis of human tumor cells and their products. Monoclonal antibodies are currently gaining use not only in the detection of antigens and products associated with the presence of tumor cells but also in the localization and imaging of tumors. Injection of radiolabeled tumor-specific antibodies (radioimmunoconjugates) into the tumor-bearing individual permits visualization of the radiolabeled anti-bodies attached to the tumor by computer-assisted tomography (CAT). This method allows the detection of small metastases as well as the primary tumor mass. Some of the most widely used and reliable immunodiagnostic procedures for the detection of malignancies are described below.

Detection of Myeloma Proteins Produced by Plasma Cell Tumors

Abnormally high serum concentrations of monoclonal immunoglobulins of a certain Ig isotype or the presence of light chains of these immunoglobulins (Bence Jones proteins) in the urine is indicative of plasma cell tumors. The concentration of these myeloma proteins in the blood or urine is a reflection of the mass of the tumor. Consequently, the effectiveness and duration of tumor therapy may be monitored by periodic measurement of the concentration of myeloma proteins in the serum and urine.

Detection of α-Fetoprotein

α-Fetoprotein (AFP) is a major protein produced by fetal liver cells and found in fetal serum. After birth, the level of AFP falls to approximately 20 ng/mL. Levels of AFP are elevated in patients with liver cancer (hepatomas), but they are also elevated in ovarian or testicular embryonal carcinomas as well as noncancerous hepatic disorders such as cirrhosis and hepatitis. Serum AFP concentrations of 500–1000 ng/mL are generally indicative of the presence of an AFP-producing tumor, and monitoring of AFP levels is indicative of regression or progression of the tumor.

Carcinoembryonic Antigen

Carcinoembryonic antigen (CEA) is a term applied to a glycoprotein produced normally by cells that line the gastrointestinal tract, particularly the colon. If the cells become malignant, their polarity may change, so that CEA is released into the blood instead of the colon. Blood concentrations of CEA exceeding 2.5 ng/mL are generally indicative of malignancy, and monitoring CEA levels is helpful in monitoring tumor growth or regression. Here again, however, higher than normal levels of CEA in blood may be due to noncancerous disease, such as cirrhosis of the liver, or inflammatory diseases of the intestinal tract and lung.

Detection of Prostate-Specific Antigen

Prostate-specific antigen (PSA) is a glycoprotein located in ductal epithelial cells of the prostate gland that can be detected in low concentrations in the sera of healthy men. Levels above 8–10 ng/mL blood are suggestive of prostate cancer. Confirmatory tests are required, because prostatitis and benign prostate hypertrophy may also release PSA derived from glandular prostate epithelium into the bloodstream. The test is especially useful for monitoring significant increases or decreases of blood levels of PSA, which correlate with increases or decreases in tumor size.

Cancer Antigen-125

A clinically useful tool for diagnosing and monitoring ther-apy for ovarian cancer involves the immunodiagnostic mea-surement of serum levels of cancer antigen-125 (CA-125). However, circulating levels of CA-125 also increase during peritoneal inflammatory processes.

Radiolabeled Monoclonal Antibody B72.3

B72.3 is a monoclonal antibody that recognizes all carci-nomas in humans (pancarcinoma antigen). This reagent is being used in tumor localization studies to find occult tumor deposits.

There are other markers associated with malignancies, such as enzymes and hormones that can be detected by immunologic methods. Qualitative as well as quantitative determinations of all tumor markers are useful in monitor-ing the extent of malignancy and the effect of therapy.

TUMOR IMMUNOPROPHYLAXIS

A major recent development in tumor immunoprophylaxis concerns the approved use of recombinant HPV capsid protein L1 to prevent cervical cancer in women. A wealth of epidemiologic and molecular evidence has led to the conclusion that virtually all cases of cervical cancer and its precursor intraepithelial lesions are a result of infection with one or other of a subset of genital HPVs. Although the duration of protection provided by this vaccine is unknown, because the antibody responses induced are probably HPV-type specific, immunization should occur prior to exposure to the virus. Second-generation vaccines under development are focused on future immunization strategies that may offer protection post-HPV exposure.

Other tumor antigens that have been characterized molecularly have also been used in concert with viral vectors (such as vaccinia) to actively vaccinate the host. Active immunization has also been studied by intramuscular injection of naked DNA plasmid constructs (**DNA vaccines**), with the goal of muscle cell expression of the unique tumor antigen. In some studies, the genes encoding cytokines such as GM-CSF, IL-2. and IL-12 are also introduced to improve the presentation of the tumor antigen by dendritic cells at the site of injection.

An immunization strategy focused on oncogenic viruses is also expected to provide prophylaxis against virus-associated cancers. Experimentally, this approach has been successful in the protection of chickens against Marek's disease, and a significant degree of protection against feline leukemia and feline sarcoma has been achieved by immunizing cats with the respective oncogenic viruses. Immunization against the tumor itself requires that the tumor possess specific antigens and that these antigens cross-react immunologically with any prepared vaccine. There are literally thousands of reports of effective immunization against transplantable animal tumors using as immunogens (1) sublethal doses of live tumor cells, (2) tumor cells in which replication has been blocked, (3) tumor cells with enzymatically or chemically modified

surface membranes, and (4) extracts of unmodified or chemically modified antigens from the surfaces of tumor cells. Despite these reported successes in protecting experimental animals against transplantable tumors, the efficacy of immunoprophylaxis against spontaneous tumors has not been sufficiently evaluated in humans. This gap relates to the need for appropriate immunogens and to the danger of inducing the production of immunologic elements that may, in fact, enhance metastasis and thus be detrimental to the host.

IMMUNOTHERAPY

Leonardo da Vinci (1452–1519) wrote that "the supreme misfortune is when theory outstrips performance." Unfortunately, this is a fairly accurate characterization of the current state of cancer immunotherapy. Immunotherapy encompasses a variety of interventions and techniques with the common goal of eliciting immune responses that are destructive to tumor cells. Numerous attempts have been made to treat cancers in animals and humans by immunologic means. Although reports of successful immunotherapy in human cancers are increasing in the literature, to date, immunotherapy has not been proved to be an effective treatment of cancer, when used either as the sole treatment or as an adjunct to other therapies such as chemotherapy, radiotherapy, or surgery.

Currently, a wide range of strategies are being used in the experimental immunotherapy of tumors (see Fig. 19.4). *Tumor-specific monoclonal antibodies* can mediate cytolysis, either by engaging NK cells via Fc receptors (ADCC) or by complement activation. Rituximab (anti-CD20) is the first monoclonal antibody to be registered for the treatment of B-cell lymphomas. Randomized studies have demonstrated its activity in

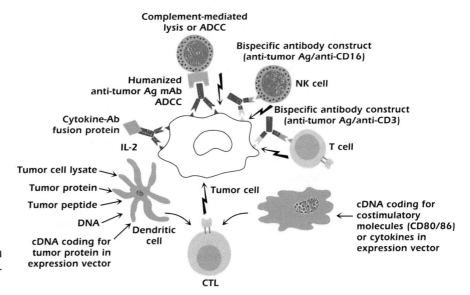

Figure 19.4. Current strategies in experimental immunotherapy: Ag, antigen; mAB, monoclonal antibody.

follicular lymphoma, mantle cell lymphoma, and diffuse large B-cell lymphoma in untreated or relapsing patients.

Follicular Lymphoma

Because of its high activity and low toxicity ratio, rituximab has transformed the outcome of patients with B-cell lymphoma. Other examples of tumor-targeted monoclonal antibodies in use today are anti-CD20 for the treatment of certain lymphomas and anti-Her2/neu-1 for the treatment of certain patients with breast and ovarian cancers. Trials of cancer immunotherapy are underway in which toxins (such as ricin) or radioactive isotopes attached to tumor-specific antibodies are delivered specifically to the tumor cells for direct killing. The extent to which these *immunotoxins* will prove effective in the treatment of cancer remains to be established. Xenogeneic antibodies (such as mouse anti-human monoclonal antibodies) that have been molecularly engineered using recombinant DNA technology to humanize their constant regions (see Chapter 5) are also being tested as candidates for immunotherapy. *Bispecific antibody* constructs designed to bring immune effector cells into contact with tumor cells and to simultaneously stimulate the cytotoxic activity of effector cells are also under investigation. Examples include antibodies that recognize unique tumor antigens and IgG Fc receptors (CD16) that activate NK cells. Similarly, bispecific antibody constructs containing Fab specific for tumor antigens and CD3 have also been studied. A relatively new approach involves the creation of recombinant fusion proteins consisting of anti-tumor antibodies and cytokines (*immunocytokines*). Such fusion proteins are designed to concentrate cytokine-mediated immune effector functions at the tumor site. Several approaches are designed to stimulate or bolster the function of tumor-specific CTLs. CTLs can be activated against tumor antigens by tumor cells rendered immunologic by expression of cytokines or costimulatory molecules such as CD80/CD86. A highly effective method for stimulating tumor-specific CTLs involves the presentation of MHC class I tumor antigen peptides by *dendritic cells*. These highly efficient APC normally express high levels of cell surface costimulatory molecules, thereby enhancing their ability to present tumor antigens to effector T cells (see Chapters 8 and 10). Dendritic cells can be loaded directly with peptides. Alternatively, they can be exposed to tumor cell lysates, tumor proteins, or transfection of tumor-derived cDNA in an expression vector and then adoptively transferred to the tumor-bearing host in hopes of activating cytotoxic T cells to kill the tumor cells.

Immunostimulatory monoclonal antibodies and, in particular, anti-CTLA-4 have also been used with tumor vaccines to potentiate antitumor responses. Because CTLA-4 is a negative regulator of T-cell responses, it can restrict antitumor immune responses. Ipilimumab is a fully human, monoclonal anti-CTLA-4 antibody that overcomes CTLA-4-mediated T-cell suppression to enhance the immune response against tumors. Preclinical and early clinical studies of patients with advanced melanoma show that ipilimumab promotes antitumor activity when used as monotherapy and when utilized in combination with other treatments, such as chemotherapy, vaccines, or cytokines.

Attempts at immunotherapy of animal and human malignancies have also been aimed at the augmentation of specific anticancer immunity, utilizing nonspecific enhancement of the immune response. In particular, stimulation of macrophages using BCG or *Corynebacterium parvum* has been used with some success. One example is the use of BCG for treating patients with residual superficial urinary bladder cancer. Repeated instillation of live mycobacteria into the bladder via catheter after surgery has become the treatment of choice for superficial bladder cancer. Finally, the use of anti-CTLA-4 monoclonal antibody with certain tumor vaccination protocols is showing promise.

Trials are also in progress investigating the effects on tumor regression of various cytokines, such as IFN-α, IFN-β, IFN-γ, IL-1, IL-2, IL-4, IL-5, IL-12, TNF, and others either singly or in combination. To date, these trials are mostly inconclusive. LAK cells and TIL have also been applied clinically to the treatment of cancer with variable results. LAK cells are produced *in vitro* by cultivation of the patient's own peripheral lymphocytes with IL-2. Upon reinfusion into the patient, dramatic improvement has been recorded in a number of cases. Success has been documented in using TIL adoptively transferred to patients with melanoma. These lymphocytes are removed from a tumor biopsy and expanded *in vitro* with IL-2; when given back to the tumor-bearing individual, their anti-tumor activity was many times higher than LAK cells, thus decreasing the amount needed for therapy.

Our growing understanding of cancer and of the immune system continues to fuel the development of new immunotherapeutic strategies. In all cases, such strategies must be evaluated carefully in preclinical models to assess their potential. The great promise of the exploitation of the immune system for the treatment and prevention of cancer must be tempered by the few examples of documented efficacy that have emerged as well as the risks involved. Nevertheless, given the rapid advances in biotechnology and the molecular identification of human tumor antigens, we are entering a new era of cancer immunotherapy. At the present time, tumor immunology has clearly yielded significant improvements in the diagnosis of cancer, and it is likely that immune-based diagnostic methods will continue to offer useful new ways to detect tumor cells and monitor their growth.

SUMMARY

1. Tumor immunology deals with (a) the immunologic aspects of the host–tumor relationship and (b) the utilization of the immune response for diagnosis, prophylaxis, and treatment of cancer.

2. Tumor antigens induced by carcinogens do not cross-react immunologically. On the other hand, extensive cross-reactivity is exhibited with virally induced tumor antigens. Several types of tumors produce oncofetal substances, which are normally present during embryonic development.

3. The immune response to tumors involves both humoral and cellular immune responses. Destruction of tumor cells may be achieved by (a) antibodies and complement, (b) phagocytes, (c) loss of the adhesive properties of tumor cells caused by antibodies, (d) cytotoxic and helper T lymphocytes, (e) ADCC, and (f) activated macrophages, neutrophils, NK cells, NK/T cells, and LAK cells.

4. The immune response to tumors appears to be important, as indicated by the increased incidence of tumors in immunosuppressed hosts and the presence of immune components at sites of tumor regression. However, the immune response to a tumor may not be effective in eliminating the tumor because of a variety of tumor- and host-related mechanisms.

5. Immunodiagnosis may be directed toward the detection of tumor antigens or may target the host's immune response to the tumor.

6. Immunoprophylaxis may be directed against oncogenic viruses or against the tumor itself.

7. Immunotherapy of malignancy employs various preparations for the augmentation of tumor-specific and tumor-nonspecific immune responses. Approaches include (a) active immunization, (b) passive therapy with antibodies, (c) local application of live bacterial vaccines (BCG), (d) use of cytokines, and (e) adoptive transfer of effector cells.

REFERENCES

Bui JD, Schreiober RD (2007): Cancer immunosurveillance, immunoediting and inflammation: Independent or interdependent processes? *Curr Opin Immunol* 19:203.

Coiffier B (2007): Rituximab therapy in malignant lymphoma. *Oncogene* 26:3603.

Dunn GP, Old, LJ, Schreiber RD (2004): The immunobiology of cancer immunosurveillance and immunoediting. *Immunity* 21:137.

Haupt K, Roggendorf M, Mann K (2002): The potential of DNA vaccination against tumor-associated antigens for antitumor therapy. *Exp Biol Med* 227:227.

Herrera L, Stanciu-Herrera C, Morgan C, Ghetie V, Vitetta ES (2006): Anti-CD19 immunotoxin enhances the activity of chemotherapy in severe combined immunodeficient mice with human pre-B acute lymphoblastic leukemia. *Leuk Lymph* 47:2380.

Jager E, Chen YT, Drifhout JW (1998): Simultaneous humoral and cellular immune response against cancer-testis antigen NY-ESO-1: Definition of human histocompatibility leukocyte antigen (HLA)-A2-binding peptide epitopes. *J Exp Med* 187:265.

Ljunggren H-G, Malmberg K-J. (2007): Prospects for the use of NK cells in immunotherapy of human cancer. *Nature Rev Immunol* 7:329.

Meklat F, Li W, Wang Z, Zhang, Y, Zhang J, Jewell A, Lim SH (2007): Cancer-testis antigens in haematological malignancies. *Br J Haematol* 136:769.

Melief CJ, Offringa R, Toes RE, Kast WM (1996): Peptide-based cancer vaccines. *Curr Opin Immunol* 8:651.

Noguchi Y, Richards EC, Chen YT, Old LJ (1995): Influence of interleukin-12 on p53 peptide vaccination against established Meth A sarcoma. *Proc Natl Acad Sci USA* 92:2219.

Ottmann OG, Druker BJ, Sawers CL, Goldman JM, et al (2002): A phase two study of imatinib in patients with relapsed or refractory Philadelphia chromosome-positive acute lymphoid leukemias. *Blood* 15:1965.

Rosenberg SA (1999): A new era for cancer immunotherapy based on the genes that encode cancer antigens. *Immunity* 10:281.

Schmitt A, Hus I, Schmitt M (2007): Dendritic cell vaccines for leukemia patients. *Exp Rev Anticancer Ther* 7:275.

Tan, T-T Coussens LM (2007): Humoral immunity, inflammation and cancer. *Curr Opin Immunol* 19:209.

Weber, J (2002): Peptide vaccines for cancer. *Cancer Invest* 20:208.

Weber J (2007): Review: Anti-CTLA-4 antibody ipilimumab: Case studies of clinical response and immune-related adverse events. *Oncologist* 12:864.

REVIEW QUESTIONS

For each question, choose the ONE BEST answer.

1. Impairment in which of the following immune mechanisms is associated with the appearance of many primary lymphoreticular tumors in humans?
A) humoral immunity
B) NK-cell activity
C) NK/T-cell activity
D) neutrophil function
E) cell-mediated immunity

2. Tumor antigens have been shown to cross-react immunologically in cases of:
A) tumors induced by chemical carcinogens
B) tumors induced by RNA viruses
C) all tumors
D) tumors induced by irradiation with ultraviolet light
E) tumors induced by the same chemical carcinogen on two separate sites on the same individual

3. Which of the following is *not* considered a mechanism by which cytokines mediate antitumor effects?
A) They enhance the expression of MHC class I molecules.
B) They activate tumor-infiltrating lymphocytes (TILs).
C) They have direct anti-tumor activity.
D) They induce complement-mediated cytolysis.
E) They increase activity of cytotoxic T cells, macrophages, and NK cells.

4. Rejection of a tumor may involve which of the following?
A) T-cell-mediated cytotoxicity
B) ADCC
C) complement-dependent cytotoxicity
D) destruction of tumor cells by phagocytic cells
E) all of the above

5. Which of the following best defines immunotoxins?
A) toxic substances released by macrophages
B) cytokines
C) toxins completed with the corresponding antitoxins
D) toxins coupled to antigen-specific immunoglobulins
E) toxins released by cytotoxic T cells

6. It has been shown that a B-cell lymphoma could be eliminated with anti-idiotypic antibodies. The use of this approach to treat a plasma cell tumor would not be warranted because:
A) Plasma cell tumors have no tumor-specific antigens.
B) Plasma cell tumors are not expected to be susceptible to ADCC.
C) Plasma cell tumors can be killed *in vivo* only by cytotoxic T lymphocytes that bear the same A, B, and C transplantation antigens.
D) The plasma cells do not have surface Ig.
E) The idiotype on the plasma cell surface is different from that on the B-cell surface.

ANSWERS TO REVIEW QUESTIONS

1. *E* There is a nearly 100-fold increase in the incidence of lymphoproliferative tumors in individuals with impaired immunity, particularly those with impaired cell-mediated immunity.

2. *B* Immunologic cross-reactivity has been demonstrated only in cases of virally induced tumors (caused by either RNA or DNA viruses). Tumors induced by chemical or physical carcinogens do not exhibit cross-reactivity, even if induced by the same carcinogen on separate sites on the same individual.

3. *D* Interferon-α, β, and γ enhance the expression of class I MHC molecules on tumor cells, which makes them more vulnerable to killing by CTLs. IL-2 activates LAK and TIL cells. TNF-α and β both have direct antitumor activity. IFN-γ increases the activity of CTLs, macrophages, and NK cells, each of which plays an important role in tumor cell destruction. Because cytokines play no role in the activation of complement, D is incorrect.

4. *E* All are correct. Destruction of tumor cells may be mediated by T-cell-mediated cytotoxicity, by ADCC, by complement-mediated cytotoxicity, and by phagocytic cells, which are attracted to the tumor by T-cell lymphokines and/or complement components and become activated by the lymphokines or perform enhanced phagocytosis as a result of the presence of opsonins on the target cells.

5. *D* Immunotoxins consist of toxic substances (or radioactive atoms) conjugated to immunoglobulin molecules specific for tumor cells or other target cells.

6. *D* The only relevant statement is that plasma cells do not have surface immunoglobulins and would therefore not be susceptible to treatment with anti-idiotypic antibodies. Plasma cell tumors do have tumor-specific antigens and would be susceptible to ADCC having antibodies to these antigens, so statements A and B are incorrect. Statements C and E are also incorrect.

20

RESISTANCE AND IMMUNIZATION TO INFECTIOUS DISEASES

⬤ INTRODUCTION

By now, you should fully appreciate the primary function of the immune system: the defense of the body against diseases caused by pathogens. Historically, infectious diseases have been the leading cause of death for human populations, with most deaths occurring in infancy and childhood. There have been many catastrophic epidemics of infectious diseases throughout history. For example, the bubonic plague caused by the bacterium *Yersinia pestis* killed one-quarter of the European population in the mid-1300s. Infectious diseases have provided tremendous selective pressures for the evolution of the immune system. As we have discussed in the early chapters of this book, host defenses are characterized by a considerable amount of layering and redundancy. *Layering* refers to defense in depth and includes physical barriers, such as the skin and mucosal membranes, and innate and adaptive immune mechanisms. *Redundancy* is exemplified by the existence of several types of phagocytic cells, APC, cytokine-producing cells, opsonins, and so on, so many that multiple mechanisms for many immune functions are in place. The redundancy of the immune system allows the host to survive for a prolonged period of time, even in cases of severe immune impairment. For example, individuals with deficiencies in immunoglobulin isotypes such as IgA, the most common Ig deficiency, are thought to live a normal existence because other immunoglobulin classes compensate for the immune deficit.

Microbes differ in their pathogenicity and virulence. Only a small minority of all microorganisms on earth serve as human pathogens. *Pathogens* are defined as microbes capable of causing host damage at the cellular, tissue, or organ level. When host damage reaches a certain threshold, it can manifest itself as disease, and if sufficient damage occurs, death of the host can be the outcome. Host damage can result from a variety of mechanisms and can be mediated by the microbe, the host, or both. Mechanisms of microbe-mediated damage include the production of toxins, cellular apoptosis resulting in depletion of immune cells, and the elaboration of enzymes that cause tissue necrosis. Mechanisms of host-mediated damage include destructive inflammation, fibrosis, and autoimmunity. The realization that host damage is the relevant parameter characterizing the outcome of the host–pathogen interaction is the basis of the recently proposed *damage–response framework* of microbial pathogenesis. In the damage–response framework, disease occurs when the presence of the microbe in the host results in sufficient damage to manifest clinical symptoms. According to this conceptual framework, the term *pathogenicity* is defined as the capacity of a microbe to cause damage in a host, and *virulence* is the relative capacity of a microbe to cause damage in a host. Virulence and pathogenicity are not singular microbial properties, because they can be expressed in only susceptible hosts and reflect complex interactions among hosts, microbes, and myriad environmental, social, and human factors.

Humans harbor many species of microbes. When a human host encounters a microbe, the interaction can result in one of two outcomes: elimination or infection. *Elimination* of the pathogen from the body can occur when the host–microbe encounter does not result in the establishment of the microbe in the host. *Infection* is the acquisition of a microbe by a host. Note that although the term infection is often used synonymously with the word disease, the two are not the same. Infection is followed by one of five outcomes: elimination, commensalism, colonization, persistence (or latency), and disease. In the latter four outcomes, the relationship between the host and microbe is maintained but the amount of damage sustained by the host differs (Fig. 20.1). Elimination can follow infection as a result of action by host defense mechanisms or therapeutic intervention. Neither commensalism nor colonization rarely, if ever, results in symptomatic or clinically evident host damage, but these states can differ in the amount of host damage and in the ability to progress to disease. When there is no host damage, commensalism and colonization are essentially indistinguishable states.

Colonization is a term that is usually used for microbes with significant pathogenic potential that establish themselves in the host without causing symptoms. Colonization can lead to elimination, persistence, or disease, depending on the competency of host defenses, the virulence of the

microbe, and the effectiveness of the immune response. Many colonizing events stimulate immune responses and prevent future infection and/or disease caused by the relevant microbe. For example, a microbe with high pathogenic potential may establish itself on a mucous membrane, cause an amount of damage insufficient to cause clinical symptoms, and elicit an immune response that eradicates it. Thus, colonization has immunized the host against reacquisition of the microbe.

In *persistence* (or latency), microbes take up residence in the host and cannot be eradicated, despite causing host damage. For example, in many humans, *Mycobacterium tuberculosis* infection is not symptomatic, even when the microbe has established itself in the host and is able to survive for long periods of time in a granuloma (see Chapter 16). In this state of persistence, local tissue damage and alterations in normal tissue occur due to granuloma formation, but the damage is not sufficient to produce clinical disease. However, unlike colonization, the host defense mechanisms cannot eradicate the mycobacteria and the infection becomes persistent. In most individuals, this state is maintained with the infection confined to a granuloma. However, in some individuals, this state progresses to tuberculosis, the disease caused by *M. tuberculosis*.

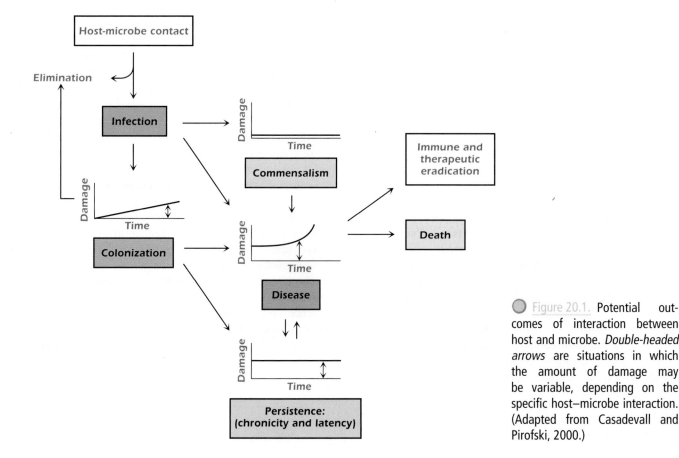

Figure 20.1. Potential outcomes of interaction between host and microbe. *Double-headed arrows* are situations in which the amount of damage may be variable, depending on the specific host–microbe interaction. (Adapted from Casadevall and Pirofski, 2000.)

In individuals with intact immune systems, microbes must be sufficiently virulent to establish themselves and cause infection. However, in individuals with compromised immune systems, low-virulence microbes can cause serious infections. Microbes that are pathogenic in individuals with weakened immune systems are often referred to as *opportunistic pathogens*. Hence, the microbial properties of pathogenicity and virulence are associated with, and partially depend upon, the immune status of the host. In circumstances of normal immune function, commensal microorganisms are not harmful and can serve important roles for the host, such as the production of vitamin K by gut bacteria. However, commensals can become pathogens when normal host defenses are breached. For example, both *Staphylococcus epidermitis* and *Candida albicans* are part of the normal skin flora but can cause life-threatening infections in patients with intravenous catheters, which provide inappropriate circulatory system access due to a break in the skin. Some therapies for cancer produce immune suppression, which leaves patients at risk for serious infections with low-virulence microbes, such as commensals.

In this chapter, we will discuss how mammalian hosts protect themselves against various types of pathogens and how the immune system can be primed for antimicrobial defense through active and passive immunization.

HOST DEFENSE AGAINST VARIOUS CLASSES OF MICROBIAL PATHOGENS

The most effective immune response to a particular microbe varies with the type of pathogen and the microbial strategy for pathogenesis. Because viruses, bacteria, parasites, and fungi each use different strategies to establish themselves in the host, the effective immune response for each class is different. However, certain common themes do emerge.

Immunity to Viruses

All viruses are *obligate intracellular pathogens*. As such, they can only exist and reproduce within the cells they infect. Many viruses have evolved highly sophisticated mechanisms for cellular invasion, replication, and evasion of the immune system. Host defenses against viral infections aim first to slow viral replication and then to eradicate infection. The antiviral response can be complex; several factors affect the outcome of the host–pathogen interaction, including the route of entry, site of attachment, aspects of pathogenesis by the infecting virus, induction of cytokines, antibody response, and cell-mediated immunity. An important early defense mechanism consists of the production of various types of interferons including IFN-α by leucocytes, IFN-β by fibroblasts, and INF-γ by T and NK cells. Interferons are antiviral proteins produced by several different types of cells in the mammalian host in response to viral infection. Interferons serve as an early protective mechanism. IFN-α and IFN-β produced by virally infected cells diffuse to adjoining cells and activate genes that interfere with viral replication. These interferons also stimulate production of MHC class I molecules and proteasome proteins, which enhance the ability of virally infected cells to present viral peptides to T cells. IFN-α and IFN-β also activate NK cells that recognize and kill host cells infected with viruses, thus limiting viral production.

NK cells, which are characterized by their ability to kill certain tumor cells *in vitro* without prior sensitization, constitute an early cellular defense against viruses. Later in the course of infection, when antibodies to viral antigens are available, NK cells can eliminate host cells infected with virus through ADCC. NK cells also produce INF-γ, a potent activator of macrophage function that helps prime the immune system to produce an adaptive immune response. Complement system proteins damage the envelope of some viruses, which may also provide some measure of protection against certain viral infections.

Despite the activities of the innate immune mechanisms, which slow and partially contain many viral infections, the infection may progress, with viral replication and damage triggering an adaptive immune response. The humoral response results in the production of antibodies to viral proteins. Some antibodies, called *neutralizing antibodies*, can prevent viruses from invading other cells. IgG appears to be the neutralizing antibody most active against viruses. Opsonization represents a convergence of humoral and cellular immune mechanisms. IgG, which combines with viral antigens on the surface of infected host cells through its Fab region, also links to Fc receptors on several cell populations, including NK cells, macrophages, and PMN cells. These cells can then phagocytose and/or damage the virus-infected cell through ADCC.

Antibodies to viral proteins can prevent infection by interfering with the binding of virus to host cells. The production of secretory IgA can protect the host by preventing infection of epithelial cells in mucosal surfaces. Antibodies can also interfere with the progression of viral infection by agglutinating viral particles, activating complement on viral surfaces, and promoting phagocytosis of viral particles by macrophages. The production of an antibody response limits viral spread and facilitates the destruction of infected host cells by ADCC. In summary, the effective antibody responses to viruses include the production of antibodies that do the following:

- Neutralize (or impede) the infectivity of viruses for susceptible host cells
- Fix complement and promote complement damage to virions
- Inhibit viral enzymes

- Promote opsonization of viral particles
- Promote ADCC of virus-infected cells

Different types of antibodies may be necessary for the control of specific types of viral infections. Consider infections with the influenza and measles viruses. Infection of the epithelium of the respiratory tract by the influenza virus leads to production of virus in epithelial cells and spread of the virus to adjacent epithelial cells. An appropriate and sufficient immune response would involve the action of antibody at the epithelial surface. This action might be effected through locally secreted IgA or local extravasation of IgG or IgM. On the other hand, viral diseases such as measles begin by infection at a mucosal epithelium (respiratory and intestinal, respectively) but exhibit their major pathogenic effects after being spread hematogenously to other target tissues. In this case, both antibody at the epithelial surface and circulating antibody could protect against the virus.

However, once a virus has attached to a host cell, it is usually not displaced by antibody. Hence, an effective antibody response is usually not sufficient to eliminate a viral infection, particularly when the virus has established itself inside host cells. The eradication of an established viral infection usually requires an effective cell-mediated response. The adaptive cellular response results in the production of specific CD4$^+$ and CD8$^+$ T cells that are essential for clearance of viral infections. CD4$^+$ T cells are believed to be intimately involved in the generation of effective antibody responses by facilitating isotype class switching and affinity maturation (see Chapter 7). CD4$^+$ T cells also produce important cytokines to stimulate inflammatory responses at sites of viral infection and activate macrophage function. Cytotoxic CD8$^+$ T cells (CTLs) are the principal effector T cells against viruses. They are generated early in viral infection and usually appear before neutralizing antibody. CD8$^+$ T cells can recognize viral antigens in the context of MHC class I molecules and can kill host cells harboring viruses. Since MHC class I molecules are expressed by most cell types in the host, CD8$^+$ T cells can recognize many types of infected cells and thus represent a critically important component of the host adaptive response against viral infections. However, for certain noncytopathic viruses, such as hepatitis B, CD8$^+$ T cells can be responsible for tissue injury. Chronic hepatitis B infection results in persistent inflammation and damage to liver cells, resulting in fibrosis that can progress to organ failure.

In summary, innate immune mechanisms initially interfere with viral infection through the production of IFNs and the killing of infected cells by NK cells. These early defenses buy time until powerful, pathogen-specific adaptive immune responses are generated. The adaptive immune responses produce neutralizing antibodies that reduce the number of viral particles and CTLs that kill infected cells.

The presence of neutralizing antibody would then protect against subsequent exposure to the same virus.

Immunity to Bacteria

Host protection against bacterial pathogens is achieved through a variety of mechanisms that include both humoral and cell-mediated immunity. Antibacterial defenses include bacterial lysis via antibody and complement, opsonization, and phagocytosis, with elimination of phagocytosed bacteria by the liver, spleen, and other components of the reticuloendothelial system. Bacteria and their products are internalized by APC such as macrophages and dendritic cells and processed for antigen presentation to T cells. Peptides resulting from such processing are presented to CD4$^+$ T cells in the context of MHC class II molecules (Chapter 8). The host response as T cells produce cytokines that activate macrophages and facilitate recruitment of additional inflammatory cells. The relative efficacy of the various immune mechanisms depends on the type of bacterium and its cell surface properties. Bacterial pathogens can be roughly divided into four classes—*Gram positive, Gram negative, mycobacteria*, and *spirochetes*—depending on the compositions of their cell walls and cell membranes. Some Gram-positive and Gram-negative bacteria have polysaccharide capsules. It is believed that this evolutionary adaptation emerged as a defense mechanism, since bacteria with capsules are resistant to phagocytosis. However, as you have already learned, when such bacterial pathogens induce opsonizing anticapsular antibody responses, the bacteria are readily phagocytized. Another crucial distinction between bacterial pathogens is whether they are intracellular or extracellular pathogens. *Intracellular* bacterial pathogens reside in cells and are partially shielded from the full array of host immune defenses. *Extracellular* bacterial pathogens are found outside cells. In general, humoral immunity is very important for protection against extracellular bacteria, and cellular immunity is the primary immune mechanism for the control and eradication of intracellular bacteria. Recently identified T$_H$17 T cells are believed to play a crucial role in this host defense mechanism.

Gram-Positive Bacteria. Gram-positive bacteria have thick electron-dense cell walls composed of complex cross-linked *peptidoglycan* that allow them to retain the stain crystal violet (hence the name Gram positive). In addition to a thick layer of peptidoglycan, the cell wall of Gram-positive bacteria contains teichoic acids, carbohydrates, and proteins. *Teichoic acids* are immunogenic and constitute major antigenic determinants of Gram-positive bacteria. This type of cell wall provides the Gram-positive bacteria with a thick layer of protection that makes them *resistant to lysis by the complement system*. Defenses against Gram-positive bacteria include the production of opsonins and phagocytic cells, such as neutrophils and macrophages, which ingest and kill them. **Opsonization** and **phagocytosis** involve the action of IgG and IgM, alone or in concert with C3b. The alternative complement pathway may be triggered directly by the Gram-positive bacterial cell wall, resulting in the deposition of complement opsonins in the cell surface and the production of mediators of the inflammatory response. Although the complement system does not lyse Gram-positive bacteria directly, it provides opsonins and mediators of inflammation that are critical for host defense.

Gram-Negative Bacteria.
Gram-positive and Gram-negative bacteria have major differences in their cell wall structure. Gram-negative bacteria do not retain crystal violet stain and have a layered cell wall structure composed of outer and inner membranes separated by a thin layer of peptidoglycan in the periplasmic space. The outer membrane of Gram-negative bacteria contains LPS, which is also known as **endotoxin**. The polysaccharide portion of LPS has antigenic determinants that confer antigenic specificity. Many Gram-negative bacterial species include variants with different LPS structure that can be identified serologically as serotypes. LPS is highly toxic to humans and can produce cardiovascular collapse, hypotension, and shock. The alternative complement pathway may be activated directly by the LPS found in the walls of Gram-negative bacteria or by the polysaccharide capsule of Gram-negative bacteria acting on C3. Activation of the alternative pathway leads to the generation of the chemotactic molecules C3a and C5a and the opsonin C3b, which can result in bacteriolytic action by the C5C9 membrane attack complex (see Chapter 13). In contrast to Gram-positive bacteria, which are impervious to complement-mediated lysis because of the thick peptidoglycan layer, the complement system can lyse some Gram-negative bacteria directly. Defenses against Gram-negative bacteria include the **complement system, specific antibody**, and **phagocytic cells**.

Mycobacteria.
Mycobacteria have cell walls distinct from Gram-positive and Gram-negative bacteria. Mycobacterial cell walls are characterized by a high lipid content, which makes the bacteria difficult to stain. A useful diagnostic microbiologic property of the mycobacterial cell wall is **acid fastness**, the retention of certain dyes after treatment with acid. Mycobacteria grow slowly and have hydrophobic surfaces that make them clump together. Mycobacterial cell wall components elicit strong immune responses during infection, including DTH reactions that form the basis for the **tuberculin test** (Chapter 16). Hypersensitivity reactions to mycobacterial proteins may be involved in the pathogenesis of mycobacterial infections. Mycobacteria elicit strong antibody responses, but the protective role of humoral immunity is uncertain. The primary defense mechanisms against mycobacteria are **macrophages** and **cell-mediated immunity**.

Spirochetes.
Spirochetes, thin helical microorganisms, include the etiologic agents of syphilis (*Treponema pallidum*) and Lyme disease (*Borrelia burgdorferi*). Spirochetes lack cell walls such as those found in Gram-positive bacteria, Gram-negative bacteria, and mycobacteria. Instead, they have a thin outer membrane that contains few proteins. Spirochetes are thin and fragile, requiring special techniques for visualization in the microscope, such as dark-field microscopy and immunofluorescence. Important host defenses against spirochetes include complement, specific antibody, and cell-mediated immunity.

Immunity to Parasites

The parasites are a diverse group of complex pathogens that include the multicellular **helminths** and single-celled **protozoa**. Many parasites have a variety of tissue stages that may differ in cellular location and antigenic composition, making the immune system's task more difficult. Because of the diversity of parasites, it is difficult to make generalizations about effective host mechanisms that protect against parasitic diseases. However, it is clear that both **innate** and **adaptive defense mechanisms** are critically important for protection against parasitic infections.

Protozoa.
Protozoa may exist in a metabolically active form called a **trophozoite** or a dormant tissue form known as a **cyst**. The protozoal diseases include amebiasis, malaria, leishmaniasis, trypanosomiasis, and toxoplasmosis. Host defenses against protozoa include both innate and adaptive humoral and cellular mechanisms, but their relative importance may vary with the individual pathogen. Some protozoal parasites, such as trypanosomes, are able to activate the complement system through the alternative pathway.

Complement activation combined with **phagocytosis** by neutrophils and macrophages of the innate immune system provide important lines of defense again many parasitic pathogens. For some protozoal infections—such as amebiasis, malaria, and trypanosomiasis—humoral immunity in the form of antibody has been shown to mediate protection against infection. However, for other protozoal infections—such as leishmaniasis and toxoplasmosis—cellular immunity is more important.

Helminths.
Unlike the pathogenic protozoan microorganisms, the multicellular worms called helminths are large macroscopic pathogens that can range in size from 1 to 10 m. Because of their large size, which poses particular problems for host defenses, the control of helminth infections requires a complex interplay

between tissue and immune responses. The helminths are notorious for causing chronic infections that can elicit intense immune responses to the worm antigens. There is general agreement that components of the innate immune system such as *eosinophils* and *mast cells* are important effector cells against helminths, but many aspects of the host response to worms remain obscure. IgE specific for helminth antigens is believed to be important for host defense by priming eosinophils for ADCC (see Fig. 14.8). Worm infections are often accompanied by an increase in blood eosinophils and serum IgE levels.

Immunity to Fungi

Fungal pathogens are eukaryotes that tend to cause serious infections in individuals with impaired immunity. Fungi cause tissue damage by the elaboration of proteolytic enzymes, inducing inflammatory responses. The most common fungal pathogen is *C. albicans*. This organism is usually a harmless commensal but can cause disease when normal defense mechanisms are compromised, such as breaks in skin resulting from intravenous catheters or surgery. Another group at risk for serious *C. albicans*–related diseases are individuals who have transient depletion of neutrophils as a result of chemotherapy. The fact that most cases of serious *Candida* infection require a break in the skin or a depletion in neutrophils suggests that innate defense mechanisms are largely responsible for preventing systemic fungal diseases. However, patients with advanced HIV infection suffer from mucosal candidiasis, highlighting the importance of cell-mediated immunity in protection against this organism at the mucosal surfaces.

Other fungi, such as *Histoplasma capsulatum* and *Cryptococcus neoformans*, are acquired from the environment by inhalation in regions where the organism is found in soils. *Cryptococcus neoformans* has a polysaccharide capsule that is required for virulence. Prevalence studies of asymptomatic individuals in such regions have shown a high incidence of infection with a very low incidence of disease, as evidenced by antibody responses or positive skin testing. In such cases, it is likely that initial acquisition of the microbe results in an adaptive immune response that controls the infection. Some fungi, such as *H. capsulatum*, survive inside macrophages and serve as intracellular pathogens. The T_H17 lineage of $CD4^+$ T cells is believed to play an important role in host defenses against intracellular fungal infections.

The cell walls of fungi, composed of cross-linked polysaccharides, differ from those of bacteria. Fungal cells are generally impervious to lysis by the complement system. The host response to fungal infections includes both humoral and cellular responses. The primary form of host defense against fungal pathogens is widely acknowledged to be cell-mediated immunity. The need for intact T-cell function is particularly evident in the predisposition of patients with AIDS to life-threatening infections with such fungi as *H. capsulatum* and *C. neoformans*. Historically, antibody-mediated immunity was not thought to be very important against fungi, but several protective monoclonal antibodies have been described in recent years against *C. albicans* and *C. neoformans*. Hence it is likely that both *cellular* and *humoral immune mechanisms* contribute to protection against fungi.

MECHANISMS BY WHICH PATHOGENS EVADE IMMUNE RESPONSES

Some microorganisms manage to establish themselves in the host and cause life-threatening infections despite the formidable defense mechanisms of the immune system. Learning about the mechanisms used by microbial pathogens to evade the host immune response is important because it can teach us about the efficacy and limitations of host defense mechanisms. In addition, a better understanding of the strategies used by microbes to survive immune attack can be used to design new therapies and vaccines to fight infection.

Encapsulated Bacteria

Polysaccharide capsules are important virulence factors for several human pathogens, including *Streptococcus pneumoniae* (pneumococcus), *Haemophilus influenzae, Neisseria meningitidis* (meningococcus), and *C. neoformans*. These capsules are antiphagocytic and thus protect the pathogen from ingestion and killing by host phagocytic cells. Some capsules also interfere with the action of the complement system. Polysaccharide molecules are often weakly immunogenic, and infection by encapsulated pathogens may not necessarily elicit high titer antibody responses. Infants and young children are particularly vulnerable to life-threatening infections with encapsulated bacteria because their immature immune systems do not mount adequate antibody responses. Other individuals at high risk are those with inherited or acquired deficiencies in antibody production and those who lack normal spleen function. Because the bacteria are cleared by the reticuloendothelial system in the spleen and liver, these organs are critical for protection against encapsulated pathogens. Individuals with compromised reticuloendothelial function as a result of disease (e.g., sickle cell anemia) or surgical removal of the spleen are particularly vulnerable to encapsulated bacteria. The mechanism of antibody action against encapsulated pathogens involves opsonins for phagocytosis and killing by neutrophils and macrophages. Antibodies to capsular polysaccharide function by promoting phagocytosis, either directly through Fc receptors or indirectly by the activation of complement. The generation of C3b following complement activation also facilitates opsonization for phagocytosis—another example of the redundancy of host defenses.

Toxins

In some bacterial infections, the disease is manifested by virulence factors called *toxins*. Bacterial toxins are proteins that produce their physiologic effects at minute concentrations. Examples of toxin-producing bacteria are *Corynebacterium dipththeriae*, *Vibrio cholerae*, and *Clostridium tetani*, which cause diphtheria, cholera, and tetanus, respectively. In diphtheria, *C. dipththeria* replication and toxin production in the nasopharynx results in the formation of a tenacious membrane in the throat that can asphyxiate the patient. Cholera is a diarrheal illness caused by *V. cholerae*, resulting from toxin-mediated alteration of water resorption in the cells of the intestinal mucosa. In tetanus, toxin produced by *C. tetani* produces unchecked excitation of peripheral muscles, resulting in titanic spasms. The relationship of the toxin to bacterial invasion and its evasion of the immune response are variable and may differ for each pathogen. Some toxins, such as tetanus and botulinum toxin, do not appear to injure the immune system directly. Diphtheria toxin may promote bacterial infection by damaging the mucosa. *Bacillus anthracis*, the causative agent of anthrax, produces pathogenic toxins that cause apoptosis in macrophages. The principal mechanism for the immune evasion occurring in anthrax involves a toxin called lethal toxin (LT). LT inhibits a macrophage protein kinase that is required for the transcription of antiapoptotic genes following cell activation.

Most toxins are highly immunogenic and elicit strong humoral and cellular immune responses. Specific antibodies can bind to and neutralize bacterial toxins. Protection against toxins is predominantly associated with IgG, although IgA may also be important in neutralization of certain exotoxins (e.g., secreted toxins) such as cholera enterotoxin. Because the exotoxins bind firmly to their target tissues, they generally cannot be displaced by subsequent administration of *antitoxin* (passive immunization using toxin-specific antibody; discussed later in this chapter). Hence, in toxin-mediated diseases (e.g., diphtheria) prompt administration of antitoxin is necessary to prevent attachment of (additional) exotoxin and to minimize the damage caused by the toxin. For example, the efficacy of diphtheria antitoxin varies depending on when it is administered (Table 20.1); as the infection progresses, the effectiveness of diphtheria antitoxin is reduced significantly. Some bacterial toxins are enzymes, such as the lecithinase of the bacterium *Clostridium perfringens* and snake venom. However,

TABLE 20.1. Protection of Humans by Diphtheria Antitoxin Given on Indicated Day of Disease

Day	Number of Cases	Fatality Rate
1	225	9.0
2	1445	4.2
3	1600	11.1
4	1276	17.3
5 (or later)	1645	18.7

Source: From Pappenheimer (1965).

antibodies that bind the toxin may not necessarily inhibit the enzymatically active sites of the toxin. When this occurs, the toxin preserves its toxic activity.

Superantigens

The interaction of certain toxins with the TCRs of large numbers of T cells can have major immunologic consequences. These toxins, known as *superantigens*, include the staphylococcal *toxic shock syndrome* toxin (see Chapter 10). In the early 1980s, many cases of staphylococcal toxic shock syndrome were associated with tampon use in menstruating women. Since then, the frequency of the disease has decreased significantly in response to changes in tampon manufacture. Superantigens stimulate large numbers of T cells to proliferate, synthesize cytokines, and then die by apoptosis, resulting in the loss of important immune cells. This phenomenon is associated with *hypotension, hypolemia*, and *organ failure*, which can lead to death. B-cell superantigens that bind to and alter the expression of certain immunoglobulin gene families have also been described.

Antigenic Variation

Pathogens can escape the immune system by generating variants with different antigenic composition. This mechanism for evasion of host defenses is known as *antigenic variation*. Classical examples of pathogens that evade the host response by antigenic variation are influenza virus, HIV, *S. pneumonia*, trypanosomes, and group A *Streptococcus*. Each of these pathogens illustrates a mechanism for antigenic variation. In the case of group A *Streptococcus*, the M protein is required for virulence and prevents phagocytosis through deposition of fibrinogen on the bacterial surface. M proteins elicit protective antibody but are antigenically variable, so that streptococcal infection with one strain does not elicit resistance to other strains.

Influenza virus has a segmented RNA genome that can be resorted to yield virions expressing new combinations of the two main surface antigens: the hemagglutinin and neuraminidase surface proteins. Antigenic variation for influenza virus occurs through both antigenic drift and antigenic shift. ***Antigenic drift*** is the result of point mutations in the influenza virus genome, which produce antigenic changes in the hemagglutinin and neuraminidase. ***Antigenic shift*** occurs when influenza virus expresses a new allele of hemagglutin or neuraminidase protein that results in a major antigenic change and the emergence of a new viral strain. The result of antigenic drift and shift for the influenza virus is that the virus changes rapidly, and one influenza infection does not confer protection against subsequent infection. Furthermore, since each epidemic is antigenically different, a new vaccine against influenza must be reformulated every year.

HIV undergoes rapid antigenic variation *in vivo* because it has an error-prone reverse transcriptase that produces mutations, which translates into antigenic changes in surface proteins. The problem of antigenic variation in HIV has been a major barrier to the development of an effective vaccine.

Other pathogens, such as *S. pneumoniae* (pneumococcus), exist in multiple serotypes, each of which has a different antigenic composition. There are 80 known pneumococcal serotypes, and infection with one serotype does not confer protection against infection with a different serotype. Hence the host must deal with infection by each pneumococcal serotype as if it were an infection by a different microbe.

Pathogens may also encode for antigenic variation in their genomes. ***Trypanosomes*** cause chronic infections because new antigenic types emerge during infection, each of which expresses different variant surface glycoproteins (VSGs). In a trypanosome infection, the host mounts an antibody response to the VSG being expressed by the majority of parasites, which clears most of them. However, in every trypanosome infection there are small numbers of organisms that express a different VSG antigen that is not recognized by the antibody response. As the antibody response helps clear the original population, the organisms expressing a different VSG proliferate and generate a new subpopulation of antigenic variants that can survive the new antibody response. This cycle is repeated over and over because of the large number of VSG genes.

Intracellular Survival

Some microorganisms are taken up by ***phagocytic cells*** but manage to survive in the intracellular environment. These pathogens include the bacteria *M. tuberculosis* and *Listeria monocytogenes*, the fungus *H. capsulatum*, and the protozoan *Toxoplasma gondii*. *Mycobacterium tuberculosis* is the cause of tuberculosis, a pulmonary infection. *Listeria monocytogenes* is a food-borne microbe that can cause meningitis in individuals with immune suppression. *Histoplasma capsulatum* is a fungus common in the soil of the Ohio and Mississippi River valleys that usually causes a self-limited

pneumonia in normal individuals. However, in individuals with impaired immunity, *H. capsulatum* can cause disseminated, life-threatening infections. *Toxoplasma gondii* is a parasite acquired from eating undercooked food, which usually causes asymptomatic infections. However, in pregnant women *T. gondii* can infect the fetus, causing severe birth defects. Patients with advanced HIV infection are particularly vulnerable to toxoplasmosis. These organisms cause very different types of diseases, but each has in common the ability to survive inside host cells.

Intracellular residence of pathogens provides a nutrient-rich environment that is outside the reach of humoral factors and neutrophils. In general, protection against intracellular microorganisms is the domain of cell-mediated immunity, although for several pathogens antibody responses also contribute to host defense. This concept is illustrated by the fact that *M. tuberculosis*, *L. monocytogenes*, *H. capsulatum*, and *T. gondii* cause serious diseases in individuals with impaired T-cell function, such as patients with AIDS. Furthermore, NK cells may play an important role during early stages of infection by destroying infected cells before the development of specific resistance. Granulomatous inflammation is a tissue manifestation of cell-mediated immunity associated with containment of several intracellular pathogens.

Although the antimicrobial function of phagocytic cells is generally effective, microbes capable of intracellular survival use any of several strategies to avoid being killed after phagocytosis. *Mycobacterium tuberculosis* blocks the fusion of lysosomes with the phagocytic vacuole, thus preventing delivery of antimicrobial substances to the phagosome (see Chapter 2). *Histoplasma capsulatum* interferes with acidification of the phagolysosomal vacuole, a phenomenon that is believed to interfere with killing of yeast cells inside macrophages. *Listeria monocytogenes* produces bacterial products that allow it to escape from the phagolysosomal vacuole to the cell cytoplasm, defeating intracellular antimicrobial mechanisms and providing a niche that is presumably more nutritionally favorable. *Toxoplasma gondii* generates its own vacuole to insulate it from host lysosomes; this avoids triggering recognition of infected cells by the immune system. Other bacteria—such as *Shigella flexneri*, a microbe that causes a diarrheal illness—may promote their survival inside phagocytic cells by triggering apoptosis and death of the phagocytic cell.

Suppression of the Immune System

Some pathogens ensure their survival in a mammalian host by active suppression of the immune response. Many viruses include genes capable of modulating the immune response. For example, a gene encoded by EBV, which infects B cells, produces a protein homolog of IL-10 that down-regulates the immune response. Other viruses, such as the herpes simplex virus, have virally encoded proteins that resemble Ig Fc regions and complement receptors that interfere with the function of antibody and complement. Herpes simplex virus can also interfere with recognition of infected cells by the immune system through inhibition of MHC class I expression on the infected cell, thwarting the host cell's ability to present virally derived peptides. Adenoviruses encode genes that down-regulate the host inflammatory response. The fungus *C. neoformans* sheds large amounts of capsular polysaccharide, which interferes with the formation of inflammatory responses in tissue. Because HIV infects a variety of cells, including CD4$^+$ T cells, it is able to interfere directly with the cells needed for an effective immune response. HIV-induced CD4$^+$ T-cell depletion produces a spiraling deterioration of immune function that culminates in AIDS and leaves the patient vulnerable to many opportunistic infections.

Extracellular Enzymes

Some bacteria produce enzymes that degrade immune molecules. For example, *N. meningitidis* and *Neisseria gonorrhoeae*, the causes of meningococcal meningitis and gonorrhea, respectively, produce IgA proteases that destroy IgA in mucosal surfaces. Streptococci, such as group A *Streptococcus* (which causes strep throat), produce hemolysins, which are believed to aid the organism in dissemination; some elaborate a peptidase that cleaves the C5a complement protein.

Expression of Antibody-Binding Proteins

Some bacteria, such as *Staphylococcus aureus*, express cell surface proteins that can bind immunoglobulins through their Fc region. Examples of these ***Fc-binding proteins*** are ***protein A*** and ***protein G***. The ability of these proteins to bind immunoglobulin molecules is exploited in immunologic research by using them to purify IgG in affinity chromatography (see Chapter 5).

PRINCIPLES OF IMMUNIZATION

Protection against infectious diseases by the use of vaccines represents an immense, if not the greatest, accomplishment of biomedical science. One disease, smallpox, has been totally eliminated by the use of vaccination, and the incidence of other diseases has been reduced significantly—at least in areas of the world where vaccines are available and administered properly.

If a large enough number of individuals can be immunized, ***herd immunity*** is achieved, and the transmission of communicable diseases among people is interrupted. Although deliberate immunization alone can sometimes reduce the incidence of a disease to a very low level, successful immunization programs require the intelligent

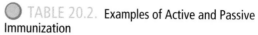 TABLE 20.2. Examples of Active and Passive Immunization

Type of Immunity	How Acquired
Active	
Natural (unintended)	Infection
Artificial (deliberate)	Vaccination
Passive	
Natural	Transfer of antibody from mother to infant in placental circulation or colostrum
Artificial	Passive antibody therapy (serum therapy, administration of immune human globulin)

practice of other measures, both hygienic and sanitary, which contribute to general improvements in public health.

Immunization can be either active or passive. ***Active immunization*** generally refers to the administration of a vaccine that can elicit a protective immune response. ***Passive immunization*** refers to the administration of antibodies or lymphocytes, which then provide protection in the recipient host (Table 20.2).

OBJECTIVES OF IMMUNIZATION

The objective of active immunization is to provide the individual with long-lasting immunologic protection against exposure to infectious agents. Many vaccines are given in childhood to protect against infections that are usually acquired early in life. The objective of passive immunization is to provide transient protection against a particular infection. For example, an individual bitten by a rabid animal may be given an injection of immune globulin to rabies virus. Protection against the development of disease can also be conferred by postexposure immunization. For example, an individual exposed to the rabies virus can be protected against this lethal infection by administration of both rabies vaccine and immune globulin against rabies virus. Other examples of postexposure immunization include the use of toxoid and antitoxin against diphtheria, vaccination with tetanus toxoid after trauma, and administration of immune serum globulins against hepatitis A virus (HAV) and hepatitis B virus (HBV) after exposure. Great effort is currently aimed at the development of therapeutic vaccines that will forestall the relentless progression of AIDS in HIV-infected individuals.

The potential for use of vaccines to prevent certain cancers in humans was discussed in Chapter 19. Some cancers may be prevented by vaccines that prevent infections associated with the subsequent development of carcinoma. For example, there is a strong association between primary carcinoma of the liver and infection by HBV. Therefore, the use of the recombinant HBV vaccine in high-risk groups may provide protection against both hepatitis and the subsequent development of hepatoma.

 ## ACTIVE IMMUNIZATIONS

As discussed in Chapter 1, the terms vaccination and vaccine derive from the work of Edward Jenner who, more than 200 years ago, showed that inoculating people with fluid obtained from the skin lesions of cows infected with cowpox virus protected them from smallpox, a highly contagious and frequently fatal disease. Jenner's process came to be called vaccination, after *vacca*, the Latin word for "cow," and the substance used to vaccinate was called a vaccine. Cowpox (vaccinia virus) induces protective immune responses to smallpox virus because the two viruses share antigenic epitopes, thus inducing a protective immune response. Table 20.3 lists some of the different kinds of vaccines currently in use. Later in this chapter, we discuss more recent approaches to vaccine development.

Recommended Immunizations

The usual recommended schedule in the United States for active immunization at various ages is given in Table 20.4. It is important to note that in other parts of the world the immunization schedule may be different. Recently, a *H. influenzae* type b polysaccharide diphtheria toxoid conjugate was added to the vaccination schedule of young children (first dose at two months of age). *Haemophilus influnzae* type b is a major cause of meningitis in nonimmunized children. The use of this vaccine has resulted in a dramatic reduction in *H. influenzae* type b infections in vaccinated children. Recently, a heptavalent pneumococcal conjugate vaccine was approved for use in children for the prevention of invasive disease, including otitis media.

Recombinant DNA technology has contributed significantly to the development of safe, effective vaccines. These include vaccines to prevent infections with HBV and oncogenic forms of HPVs. The HPV vaccine is also known as the *cervical cancer vaccine*.

Use of Vaccines in Selected Populations

In addition to the usual schedule of immunizations given in Table 20.4, some individuals receive additional vaccinations (listed in Table 20.5). Influenza virus (inactivated) is given to children beginning at six months of age. Annual immunization in adults is recommended and strongly encouraged in persons aged 50 years or older. Hepatitis B vaccine (viral protein produced by recombinant DNA technology) is given to health care and emergency workers who are exposed to human blood. Hepatitis A (inactivated) virus has been approved for use in children and adults. Adenovirus vaccines are used to prevent outbreaks of respiratory infections in military recruits. Anthrax vaccine is used in military personnel, given the threat posed by the use of *B. anthracis*

TABLE 20.3. Vaccines Used in Active Immunization

Vaccine Type	Vaccine Composition	Examples
Killed whole organisms	Made from entire organism, killed to make it harmless	Typhoid
Attenuated bacteria	Organism cultured to reduce its pathogenicity but still retain some of the antigens of virulent form	Bacille Calmette-Guérin (BCG), vaccine against *M. tuberculosis* used in many European countries but rarely used in United States
Toxoids	Bacterial toxins treated (e.g., with formaldehyde) to denature protein so that it is no longer dangerous but still retains some epitopes that will elicit protective antibodies	Diphtheria, tetanus
Surface molecules	Purified surface molecules isolated from various pathogens (e.g., hemagglutinins from influenza virus)	Influenza, hepatitis B surface antigen, *S. pneumoniae* capsular polysaccharides, and *H. influenzae* type b capsular oligosaccharides (the latter are formulated as protein conjugates)
Inactivated virus	Whole virus particles treated (e.g., with formaldehyde) so that they cannot infect host's cells but still retain some unaltered epitopes	Salk vaccine for polio
Attenuated virus	Live viruses that are weakened and nonpathogenic	Sabin oral polio vaccine, measles, mumps, rubella vaccines
Recombinant viral proteins	Major capsid proteins	Hepatitis B, HPV

TABLE 20.4. Schedule for Active Immunization in U.S. Children

Age	Vaccine
Birth	Hepatitis B (Hep B), first dose
14 months	Hep B, second dose
2 months	Dipththeria, tetanus toxoids, acellular pertussis vaccine (DTP); *H. influenzae* type b (Hib); inactivated polio vaccine (IPV); and pneumococcal conjugate vaccine (PCV), first doses
4 months	DTP, Hib, IPV, and PCV, second doses
6 months	DTP, Hib, and PCV, third doses
6–18 months	Hep B and IPV, third doses
12–15 months	Measles, mumps, rubella (MMR), first doses; varicella vaccine
15–18 months	DTP, fourth dose
4–6 years	DTP, fifth dose; IPV, fourth dose; MMR, second dose
11–12 years	Tetanus toxoid booster
11–12 years (girls)	HPV

Source: Adapted from Centers for Disease Control and Prevention (www.cdc.gov/vaccines).

TABLE 20.5. Additional Vaccinations

Vaccine	Population(s)
Anthrax	Military personnel; handlers of animal hides, furs, bone meal, wool, and animal bristles; researchers who work with *B. anthracis;* veterinarians likely to be exposed
Bacille Calmette-Guérin	Health care personnel in close contact with tuberculosis patients
Hepatitis A	Children and adults in high-risk areas
Hepatitis B	All children, susceptible health care workers, homosexual males, intravenous drug users, individuals exposed to blood products
Japanese B encephalitis	Travelers to high-risk areas
Influenzae	Infants >6-months old, adults (especially >50 years of age)
Measles, mumps, influenza, varicella, rubella	Susceptible health care personnel
Meningococcus	Military personnel, young adults living in college dormitories
Plague	Persons in regular contact with rodents, investigators working with *Yersinia pestis*
Rabies	Veterinarians, animal handlers, animal bite victims
Typhoid	Travelers to high-risk areas
Yellow fever	Travelers to high-risk areas

Source: Adapted from Centers for Disease Control and Prevention (www.cdc.gov/vaccines).

spores in biologic warfare. Vaccination against smallpox is no longer recommended for civilians but is still given to selected military personnel. However, there is currently a great deal of debate about expanding the use of this vaccine given heightened concerns about the use of smallpox as a biologic weapon.

Several vaccines against bacterial infections are also used in specific populations. A polyvalent vaccine consisting of several antigenic types of capsular polysaccharides from *S. pneumoniae* is given to individuals with cardiorespiratory ailments, to anatomically or functionally asplenic individuals, and to patients with sickle-cell anemia, renal failure, alcoholic cirrhosis, or diabetes mellitus. These individuals have limited capability to mount the antibody/complement/phagocytic activity required against encapsulated bacteria such as *S. pneumoniae*. Unfortunately, this vaccine may not be as effective in persons at high risk for pneumococcal pneumonia as in normal individuals because the immune defects preclude the generation of strong antibody responses. *Neisseria meningitidis* vaccine (several serogroups of capsular polysaccharide) is given to military recruits and to children in high-risk regions. This vaccine is also recommended for young adults living in college dormitories, who are at high risk for meningococcal meningitis. Both live attenuated and polysaccharide vaccines are available for protection against *Salmonella typhi*, the cause of typhoid fever. Because of unique needs or limited efficacy, some vaccines are only recommended in certain limited circumstances. These vaccines and appropriate circumstances are listed in Table 20.5.

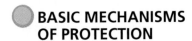

BASIC MECHANISMS OF PROTECTION

Significance of Primary and Secondary Immune Responses

The rapidity of the anamnestic response (see Chapter 14) to a subsequent encounter with antigen provides the host with potential protection from repeated exposures to an infectious agent. The relevance of the anamnestic response in the application of immunoprophylaxis is twofold. First, it may be of particular importance in infections with a relatively long incubation period (>7 days), as shown in Figure 20.2. An individual infected by agent A, which causes disease after a 3-day incubation period, would produce a primary immune response some time (say, 7–14 days) after onset of the infection. On a second encounter with agent A, the individual may again develop disease, because the anamnestic response occurs after the incubation period. The individual infected with agent B, which causes disease after a 14-day incubation period, would also produce a primary response, again 7–14 days after infection. On a second encounter with agent B, the anamnestic response occurring within 7 days would be sufficient to reduce the severity of the disease or prevent it entirely within the 14-day incubation period.

The second influence of the anamnestic response concerns the level to which the immune response has been raised. In the example cited above, agent A, which causes disease in 3 days, may be prevented from causing disease after reexposure if there is a persisting high enough level of antibody. Such a level can be achieved deliberately by a series of immunizations (especially applicable with nonviable antigens). Thus, it is customary to give several injections of tetanus toxoid (as the combined DTP vaccine) over a period of 6 months in childhood immunizations. Such a primary series of injections generates anamnestic secondary responses that successively raise the concentration of antitoxin to protective levels, which are sustained in the serum for 10–20 years.

Age and Timing of Immunizations

The various mechanisms involved in protection via immunization can be affected by several factors, including nutritional status, presence of underlying disease (which affects levels of globulin and cell-mediated immunity), and age. The timing of childhood immunization is driven largely by the fact that the efficacy of certain vaccines depends on the age of the child.

In utero, the human fetus normally appears well insulated from antigens and most infectious agents, although certain pathogens (such as the rubella virus and *T. gondii*) can infect the mother and seriously injure the fetus. The immunity of the mother protects the fetus by permitting interception and removal of infectious agents before they can enter the uterus; it can also protect the newborn by virtue of transplacental or mammary gland antibody.

The fetus and neonate have poorly developed lymphoid organs, with the exception of the thymus, which at the time

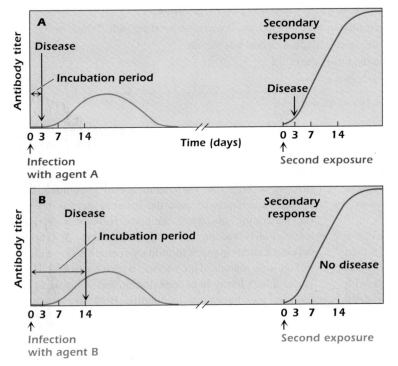

Figure 20.2. Relationship between primary and secondary immune responses and disease produced by infection with agent A or B. Infection caused by agent A has shorter incubation period than infection caused by agent B.

of birth is larger relative to body size than it will be at any subsequent age. The fetus appears capable of synthesizing primarily IgM, which becomes apparent after 6 months of gestation. Levels of IgM gradually increase to about 10% of the adult level at the time of birth.

IgG of maternal origin becomes detectable in the fetus at about the second month of gestation. There is a signficant increase in the level of Ig at about 4 months of gestation and again in the last trimester. At the time of birth, the concentration of IgG slightly exceeds the maternal concentration of IgG. Thus, the fetus is provided with maternally synthesized IgG antibodies, which can provide antitoxic, antiviral, and some antibacterial protection. The levels of these maternal antibodies gradually decline as the infant begins to synthesize its own antibodies, so that total IgG at 23 months of age is <50% of the level at birth. The serum concentrations of immunoglobulins during human development are shown in Figure 20.3.

Some aspects of the immune response of the newborn are not well developed, such as those against some infectious agents (*T. gondii, L. monocytogenes*, HSV) in which cell-mediated immunity is critical. But the newborn can produce antibody to various antigens, such as parenterally administered toxoid, inactivated poliomyelitis virus, hepatitis B antigens, and others. However, administration of pertussis vaccine very soon after birth not only fails to induce a protective response but also creates an impaired response (tolerance) to the vaccine when it is given again later in infancy. Therefore, with the exception of HBV, which is given shortly after birth, in most industrialized countries the initial administration of vaccines is deferred until the child is two months old. However, in developing countries earlier commencement of immunization (at 6 weeks) is recommended by the World Health Organization (WHO).

While capable of providing protection to the neonate against a variety of infectious agents or their toxins, maternal antibody may also reduce the response to antigen. For example, because a sufficient quantity of maternal measles antibody persists in the 1-year-old infant to interfere with the active response of the infant to the vaccine, vaccination against measles is usually delayed until the child is at least 1 year of age.

Children less than 2 years of age have a general inability to produce adequate levels of antibody in response to injection of bacterial capsular polysaccharides, such as those of *H. influenzae* type b, various serogroups *of N. meningitidis*, and *S. pneumoniae* serotypes. It has been suggested that this inability arises because infants do not respond to T-independent antigens, despite their early (*in utero*) capacity to generate IgM. Chemical linkage of polysaccharide to T-dependent antigens (e.g., diphtheria toxoid) or to *N. meningitidis* outer membrane protein has improved immunogenicity so that children younger than 2 years of age respond to polysaccharides. An effective conjugate vaccine is already available against *H. influenzae*, which has virtually eliminated this infection in vaccinated children. For *S. pneumoniae*, a heptavalent vaccine containing polysaccharides of pneumococcal serotypes common in childhood infections is now in routine use.

At the other end of the age spectrum (people older than 60 years of age), there also appears to be a reduced capability to mount a primary response to some antigens, such as influenza virus vaccine; however, the elderly retain the ability to mount a secondary response to previously encountered antigens. The healthy elderly also respond well to bacterial polysaccharides, so that administration of pneumococcal polysaccharide vaccine can usually induce protective levels of antibody. Other groups that are especially susceptible to pneumococcal pneumonia (see coverage earlier in this chapter) should also be immunized. Groups that have enhanced susceptibility to the encapsulated respiratory pathogen *S. pneumoniae* and those at high risk of exposure (e.g., residents of nursing homes and medical personnel) should also receive influenza virus vaccines.

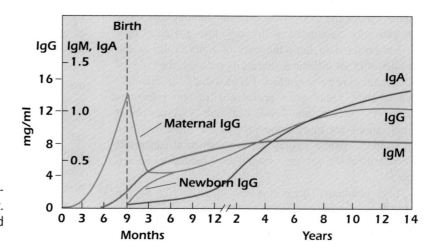

Figure 20.3. Concentration of immunoglobulin in serum during human development. (Reprinted with permission from Benich and Johanssen, 1971.)

VACCINE PRECAUTIONS

Site of Administration of Antigen

The usual site of parenteral administration of vaccines in adults (whether intradermal, subcutaneous, or intramuscular) is the arm, in particular the deltoid muscle. In children, the thigh is routinely used. Studies have shown a suboptimal response to hepatitis B vaccine when given by intragluteal injection rather than by injection in the arm. The parenteral administration of inactivated polio vaccine (Salk) may induce a higher antibody response in the serum than the attenuated oral polio vaccine (Sabin) but the response to the latter, which includes secretory IgA, affords adequate protection. However, use of the attenuated oral polio vaccine has been discontinued because the live virus can, in exceptionally rare circumstances, cause disease.

Some vaccines may provide a greater antibody response when given by the respiratory route than when given by injection (such as the attenuated measles vaccine), but administration via the respiratory route remains an experimental method.

Hazards

There are potential hazards associated with the use of some vaccines. Vaccines made from attenuated agents (such as measles, mumps, rubella, oral polio, and BCG) have the potential for causing progressive disease in the *immunocompromised patient* or in the patient on *immunosuppressive therapy*. In rare cases, reversion to virulence of attenuated poliovirus in the intestine of the vaccinated individual has caused paralytic polio. Concern about vaccine-associated paralytic polio has resulted in a change in recommendations for vaccination; the inactivated poliovirus vaccine is now the recommended vaccine in the United States. This situation illustrates the need for vigilant monitoring of the prevalence of infectious disease in a given population and for balancing the risks of disease against the risks of vaccination. Although vaccines are generally associated with very low toxicity, they are administered to large numbers of individuals; as the prevalence of an infectious disease is reduced, the risks of vaccination may be magnified. Paradoxically, an effective vaccine may reduce the prevalence of an infectious disease to such a low level that rare vaccine-related complications are more frequent than the disease. When that happens, public anxiety about vaccination can result in concerns about vaccine use and may reduce its acceptance.

Live attenuated organisms should ordinarily not be given to *pregnant women* because of potential damage to the fetus. It has been shown that the virions in rubella vaccine are transmitted to the fetus, although without any recognized injurious effect. In addition, live attenuated vaccines are generally contraindicated for *patients with severe immune disorders* who may not be able to control the weakened pathogen in the vaccine preparation. Vaccination against smallpox is no longer practiced (except in some military personnel) since the disease has essentially been eradicated. However, as we noted above, concerns about the potential of variola virus as a biologic weapon have led to debate as to whether universal vaccination should be reintroduced. At this time, the plan is to vaccinate only individuals who are likely to respond or be exposed to a potential biologic attack. Additional stocks of this virus are reserved for use in postexposure prophylaxis. One argument against universal vaccination is that vaccinia virus inoculation carries significant risks, not only in immunocompromised individuals but also in individuals with certain cutaneous lesions. Contact between vaccinated and vulnerable individuals must be avoided until the vaccinia lesions have healed.

Arthritis and *arthralgia* are common but transient complications following vaccination with attenuated rubella virus, particularly in adult women. Of the inactivated vaccines, the killed *Bordetella pertussis* bacterial vaccine in DTP has been associated with some serious side effects, including *encephalopathy* in the infant. Although serious side effects were relatively rare and the benefits of the pertussis vaccine outweighed any alleged risks, the killed bacteria vaccine was replaced by an acellular vaccine containing inactivated pertussis toxin and one or more antigenic components (e.g., filamentous hemagglutinin and fimbriae). The acellular pertussis vaccine retains the efficacy of the earlier vaccine but has significantly fewer side effects.

Tetanus and diphtheria toxoids may provoke *local hypersensitivity reactions*. Because an adequate initial series of immunizations in childhood appears to give immunity that lasts some 10 years, the use of booster injections of tetanus toxoid should be guided by the nature of an injury and the history of immunization. Increased hypersensitivity to diphtheria toxoid in adolescents and adults necessitates the use of a smaller dose of diphtheria toxoid than that given to children. Because influenza virus is cultivated in chick embryos, allergy to egg protein is a contraindication to flu vaccination. Because whole influenza virus vaccine gives side effects in children, a split-virus component vaccine is recommended for children younger than 13 years of age. Some vaccines contain preservatives, such as the organomercurial compound thimerosal (Merthiolate), or antibiotics, such as neomycin or streptomycin, to which the vaccinated individual may be allergic.

RECENT APPROACHES TO PRODUCTION OF VACCINES

Advances in recombinant DNA technology, the rapid, automated synthesis of proteins, and other areas of bioengineering (such as monoclonal antibodies) hold promise for improvements in available vaccines and new approaches to vaccine production.

Vaccines Produced by Recombinant DNA

Recombinant DNA technology provides the means for expressing protein antigens in large amounts for vaccine use. As noted earlier, one example of the successful application of recombinant DNA technology to vaccine production is the hepatitis B vaccine. Hepatitis B, a major cause of liver infection, is associated with a long-term risk of hepatocellular carcinoma. An effective vaccine against hepatitis B was developed in the 1970s by purifying viral antigen from the blood of chronically infected donors. In the 1980s, the HIV epidemic heightened awareness about transmission of blood-borne pathogens, and there were concerns that this vaccine could transmit disease. Although several studies showed that the plasma-derived vaccine was safe, an alternative was developed; using recombinant DNA technology, the hepatitis B antigen was expressed in yeast. This recombinant vaccine simplified the production of antigen by avoiding reliance on human blood plasma and eliminated any potential hazard arising from inadvertent contamination of vaccine antigen with blood-borne pathogens.

In 2006, the first recombinant vaccine against HPV was approved for use in girls 11–12 years of age. This was the first vaccine developed to prevent cervical cancer and other diseases in females caused by HPV. Another effective recombinant vaccine has been developed against Lyme disease. Other vaccines produced by recombinant DNA technology are in various stages of clinical testing, some of which may provide practical, safer, and more effective means of immunization than are currently available.

Conjugated Polysaccharides

Conjugated polysaccharide vaccines have revolutionized the approach to vaccination against encapsulated bacterial pathogens. Humoral immunity is critical for protection against encapsulated pathogens, but most microbial polysaccharides are T-independent antigens, which are usually poorly immunogenic. Another problem with polysaccharide vaccines is that young children tend not to mount antibody responses to polysaccharide antigens. Children are at high risk for infection with encapsulated bacteria such as *S. pneumoniae* and *H. influenzae*. Conjugation of polysaccharide to a protein (such as tetanus or diphtheria toxoid) results in a molecule that behaves as a T-dependent antigen and elicits strong antibody responses to the polysaccharide moiety. Conjugation has provided vaccines that are effective in this age group. Conjugated polysaccharide vaccines are currently available against *H. influenzae* type b and certain serotypes of *S. pneumoniae*. Conjugated polysaccharide vaccines are under development for other pathogens, including meningococci, group B streptococci, *S. typhi*, and *Shigella* spp.

Synthetic Peptide Vaccines

The premise underlying the development of synthetic peptide vaccines is to use immunogenic peptides to elicit a protective immune response. Synthetic peptide vaccines are designed using the knowledge of the amino acid sequence of the antigen eliciting the protective immune response. In theory, highly purified peptides may be made in large quantities and their simpler antigenic composition may afford protection with fewer side effects. The general approach is to identify potential epitopes in a protective protein antigen using various algorithms, synthesize a series of peptides corresponding to the amino acid sequence, and test these for immunologic activity. One problem with peptide vaccines is that peptides are poorly immunogenic due to their small size and require conjugation to carrier proteins. Several synthetic peptide vaccines are currently in clinical testing. Peptide vaccines have shown promise against foot-and-mouth disease virus and malaria.

Anti-Idiotype Vaccines

An antibody induced to a specific epitope of an antigen has a combining site (idiotype) that structurally fits the epitope. If that antibody in turn is used as an immunogen to induce another antibody (an anti-idiotype) to react with the antigen-combining site of the idiotype, the anti-idiotype may structurally mimic the epitope. This structural mimicry is referred to as an ***internal image***. Because of the resemblance of the anti-idiotype and the original antigen epitope, its internal image (anti-idiotypic antibody) can be used as an immunogen to induce antibodies against the original epitope (Fig. 20.4). Several anti-idiotypic vaccines are currently being investigated for their effectiveness in treating human cancers.

One example is an immunogen consisting of antibodies against a monoclonal mouse antibody to hepatitis B surface antigen. Immunization with these anti-idiotypic antibodies, which contain the internal image of an epitope on the hepatitis B surface antigen, induces antibodies to that epitope. When the negative effects of certain biologic toxins preclude their use as antigens, anti-idiotypic antibodies can be used to elicit an antitoxic response.

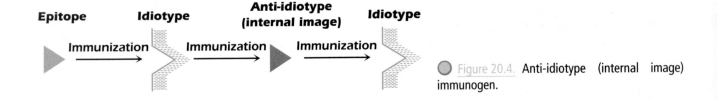

Figure 20.4. Anti-idiotype (internal image) immunogen.

Virus-Carrier Vaccine

It is possible to introduce into a live virus (such as vaccinia, adenovirus, or poliovirus) a gene from another organism that codes for a desired antigen by means of a vector. The vaccinia virus constructs replicates in the host, expresses the foreign gene, and then serves as a vaccine to that particular antigen. This approach is useful if the vaccinia virus is not hazardous to the host (as it may be to an immunocompromised individual). This virus-carrier vaccine has the additional advantage of potentially inducing both cell-mediated immunity and antibody-mediated immunity to the incorporated antigen.

Bacterium-Carrier Vaccine

Attenuated bacteria such as strains of *Salmonella typhimurium, Escherichia coli*, and BCG can also serve as carriers for pathogen genes in an effort to elicit pathogen-specific responses. These bacteria are altered by recombinant techniques, which introduce a foreign gene that can express the antigens of pathogenic microbes and induce immune responses. In the future, *S. typhimurium*, an intestinal pathogen, could be used to induce mucosal immunity to the foreign antigens.

DNA Vaccines

Vaccination with a plasmid encoding the DNA sequence for a protective antigen linked to a strong mammalian promoter can elicit an immune response to the protein. DNA vaccines are thought to work by allowing the expression of the microbial antigen inside host cells that take up the plasmid. DNA vaccines function by generating the desired antigen inside cells, which may facilitate MHC presentation. Other advantages of DNA vaccines include the absence of infection risk, greater stability relative to protein vaccines, and the possibility of delivering the antigen to cells that are not usually infected by the pathogen for better modulation of the immune response. DNA vaccines could be useful for immunizing young children who still have maternal antibody. The feasibility of DNA immunization has now been demonstrated against several viral, bacterial, and protozoal infections in laboratory animals. Several DNA vaccines are undergoing testing in humans to determine their usefulness in prevention or treatment of malaria and hepatitis B infection. However, no DNA vaccines are currently in use in

humans. A recent clinical trial to examine the efficacy of a DNA-based HIV vaccine comprised of a nonreplicating adenovirus vector and the HIV *gag, pol*, and *nef* genes unfortunately had to be terminated abruptly. It was found that administration of the vaccine to uninfected people was associated with significant increases in HIV infection compared to individuals given a placebo control vaccine. The apparent explanation for this disappointing outcome was that an earlier infection with adenovirus (common cold virus) activated memory CD4$^+$ T cells—the ideal targets of HIV. Another, unrelated concern is the possibility that DNA vaccines could be mutagenic if they integrate in host DNA. At this time, DNA vaccines continue to be the subject of intense experimental study.

Toxoids

Toxins can be inactivated to produce nonpathogenic toxoids that can be used for vaccination. Toxoids are among the earliest and most successful vaccines. Administration of toxoids prepared from inactivated tetanus, botulism, or diphtheria toxin elicits antibody responses that prevent disease. Despite the fact that natural infection does not always confer long-lasting immunity, toxoids are effective, presumably because the amount of toxin produced in infection may not be sufficient to elicit a strong immune response. That is why a bout of tetanus or diphtheria does not confer immunity to recurrent infection, but vaccination with a toxoid provides full protection.

PASSIVE IMMUNIZATION

Passive immunization results from the transfer of antibody or immune cells to an individual from another individual who has already responded to direct stimulation by antigen. Unlike active immunization, passive immunization does not rely on the ability of the host's immune system to make the appropriate response. Hence, passive immunization results in the immediate availability of antibodies that can mediate protection against pathogens. Passive immunization can occur naturally, when antibodies are transferred through the placenta or colostrum, or therapeutically, when preformed antibody is administered for the prophylaxis or therapy of infectious diseases.

Passive Immunization Through Placental Antibody Transfer

The developing fetus is passively immunized with maternal IgG as a result of placental transfer of antibody. Such antibodies are present at birth and protect the infant against those infections for which IgG is sufficient and for which the mother had immunity. For example, transfer of antibody to toxins (tetanus, diphtheria), viruses (measles, poliovirus, mumps, etc.), and certain bacteria (*H. influenzae* or *Streptococcus agalactiae* group B) can provide protection to the child in the first months of life. Thus, adequate active immunization of the mother is a simple and effective means of providing passive protection to the fetus and infant. (Note, however, that some premature infants may not acquire the maternal antibodies to the extent that full-term infants do.) Toxoid vaccination can elicit IgG responses that cross the placenta to provide protection to the fetus and newborn. This protection is extremely important in areas of the world where an unclean obstetric environment can lead to **tetanus neonatorum** (tetanus of the newborn).

Passive Immunization via Colostrum

Human milk contains a variety of factors that may influence the response of the nursing infant to infectious agents. Some of these factors are natural selective factors that can affect the intestinal microflora. This is accomplished by enhancement of the growth of desirable bacteria and by nonspecific inhibition of some microbes—through the action of lysozyme, lactoferrin, interferon, and leukocytes (including macrophages, T cells, B cells, and granulocytes). During the first two-three weeks post-partum, antibodies (IgA, IgM, and IgG) are found in breast milk; IgA concentration is higher in the colostrum (first milk) produced immediately postpartum (Table 20.6). Antibody is produced from B cells that are stimulated by intestinal antigens and migrate to the breast where they produce immunoglobulin (the enteromammary system). Thus, if organisms colonize or infect the mother's alimentary tract, it may lead to production of colostral antibody, which affords mucosal protection to the nursing infant against pathogens that enter via the intestinal tract. Antibodies to the enteropathogens *E. coli, S. typhi, Shigella* spp., poliomyelitis virus, coxsackievirus, and echovirus have been demonstrated. Feeding a mixture of IgA (73%) and IgG (26%) derived from human serum to low-birth-weight infants who did not have access to mothers' breast milk protected them against necrotizing enterocolitis. Antibodies to nonalimentary pathogens have also been demonstrated in colostrum—for example, tetanus and diphtheria antitoxins and antistreptococcal hemolysin.

Tuberculin-sensitive T lymphocytes are also transmitted to the infant through the colostrum, but the role of such cells in passive transfer of cell-mediated immunity is uncertain.

Passive Antibody Therapy and Serum Therapy

The administration of specific antibody preparations was one of the first effective antimicrobial therapies. Antibody against particular pathogens could be raised in animals, such as horses and rabbits (heterologous antibody), and administered to humans for treatment of various infections as serum therapy. Serum from individuals recovering from infection is rich in antibodies and can also be used for passive antibody therapy (homologous antibody). In recent years, some monoclonal antibodies made in the laboratory have been used for passive antibody therapy of infectious diseases. This is an area of great research interest, and it is likely that more antimicrobial therapies based on antibody administration will be developed in the future.

The active agent in serum therapy is specific antibody. In the preantibiotic era (before 1935), serum therapy was often the only therapy available for the treatment of infection. Serum therapy was used for the treatment of diphtheria, tetanus, pneumococcal pneumonia, meningococcal meningitis, scarlet fever, and other serious infections. For example, during World War I, tetanus antitoxin produced in horses injected with tetanus toxoid was used to treat wounded British troops and resulted in prompt reduction in cases of tetanus. This experience allowed the determination of the minimum concentration of antitoxin needed to provide protection and showed that the period of protection

TABLE 20.6. Levels of Immunoglobulin in Colostrum[a]

Class	Day postpartum				Approximate normal adult
	1	2	3	4	
IgA[b]	600	260	200	80	200
IgG[c]	80	45	30	16	1000
IgM	125	65	58	30	120

[a] After Michael et al. (1971). Values given are mg/100 mL.
[b] Approximately 80% is secretory IgA.
[c] IgG$_4$ represents 15% of colostral IgG and 3.5% of serum IgG.

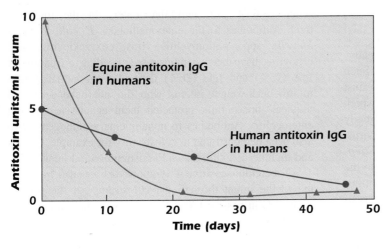

Figure 20.5. Serum concentration of human and equine IgG antitoxin following administration into humans.

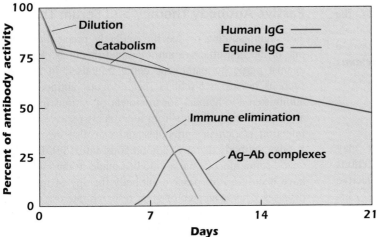

Figure 20.6. Fate of human and equine IgG following administration into humans.

in the human was brief (see Figs. 20.5 and 20.6). The heterologous equine antibody undergoes dilution, catabolism, immune complex formation, and immune elimination in the human. By contrast, the homologous human antibody, which reaches a peak level in the serum about 2 days after subcutaneous injection, undergoes dilution and catabolism with a reduction to half the maximal concentration in about 23 days (the half-life of human IgG_1, IgG_2, and IgG_4 is 23 days; that of IgG_3 is 7 days). The protective level of the human antibody is thus sustained considerably longer. Heterologous antibody, such as that from the horse, can cause at least two types of hypersensitivity reaction: type I (immediate, anaphylaxis; see Chapter 14) or type III (serum sickness from immune complexes; see Chapter 15). If no other treatment is available, it is possible to use the heterologous antiserum in an individual with type I sensitivity by administration of gradually increasing but minute amounts of the foreign serum given repeatedly over several hours. Some preparations of heterologous antibody [e.g., equine diphtheria antitoxin and antilymphocyte serum (ALS)] are still used in humans. In recent years, advances in hybridoma and recombinant DNA technology have allowed the synthesis of human immunoglobulins for therapy, so we no longer depend on animal sources for therapeutic antibodies. In addition to the significantly longer half-life, human antibodies have reduced toxicity.

Monoclonal and Polyclonal Antibodies

Hybridoma technology, which allows the production of monoclonal antibodies, was developed in 1975 (see Chapter 5). Polyclonal preparations result from the antibody response to immunization or recovery from infection in a host. In general, antibody to a specific agent is only a small fraction of the total antibody in a polyclonal preparation. Furthermore, polyclonal preparations usually contain antibodies to multiple antigens and include antibodies of various isotypes. Unlike their polyclonal counterparts, a monoclonal antibody preparation has one specificity and one isotype. As a result, the activity of monoclonal antibody preparations is considerably greater in proportion to the amount of protein present. Another advantage of monoclonal preparations is that they are invariant and do not have the lot-to-lot variability associated with polyclonal preparations, which depend on quantitative and qualitative aspects of the immune response for their potency. However, because they include antibodies with multiple specificities and isotypes, polyclonal preparations encompass a higher biologic diversity. In the past five years at least a dozen monoclonal antibodies have been licensed for clinical use. Most of them have been developed for the treatment of cancer, although one is now licensed for the prevention of infection by respiratory syncytial virus in young children. Several monoclonal and polyclonal antibody preparations are currently used for human therapy.

Preparation and Properties of Human Immune Serum Globulin

The use of immune globulin from human serum began in the early 1900s, when the serum of patients convalescing from measles was given to children who had been exposed to measles but had not yet developed symptoms. Additional attempts in 1916 and later showed that early administration of serum from recovered patients could protect against the emergence of clinically apparent measles. In 1933, human placentae were also recognized as a source of measles antibody. A problem with using serum for passive therapy is that it contains relatively little antibody in a large volume. In the early 1940s, Cohn and co-workers devised a method for the separation of the γ-globulin fraction from human serum by precipitation with cold ethanol. This so-called *Cohn fractionation* represented a practical and safe method for production of homologous human antibody for clinical use.

Plasma or serum is collected from healthy donors is pooled and used to prepare immune serum globulin (ISG) or human normal immunoglobulin (HNI). If the plasma or serum comes from donors who are specially selected after an immunizing or booster dose of antigen or after convalescence from a specific infection, the specific immune globulin preparation is designated accordingly: tetanus immune globulin (TIG), hepatitis B immune globulin (HBIG), varicella-zoster immune globulin (VZIG), and rabies immune globulin (RIG). Large quantities can be obtained by *plasmapheresis*, removal of the plasma and return of the blood cells to the donor. The fraction containing antibody globulin(s) is precipitated by cold ethanol. The resultant preparation (1) is theoretically free of viruses such as hepatitis virus and HIV, (2) concentrates many of the IgG antibodies about 25-fold, (3) is stable for years, and (4) can provide peak levels in blood approximately two days after intramuscular injection. Preparations that are safe when administered intravenously (called IVIG or IVGG) involve cold alcohol precipitation followed by various other treatments, including fractionation using polyethylene glycol or ion exchangers; acidification to pH 4–4.5; exposure to pepsin or trypsin; and stabilization with maltose, sucrose, glucose, or glycine. Such stabilization

reduces aggregation of the globulins that can trigger anaphylactoid reactions (see below). In these newer intravenous preparations, IgG is present in one-third to one-fourth its concentration in the intramuscular immune globulin preparations, and there is only a trace of IgA and IgM (Table 20.7).

Indications for Use of Immune Globulin

Antibody to RhD antigen (*Rhogam*) is given to Rh$^-$ mothers within a 72-h perinatal period to prevent their immunization by fetal Rh$^+$ erythrocytes that could affect future pregnancies. As discussed in Chapter 15, Rhogam administration promotes the removal of Rh$^+$ fetal cells to which the mother is exposed during parturition and thus avoids the sensitizing of the Rh$^-$ mother by Rh$^+$ antigens. TIG (antitoxin) is used to provide passive protection after certain wounds and in the absence of adequate active immunization with tetanus toxoid. Varicella zoster Ig (VZIG) is given to patients with leukemia who are highly vulnerable to the varicella-zoster (chickenpox) virus and to pregnant women and their infants exposed to or infected with varicella virus. Cytomegalovirus human immune globulin (CMV-IGIV) is used prophylactically for recipients of bone marrow or renal transplants. Rabies Ig (RIG) is given together with active immunization with human diploid cell rabies vaccine to individuals bitten by potentially rabid animals (human RIG is not universally available, so equine antibody may be necessary in some areas). Hepatitis B Ig (HBIG) may be given to a newborn child of a mother who has evidence of hepatitis B infection, to medical personnel after an accidental stick with a hypodermic needle, or after sexual contact with an individual with hepatitis B. Vaccinia immune globulin is given to eczematous or immunocompromised individuals with intimate exposure to others who have been vaccinated against smallpox by live attenuated vaccinia vaccine. Such compromised individuals can develop destructive progressive disease from the attenuated vaccine. IVIG has been used in certain circumstances for its antimicrobial properties and has had significant success against group B streptococcal infections in premature neonates, echovirus-induced chronic meningoencephalitis, and Kawasaki disease (a condition of unknown cause). Intravenous administration of immune globulin can reduce bacterial infections in patients with hematopoietic malignancies, such as chronic B-cell lymphocytic leukemia and multiple myeloma. Chronic IVIG administration has been useful in children who have immunosuppressive conditions and in premature infants; in hypogamma-globulinemia and primary immune deficiency disease, repeated injections of IVIG are required. IVIG also has therapeutic value in a variety of autoimmune conditions. For example, in immune idiopathic thrombocytopenic purpura (ITP), IVIG presumably blocks the Fc receptors

TABLE 20.7. Comparison of Human Immune Serum Globulin

Source	Immunoglobulin (mg/100 mL)		
	IgG	IgA	IgM
Whole serum	1,200	180	200
Immune serum globulin	16,500	100,500	25,200
Intravenous immunoglobulin	3,0005,000	Trace	Trace
Placental immune serum globulin	16,500	200,700	150,400

on phagocytic cells and prevents them from phagocytosing and destroying platelets coated with autoantibodies. IVIG has also been used with varying success in other immune cytopenias.

Precautions About Uses of Human Immune Serum Globulin Therapy

The preparations of globulin other than IVIG must be given by the intramuscular route; intravenous administration is contraindicated because of possible anaphylactoid reactions. These are probably due to aggregates of immunoglobulin formed during the fractionation by ethanol precipitation. These aggregates activate complement to yield anaphylatoxins (IgG_1, IgG_2, IgG_3, and IgM by the classical pathway; IgG4 and IgA by the alternative pathway) or cross-link Fc receptors directly, leading to the release of inflammatory mediators. An IVIG safe for intravenous administration has been used increasingly, particularly when repeated administration is required, as in agammaglobulinemia.

One unique contraindication to the use of the usual immune globulin preparations is in cases of congenital deficiency of IgA. Since these patients lack IgA, they recognize it as a foreign protein and respond by making antibodies against it, including IgE antibodies, which can lead to a subsequent anaphylactic reaction. The IVIG preparations with only a trace of IgA may pose less of a problem.

Colony-Stimulating Factors

As discussed in Chapter 11, colony-stimulating factors are cytokines that stimulate the development and maturation of WBCs. Granulocyte colony-stimulating factor (G-CSF), granulocyte–macrophage colony-stimulating factor (GM-CSF), and macrophage colony-stimulating factor (M-CSF) have been cloned by recombinant DNA technology and are now available for clinical use. CSFs have proven useful in accelerating the recovery of bone marrow cells in patients who have undergone myelosuppressive therapy for cancer or organ transplantation. In these patients, neutrophil depletion (neutropenia) is a major predisposing factor for severe infection. By shortening the period of neutropenia, CSFs can reduce the incidence of serious infections in patients receiving myelosuppressive therapy. CSFs also enhance leukocyte function, and there is encouraging preliminary information suggesting that these proteins may be useful in enhancing host defenses against various pathogens.

Several other cytokines are powerful activators of the immune system, and there is great interest in learning how to use them as adjunctive therapy against infectious diseases. IFN-γ is a powerful activator of macrophage function, which has been shown to reduce the incidence of severe infections in patients with chronic granulomatous disease. IFN-γ has shown encouraging results as adjunctive therapy for some infections, including drug-resistant *M. tuberculosis* infection and several unusual fungal infections.

SUMMARY

1. To cause disease, microbes must cause damage to the host.

2. The effective host defenses against individual pathogens depend on the type of pathogen. In general, successful protection against most pathogens involves both humoral and cellular components of the innate and adaptive immune systems.

3. Pathogens use a variety of strategies to escape host defenses, including polysaccharide capsules, antigenic variation, intracellular survival, proteolytic enzymes, and active suppression of the immune response.

4. In general, an effective host response to a pathogen uses components of both humoral and cellular immunity. However, for some pathogens, one arm of the immune system may provide the primary protection.

5. Protection against infectious diseases may be achieved by active as well as passive immunization.

6. Active immunization may result from previous infection or from vaccination, while passive immunization may occur by natural means (such as the transfer of antibodies from mother to fetus via the placenta or to an infant via the colostrum) or by artificial means (such as by the administration of immune globulins).

7. Active immunization may be achieved by administration of one immunogen or a combination of immunogens.

8. The incubation period of a disease and the rapidity with which protective antibody titers develop influence both the efficacy of vaccination and the anamnestic effect of a booster injection.

9. The site of administration of a vaccine may be of great importance; many routes of immunization lead to the synthesis of serum IgM and IgG; oral administration of some vaccines leads to the induction of secretory IgA in the digestive tract.

10. Immunoprophylaxis has had striking success against subsequent infection; immunotherapy has had limited success in infectious diseases.

REFERENCES

Barr E, Tamms G (2007): Quadrivalent human papillomavirus vaccine. *Clin Infect Dis* 45:609.

Bijker MS, Melief CJ, Offringa R, van der Burg SH (2007): Design and development of synthetic peptide vaccines: Past, present and future. *Exp Rev Vaccines* 6:591.

Carruthers VB, Cotter PA, Kumamoto CA (2007): Microbial pathogenesis: Mechanisms of infectious disease. *Cell Host Microbe* 2:214.

Casadevall A, Pirofski L (2000): Host-pathogen interactions: Basic concepts of microbial commensalism, colonization, infection, and disease. *Infect Immun* 68:6511.

Casadevall A, Scharff MD (1994): "Serum therapy" revisited: Animal models of infection and the development of passive antibody therapy. *Antimicrob Agents Chemother* 38:1695.

Centers of Disease Control and Prevention (2006): Recommended childhood immunization schedule—United States. *Ann Pharmacother* 40: 369.

Deitsch KW, Moxon ER, Wellems TE (1997): Shared themes of antigenic variation and virulence in bacterial, protozoal, and fungal infections. *Microbiol Molec Biol Rev* 61:283.

Doherty PC, Turner SJ (2007): The challenge of viral immunity. *Immunity* 27: 363.

Hanke T (2006): On DNA vaccines and prolonged expression of immunogens. *Eur J Immunol* 36: 806.

Hemming VG (2001): Use of intravenous immunoglobulins for prophylaxis and treatment of infectious diseases. *Clin Diag Lab Immunol* 8: 85963.

Hubel K, Dale DC, Liles WC (2002): Therapeutic uses of cytokines to modulate cytokine function for the treatment of infectious diseases: Current status of granulocyte colony-stimulating factor, granulocyte-macrophage colony-stimulating factor, macrophage colony-stimulating factor, and interferon-gamma. *J Infect Dis* 185:1490.

Letvin NL (2007): Correlates of immune protection and the development of a human immunodeficiency virus vaccine. *Immunity* 27:366.

Mirza A, Rathore MH (2007): Immunization update. *Adv Pediat* 54:135.

Park JM, Greten FR, Li ZW, Karin M (2002): Macrophage apoptosis by anthrax lethal factor through p38 MAP kinase inhibition. *Science* 297:2048.

Reichert JM (2001): Monoclonal antibodies and the clinic. *Nat Biotech* 19:819.

Robinson HL (2007): HIV/AIDS vaccines. *Clin Pharmacol Ther* 82:686.

Schiffman M, Castle PE, Jeronimo J, Rodriguez AC, Wacholder S (2007): Human papillomavirus and cervical cancer. *Lancet* 370:890.

REVIEW QUESTIONS

For each question, choose the ONE BEST answer.

1. The usual sequence of events in the development of an effective immune response to a viral infection is:

   A) interferon secretion, antibody synthesis, cellular immune response, NK-cell ADCC

   B) antibody synthesis, interferon secretion, NK-cell ADCC, cellular immune response

   C) NK-cell ADCC, interferon secretion, antibody synthesis, cellular immune response

   D) interferon secretion, cellular immune response, antibody synthesis, NK-cell ADCC

   E) cellular immune response, interferon secretion, antibody synthesis, NK-cell ADCC

2. Differences between Gram-positive and Gram-negative bacteria include:
   A) staining with crystal violet
   B) ability of complement to lyse cells
   C) thickness of the peptidoglycan layer
   D) endotoxin in the cell walls of Gram-negative bacteria
   E) all of the above

3. Antigenic variation is a mechanism of immune evasion that results in:
   A) interference with attachment to host receptors
   B) induction of immune suppression
   C) alterations in important surface antigens so that escape variants arise as a result of immune selection
   D) mutations in surface antigens
   E) destruction of antigens by proteolytic enzymes

4. The best way to provide immunologic protection against tetanus neonatorum (tetanus of the newborn) is to:
   A) inject the infant with human tetanus antitoxin
   B) inject the newborn with tetanus toxoid
   C) inject the mother with toxoid within 72 h of the birth of her child
   D) immunize the mother with tetanus toxoid before or early in pregnancy
   E) give the child antitoxin and toxoid for both passive and active immunization

5. Active, durable immunization against poliomyelitis can be accomplished by oral administration of attenuated vaccine (Sabin) or by parenteral injection of inactivated (Salk) vaccine. These vaccines are equally effective in preventing disease because:
   A) both induce adequate IgA at the intestinal mucosa, the site of entry of the virus
   B) antibody in the serum protects against the viremia that leads to disease
   C) viral antigen attaches to the anterior horn cells in the spinal cord, preventing attachment of virulent virus
   D) both vaccines induce formation of interferon
   E) both vaccines establish a mild infection that can lead to formation of antibody

6. The administration of vaccines is not without hazard. Of the following, which is least likely to adversely affect an immunocompromised host?
   A) measles vaccine
   B) pneumococcal vaccine
   C) bacille Calmette-Guérin (BCG)
   D) mumps vaccine
   E) Sabin poliomyelitis vaccine

7. The administration of foreign (e.g., equine) antitoxin for passive protection in humans can lead to serum sickness, which is characterized by all of the following except:
   A) production by host of antibody to foreign antibody
   B) onset in 24–48 h
   C) use of homologous antitoxin
   D) deposition of antigen–antibody complexes at various sites in the host
   E) although delayed, a reaction that is not a cell-mediated delayed, type IV immune response

8. The pneumococcal polysaccharide vaccine should be administered to all of the following except:
   A) individuals with chronic cardiorespiratory disease
   B) the elderly (>60 years of age)
   C) children (<2 years of age)
   D) persons with chronic renal failure
   E) individuals with sickle cell disease

9. Which of the following statements about human immune serum globulin is *false*?
   A) The source is human placenta.
   B) The globulins are obtained by precipitation with cold ethanol.
   C) The concentration of IgG is more than 10-fold greater than in plasma.
   D) IgA and IgM are present in concentrations slightly lower than in plasma.
   E) The ethanol precipitation does not render preparation of globulin free of hepatitis virus.

ANSWERS TO REVIEW QUESTIONS

1. *D* The usual sequence of events in the host immune response to a viral infection is interferon secretion, cellular immune response, and antibody synthesis followed by NK-cell ADCC. Interferon is produced early in the course of viral infection and serves to slow the infection of adjoining cells. Cellular immune responses in the form of cytotoxic CD8$^+$ T cells occur early in viral infection and usually precede the appearance of serum-neutralizing antibody or NK-cell-mediated ADCC (which requires specific antibody).

2. *E* Differences between Gram-positive and Gram-negative bacteria include staining with crystal violet. Gram-negative cells can be lysed by complement, but Gram-positive cells are complement resistant because of a thick peptidoglycan layer. Gram-negative bacteria have endotoxin in their cell walls that can cause hemodynamic compromise and septic shock in patients with Gram-negative sepsis. Gram-positive bacteria lack endotoxin but have immunogenic teichoic acids.

3. *C* Antigenic variation is common to many pathogens and is a mechanism by which they are able to escape the immune system. Antigenic variation can be the result of various mechanisms including mutation, changes in surface protein expression, and natural variation among strains such as occurs in the pneumococci. The potential of a microorganism for antigenic variation is a major consideration in vaccine design.

4. *D* The simplest and most effective way to protect the newborn infant against exotoxic disease, such as tetanus and diphtheria, is to induce antibody in the mother. The antitoxic IgG passing through the placenta will provide the necessary protection. While tetanus antitoxin could be used to provide short-term passive protection, it would be more costly and require an otherwise unnecessary and painful injection. Injection of toxoid in the mother within 72 h of delivery of the child would not allow time for induction of antibody. While antitoxin and toxoid could provide immediate passive and future active protection, the latter would have to be accompanied by future injections of toxoid and the former is expensive; both would require undesirable injections.

5. *B* Both attenuated and inactivated vaccines lead to formation of circulating antibody, which would provide protection by intercepting the infecting virus before it reaches the target tissue in the central nervous system. While the Sabin vaccine induces mucosal gut IgA that may intercept virus at the portal of entry, the parenterally injected Salk vaccine is not effective in inducing mucosal IgA. Viral antigen in the vaccine might attach to the anterior horn cells in the nervous system, but it probably would not provide durable immunity. Induction of interferon would represent potentially only brief protection. Only the Sabin vaccine, being attenuated and live, would induce a mild infection.

6. *B* The pneumococcal vaccine consists of capsular polysaccharides from *S. pneumoniae* and represents a nonviable vaccine that cannot lead to infection. Measles, mumps, and Sabin polio vaccines contain attenuated viruses, and bacille Calmette-Guérin is an attenuated bacterium. These attenuated organisms are capable of proliferating in the human host. The normal host limits their replication, but the immunocompromised host may not be able to do so, and progressive infection may occur.

7. *B* The reactions that constitute serum sickness follow administration of the foreign substance within 6–12 days. During this time, the host produces antibody that reacts with the foreign substance(s), which persists in the host and leads to antigen–antibody complexes that can be deposited in joints, lymph nodes, skin, and elsewhere. The manifestations of the immune reaction, although appearing later, nevertheless are classified as type III rather than cell-mediated delayed (type IV) hypersensitivity because they involve antibodies rather than T cells.

8. *C* Children younger than two years of age do not respond adequately to immunization with pure bacterial capsule polysaccharide vaccine. Therefore, vaccinating them may be useless. The various other individuals listed are particularly vulnerable to infection with *S. pneumoniae*. While some of them may mount a suboptimal response to the vaccine, they should nevertheless be vaccinated.

9. *E* The potential hazard of hepatitis viruses in human plasma is overcome by the separation of ethanol-precipitated globulins. The concentration of IgG is about 16,500 mg/dL, compared to 1200 mg/dL in plasma. The IgG thus becomes highly concentrated in immune serum globulin, but IgA and IgM are relatively depleted, and their concentrations in the ethanol-precipitated immune serum globulin are close to their original concentrations in the plasma.

GLOSSARY

ABO blood group system Antigens expressed on red blood cells used for typing human blood for transfusion. Individuals who do not express A or B antigens on their red blood cells naturally form antibodies that interact with them.

accessory cell A cell required to initiate immune responses, often used to describe an antigen-presenting cell. See also antigen-presenting cell.

accessory molecules Molecules other than the antigen receptor and the major histocompatibility complex (MHC) that participate in activation and effector functions of T-lymphocytes.

acquired immune response The response of antigen-specific lymphocytes to antigen, including the development of immunologic memory; also known as adaptive immune response.

acquired immunodeficiency syndrome (AIDS) A disease caused by human immunodeficiency virus (HIV) infection that is characterized by depletion of CD4$^+$ T cells leading to a profound defect in cell-mediated immunity. Clinically, AIDS manifests with opportunistic infections, malignant tumors, encephalopathy, and wasting.

activation-induced cytidine deaminase (AID) Enzyme that plays a key role in initiating the three major pathways that generate diversity of antibodies: class switch recombination, somatic hypermutation, and gene conversion. It removes cytidine groups from the DNA in activated B cells to form uridine.

activation protein 1 (AP-1) A family of DNA-binding transcription factors that binds to one another through a shared structural motif called a leucine zipper. Important members of the AP-1 family include Fos and Jun.

acute-phase proteins Found in the blood after the onset of an infection, they participate in the early phases of host defense. Include cytokines such as IL-1, IL-6, TNF and interferons as well as C-reactive protein.

acute-phase response (APR) Early phase (within hours) of systemic response to infection (see also acute-phase proteins.)

acute rejection A form of graft rejection involving injury mediated by T cells, macrophages, and antibodies that usually begins after the first week following transplantation.

adaptive immune response See acquired immune response.

adaptor proteins Key linkers between receptors and downstream members of signaling pathways. All use a similar domain known as an SH2 domain.

ADCC See antibody-dependent, cell-mediated cytotoxicity.

addressins Glycoproteins expressed on high endothelial venules of the vascular endothelium at the boundary of the nodes that bind adhesion molecules expressed on leukocytes.

Immunology: A Short Course, Sixth Edition, By Richard Coico and Geoffrey Sunshine
Copyright © 2009 John Wiley & Sons, Inc.

adenosine deaminase (ADA) deficiency A form of severe combined immunodeficiency (SCID) in which B and T cells fail to develop. Affected individuals lack an enzyme, adenosine deaminase (ADA), which catalyzes the deamination of adenosine as well as deoxyadenosine to produce inosine and deoxyinosine, respectively.

adhesion molecules Mediate the binding of one cell to another or to extracellular matrix proteins. They include integrins, selectins, and members of the immunoglobulin gene superfamily.

adjuvant A substance given with antigen that enhances the response to the antigen.

adoptive transfer The transfer of the capacity to make an immune response by transplantation of immunocompetent cells.

affinity A measure of the binding constant of a single antigen-combining site with a monovalent antigenic determinant.

affinity chromatography The purification of a substance by means of its affinity for another substance immobilized on a solid support; for example, an antigen can be purified by affinity chromatography on a column of antigen-specific antibody molecules covalently linked to beads.

affinity maturation The sustained increase in affinity of antibodies for an antigen with time following immunization. The genes encoding the antibody variable regions undergo somatic hypermutation with concomitant selection of B lymphocytes whose receptors express high affinity for the antigen.

agammaglobulinemia See X-linked agammaglobulinemia.

agglutination The aggregation of particulate antigen by antibodies.

agonist peptides Peptide antigens that activate T cells with specific TCRs, inducing them to make cytokines and to proliferate.

AIRE See autoimmune regulator.

alleles Two or more alternate forms of a gene that occupy the same position or locus on a specific chromosome.

allelic exclusion The ability of heterozygous lymphoid cells to produce only one allelic form of antigen-specific receptor (Ig or TCR) when they have the genetic endowment to produce both. Genes other than those for the antigen-specific receptors are usually expressed codominantly.

allergen An antigen responsible for producing allergic reactions by inducing IgE synthesis.

allergic asthma A clinical phenomenon caused by constriction of the bronchial tree due to an allergic reaction to inhaled antigen.

allergic reaction A response to environmental antigens, or allergens, which most commonly involves responses mediated by IgE and $CD4^+$ T_H2 cells.

allergic rhinitis An allergic reaction in the nasal mucosa, also known as hay fever, that causes runny nose, sneezing, and tears.

allergy Reaction to nonpathogenic antigens in the environment. See allergic reaction.

alloantigens MHC antigens expressed on the cells of one individual that differ from the MHC antigens expressed by the cells of a genetically distinct individual. These alloantigen differences stimulate a powerful T cell responses when a tissue is transplanted from one individual to another. Polymorphisms at the MHC locus stimulate intense reactions to allografted tissues.

allogeneic An adjective that describes genetic variations or differences among members or strains of the same species. The term refers to organ or tissue grafts between genetically dissimilar humans or between unrelated members of the same species.

allograft A tissue transplant (graft) between two genetically nonidentical members of a species.

allotypes Antigenic determinants that are present in allelic (alternate) forms. When used in association with immunoglobulin, describes allelic variants of immunoglobulins detected by antibodies raised between members of the same species.

alternative complement pathway The mechanism of complement activation by nearly all foreign substances in the absence of antibody. Initiated by deposition of C3b on cell surface.

alveolar macrophage A macrophage found in the lung alveoli that may remove inhaled material.

anamnestic A term used to describe immunologic memory, which leads to a rapid increase in response after reexposure to antigen.

anaphylatoxin Substance such as C3a or C5a capable of releasing histamine from mast cells and basophils and inducing inflammatory responses.

anaphylaxis Immediate hypersensitivity response to antigenic challenge, mediated by IgE and mast cells. Anaphylaxis is a life-threatening allergic reaction caused by the release of pharmacologically active agents.

anchor residues The amino acid residues of a peptide whose side chains fit into pockets in the peptide-binding cleft of an MHC molecule. The side chains bind to complementary amino acids in the MHC molecule and therefore serve to anchor the peptide in the cleft of the MHC molecule.

anergy A state of antigen-specific nonresponsiveness in which a T or B cell is present but functionally unable to respond to antigen.

ankylosing spondylitis A chronic inflammatory disease affecting the spine, sacroiliac joints, and large peripheral joints. There is a major genetic predisposition, approximately 90% of patients with ankylosing spondylitis are positive for HLA-B27 as compared with 8% among individuals who are negative for this HLA determinant in the United States.

antibody Serum protein formed in response to immunization; antibodies are typically defined in terms of their specific binding to the immunogen.

antibody-dependent, cell-mediated cytotoxicity (ADCC) A phenomenon in which target cells, coated with IgG antibody, are destroyed by specialized killer cells (NK cells and macrophages) which bear receptors for the Fc portion of the coating antibody (Fc receptors). These receptors allow the killer cells to bind to the antibody-coated target.

antigen Any foreign material that is specifically bound by antibody or lymphocytes; also used loosely to describe materials used for immunization.

antigen-binding site The location on an antibody molecule where an antigenic determinant or epitope is bound. The antigen-binding site is located in a cleft bordered by the N-terminal variable regions of heavy- and light-chain parts of the Fab region.

antigen capture assay Antigen binds to a specific antibody and its presence is detected using a second antibody that binds to a different epitope.

antigenic determinant A single antigenic site or epitope on a complex antigenic molecule or particle.

antigenic drift Variations in antigenicity of microorganisms (e.g., viruses, parasites) resulting from point mutations of genes causing small differences in surface antigen expression.

antigenic shift Reassortment of segmented influenza virus genome with another influenza virus, causing surface antigens to change radically.

antigen presentation The display of antigen as peptide fragments bound to MHC molecules on the surface of a cell; T cells recognize antigen only when it is presented in this way.

antigen-presenting cell (APC) Cells such as dendritic cells, macrophages and B cells that express MHC class II molecules and are involved in presentation of antigen to T cells.

antigen processing The degradation of proteins into peptides that can bind to MHC molecules for presentation to T cells.

antigen receptor The specific antigen-binding receptor on T or B lymphocytes; these receptors are transcribed and translated from rearrangements and translocation of V, D, and J genes.

anti-immunoglobulin antibodies Antibodies specific for immunoglobulin constant domains that are useful for detecting bound antibody molecules in immunoassays and other applications.

antiserum (plural: *antisera*) The fluid component of clotted blood from an immune individual that contains a heterogeneous collection of antibodies against the molecule used for immunization. Such antibodies bind the antigen used for immunization. Each has its own structure, its own epitope on the antigen, and its own set of cross-reactions. This heterogeneity makes each antiserum unique.

antitoxin Antibody specific for exotoxins produced by certain microorganisms such as the causative agents of diphtheria and tetanus.

APC See antigen-presenting cell.

apoptosis A form of programmed cell death caused by activation of endogenous molecules leading to the fragmentation of DNA.

appendix A gut-associated lymphoid tissue located at the beginning of the colon.

Arthus reaction A hypersensitivity reaction produced by local formation of antigen-antibody aggregates that activate the complement cascade and cause thrombosis, hemorrhage, and acute inflammation.

asthma A disease of the lungs characterized (in most cases) by reversible airway obstruction, inflammation of the airway with prominent eosinophil participation, and increased responsiveness by the airway to various stimuli. Some cases of asthma are allergic (see allergic asthma) and are mediated, in part, by IgE antibody to environmental allergens. Other cases are provoked by no allergic factors.

ataxia telangiectasia A disorder characterized by cerebellar ataxia, oculocutaneous telangiectasis, and variable immunodeficiency that affects the function of both T and B lymphocytes, the development of lymphoid malignancies, and recurrent sinopulmonary infections.

atopic allergy or atopy A term used to describe IgE-mediated allergic responses in humans, usually showing a genetic predisposition.

autoantibody An antibody produced in an individual that is specific for a self-antigen. Autoantibodies can cause damage to cells and tissues.

autochthonous Pertaining to self.

autograft A tissue transplant from one area to another on a single individual.

autoimmune disease A disease caused by a breakdown of self-tolerance such that the adaptive immune system responds to self-antigens and mediates cell and tissue damage. Autoimmune diseases can be systemic (e.g., systemic lupus erythematosus) or organ specific (e.g., thyroiditis or diabetes).

autoimmunity An immune response to self tissues or components. Such immune responses may have pathologic consequences leading to autoimmune diseases.

autoimmune regulator (AIRE) AIRE gene product codes for a protein that at least partly controls the expression of self-molecules in thymic medullary epithelial cells. If the AIRE gene product is lacking, deletion of autoreactive lymphocytes is impaired, resulting in incomplete and autoimmune responses in several tissues.

autologous Derived from the same individual, self.

autophagy Pathway that transports proteins from the cytoplasm into lysosomes for degradation and possible association with MHC class II molecules.

avidity The summation of multiple affinities, for example, when a polyvalent antibody binds to a polyvalent antigen.

azathioprine A potent immunosuppressive drug that is converted to its active form *in vivo* and then kills rapidly proliferating cells, including lymphocytes responding to grafted tissues.

B7 A costimulatory immunoglobulin superfamily protein whose expression is restricted to the surface of T lymphocytes of APC activate (e.g., dendritic cells, B cells, macrophages). The ligand for B7 is CD28.

β$_2$ microglobulin The extracellular light chain of the class I MHC molecule that associates with the transmembrane α chain.

BALT See bronchus-associated lymphoid tissue.

bare lymphocyte syndrome An immunodeficiency condition characterized by failure to express either HLA class I or class II gene products.

basophils White blood cells containing granules that stain with basic dyes. They are thought to have a function similar to mast cells.

B cell See B lymphocyte.

B-cell receptor (BCR) The cell surface receptor of B cells for a specific antigen composed of a transmembrane immunoglobulin molecule associated with the invariant Igα and Igβ chains in a noncovalent complex.

B-cell tyrosine kinase (Btk) A Src family tyrosine kinase involved in B-cell maturation. Mutations in the gene expressing Btk cause X-linked agammaglobulinemia, in which B cells fail to develop beyond the pre-B-cell stage.

BCG (bacille Calmette-Guerin) A *Mycobacterium bovis* strain that has long been used outside the United States as a vaccine against tuberculosis.

BCR See B-cell receptor.

Bence Jones protein Dimers of immunoglobulin light chains in the urine of patients with multiple myeloma.

Blk See tyrosine kinases.

blocking antibody A functional term for an antibody molecule capable of blocking the interaction of antigen with other antibodies or with cells.

Bloom's syndrome A disease caused by mutations in DNA helicase and characterized by low T-cell numbers, reduced antibody levels, and increased susceptibility to respiratory infections, cancer, and radiation damage.

B lymphocyte Lymphocyte that expresses immunoglobulin on its surface. It is the precursor of the plasma cell that synthesizes and secretes antibodies and is thus the central cellular component of humoral immune responses. B lymphocytes develop in the bone marrow, and mature B cells are found mainly in lymphoid follicles in secondary lymphoid tissues, in bone marrow, and in low numbers in the circulation.

bone marrow The site of hematopoiesis, in which stem cells give rise to the cellular elements of blood, including red blood cells, monocytes, polymorphonuclear leukocytes, platelets, and lymphocytes.

bone marrow transplantation A procedure used to treat a variety of conditions including neoplasia that are not amenable to other forms of therapy. It has been especially used in cases of aplastic anemia, acute lymphocytic leukemia, and acute nonlymphocytic leukemia.

bradykinin A vasoactive peptide that is produced as a result of tissue damage and acts as an inflammatory mediator.

bronchus-associated lymphoid tissue (BALT) Secondary lymphoid organs connected to the bronchial tree.

Bruton's agammaglobulinemia See X-linked agammaglobulinemia.

bursa of Fabricius Site of development of B cells in birds; an outpouching of the cloaca.

C (constant region) The DNA sequence in an immunoglobulin or T-cell receptor gene that encodes the nonvariable portion of an Ig light or heavy chain or TCR chain.

C1 A complement component that initiates the classical complement pathway by attaching to the Fc regions of IgG or IgM.

C1 deficiencies Patients with C1 defects may manifest systemic lupus erythematosus, glomerulonephritis, or pyogenic infections as well as an increased incidence of type III (immune complex) hypersensitivity diseases. Only a few cases of C1q, C1r, or C1r and C1s deficiencies have been reported.

C1 esterase inhibitor A serum protein that counteracts activated C1. This diminishes the generation of C2b, which facilitates development of edema.

C1 inhibitor (C1 INH) A serum protein that blocks C1r activation, prevents C1r cleavage of C1s, and inhibits C1s splitting of C4 and C2.

C1 inhibitor (C1 INH) deficiency The most frequently found deficiency of the classic complement pathway characterized by the absence of C1 INH; may be seen in patients with hereditary angioedema.

C1q An 18-polypeptide-chain subcomponent of C1, the first component of the classical complement pathway.

C1q deficiency Deficiency of C1q may be found in association with lupus-like syndromes.

C1r A subcomponent of C1, the first component of complement in the classical activation pathway. A serine esterase.

C1s A serine esterase that is a subcomponent of C1. Ca^{2+} binds two C1s molecules to the C1q stalk.

C2 The third complement protein in the classical complement pathway activation. C2 is a single polypeptide chain that unites with C4b molecules on the cell surface in the presence of magnesium.

C2 deficiency Rare deficiency; in general, no symptoms are exhibited. It has an autosomal recessive mode of inheritance; autoimmune-like manifestations that resemble features of certain collagen-vascular diseases, such as systemic lupus erythematosus, may appear.

C3 A glycoprotein heterodimeric complement component that is linked by disulfide bonds. It is the fourth complement component to react in the classical pathway, and it is also a reactant in the alternative complement pathway. C3 contains alpha and beta polypeptide chains and has an internal thioester bond which permits it to link covalently with surfaces of cells and proteins.

C3a A low-molecular-weight (9-kDa) peptide fragment of complement component C3; it is an anaphylatoxin.

C3b The principal fragment produced when complement component C3 is split by either classical or alternative pathway convertases, i.e., C4b2a or C3bBb, respectively. It results from C3 convertase digestion of C3. A key opsonin.

C3 convertase An enzyme that splits C3 into C3b and C3a. There are two types: one in the classical pathway designated C4b2a and one in the alternative pathway of complement activation termed C3bBb.

C3 tickover Alternative pathway C3 convertase perpetually generates C3b. C3 internal thioester bond hydrolysis is the initiating event.

C4 C4 reacts immediately following C1 in the classical pathway of complement activation.

C5 Component in the complement cascade that binds to the C5 convertase in the classical and alternative pathways.

C5a Small peptide fragment released into the fluid after cleavage of C5; an anaphylatoxin.

C5b The larger molecular species that remains after C5 convertase splits C5. It has a binding site for complement component C6 and complexes with it on the cell surface to begin generation of the membrane attack complex (MAC).

C5 convertase A molecular complex that splits C5 into C5a and C5b in both the classical and the alternative pathways of complement activation.

C5 deficiency A very uncommon genetic disorder that has an autosomal recessive mode of inheritance. Individuals with this deficiency have a defective ability to form the membrane attack complex (MAC), which is necessary for the efficient lysis of invading microorganisms. They have an increased susceptibility to disseminated infections by *Neisseria* microorganisms.

C6 A complement component that participates in the membrane attack complex (MAC).

C6 deficiency Very uncommon genetic defect. Has an autosomal recessive mode of inheritance. Affected individuals have only trace amounts of C6 in their plasma and have defective ability to form a membrane attack complex (MAC) with increased susceptibility to disseminated infections by *Neisseria* microorganisms.

C7 A complement component that binds to C5b and C6 to form C5b67 on the surface of a cell as part of the MAC. The complex has the appearance of a stalk with a leaf type of structure.

C7 deficiency Rare genetic disorder, with an autosomal recessive mode of inheritance, associated with a defective ability to form a membrane attack complex (MAC) and increased incidence of disseminated infections caused by *Neisseria* microorganisms.

C8 A complement component that binds to C5bC6C7 and participates in the membrane attack complex (MAC).

C8 deficiency Rare genetic disorder with an autosomal recessive mode of inheritance; associated with a defective ability to form a membrane attack complex (MAC) and an increased propensity to develop disseminated infections caused by *Neisseria* microorganisms such as meningococci.

C9 A complement component that binds to the C5b678 complex on the cell surface. The interaction of 12–15 C9 molecules with one C5b678 complex is the final step in the production of the membrane attack complex (MAC).

C9 deficiency Rare genetic disorder with an autosomal recessive mode of inheritance. There is a defective ability to form the membrane attack complex (MAC).

calcineurin Cytosolic serine/threonine phosphatase that plays a crucial role in signaling via the TCR. The immunosuppressive drugs cyclosporine A and tracolimus (FK506) form complexes with cellular proteins called immunophilins that inactivate calcineurin, thereby suppressing T-cell responses.

calnexin An endoplasmic reticulum (ER) protein that binds partly folded molecules of the Ig superfamily of proteins and returns them to the ER until folding is completed.

calreticulin A molecular chaperone that binds initially to MHC class I, class II, and other proteins containing immunoglobulin-like domains such as the TCR and BCR.

CAM Cell-surface adhesion molecule. See adhesion molecules.

carcinoembryonic antigen (CEA) A membrane glycoprotein epitope that is present in the fetal gastrointestinal tract in normal conditions. CEA levels are elevated in almost one third of patients with colorectal, liver, pancreatic, lung, breast, head and neck, cervical, bladder, medullarythyroid, and prostatic carcinomas.

carrier A large immunogenic molecule or particle to which a hapten or other nonimmunogenic, epitope-bearing molecule may attach, allowing it to become immunogenic.

caspases A family of closely related cysteine proteases that cleave proteins at aspartic acid residues. They have important roles in apoptosis.

CD See cluster of differentiation.

CDR See complementarity-determining regions.

CEA See carcinoembryonic antigen.

cell-mediated cytotoxicity Killing (lysis) of a target cell by an effector lymphocyte.

cell-mediated immunity (CMI) Immune reaction mediated by T cells, in contrast to humoral immunity, which is antibody mediated. Also referred to as delayed-type hypersensitivity.

central lymphoid organs Sites of lymphocyte development. In humans, B lymphocytes develop in bone marrow, whereas T lymphocytes develop with the thymus from bone-marrow-derived progenitors.

central tolerance Self-tolerance induced in central lymphoid organs as a consequence of immature self-reactive lymphocytes recognizing self-antigens and subsequently leading to their death or inactivation. Central tolerance prevents the emergence of lymphocytes with high-affinity receptors for the ubiquitous self-antigens that are likely to be present in the bone marrow or thymus.

centroblasts Large, rapidly dividing cells found in germinal centers that undergo somatic hyperrmutation and give rise to antibody-secreting and memory B cells.

CFU See colony-forming unit.

CH50 unit The amount of complement (serum dilution) that induces lysis of 50% of erythrocytes coated with specific antibody.

chaperone A molecule that binds to a newly synthesized molecule and ensures that it traffics to the correct compartment inside a cell.

Chediak–Higashi syndrome A childhood disorder with a defect in lysosomal fusion that leads to impaired intracellular killing of microorganisms.

chemokines Cytokines of relatively low molecular weight, released by a variety of cells, and involved in inflammatory responses and the migration and activation of primarily phagocytic cells and lymphocytes.

chemotaxis Migration of cells along a concentration gradient of an attractant.

chimera A mythical animal possessing the head of a lion, the body of a goat, and the tail of a snake. Refers to an individual containing cellular components derived from another genetically distinct individual.

chromosomal translocation A chromosomal abnormality in which a segment of one chromosome is transferred to another. Malignant diseases of lymphocytes are associated with chromosomal translocations involving an Ig or TCR locus and a chromosomal segment containing a cellular oncogene.

chronic granulomatous disease (CGD) A disorder that is inherited as an X-linked trait characterized by an enzyme defect associated with NADPH oxidase. This enzyme deficiency causes neutrophils and monocytes to have decreased consumption of oxygen and diminished glucose utilization by the hexose monophosphate shunt.

chronic lymphocytic leukemia (CLL) A B-cell leukemia in which long-lived small lymphocytes continually collect in the spleen, lymph nodes, bone marrow, and blood. Most are transformed B-1 cells and express CD5.

chronic rejection A form of allograft rejection characterized by fibrosis with loss of normal organ structures occurring during a prolonged period. In many cases, the major pathologic event in chronic rejection is graft arterial occlusion.

class-II-associated invariant chain peptide (CLIP) A peptide of variable length cleaved from the invariant chain by proteases. CLIP remains associated with the class II MHC molecules in an unstable form until it is removed by the HLA-DM protein.

classical complement pathway The mechanism of complement activation initiated initiated by component C1 binding to antigen–antibody aggregates.

class switch See isotype switch.

clonal deletion The removal of lymphocytes of a particular specificity after contact with either self- or foreign antigen.

clonal expansion The increase in number of lymphocytes specific for an antigen that results from antigen stimulation and proliferation of naïve T cells. Clonal expansion occurs in lymphoid tissues and is required to generate enough antigen-specific effector lymphocytes from rare naïve precursors to eradicate infections.

clonal ignorance A form of lymphocyte unresponsiveness in which self-antigens are ignored by the immune system even though lymphocytes with receptors specific for those antigens remain viable and functional.

clonal selection theory The prevalent concept that specificity and diversity of an immune response are the result of selection by antigen of specifically reactive clones from a large repertoire of preformed lymphocytes, each with individual specificities.

cluster of differentiation (CD) Cluster of antigens with which antibodies react that characterize cell surface molecules.

c-myc A cellular protooncogene that encodes a nuclear factor involved in cell cycle regulation. Translocations of the c-*myc* gene into Ig loci are associated with B-cell malignant neoplasms.

cold agglutinin An antibody that agglutinates particulate antigen, such as bacteria or red cells, optimally at temperatures less than 37°C. In clinical medicine, the term usually refers to antibodies against red blood cell antigens as in the cold agglutinin syndrome.

colony-forming unit (CFU) The hematopoietic stem cell and the progeny cells that derive from it. Mature hematopoietic cells in the blood are considered to develop from one CFU.

colony-stimulating factors (CSFs) Glycoproteins that govern the formation, differentiation, and function of hematopoietic progenitor cells. CSFs promote the growth, maturation, and differentiation of stem cells to produce progenitor cell colonies *in vitro*.

combinatorial joining The joining of V, D, and J segments of Ig and TCR genes to generate essentially new genetic information during the development of B and T cells. Combinatorial joining allows multiple opportunities for two sets of genes to combine in different ways.

common leukocyte antigen (LCA) (CD45) An antigen shared in common by both T and B lymphocytes.

common lymphoid progenitors Stem cells that give rise to all lymphocytes.

common variable immunodeficiency (CVID) A relatively common congenital or acquired immunodeficiency that may be either familial or sporadic. The familial form may have a variable mode of inheritance. Hypogammaglobulinemia is common to all of these patients and usually affects all classes of immunoglobulin, but in some cases only IgG is affected.

complement A key effector mechanism in both innate and adaptive immunity for the elimination of microbial pathogens.

complementarity-determining regions (CDRs) Hypervariable regions of immunoglobulins and T-cell receptors that determine their specificity and make contact with specific ligand. The CDRs are the most variable part of the molecule and contribute to the diversity of these molecules. There are three such regions (CDR1, CDR2, and CDR3) in each V domain.

complement receptors (CRs) Cell-surface proteins on a variety of cells that recognize and bind complement proteins that have bound pathogens or other antigens. CRs on phagocytes allow them to identify pathogens coated with complement proteins for uptake and destruction. Complement receptors include CR1, the receptor for C1q, CR2, CR3, and CR4.

complete Freund's adjuvant (CFA) See Freund's complete adjuvant.

concanavalin A (Con A) A jack bean (*Canavalia ensiformis*) lectin that induces erythrocyte agglutination and is mitogenic for T lymphocytes; that is, they undergo mitosis and proliferate.

conformational epitopes Discontinuous epitopes on a protein antigen that are formed from several separate regions in the primary sequence of a protein that are brought together by protein folding. Antibodies that bind conformational epitopes bind only native-folded not denatured proteins.

congenic (also coisogenic) Describes two individuals who differ only in the genes at a particular locus and are identical at all other loci.

constant (C) region The invariant carboxyl-terminal portion of an Ig or TCR molecule, as distinct from the variable region at the amino terminus of the chain.

contact dermatitis A type IV, T-lymphocyte-mediated hypersensitivity reaction of the delayed type that develops in response to an allergen applied in the skin.

contact hypersensitivity A form of delayed-type hypersensitivity in which T cells respond to antigens introduced by contact with the skin. Poison ivy hypersensitivity is a contact hypersensitivity reaction that results from exposure to pentadecacatechol found in poison ivy leaves. Chemicals eliciting contact hypersensitivity typically bind to and modify self-proteins or molecules on the surfaces of APC, which are then recognized by CD4$^+$ or CD8$^+$ T cells.

convertase An enzymatic activity that converts a complement protein into its reactive form by cleaving it. Generation of the C3/C5 convertase is the pivotal event in complement activation.

Coombs test Named for its originator, R. R. A. Coombs, and used to detect antibodies by addition of an anti-immunoglobulin antibody.

coreceptor A cell surface specific protein that increases the sensitivity of the antigen-receptor to antigen; it enhances signaling through the BCR or TCR complex.

cortex Outer region of a gland, such as the adrenal gland or thymus.

corticosteroids Steroid hormones that are lympholytic and derived from the adrenal cortex. Glucocorticoids (e.g. prednisone, dexamethasone) can diminish the size and lymphocyte content of lymph nodes and spleen, while sparing proliferating myeloid or erythroid stem cells of the bone marrow.

costimulator molecules Membrane-bound molecules expressed by APC that interact with the T cell surface and provide a stimulus (second signal) in addition to antigen required for the full activation of naïve T cells. The best defined costimulators are the B7 molecules expressed on professional APC that bind to the CD28 molecule expressed on T cells. They activate signal transduction events in addition to those induced by MHC/TCR interactions.

cowpox The common name for the disease in cows caused by vaccinia virus; used by Edward Jenner in the successful vaccination against smallpox.

CpG nucleotides Unmethylated cytidine–guanine sequences found in microbial DNA that stimulate innate immune responses. CpG nucleotides are recognized by TLR-9 and have adjuvant properties in the mammalian immune system.

CR See complement receptors.

C-reactive protein A protein found in serum; produced by hepatocytes as part of the acute-phase response. Inflammation induced by bacterial infection, necrosis of tissue, trauma, or malignant tumors may cause an increase in the serum concentration within 48 h of the inducing condition.

C region See constant region.

cromolyn sodium A drug that blocks the release of pharmacologic mediators from mast cells and diminishes the symptoms and tissue reactions of type I hypersensitivity (i.e., anaphylaxis) mediated by IgE.

cross-presentation A pathway in APC, particularly dendritic cells, for generating peptides derived from exogenous protein antigens and presenting them to CD8$^+$ T cells.

cross-reactivity The ability of an antibody specific for one antigen to react with a second antigen; a measure of relatedness between two different antigenic substances.

CTLA-4 The high-affinity receptor for B7 molecules expressed on T cells.

cutaneous lymphocyte antigen (CLA) A cell surface molecule involved in lymphocyte homing to the skin in humans.

cyclophosphamide An immunosuppressive drug that is more toxic for B lymphocytes than T lymphocytes. Consequently, it is a more effective suppressor of humoral antibody synthesis than of cell-mediated immune reactions.

cyclosporine An immunosuppressive drug that inhibits signaling in T cells, thus preventing T-cell activation and effector function. It acts by binding to cyclophilin to create a complex that binds to and inactivates the serine/threonine phosphatase calcineurin.

cytokine receptors Cellular receptors for cytokines. Binding of the cytokine to the cytokine receptor stimulates signal transduction, resulting in new activities in the cell, such as growth, differentiation, or death.

cytokines Soluble substances secreted by cells which have a variety of effects on other cells.

cytophilic antibody An antibody that attaches via its FcR region to a cell expressing an Fc receptor; for example, IgE molecules binding to the FCε receptor expressed on the surface of mast cells and basophils.

cytotoxic (or cytolytic) T lymphocyte (CTL) A type of T lymphocyte whose major effector function is to recognize and kill host cells infected with viruses or other intracellular microbes. CTLs usually express CD8 and recognize microbial peptides displayed by class I MHC molecules. CTL killing of infected cells involves the release of cytoplasmic granules whose contents include membrane pore-forming proteins and enzymes that initiate apoptosis of the infected cell.

cytotoxins Proteins made by cytotoxic T cells that participate in the destruction of target cells. Perforins and granzymes or fragmentins are the major defined cytotoxins.

death domain Originally defined in proteins encoded by genes involved in programmed cell death but now known to be involved in protein–protein interactions.

decay-accelerating factor (DAF) A membrane glycoprotein of normal human erythrocytes, leukocytes, and platelets that is absent from the red blood cells of paroxysmal nocturnal hemoglobulinuria patients. It facilitates dissociation of classical complement pathway C3 convertase (C4b2a) into C4b and C2a.

D gene A small segment of immunoglobulin heavy-chain and T-cell receptor DNA, coding for the third hypervariable region of most receptors.

degranulation A mechanism whereby cytoplasmic granules in cells fuse with the cell membrane to discharge the contents from the cell. A classic example is degranulation of the mast cell or basophil in immediate (type I) hypersensitivity

delayed-type hypersensitivity (DTH) A form of cell-mediated immunity elicited by antigen present in the skin. Reaction is mediated by CD4-positive T_H1 cells and involves release of cytokines and recruitment of monocytes and macrophages. It is called DTH because the reaction appears hours to days after antigen is injected.

dendritic cells Interdigitating reticular cells, derived from bone marrow precursors that are found in T-cell areas of lymphoid tissues. They have a branched or dendritic morphology and are the most potent activators of naïve T-cell responses. Dendritic cells present in nonlymphoid tissues do not appear to stimulate T-cell responses until they are activated and migrate to lymphoid tissues.

desensitization A procedure in which an allergic individual is exposed to increasing doses of allergens with the goal of inhibiting his or her allergic reactions. The mechanism involves shifting the pattern of response away from $CD4^+$ T_H2 responses to T_H1 or T_{reg} types and thus changing the antibody produced from IgE to IgG.

determinant Part of the antigen molecule that binds to an antibody-combining site or to a receptor on T cells; also termed epitope (see hapten and epitope).

diapedesis The movement of blood cells, particularly leukocytes, from the blood across blood vessel walls into tissues.

differentiation antigen A cell surface antigenic determinant found only on cells of a certain lineage and at a particular developmental stage; used as an immunologic marker.

DiGeorge syndrome An immunodeficiency condition in which there is a failure to develop thymic epithelium and so T cells do not develop; associated with absent parathyroid glands and large-vessel anomalies.

diphtheria toxoid An immunizing preparation generated by formalin inactivation of *Corynebacterium diphtheriae* exotoxins. This toxoid, used in the immunization of children against diphtheria, is usually administered as a triple vaccine, together with pertussis microorganisms and tetanus toxoid (DPT).

diversity The existence of a large number of lymphocytes with different antigenic specificities in any individual. Diversity is a fundamental property of the adaptive immune system and is the result of variability in the structures of the antigen-binding sites of lymphocyte receptors for antigens (antibodies and TCRs).

diversity gene segments See D gene.

DNA vaccination A vaccination procedure in which plasmid DNA is used to initiate an adaptive immune response to the encoded protein.

domain A compact segment of an immunoglobulin or TCR chain, made up of amino acids around an S–S bond.

double-negative thymocyte Immature T cells within the thymus that lack expression of the CD4 and CD8.

double-positive thymocyte An intermediate stage in T-cell development in the thymus characterized by expression of both CD4 and CD8.

DP, DQ, and DR molecules MHC class II molecules of humans expressed on B cells and APC.

draining lymph node Any lymph node downstream of an infection or site of antigen injection that receives microbes and antigens from the site via the lymphatic system. Draining nodes often enlarge during an immune response and can be palpated (a phenomenon originally called "swollen glands").

DTH See delayed-type hypersensitivity.

ECAM Endothelial cell adhesion molecule; see adhesion molecules.

effector cells Lymphocytes that can mediate the removal of pathogens or antigens from the body without the need for further differentiation. Effectors are distinct from naïve lymphocytes, which must proliferate and differentiate before they can mediate effector cell functions. Effector cells are distinct from memory cells, which must differentiate and sometimes proliferate before they become effector cells.

ELISA See enzyme-linked immunosorbent assay.

ELISPOT assay An adaptation of ELISA in which cells are placed over antibodies or antigens attached to a surface. The antigen or antibody traps the cells' secreted products, which can then be detected using an enzyme-coupled antibody that cleaves a substrate to make a localized colored spot.

encapsulated bacteria Bacteria with thick carbohydrate coats that protect them from phagocytosis. They can cause extracellular infections and are effectively engulfed and destroyed by phagocytes only if they are first coated with antibody and/or complement components produced in an adaptive immune response.

endocytosis A mechanism whereby substances are taken into a cell from the extracellular fluid through plasma membrane vesicles. This is accomplished by either pinocytosis or receptor-facilitated endocytosis.

endogenous antigen An antigen that is synthesized inside host cells.

endogenous pyrogens Cytokines (e.g., IL-1, TNF-α) that can induce a rise in body temperature. They are distinct from exogenous substances such as endotoxin from Gram-negative bacteria that induce fever by triggering endogenous pyrogen synthesis.

endosome An intracellular membrane-bound acidic vesicle into which extracellular proteins are internalized during antigen processing. Endosomes contain proteolytic enzymes that degrade proteins into peptides (epitopes) allowing these peptides to bind to class II MHC molecules.

endotoxins Bacterial toxins that are released when bacterial cells are damaged or destroyed. The most important endotoxin is the lipopolysaccharide of Gram-negative bacteria, which induces cytokine synthesis.

enzyme-linked immunosorbent assay (ELISA) An assay in which an enzyme is linked to an antibody and a colored substrate is used to measure the activity of bound enzyme and hence the amount of bound antibody.

eosinophils Bone-marrow-derived granulocytes important in defense against parasitic infections, including helminths. Found in abundance in inflammatory infiltrates of immediate hypersensitivity late-phase reactions, eosinophils contribute to many of the pathologic consequences of allergic diseases.

epitope The specific portion of a macromolecular antigen to which antibody or the TCR binds. An alternative term for antigenic determinant.

exocytosis The release of intracellular vesicle content to the exterior of the cell. The vesicles make their way to the plasma membrane, with which they fuse to permit the contents to be released to the external environment.

exogenous antigen An antigen that is taken into a cell, particularly an APC.

exon The region of DNA coding for a protein or a segment of a protein.

experimental allergic encephalomyelitis (EAE) An experimental inflammatory disease of the central nervous system that develops after rodents are immunized with antigens of the nervous system together with an adjuvant. Used as a model of multiple sclerosis.

extravasation Escape of the fluid and cellular components of blood from a blood vessel into tissues.

Fab Fragment of antibody containing one antigen-binding site; generated by cleavage of the antibody with the enzyme papain, which cuts at the hinge region N terminally to the inter-heavy-chain disulfide bond and generates two Fab fragments from one antibody molecule.

F(ab′)₂ A fragment of an antibody containing two antigen-binding sites; generated by cleavage of the antibody molecule with the enzyme pepsin, which cuts at the hinge region C-terminally to the inter-heavy-chain disulfide bond.

FACS See fluorescence-activated cell sorter.

factor B Alternative complement pathway component which combines with C3b and is cleaved by factor D to produce alternative pathway C3 convertase.

factor H A key regulator of complement activation: it competes with factor B for binding to C3b on a cell surface; it also binds to C3b when it is part of the C3b convertase, C3bBb, and promotes the dissociation of the convertase.

factor I A regulator of both classical and alternative complement pathways; A serine protease that splits C3b and C4b.

factor P (properdin) A key participant in the alternative pathway of complement activation that combines with C3b and stabilizes alternative pathway C3 convertase (C3bB) to produce C3bBbP.

farmer's lung A hypersensitivity disease caused by the interaction of IgG antibodies with large amounts of an inhaled allergen in the alveolar wall of the lung, causing alveolar wall inflammation and compromising gas exchange.

Fas (CD95) A member of the TNF receptor family that is expressed on many types of cell and makes them susceptible to killing by cells expressing Fas ligand. Binding of Fas ligand to Fas triggers apoptosis in the Fas-expressing cells.

Fas ligand (CD95 ligand) A cell surface member of the TNF family of proteins (CD178). Binding of Fas ligand to Fas triggers apoptosis in the Fas-expressing cell.

Fc Fragment of antibody without antigen-binding sites, generated by cleavage with papain; the Fc fragment contains the C-terminal domains of the immunoglobulin heavy chains.

Fc receptor (FcR) A receptor on a cell surface with specific binding affinity for the Fc portion of an antibody molecule. Fc receptors are found on many types of cells.

FITC See fluorescein isothiocyanate.

FK506 See tacrolimus. An immunosuppressive polypeptide drug that inactivates T cells by inhibiting signal transduction from the T-cell receptor.

fluorescein isothiocyanate (FITC) A fluorescent dye which emits a yellow-green color and can be conjugated to antibody or other proteins.

fluorescence-activated cell sorter (FACS) An instrument that uses a laser to differentially deflect cells bound to fluorochrome-linked antibodies, thus sorting the cells into fluorescent-positive and fluorescent-negative populations.

fluorescence microscopy A microscope method that uses ultraviolet light to illuminate a tissue or cell stained with a fluorochrome-labeled substance such as an antibody against an antigen of interest in the tissue.

fluorescent antibody An antibody coupled with a fluorescent dye used to detect antigen on cells, tissues, or microorganisms.

follicles Circular or oval areas of lymphocytes in lymphoid tissue rich in B cells. They are present in the cortex of lymph nodes and in the splenic white pulp. Primary follicles contain B lymphocytes that are small and medium sized. Antigen stimulation causes development of secondary follicles which contain large B lymphocytes in the germinal centers where tingible body macrophages (those phagocytizing nuclear particles) and follicular dendritic cells are present.

follicular dendritic cells Cells within lymphoid follicles that are crucial in selecting antigen-binding B cells during antibody responses. They have Fc receptors that are not internalized by receptor-mediated endocytosis; thus they hold antigen–antibody complexes on their surface for long periods.

Freund's complete adjuvant An oil containing killed mycobacteria and an emulsifier that, forms an emulsion when mixed with an immunogen in aqueous solution. Injection of the emulsion enhances the immune response to the immunogen. Termed incomplete Freund's adjuvant if mycobacteria are not included.

FYN See tyrosine kinases.

γδ T-cell receptor (TCR) A form of TCR distinct from the more common αβ TCR and expressed on a subset of T cells found mostly in epithelial barrier tissues.

GALT See gut-associated lymphoid tissue.

gene knockout Term for gene disruption by homologous recombination.

gene therapy Correction of a genetic defect by the introduction of a normal gene into bone marrow or other cells. Also known as somatic gene therapy because it does not affect the germline genes of the individual.

genetic immunization A novel technique for inducing adaptive immune responses by injecting a plasmid DNA encoding a protein of interest, usually into muscle; the protein is then expressed *in vivo* and elicits antibody and T-cell responses.

genotype All the genes possessed by an individual; in practice it refers to the particular alleles present at the loci in question.

germinal centers Secondary lymphoid structures that are sites of intense B-cell proliferation, selection, maturation, and death during antibody responses. They form around follicular dendritic cell networks after migration of B cells and helper T cells into lymphoid follicles.

germline Refers to genes in germ cells as opposed to somatic cells. In immunology, it refers to immunoglobulin or TCR genes in their unrearranged state.

glomerulonephritis Group of diseases characterized by glomerular injury. Patients usually have glomerular deposits of immunoglobulins frequently associated with complement components.

Goodpasture's syndrome An autoimmune disease in which autoantibodies against basement membrane or type IV collagen are produced and cause extensive vasculitis. It is rapidly fatal.

G proteins Proteins that bind GTP and convert it to GDP in the process of cell signal transduction.

graft-versus-host reaction (GVH) The pathologic consequences of a response generally initiated by transplanted immunocompetent T lymphocytes into an allogeneic, immunologically incompetent host. The host is unable to reject the grafted T cells and becomes their target. The emerging graft-versus-host disease (GVHD) most often affects skin, liver, and intestines.

granulocyte See polymorphonuclear leukocytes.

granulocyte–macrophage colony-stimulating factor (GM-CSF) A cytokine involved in the growth and differentiation of myeloid and monocytic lineage cells, including dendritic cells, monocytes and tissue macrophages, and cells of the granulocyte lineage.

granuloma A structure in the form of a mass of mononuclear cells at the site of a persisting inflammation; the cells are mostly macrophages with some T lymphocytes at the periphery. A common delayed hypersensitivity reaction associated with continuous presence of a foreign body or infection.

granzyme A serine protease enzyme found in the granules of CTLs and NK cells that is released by exocytosis, enters target cells, and proteolytically cleaves and activates caspases to induce apoptosis.

Graves disease An autoimmune disease in which antibodies against the thyroid-stimulating hormone receptor cause overproduction of thyroid hormone and thus hyperthyroidism.

Guillain-Barre syndrome A type of idiopathic polyneuritis in which autoimmunity to peripheral nerve myelin leads to a condition characterized by chronic demyelination of the spinal cord and peripheral nerves.

gut-associated lymphoid tissue (GALT) Lymphoid tissue situated in the gastrointestinal mucosa and submucosa which constitutes the gastrointestinal immune system. GALT is present in the Peyer's patches, appendix, and tonsils.

GVH See graft-versus-host reaction.

H-2 The major histocompatibility complex of the mouse, situated on chromosome 17. Haplotypes are designated by a lowercase superscript, as in H-2^b. H-2 contains the subregions K, I, D, and L.

haplotype A linked set of genes associated with one haploid genome. The term is used mainly in connection with the linked genes of the major histocompatibility complex (MHC), which are usually inherited as one haplotype contributed by each parent. Some MHC haplotypes are overrepresented in the population, a phenomenon known as linkage disequilibrium.

hapten A compound, usually of low molecular weight, that is not itself immunogenic but that, after conjugation to a carrier protein or cells, becomes immunogenic and induces an antibody response. The hapten alone can bind to the antibody in the absence of carrier.

Hashimoto's thyroiditis An autoimmune disease characterized by persistent high levels of antibody against thyroid-specific antigens. These antibodies recruit NK cells to the tissue, leading to damage and inflammation.

HAT Hypoxanthine–aminopterin–thymidine, commonly used as a selective media cocktail in cell cultures to generate hybridomas.

H chain See heavy chain.

heavy (H) chain The larger of the two types of chains that comprise a normal immunoglobulin or antibody molecule.

helper T cells A class of T cells that cooperates with B cells to make antibody in responses to thymus-dependent antigens.

hemagglutinin Any substance that causes red blood cells to agglutinate. The hemagglutinins in human blood are antibodies that recognize the ABO blood group antigens. Influenza and some other viruses have hemagglutinins that bind to glycoproteins on host cells to initiate the infectious process.

hematopoiesis The generation of the cellular elements of blood, including the red blood cells, leukocytes, and platelets.

hematopoietic stem cell (HSC) A bone marrow cell that is undifferentiated and serves as a precursor for multiple hematopoietic cell lineages. These cells are also demonstrable in the yolk sac and later in the liver in the fetus.

hemolytic disease of the newborn (HDN) Also called erythroblastosis fetalis, HDN is caused by a maternal IgG antibody response to paternal antigens expressed on fetal RBCs. The usual target of this response is the Rh blood group antigen. The maternal anti-Rh IgG antibodies cross the placenta, bind to fetal RBC, and trigger their destruction.

herd immunity Protection afforded to non-vaccinated individuals in a population when the majority have been successfully vaccinated.

hereditary angioedema A disorder in which recurrent attacks of edema occur in the skin and gastrointestinal and respiratory tracts. It is due to decreased or absent C1 inhibitor (C1 INH). The most serious consequence of this disorder is epiglottal swelling leading to suffocation.

heterodimer A molecule comprised of two components that are different but closely joined structures, such as a protein comprised of two separate chains. Examples include the TCR comprised of either α or β chains or of γ and δ chains and MHC class I or class II molecules.

heterophile antigen A cross-reacting antigen expressed by widely different species such as humans and bacteria.

heterozygous Refers to individuals with two different alleles of a particular gene.

HEV See high endothelial venules.

high endothelial venules (HEV) Specialized venules found in lymphoid tissues. Lymphocytes migrate from blood into lymphoid tissues by attaching to and migrating across the high endothelial cells of these vessels.

highly active antiretroviral therapy (HAART) Combination chemotherapy for HIV infection consisting of a viral protease inhibitor and reverse transcriptase inhibitors. HAART can reduce plasma virus titers to below detectable levels and slow the progression of HIV disease.

hinge region A flexible, open segment of an antibody molecule that allows bending of the molecule. The hinge region is located between the Fab and Fc regions of an antibody molecule and is susceptible to enzymatic cleavage.

histamine A vasoactive amine stored in mast cell granules that is released by antigen binding to IgE molecules on mast cells, causing dilation of local blood vessels and smooth muscle contraction. Histamine release produces some of the symptoms of immediate hypersensitivity reactions.

histocompatibility Literally, the ability of tissues to get along; in immunology, it means identity in all transplantation antigens. These antigens, in turn, are collectively referred to as histocompatibility antigens.

HIV See human immunodeficiency virus.

HLA See human leukocyte antigen.

Hodgkin's disease A malignant disease in which antigen-presenting cells that resemble dendritic cells seem to be the transformed cell type. Hodgkin's lymphoma is a form of the disease in which lymphocytes predominate.

homing The directed migration of different types of leukocytes into particular tissue sites and regulated by the selective expression of adhesion molecules and chemokine receptors. See also lymphocyte homing.

homodimer A protein comprised of two identical peptide chains.

human immunodeficiency virus (HIV) Retrovirus that infects human CD4$^+$ cells and causes AIDS.

humanization A term used to describe the genetic engineering of mouse hypervariable loops of a desired specificity into otherwise human antibodies. The DNA encoding hypervariable loops of mouse monoclonal antibodies or V regions selected in phage display libraries is inserted into the framework regions of human immunoglobulin genes. This allows the production of antibodies of a desired specificity that do not cause an immune response in humans treated with them.

Human leukocyte antigen (HLA) The human major histocompatibility complex; contains the genes coding for the polymorphic HLA class I and II molecules and many other important genes.

humoral immunity Refers to immune responses that involve antibody (contrast with cell-mediated immunity: T-cell responses in the absence of antibody). Can be transferred to another individual using antibody-containing serum.

hybridoma An immortalized hybrid cell resulting from the *in vitro* fusion of an antibody-secreting B cell with a myeloma; it secretes antibody without stimulation and proliferates continuously, both *in vivo* and *in vitro*. The term is also used for a hybrid T cell resulting from the fusion of a T lymphocyte with a thymoma (a malignant T cell); the T-cell hybridoma proliferates continuously and secretes cytokines upon activation by antigen and APC.

hyperacute rejection A form of graft rejection that begins within minutes to hours after transplantation, particularly of a xenograft, and is characterized by thrombotic occlusion of the graft vessels. It is mediated by preexisting antibodies in the host circulation that bind to donor endothelial antigens, such as blood group antigens or MHC molecules, and activate the complement system and the blood-clotting cascade, leading to an engorged, ischemic graft and rapid loss of the organ.

hypergammaglobulinemia Elevated serum immunoglobulin levels. A polyclonal increase in immunoglobulins in the serum occurs in any condition where there is continuous stimulation of the immune system, such as chronic infection, autoimmune disease, systemic lupus erythematosus, etc. Hypergammaglobulinemia may also result from a monoclonal increase in immunoglobulin production, as in multiple myeloma, Waldenstrom's macroglobulinemia, or other conditions associated with the formation of monoclonal immunoglobulins.

hyperimmune A descriptor for an animal with a high level of immunity that is induced by repeated immunization to generate large amounts of functionally effective antibodies, in comparison to animals subjected to routine immunization protocols, generally with fewer boosters.

hypersensitivity State of reactivity to antigen that is greater than normal; denotes a deleterious rather than a protective outcome. Four types are defined (see types I–IV hypersensitivity).

hypersensitivity diseases Immune-mediated diseases that include autoimmune diseases, in which immune responses are directed against self-antigens, and diseases that result from uncontrolled or excessive responses against foreign antigens, such as microbes and allergens. The tissue damage that occurs in hypersensitivity diseases is due to the same effector mechanisms used by the immune system to protect against microbes.

hypervariable regions Portions of the light and heavy immunoglobulin chains that are highly variable in amino acid sequence from one immunoglobulin molecule to another and that together constitute the antigen-binding site of an antibody molecule. Also, portions of the T-cell receptor that constitute the antigen-binding site. See also complementarity-determining region.

Ia (I region associated) An older term for mouse MHC class II I-A and I-E genes and molecules.

IDC See interdigitating dendritic cells.

idiotype The combined antigenic determinants (idiotopes) expressed in the variable region of antibodies of an individual that are directed at a particular antigen.

Ig See immunoglobulin.

Igα See B-cell receptor.

Igβ See B-cell receptor.

IgA The class of immunoglobulin characterized by α heavy chains. IgA antibodies are mainly secreted by mucosal lymphoid tissues.

IgD The class of immunoglobulin characterized by δ heavy chains. IgD is a cell surface immunoglobulin coexpressed on naïve B cells together with IgM. It may have a function as a coreceptor that binds to IgD receptors expressed on T cells.

IgE The class of immunoglobulin characterized by ε heavy chains. IgE is involved in allergic reactions.

IgG The class of immunoglobulin characterized by γ heavy chains. It is the most abundant class of immunoglobulin found in plasma.

IgM The class of immunoglobulin characterized by μ heavy chains. IgM is the first immunoglobulin to appear on the surface of B cells and the first to be secreted following B-cell stimulation with antigen.

IL See interleukins.

immature B cell IgM-positive cell in the B-cell lineage; easily tolerized by exposure to antigen.

Immature dendritic cell Antigen-presenting cell in tissue that takes up and processes antigen.

immediate-type hypersensitivity (Type I) hypersensitivity reaction occurring within minutes after the interaction of antigen and IgE antibody.

immune adherence The adherence of particulate antigen coated with C3b to cells expressing C3b receptors; results in enhanced phagocytosis of bacteria by macrophages.

immune complex Molecules formed by the interaction of a soluble (i.e., nonparticulate) antigen with antibody

molecules. Large immune complexes are cleared rapidly, but smaller complexes formed in antigen excess may deposit in tissues resulting in tissue damage (immune complex disease).

immune modulators Substances that control the level of the immune response.

immune surveillance The concept that a physiologic function of the immune system is to recognize and destroy clones of transformed cells before they grow into tumors.

immunity The general term for resistance to a pathogen.

immunodeficiency Decrease in immune responses that result from absence or defect of some component of the immune system.

immunodiffusion Identifies antigen or antibody by the formation of antigen–antibody complexes in a gel.

immunogen A substance capable of inducing an immune response (as well as reacting with the products of an immune response). Compare with antigen.

immunoglobulin (Ig) A general term for all antibody molecules (IgM, IgD, IgG, IgA, and IgE); each Ig unit is made up of two heavy chains and two light chains and has two antigen-binding sites.

immunoglobulin A See IgA.

immunoglobulin D See IgD.

immunoglobulin domain A three-dimensional globular structural motif found in many proteins in the immune system, including Igs, TCRs, and MHC molecules. Ig domains are about 110 amino acid residues in length, include an internal disulfide bond, and contain β-pleated sheets.

immunoglobulin E See IgE.

immunoglobulin G See IgG.

immunoglobulin heavy chain One of the two basic structural units of an antibody which includes two identical, disulfide-linked heavy chains and two identical light chains. Each heavy chain is composed of a variable (V) Ig domain and three or four constant (C) Ig domains that define the antibody isotype: IgM, IgD, IgG, IgA, or IgE. Each of these is distinguished by structural differences in their heavy-chain constant regions. The heavy-chain constant regions also mediate effector functions, such as phagocytes and complement activation.

immunoglobulin light chain One of the two basic structural units of an antibody molecule. An antibody includes two identical light chains, each disulfide linked to one of two identical heavy chains. Each light chain is composed of one variable (V) Ig domain and one constant (C) Ig domain. There are two light-chain isotypes, called κ and λ, both functionally identical. About 60% of human antibodies have κ light chains and 40% have λ light chains.

immunoglobulin M See IgM.

immunoglobulin superfamily Proteins involved in cellular recognition and interactions that are structurally and genetically related to immunoglobulins.

Immunologic synapse Area of contact between the surfaces of a T cell and an APC such as dendritic cells or a B cell.

immunoreceptor tyrosine-based activation motif (ITAM) A pattern of amino acids in the cytoplasmic tail of many transmembrane receptor molecules, including Igα and Igβ and CD3 chains, which are phosphorylated and then associate with intracellular molecules as an early consequence of cell activation.

immunoreceptor tyrosine-based inhibitory motif (ITIM) Motifs with opposing effects to immunoreceptor tyrosine-based activation motifs (ITAM). They recruit phosphatases to the receptor site that remove the phosphate groups added by the tyrosine kinases.

immunosuppression Inhibition of one or more components of the adaptive or innate immune system, either as a result of an underlying disease or intentionally induced by drugs for the purpose of preventing or treating graft rejection or autoimmune disease. A commonly used immunosuppressive drug is cyclosporine, which blocks T-cell cytokine production.

immunotherapy The treatment of a disease with therapeutic agents that promote or inhibit immune responses. Cancer immunotherapy, for example, involves promoting active immune response to tumor antigens or administering antitumor antibodies or T cells to establish passive immunity.

immunotoxins Antibodies that are chemically coupled to toxic proteins usually derived from plants or microorganisms. They are being tested as anticancer agents and as immunosuppressive drugs.

inflammation An acute or chronic response to tissue injury or infection involving accumulation of leukocytes, plasma proteins, and fluid.

inducible NO synthase (INOS) Produced by macrophages and many other cell types. Induced by many stimuli to activate NO synthesis, thereby playing a major role in host resistance to intracellular infection.

innate immunity The antigen-nonspecific mechanisms involved in the early phase of resistance to a pathogen, which include phagocytic cells, cytokines, and complement; not expanded by repeat stimulation with the pathogen.

integrins A family of two-chain cell surface adhesion molecules found on leukocytes; important in the adhesion of APC and lymphocytes and in leukocyte migration into tissues.

intercellular adhesion molecules (ICAMs) 1, 2, and 3 Adhesion molecules on the surface of several cell types, including APC and T cells, that interact with integrins; members of the immunoglobulin superfamily.

interdigitating dendritic cells (IDCs) Thymic bone-marrow-derived cells which play a critical role in negative selection of developing thymocytes.

interferons (IFNs) A group of proteins having antiviral activity and capable of enhancing and modifying the immune response.

interleukins (ILs) Glycoproteins secreted by a variety of leukocytes that have effects on other leukocytes.

intron A segment of DNA that does not code for protein: the intervening sequence of nucleotides between coding sequences or exons.

invariant chain (I_i) A nonpolymorphic protein that binds to newly synthesized class II MHC molecules in the endoplasmic reticulum. The invariant chain prevents loading of the class II MHC peptide-binding cleft with peptides present in the endoplasmic reticulum. The invariant chain also promotes folding and assembly of class II molecules and directs newly formed class II molecules to the specialized endosomal MHC compartment, where peptide loading takes place.

ISCOMs Immune stimulatory complexes of antigen held within a lipid matrix that acts as an adjuvant and enables the antigen to be taken up into the cytoplasm after fusion with the cytoplasmic membrane.

isoelectric focusing Protein identification technique; proteins migrate in an electric field under a pH gradient to the pH at which their net charge is zero (their isoelectric point).

isograft Tissue transplanted between two genetically identical individuals (same as syngraft).

isohemagglutinins Naturally occurring IgM antibodies specific for the red blood cell antigens of the ABO blood groups; thought to result from immunization by bacteria in the gastrointestinal and respiratory tracts.

isotypes Also known as antibody classes, isotypes are antibodies that differ in the heavy-chain constant regions: IgM, IgG, IgD, IgA, and IgE. These differences result in distinct biological activities of the antibodies; distinguishable also on the basis of reaction with antisera raised in another species.

isotype switch The switch, which occurs when a B cell stops secreting antibody of one isotype or class and starts producing antibody of a different isotype but with the same antigenic specificity; involves joining a rearranged VDJ gene unit to a different heavy-chain constant-region gene.

ITAM See immunoreceptor tyrosine-based activation motif.

ITIM See immunoreceptor tyrosine-based inhibition motif.

JAK See Janus kinases.

JAK/STAT signaling pathway A signaling pathway initiated by cytokine binding to type I and type II cytokine receptors. The JAK/STAT pathway sequentially involves activation of receptor-associated Janus kinase (JAK) tyrosine kinases, JAK-mediated tyrosine phosphorylation of the cytoplasmic tails of cytokine receptors, docking of signal transducers and activators of transcription (STATs) to the phosphorylated receptor chains, JAK-mediated tyrosine phosphorylation of the associated STATs, dimerization, nuclear translocation of the STATs, and binding of STAT to regulatory regions of specific target genes, causing transcriptional activation of those genes.

Janus kinases (JAKs) Tyrosine kinases activated by cytokines binding to their cellular receptors.

J (joining) chain A polypeptide involved in the polymerization of immunoglobulin molecules IgM and IgA.

J gene A gene segment coding for the J, or joining, segment in immunoglobulin or T-cell receptor.

Joining (J) segments Short coding sequences within Ig and TCR loci positioned between the variable (V) and constant (C) gene segments. Together with D segments, J-region segments are somatically recombined with V segments during lymphocyte development. The resulting recombined VDJ DNA codes for the carboxy-terminal ends of the antigen receptor V regions. Random use of different J segments contributes to the diversity of the antigen receptor repertoire.

junctional diversity The diversity in Ig and TCR repertoires attributed to the random addition or removal of nucleotide sequences at junctions between V, D, and J gene segments.

Kaposi's sarcoma A malignant tumor of vascular cells that frequently arises in patients with AIDS; associated with infection by the Kaposi's-sarcoma-associated herpes virus 8.

killer activatory receptor (KAR) Receptor expressed on NK or cytotoxic cells that can activate killing by these cells.

killer inhibitory receptor (KIR) Receptor expressed on NK cells that binds to MHC class I molecules on target cells; ligation of MHC class I inhibits the signaling that would otherwise lead to target cell killing.

killer T cell A T cell that kills a target cell expressing foreign antigen bound to MHC molecules on the surface of the target cell. Also called cytotoxic T cell.

KIR See killer inhibitory receptor.

knockout mouse A mouse with a targeted disruption of one or more genes that is created by homologous recombination techniques. Knockout mice lacking functional genes encoding cytokines, cell surface receptors, signaling molecules, and transcription factors have provided extensive information about the roles of these molecules in the immune system.

LAK cells See lymphokine-activated killer cells.

Langerhans cell Cell of the monocyte/dendritic cell family that takes up and processes antigens in the epidermal layer of the skin; migrates through lymphatics to lymph nodes draining the site of exposure to antigen, where it differentiates into a dendritic cell.

late-phase reaction A component of the immediate hypersensitivity reaction that develops 2 to 4 h after mast cell and basophil degranulation characterized by an inflammatory infiltrate of neutrophils, eosinophils, basophils, and lymphocytes. Reoccurring late-phase inflammatory reactions can cause tissue damage.

L chain See light chain.

Lck A Src family nonreceptor tyrosine kinase that noncovalently associates with the cytoplasmic tails of CD4 and CD8 molecules in T cells. Lck is involved in the early signaling events of antigen-induced T-cell activation and mediates tyrosine phosphorylation of the cytoplasmic tails of CD3 and ζ proteins of the TCR complex.

lectin pathway of complement activation A pathway of complement activation triggered, in the absence of antibody, by the binding of microbial polysaccharides to circulating lectins such as mannose-binding lectin (MBL). MBL is found in the circulation complexed with proteases, the mannose-associated serine proteases (MASPs). Once bound to a pathogen, one of the proteases, MASP-2, sequentially cleaves C4 and C2 to form C4b2a on the surface of the bacterium. The remaining steps of the lectin pathway, beginning with cleavage of C4, are identical to the classical complement pathway.

Leishmania An obligate intracellular protozoan parasite that infects macrophages and can cause a chronic inflammatory disease involving many tissues. T_H1 responses and associated IFN-γ production control *Leishmania major* infection, whereas T_H2 responses with IL-4 production lead to disseminated lethal disease.

leukemia Uncontrolled proliferation of a malignant leukocyte.

leukocyte adhesion deficiency (LAD) One of a rare group of immunodeficiency diseases with infectious complications; caused by defective expression of the leukocyte adhesion molecules required for tissue recruitment of phagocytes and lymphocytes.

leukocytes White blood cells; comprise monocytes/macrophages, lymphocytes, and polymorphonuclear cells.

leukotrienes A class of arachidonic-acid-derived lipid inflammatory mediators produced by the lipoxygenase pathway in many cell types. Mast cells make abundant leukotriene C_4 (LTC_4) which is degraded to LTD_4 and LTE_4, which bind to receptors on smooth muscle cells and cause prolonged bronchoconstriction. Leukotrienes contribute significantly to the pathologic processes of bronchial asthma.

ligand A molecule or part of a molecule that binds to a receptor.

ligation The binding of a molecule or a part of a molecule to a receptor.

light (L) chain The light chain of the immunoglobulin molecule, which occurs in two forms: κ or λ.

linked recognition The requirement for the T helper and B cell involved in the antibody response to a thymus-dependent antigen to interact with different epitopes physically linked in the same antigen.

lipopolysaccharide (LPS) Components of Gram-negative bacteria cell walls; also known as endotoxin.

LPS See lipopolysaccharide

Lyme disease A chronic infection with *Borrelia burgdorferi*, a spirochete that can evade the immune response.

lymph Extracellular fluid that bathes tissues; contains tissue products, antigens, antibodies, and cells (predominantly lymphocytes).

lymphatic system System of vessels through which lymph travels and which includes organized structures, with lymph nodes at the intersection of vessels. Three major functions: to concentrate antigen from all parts of the body into a few lymphoid organs; to circulate lymphocytes through lymphoid organs so that antigen can interact with rare antigen-specific cells; and to carry products of the immune response (antibody and effector cells) to the bloodstream and tissues.

lymph nodes Secondary lymphoid organs in which mature B and T lymphocytes interact with antigen and with each other.

lymphoblast A lymphocyte that has enlarged and increased its rate of RNA and protein synthesis.

lymphocyte homing The directed migration of subsets of circulating lymphocytes into particular tissue sites and regulated by the selective expression of adhesion molecules and chemokine receptors. Such homing receptors are expressed on lymphocytes and complementary ligands (addressins) expressed in tissue vascular beds. For example, some T lymphocytes preferentially home to Peyer's patches (intestinal lymphoid tissue) and others to peripheral (non-mucosa) nodes.

lymphocyte maturation The process by which bone marrow precursor cells develop into mature, antigen receptor-expressing naïve B or T lymphocytes that populate peripheral lymphoid tissues. This process takes place in the specialized environments of the bone marrow (for B cells) and the thymus (for T cells).

lymphocyte migration The movement of lymphocytes around the body (see also lymphocyte homing).

lymphocyte recirculation The continuous movement of lymphocytes through the blood and lymphatics, between the lymph nodes or spleen, and, if activated, to peripheral inflammatory sites.

lymphocyte repertoire The complete collection of antigen receptors (and therefore antigen specificities) expressed by the B and T lymphocytes of an individual.

lymphocytes Cells that express antigen-specific receptors. Small leukocytes with virtually no cytoplasm found in blood, tissues, and lymphoid organs such as lymph nodes, spleen, and Peyer's patches. Responsible for specificity, diversity, memory, and self–nonself discrimination.

lymphoid follicle A B-cell-rich region of a lymph node or the spleen that is the site of antigen-induced B-cell proliferation and differentiation. In T-cell-dependent B-cell responses to protein antigens, a germinal center forms within the follicles.

lymphokine A cytokine secreted by lymphocytes.

lymphokine-activated killer (LAK) cells The heterogeneous population of lymphocytes, including NK cells, derived from the *in vitro* cytokine-driven activation of peripheral blood lymphocytes from a tumor-bearing patient.

lymphoma Lymphocyte tumors in lymphoid tissues or other sites but not generally found in the blood.

lymphotoxin (LT, TNF-β) A cytokine produced by T_H1 and CTL cells that kills T cells and tumor cells and also has proinflammatory effects, including endothelial and neutrophil activation; also critical for the normal development of lymphoid organs.

lysosome A membrane-bound, acidic organelle abundant in phagocytic cells that contains proteolytic enzymes that degrade proteins derived both from the extracellular environment and from within the cell. Lysosomes are involved in the MHC class II pathway of antigen processing.

macrophages Large phagocytic leukocytes found in tissues; derived from blood monocytes.

major histocompatibility complex (MHC) A cluster of genes encoding polymorphic cell surface molecules (MHC class I and class II) that are involved in interactions with T cells. These molecules also play a major role in transplantation rejection. Several other nonpolymorphic proteins are encoded in this region.

MALT See mucosal-associated lymphoid tissue.

mannose-binding lectin (MBL) A plasma protein that binds to mannose residues on bacterial cell walls and activates complement in the absence of antibody.

mannose receptor A carbohydrate-binding receptor (lectin) expressed by macrophages that binds mannose and fucose residues on microbial cell walls and mediates phagocytosis of the organisms.

marginal zone A peripheral region of splenic lymphoid follicles containing macrophages. Marginal zones are associated with the trapping of polysaccharide antigens which may persist locally for prolonged periods of time within macrophages and allow them to be recognized by antigen-specific B cells or to be transported into follicles.

marginal zone B lymphocytes A subset of B lymphocytes, found exclusively in the marginal zone of the spleen, which respond rapidly to blood-borne microbial antigens by producing IgM antibodies with limited diversity.

mast cell Bone-marrow-derived granule-containing cell found in connective tissues; releases mediators such as histamine and cytokines following cell activation; plays a major role in allergic responses.

mature B cell B cells with IgM and IgD on their surface.

M cells Specialized epithelial cells overlying Peyers's patches in the gut that deliver antigens to Peyer's patches.

medulla Inner region of a gland such as the thymus or adrenal gland.

membrane attack complex Terminal components of the complement cascade (C5b–C9), which form a pore on the surface of a target cell, resulting in cell damage or death.

memory Denotes second interaction of B or T lymphocytes with antigen or antigenic peptides, leads to a more effective and more rapid response than the first interaction (primary response).

memory lymphocytes B or T lymphocytes that mediate rapid and enhanced memory responses to second and subsequent exposures to antigens. Memory B and T cells are produced by antigen stimulation of naïve lymphocytes and survive in a functionally quiescent state for long periods of time (years) after the antigen is eliminated.

MHC See major histocompatibility complex.

MHC class I molecule A molecule encoded by genes of the MHC that binds peptides in the endoplasmic reticulum and interacts with $CD8^+$ (cytotoxic) T cells.

MHC class II molecule A molecule encoded by genes of the MHC that binds peptides in acid compartments of the cell and interacts with participates in antigen presentation to $CD4^+$ T cells.

MHC class III molecules Complement components including C2, C4, and factor B that are encoded by genes in the MHC.

MHC restriction The property of T lymphocytes to respond to antigenic peptides only when they are presented in association with either self-MHC class I or class II molecules.

minor histocompatibility antigens Antigens encoded outside the MHC that stimulate graft rejection, but not as rapidly as MHC molecules.

mitogen A substance that stimulates the proliferation of many different clones of lymphocytes.

mixed-lymphocyte reaction (MLR) Proliferative response occurring when leukocytes from two individuals are mixed *in vitro*; T cells from one individual (the responder) are activated by MHC antigens expressed by APC of the other individual (the stimulator).

MLR See mixed-lymphocyte reaction.

Mls antigens Non-MHC antigens that provoke strong primary mixed-lymphocyte responses.

molecular mimicry Identity or similarity of epitopes expressed by a pathogen and by a self-molecule. Molecular mimicry may explain how autoimmune responses develop.

monoclonal Derived from a single clone, the progeny of a single cell. Generally refers to a homogeneous population of T cells, or B cells, or an antibody that is reactive to only one antigen epitope.

monoclonal antibody An antibody produced by a B-cell hybridoma (a cell line derived by the fusion of a single normal B cell and an immortal B-cell tumor line) that is specific for one antigen. Monoclonal antibodies are widely used in research, clinical diagnosis, and therapy.

monocyte Phagocytic leukocyte found in the blood; precursor to tissue macrophage.

motif A pattern of amino acids in the sequence of a molecule critical for the binding of a ligand.

mucins Highly glycosylated cell surface proteins. Mucin-like molecules are bound by L-selectin in lymphoid organs.

mucosal-associated lymphoid tissue (MALT) System that connects lymphoid structures found in the gastrointestinal and respiratory tracts; includes tonsils, appendix, and Peyer's patches of the small intestine.

mucosal immune system A part of the immune system that responds to and protects against microbes that enter the body through mucosal surfaces within the gastrointestinal and respiratory tracts. The mucosal immune system is composed of mucosa-associated lymphoid tissues composed of collections of lymphocytes and accessory cells in the epithelia and lamina propria of mucosal surfaces.

multiple myeloma A malignant tumor of antibody-producing clones of B cells that often secretes immunoglobulins or parts of Ig molecules. The monoclonal antibodies produced by multiple myelomas were critical for early biochemical analyses of antibody structure.

multiple sclerosis Disease of the central nervous system believed to be autoimmune in nature in which an inflammatory response results in demyelination and loss of neurologic function.

myasthenia gravis Autoimmune disease in which antibody specific for the acetylcholine receptor expressed in muscle blocks function at the neuromuscular junction.

myeloma A tumor of plasma cells generally secreting a single monoclonal immunoglobulin.

naïve lymphocytes Lymphocytes that have not yet encountered their specific antigen and therefore have never responded to it. All lymphocytes leaving the central lymphoid organs (bone marrow and thymus) are naïve.

natural killer (NK) cells Large granular lymphocyte-like cells that kill various tumor cells *in vitro* and may play a role in resistance to tumors; also participate in ADCC.

negative selection Step in development of B and T cells at which cells with potential reactivity to self-molecules are functionally inactivated.

neonatal immunity Immunity mediated by maternally produced antibodies transported across the placenta into the fetal circulation before birth or derived from ingested maternal milk and transported across the epithelium.

neutralization The ability of an antibody to block or inhibit the effects of a virus.

neutropenia A situation in which there are fewer neutrophils in the blood than normal.

neutrophil (polymorphonuclear leukocyte, PMN) A phagocytic cell morphologically characterized by a segmented lobular nucleus and cytoplasmic granules filled with degradative enzymes. PMNs are short-lived (<1 day) and the most abundant type of circulating white blood cells. They are the major innate immune cell type mediating acute inflammatory responses to bacterial infections.

nitric oxide A vasoactive and microbicidal effector molecule produced by macrophages from L-arginine.

nitric oxide synthase A member of a family of enzymes that synthesize nitric oxide from L-arginine. Macrophages express an inducible form of this enzyme (see INOS) following activation by various microorganisms or cytokines.

NK cells See natural killer cells.

NKT cells A small subset of T cells that express the NK1.1 marker, a molecule normally found on NK cells as well as a TCR of limited diversity. They rapidly produce cytokines in response to pathogens. They are considered to have features of both innate and adaptive immunity. Thought to play a regulatory role in several diseases and conditions.

nuclear factor κB (NF-κB) A family of transcription factors composed of homodimers or heterodimers of proteins important in the transcription of many genes in both innate and adaptive immune responses.

nuclear factor of activated T cells (NFAT) A transcription factor complex of a protein called NFATc that is held in the cytosol by serine/threonine phosphorylation and the Fos/Jun dimer called AP-1. Following cleavage of the phosphate residues of NFAT by calcineurin, it moves from the cytosol to the nucleus.

nude mice Mice in which the thymus does not develop, so they lack T cells; also hairless.

oncofetal antigen Proteins that are expressed at high levels on some types of cancer cells and in normal developing fetal tissue but not adult tissues. Antibodies specific for these proteins are used as diagnostic histologic tools to identify tumors or to monitor the progression of tumor growth in patients. CEA (CD66) and α-fetoprotein are two oncofetal antigens commonly expressed by certain carcinomas.

oncogenes Genes involved in regulating cell growth which, when defective in structure or expression, can cause cells to grow continuously to form a tumor.

opsonin A macromolecule that becomes attached to the surface of a microbe by neutrophils and macrophages, and increases the efficiency of phagocytosis of the microbe. Opsonins include IgG antibodies whose Fc regions are recognized by Fcγ receptors on phagocytes. They also include fragments of complement proteins, particularly C3b, which are recognized by CR1 (CD35) and by the leukocyte integrin Mac-1.

opsonization The coating of a particle such as a bacterium with antibody and/or a complement component (an opsonin) that leads to enhanced phagocytosis by phagocytic cells.

paracortical area (or paracortex) The T-cell area of the lymph node.

passive cutaneous anaphylaxis (PCA) The passive transfer of anaphylactic sensitivity by intradermal injection of serum from a sensitive donor.

passive hemagglutination Technique for measuring antibody in which antigen-coated red blood cells are agglutinated by adding antibody specific for the antigen.

passive immunization Immunization of an individual by the transfer of antibody synthesized in another individual.

pathogen An agent that causes disease.

pathogen-associated molecular patterns (PAMP) Molecular structures such as lipopolysaccharide, teichoic acid and double-stranded RNA that are expressed by pathogens (viruses, bacteria, fungi) but not mammalian cells and which activate cells of the innate immune system.

pattern recognition receptors Receptors expressed by cells of the innate immune system that recognize pathogen-associated molecular patterns (PAMP) expressed by microorganisms and facilitate innate immune responses against the microorganisms.

PCA See passive cutaneous anaphylaxis.

PCR See polymerase chain reaction.

peptide-binding cleft The portion of an MHC molecule that binds peptides derived from antigen processing. The cleft or groove is composed of paired α helices resting on an eight-stranded β-pleated sheet. The polymorphic residues that account for different MHC alleles are located in and around the peptide-binding cleft.

perforin A molecule synthesized by cytotoxic T cells and NK cells that polymerizes on the surface of a target cell and creates a pore in the membrane, resulting in target cell death.

periarteriolar lymphoid sheath (PALS) Part of the inner region of the white pulp of the spleen that mainly contains T cells.

peripheral lymphoid organs Lymphoid organs other than the thymus; include spleen, lymph nodes, and mucosal associated lymphoid tissue.

peripheral tolerance Physiologic unresponsiveness to antigens induced in mature lymphocytes outside the central lymphoid tissues.

Peyer's patches Clusters of lymphocytes distributed in the lining of the small intestine.

PHA See phytohemagglutinin.

phagocytosis The engulfment of a particle or a microorganism by leukocytes such as macrophages and neutrophils.

phagosome A membrane-bound intracellular vesicle that contains particulate material, including microbes, from the extracellular environment. Phagosomes are formed during the process of phagocytosis and fusion with other vesicular structures such as lysosomes. This leads to enzymatic degradation of the ingested material.

phenotype The physical expression of an individual's genotype.

phosphatase Enzyme that removes phosphate groups from the side chains of specific amino acids of proteins.

phospholipase C-γ(PLC-γ) An enzyme involved in T- and B-cell activation pathways; splits phosphatidylinositol bisphosphate into diacylglycerol (DAG) and inositol triphosphate, leading to the activation of two major signaling pathways.

phytohemagglutinin (PHA) A mitogen that polyclonally activates T cells.

pinocytosis Ingestion of liquid or very small particles by vesicle formation in a cell.

plasma Fluid component of unclotted blood.

plasma cell The antibody-producing end stage of B-cell differentiation.

platelets Bone-marrow-derived cells crucial in blood clotting.

PMN leukocytes See polymorphonuclear leukocytes.

poison ivy A plant whose leaves contain pentadecacatechol, a potent contact-sensitizing agent and a frequent cause of contact hypersensitivity.

pokeweed mitogen A mitogen that polyclonally activates B cells.

polyclonal activator A substance that induces activation of many individual clones of either T or B cells. See also mitogen.

poly-Ig receptor Binds to IgA at one surface of an epithelial cell, transports it through the cell, and releases it at the opposite lumenal surface; the IgA can then participate in protecting the mucosal system.

polymerase chain reaction (PCR) A reaction that produces large amounts of DNA from a sequence by repeated cycles of synthesis.

polymorphism Literally, having many shapes; in genetics, the existence of multiple alleles at a particular genetic locus, resulting in variants of the gene and product among different members of the species.

polymorphonuclear leukocytes (PMNs) Leukocytes containing cytoplasmic granules with characteristic multilobed nucleus; the three major types are neutrophils, eosinophils, and basophils.

polyvalency The presence of multiple identical copies of an epitope on a single antigen molecule, cell surface, or particle; examples include bacterial capsular polysaccharides. Polyvalent antigens are often capable of activating B lymphocytes independent of helper T cells.

positive selection The process by which developing B and T cells receive signals in the primary lymphoid organ in which they are developing to continue their differentiation; in the absence of these signals the cells die.

pre-B cell Cell in the B-cell lineage which has rearranged heavy- but not light-chain genes; expresses surrogate light chains and μ heavy chain at its surface in conjunction with Igα and Igβ; all these molecules comprise the pre-B-cell receptor.

pre-B-cell receptor A complex of proteins which, when expressed in pre-B cells, causes them to enter the cell cycle and turn off *RAG* genes. Once this process is completed, the pre-B cells are ready to rearrange their light chains.

precipitin reaction The mixing of soluble antigen and antibody at different proportions that can result in the precipitation of insoluble antigen–antibody complexes.

prednisone A synthetic steroid with potent anti-inflammatory and immunosuppressive activity used to treat acute graft rejection, autoimmune disease, and lymphoid tumors.

pre-T cell Cell in T-lymphocyte differentiation in the thymus that has rearranged TCR β genes and expresses TCR β polypeptide on the surface with the molecule pT-α (gp33), forming the pre-T-cell receptor.

pre-T-cell receptor Expressed on the surface of pre-T cells, consisting of TCR β chains and a surrogate α chain complexed with CD3.

primary follicle Region of a secondary lymphoid organ containing predominantly unstimulated B lymphocytes; develops into a germinal center following antigen stimulation.

primary immunodeficiency A genetic defect in which an inherited deficiency in some aspect of the innate or adaptive immune system leads to an increased susceptibility to infections. Primary immunodeficiencies are frequently manifested early in infancy and childhood but sometimes are detected clinically later in life.

primary lymphoid organs Organs in which the early stages of T- and B-lymphocyte differentiation take place and antigen-specific receptors are first expressed.

primary response The adaptive immune response resulting from first encounter with antigen; generally small in magnitude with a long induction phase or lag period. In the primary B-cell response, mainly IgM antibodies are made.

priming The activation of naïve lymphocytes by exposure to antigen.

pro-B cell Earliest stage of B-cell differentiation in which a heavy-chain D gene segment rearranges to a J gene segment.

professional antigen-presenting cells (APC) APC capable of presenting antigen to naïve helper T lymphocytes; often used to refer to dendritic cells, mononuclear phagocytes, and B lymphocytes, all of which are capable of expressing class II MHC molecules and costimulators. The most important professional APC for initiating primary T-cell responses are dendritic cells.

programmed cell death See apoptosis.

promoter A DNA sequence immediately 5′ to the transcription start site of a gene where the proteins that initiate transcription bind. The term promoter is often used to mean the entire 5′ regulatory region of a gene, including enhancers, which are additional sequences that bind transcription factors and interact with the basal transcription complex to increase the rate of transcriptional initiation. Other enhancers may be located at a significant distance from the promoter, either 5′ of the gene, in introns, or 3′ of the gene.

properdin (factor P) A positive regulator of the alternative pathway of complement activation; stabilizes C3bBb.

prophylaxis Protection.

pro-T cell A developing T cell in the thymic cortex that does not express TCR, CD3, ζ chains, or CD4 or CD8 molecules. Pro-T cells are also called double-negative (CD4$^-$, CD8$^-$) thymocytes.

protease An enzyme that cleaves peptide bonds and thereby breaks proteins down into peptides. Different kinds of proteases have different specificities for bonds between particular amino acid residues. Proteases within phagocytes are important for killing ingested microbes during innate immune responses. Within APC, proteases generate peptide fragments of protein antigens that bind to MHC molecules during T-cell-mediated immune responses. Finally, when released from phagocytes at inflammatory sites, proteases can cause tissue damage.

proteasome Multiprotein cytoplasmic complex which catabolizes proteins to peptides.

protein A A membrane component of *Staphylococcus aureus* that binds to the Fc region of IgG and is thought to protect the bacteria from IgG antibodies by inhibiting their interactions with complement and Fc receptors. It is useful in purifying IgG.

protein kinase C Enzyme activated by calcium and diacylglycerol during T- and B-lymphocyte activation.

protein tyrosine kinases (PTKs) Enzymes that mediate the phosphorylation of tyrosine residues in proteins and thereby promote phosphotyrosine-dependent protein–protein interactions. PTKs are involved in many signal transduction pathways in cells of the immune system.

prostaglandins Lipid products of metabolism of arachidonic acid which, like leukotrienes, have a variety of effects (e.g., inflammatory mediators) on a variety of tissues.

protooncogenes Cellular genes regulating growth control; mutation or aberrant expression can lead to malignant transformation of the cell.

protozoa Single-celled eukaryotic organisms, many of which are human parasites and cause disease. Examples of pathogenic protozoa include *Leishmania*, which causes leishmaniasis; *Entamoeba histolytica*, which causes amebic dysentery; and *Plasmodium*, which causes malaria.

provirus DNA form of a retrovirus integrated into the host DNA.

pseudogene Sequence of DNA resembling a gene but containing codons that prevent transcription into full-length RNA species.

pus A mixture of cell debris and dead neutrophils that is present in wounds and abscesses infected with extracellular encapsulated bacteria.

pyogenic Refers to the generation of pus at the sites of response to bacteria with large capsules.

pyrogen A substance that causes fever.

Rac A small guanine-nucleotide-binding protein that is activated by the GDP–GTP exchange factor Vav during the early events of T-cell activation. GTP·Rac triggers a three-step protein kinase cascade that culminates in activation of the stress-activated protein (SAP) kinase, c-*jun* N-terminal kinase (JNK), and p38 kinase, which are similar to the MAP kinases.

radioallergosorbent test (RAST) A solid-phase radioimmunoassay for detecting IgE antibody specific for a particular allergen.

radioimmunoassay (RIA) A technique for measuring the level of a biologic substance in a sample, by measuring the binding of antigen to radioactively labeled antibody (or vice versa).

RAG-1 **and** *RAG-2* Recombination-activating genes; their products are involved in V(D)J recombination in B and T cells.

rapamycin An immunosuppressive agent used to prevent transplantation rejection; blocks cytokine production.

Ras A member of a family of nucleotide-binding proteins with intrinsic GTPase activity that are involved in many different signal transduction pathways in diverse cells types. Mutated Ras genes are associated with neoplastic transformation. Physiologically, during T-cell activation, Ras is recruited to the plasma membrane by tyrosine-phosphorylated adaptor proteins, where it is activated by GDP–GTP exchange factors. Activated Ras then initiates the MAP kinase cascade, which leads to *fos* gene expression and assembly of the AP-1 transcription factor.

reactive oxygen intermediates (ROIs) Highly reactive metabolites of oxygen, including superoxide anion, hydrogen peroxide, and hydroxyl radical, that are produced by activated phagocytes. Phagocytes use ROIs to form oxyhalides that damage ingested bacteria. ROIs may also be released from cells and promote inflammatory responses or cause tissue damage.

reagin IgE antibody that mediates an immediate hypersensitivity reaction.

receptor Generally a transmembrane molecule that binds to a ligand on the exterior surface of the cell, leading to biochemical changes inside the cell.

receptor editing A process by which the rearranged immunoglobulin light chain genes of a cell in the B-cell lineage may undergo a secondary rearrangement, generating a different antigenic specificity.

recombination See V(D)J recombination.

recombination-activating genes See *RAG-1* and *RAG-2*.

red pulp An anatomic and functional compartment of the spleen composed of vascular sinusoids in which large numbers of erythrocytes, macrophages, dendritic cells, sparse lymphocytes, and plasma cells are scattered. Macrophages within red pulp clear the blood of microbes, other foreign particles, and damaged red blood cells.

Reed–Sternberg cells Large malignant B cells that are found in Hodgkin's disease.

regulatory T (T_{reg}) cells A population of T cells, most of which are CD4$^+$, that regulate the activation of other T cells and is necessary to maintain peripheral tolerance to self-antigens. Many T_{reg} cells constitutively express CD25, the α chain of the IL-2 receptor, and the transcription factor FoxP3.

repertoire The complete library of antigenic specificities generated by either B or T lymphocytes to respond to foreign antigen.

RES See reticuloendothelial system.

respiratory burst The process by which reactive oxygen intermediates such as superoxide anion, hydrogen peroxide, and hydroxyl radical are produced in macrophages and polymorphonuclear leukocytes. The respiratory burst is mediated by the enzyme phagocyte oxidase and often triggered by inflammatory mediators, such as TNF, LTB$_4$, and PAF, or by products uniquely produced by bacteria, such as N-formylmethionyl peptides.

reticuloendothelial system (RES) A general term for the network of phagocytic cells.

reverse transcriptase Enzyme that transcribes the RNA genome of a retrovirus into DNA; used in molecular biology to convert RNA into complementary DNA (cDNA).

Rh blood group antigens A complex system of protein alloantigens expressed on red blood cell membranes. Differences between maternal and paternal Rh antigens are the cause of transfusion reactions and hemolytic disease of the newborn.

rheumatic fever Caused by antibodies elicited by infection with some *Streptococcus* species. Some of these antibodies cross-react with kidney, joint, and heart antigens.

rheumatoid arthritis Autoimmune, inflammatory disease of the joints.

rheumatoid factor An autoantibody (usually IgM) that reacts with the individual's own IgG; present in rheumatoid arthritis.

ring vaccination A public health strategy for immunizing a select group of individuals, usually within a relatively small geographic location, who have either been exposed to or potentially exposed to an infectious microorganism that poses a public health threat such as a biologic weapon.

SCID See severe combined immunodeficiency disease.

secondary immune response An adaptive immune response that occurs on second exposure to an antigen. A secondary response is characterized by more rapid kinetics and greater magnitude relative to the primary immune response, which occurs after initial exposure to the antigen.

secondary lymphoid organs Organs such as spleen and lymph nodes in which antigen-driven proliferation and differentiation of mature B and T lymphocytes take place following antigen recognition.

second set rejection Accelerated rejection of an allograft in a primed recipient.

secretory component Cleaved component of the poly-Ig receptor that attaches to dimeric IgA and protects it from proteolytic cleavage as it is transported through an epithelial cell.

selectins A family of cell surface adhesion molecules found on leukocytes and endothelial cells; bind to sugars on glycoproteins.

selective immunoglobulin deficiency Immunodeficiencies characterized by the inability to produce one or more Ig classes or subclasses. Selective IgA deficiency is the most common selective Ig deficiency, followed by IgG$_3$ and IgG$_2$ deficiencies. Patients with these disorders may be at increased risk for bacterial infections, but many are normal.

self-MHC restriction The restriction of antigens that can be recognized by an individual's T cells to complexes of peptides bound to MHC molecules that were present in the thymus during T-cell maturation (i.e., self-MHC molecules). The T-cell repertoire is self-MHC restricted as a result of the process known as positive selection, which occurs within the thymus during T-cell development.

self-tolerance Unresponsiveness of B and T lymphocytes to self-antigens, largely as a result of inactivation or death of self-reactive lymphocytes induced by exposure to those self-antigens. Self-tolerance is a cardinal feature of the normal immune system, and failure of self-tolerance leads to autoimmune diseases.

sensitization Immunization by antigen; generally used for first encounter with allergen.

sepsis Infection of the bloodstream.

septic shock An often lethal complication of severe Gram-negative bacterial infection with spread to the bloodstream (sepsis) that is characterized by vascular collapse, disseminated intravascular coagulation, and metabolic disturbances. Septic shock is typically triggered by bacterial lipopolysaccharides (LPS, or endotoxin) which can induce a cytokine storm characterized by immune cell production of dangerous levels of specific cytokines, including IL-1, IL-12, and TNF. Septic shock is also called endotoxin shock.

seroconversion The production of detectable antibodies in the serum specific for a microorganism during the course of an infection or in response to immunization.

serology Use of antibodies to detect antigens.

serotype An antigenically distinct subset of a species or subspecies of an infectious organism that is distinguished from other subsets by serologic tests (i.e., serum antibody). Antibody responses to one serotype of microbes (e.g., influenza virus) may not be protective against another serotype.

serum Residual fluid derived from clotted blood; contains antibodies.

serum sickness A type III hypersensitivity reaction resulting from deposition of circulating, soluble, antigen–antibody complexes leading to complement and neutrophil activation in tissues such as the kidney; typically induced following therapy with large doses of antibody from a foreign source, such as monoclonal antibodies made in mice (or, originally, by treating patients with horse serum).

severe combined immunodeficiency (SCID) Disease resulting from early block in differentiation pathways of both B and T lymphocytes.

signal transducers and activators of transcription (STATs) Intracellular proteins phosphorylated by Janus kinases as a consequence of cytokine–cytokine receptor engagement.

signal transduction Processes involved in transmitting the signal received on the outer surface of the cell (e.g., by antigen binding to its receptor) into the nucleus of the cell, which leads to altered gene expression.

SLE See systemic lupus erythematosus.

slow-reacting substance of anaphylaxis (SRS-A) A group of leukotrienes released by mast cells during anaphylaxis that induce a prolonged contraction of smooth muscle.

smallpox An infectious disease caused by the virus *Variola*.

somatic gene conversion A nonreciprocal exchange of sequences between genes: Part of the donor gene or genes is copied into an acceptor gene, but only the acceptor gene is altered; mechanism for generating diverse Ig repertoire in many nonhuman species.

somatic hypermutation Change in the variable-region sequence of an antibody produced by a B cell following antigenic stimulation, resulting in increased antibody affinity for antigen.

somatic recombination The process of DNA recombination by which the functional genes encoding the variable regions of antigen receptors are formed during lymphocyte development. This process occurs only in developing B or T lymphocytes and is sometimes referred to as somatic rearrangement.

specificity A term used in the immune lexicon to indicate that adaptive immune responses are directed toward and able to distinguish between distinct antigens or small parts of antigens. This fine specificity is attributed to the ability of BCRs and TCRs on B and T cells, respectively, to bind to one molecule but not to another with only minor structural differences from the first.

spleen Largest of the secondary lymphoid organs; traps and concentrates foreign substances carried in the blood; composed of white pulp, rich in lymphoid cells and red pulp, which contains many erythrocytes and macrophages.

Src homology 2 (SH2) domain A three-dimensional domain structure of about 100 amino acid residues present in many signaling proteins that permits specific noncovalent interactions with other proteins by binding to phosphotyrosines. Each SH2 domain has a unique binding specificity that is determined by the amino acid residues adjacent to the phosphotyrosine on the target protein. Several proteins involved in early signaling events in T and B lymphocytes interact with one another through SH2 domains.

Src homology 3 (SH3) domain A structural domain of about 60 amino acid residues present in many signaling proteins that mediates protein–protein binding. SH3 domains bind to proline residues and function cooperatively with the SH2 domains of the same protein.

STATs See signal transducers and activators of transcription.

stem cell An undifferentiated cell that gives rise to additional stem cells and to cells of multiple different lineages. For example, all blood cells arise from a common hematopoietic stem cell.

strain Set of animals (particularly mice and rats) in which every animal is bred to be genetically identical.

superantigen A molecule that activates all T cells with a particular Vβ gene segment, irrespective of their Vα expression.

suppression A mechanism for producing a specific state of immunologic unresponsiveness by which one cell or its products inhibit the function of another.

surrogate light chains Nonrearranging chains ($V\lambda_5$ and V pre-B) expressed in conjunction with the μ chain in the pre-B cell; form part of the pre-BCR.

switch recombination The molecular mechanism underlying Ig isotype switching in which a rearranged VDJ gene segment in an antibody-producing B cell recombines with a downstream C gene and the intervening C genes are deleted. It involves nucleotide sequences called switch regions located in the introns at the 5′ end of each C_H locus. Switch recombination is triggered by ligation of CD40 and exposure of B cells to T-cell derived cytokines.

switch region Region of B-cell heavy-chain DNA at which recombination occurs in antigen-stimulated cell; allows isotype switch (e.g., IgM to IgE).

syngeneic Literally, genetically identical; e.g., monozygotic twins or mice of the same strain.

syngraft Same as isograft.

synthetic vaccine Vaccine composed of recombinant-DNA-derived antigens; also called recombinant vaccine. Synthetic vaccines for hepatitis B virus and herpes simplex virus are now in use.

systemic inflammatory response syndrome (SIRS) The systemic changes observed in patients who have disseminated bacterial infections ranging from mild forms characterized by neutrophilia, fever, and a rise in acute-phase reactants in the plasma to severe cases that include disseminated intravascular coagulation, adult respiratory distress syndrome, and septic shock. SIRS is stimulated by bacterial products such as LPS and mediated by cytokines of the innate immune system.

systemic lupus erythematosus (SLE) An autoimmune disease that affects many organs of the body and causes fever and joint pain. Patients produce high levels of antibodies against the components of cell nuclei, particularly DNA, and form circulating soluble antigen–antibody complexes. These complexes deposit in tissues such as the kidney, activate the complement cascade, and result in tissue damage.

tacrolimus An immunosuppressive polypeptide drug (also called FK506) that inactivates T cells by inhibiting signal transduction from the T-cell receptor.

TAP-1 and TAP-2 See transporter associated with antigen processing.

target A cell killed by one of the body's killer cells, such as a CTL or NK cell.

tapasin A TAP-associated protein that is a key molecule for the assembly of MHC class I molecules. Cells deficient in this protein are unable to express MHC class I molecules on their surface.

T-bet A T-box family transcription factor that promotes the differentiation of T_H1 cells from naïve T cells.

Tc cell Cytotoxic T cell.

T-cell receptor (TCR) Two-chain clonally distributed heterodimer on the T cell that recognizes antigen. Each chain contains one Ig-like variable (V) domain, one Ig-like constant (C) domain, a hydrophobic transmembrane region, and a short cytoplasmic region. $\alpha\beta$ is the most common form. It interacts with complexes of foreign peptides bound to self-MHC molecules on the surface of host cells. A smaller population of T cells uses γ and δ chains as their TCR. $\gamma\delta$ T cells are found mostly in epithelial barrier tissues.

T-cell receptor complex A multiprotein plasma membrane complex expressed by T lymphocytes composed of the clonally distributed, antigen-binding TCR heterodimer and the invariant signaling proteins CD3 δ, ε, and γ and the ζ chain.

T cells See T lymphocyte.

TCR See T-cell receptor.

T-dependent antigen An antigen capable of stimulating antibody responses but only when the responding B cells receive help from CD4$^+$ T cells. T-dependent antigens are protein antigens that contain epitopes recognized by B cells. Helper T cells produce cytokines and express cell surface molecules that stimulate B-cell growth and differentiation into antibody-secreting cells. Humoral immune responses to T-dependent antigens are characterized by isotype switching, affinity maturation, and memory.

terminal deoxynucleotidyl transferase (TdT) Enzyme that inserts nontemplated nucleotides at the junctions of V, D, and J gene segments of Ig and TCR locus DNA; these N-nucleotides increase the diversity of antigen-specific receptors.

T_H1 cells Subset of CD4$^+$ T cells that synthesize the signature cytokines IL-2, IFN-γ, and TNF-β and are mainly involved in activating cells of cell-mediated immunity and in stimulating B cells to produce IgG$_3$ antibody.

T_H2 cells Subset of CD4$^+$ T cells that synthesize the signature cytokines IL-4, IL-5, IL-10, and IL-13 and are mainly involved in activating effector cells involved in responses to parasitic worms and to allergens.

T_H17 cells Subset of CD4$^+$ T cells that secrete the IL-17 family of proinflammatory cytokines as well as IL-22 and other cytokines. They are protective against certain bacterial and fungal infections and also mediate pathogenic responses in autoimmune diseases.

thymic epithelial cells Epithelial cells found in the cortical and medullary stroma of the thymus that play a critical role in T-cell development. Thymic epithelial cells secrete cytokines, such as IL-7, that are required for the early stages of T-cell development. In the process of positive selection, T cells must recognize self-peptides bound to MHC molecules on the surface of thymic cortical epithelial cells to be rescued from programmed cell death. Medullary epithelial cells play a role in negative selection (see AIRE gene).

thymocytes T cells differentiating in the thymus.

thymus The primary lymphoid organ for T-cell differentiation, comprising an outer cortex and inner medulla; developing thymocytes interact with thymic epithelial cells and bone-marrow-derived macrophages, and dendritic cells.

TIL See tumor-infiltrating lymphocyte.

T-independent antigen An immunogen that induces B lymphocytes to generate antibody responses in the absence of T cells or their products; usually stimulate only IgM responses (no class switching) and no memory response.

tissue typing A laboratory method to determine the particular MHC alleles expressed by an individual for the purpose of matching allograft donors and recipients. Often called HLA typing, it can be performed by testing whether sera known to be reactive with certain MHC gene products mediate complement-dependent lysis of an individual's lymphocytes. More commonly, PCR techniques are used to determine HLA allele expression.

titer Used generally as an empirical measure of the avidity of an antibody; it is the reciprocal of the last dilution of a titration giving a measurable effect; e.g., if the last dilution of an antibody giving significant agglutination is 1:128, the titer is 128.

T lymphocyte The lymphocyte population (also called T cells) that requires the thymus for differentiation, expresses an antigen-specific receptor, the TCR, and mediates cell-mediated immune responses in the adaptive immune system. Several subsets are defined by expression of different surface markers and function: CD4$^+$ (cytokine synthesis), CD8$^+$ (cytotoxic), $\gamma\delta$, and NKT.

TNF See tumor necrosis factor.

tolerance Antigen-specific unresponsiveness of B or T cells.

Toll-like receptors (TLRs) A family of pattern-recognition receptors that recognize microorganisms and evoke a host defense response and the development of adaptive immunity through production of inflammatory cytokines and expression of costimulatory molecules.

Toll pathway A signaling pathway that activates transcription factor NF-κB by degrading its inhibitor I-κB.

toxic-shock syndrome The systemic reaction produced by the toxin derived from the bacterium *Staphylococcus aureus*; the toxin acts as a superantigen, which activates a high proportion of CD4$^+$ cells to produce cytokines.

toxoid A nontoxic derivative of a toxin used as an immunogen in vaccines to induce antibodies capable of cross-reacting with the toxin.

transfusion Transplantation of blood cells, platelets, or plasma from one individual to another. Transfusions are performed to treat blood loss from hemorrhage or to treat a deficiency in one or more blood cell types resulting from inadequate production or excess destruction.

transfusion reaction An immunologic reaction against transfused blood products, usually mediated by preformed antibodies in the recipient that bind to donor blood cell antigens, such as ABO blood group antigens or histocompatibility antigens. In severe cases, transfusion reactions can cause disseminated intravascular coagulation, kidney damage, fever, and shock.

transgenic mouse A mouse that expresses an exogenous gene that has been introduced into the genome by injection of a specific DNA sequence into the pronuclei of fertilized mouse eggs. Transgenes insert randomly at chromosomal break points and are subsequently inherited as simple Mendelian traits.

transplantation Grafting solid tissue (such as a kidney or heart) or cells (particularly bone marrow) from one individual to another. See allograft and xenograft.

transporter associated with antigen processing (TAP) Two-chain peptide transporter (TAP-1 and TAP-2) that mediates the active transport of peptides from the cytosol to the site of assembly of MHC class I molecules inside the endoplasmic reticulum.

T$_{reg}$ cells Subset of CD4$^+$ T cells that regulate or inhibit the function of other lymphocyte subsets. Synthesize inhibitory cytokines TGF-β and IL-10. See also regulatory T cells.

tuberculin test Subcutaneous injection of antigens derived from the organism causing tuberculosis; individuals who have been exposed to the organism and those who have been previously vaccinated with BCG develop a delayed hypersensitivity response at the injection site 24–48 h later.

tumor immunity A term used to describe protection by the immune system against the development of tumors.

tumor-infiltrating lymphocyte (TIL) Mononuclear cells derived from the inflammatory infiltrate of solid tumors.

tumor necrosis factor β(TNF-β) See lymphotoxin

tumor necrosis factor (TNF) Proinflammatory cytokine with functions including the selective killing of tumor cells; toxicity may be the result of the production of free radicals following the binding of high-affinity cell surface receptors.

tumor-specific transplantation antigen (TSTA) Antigens uniquely expressed by certain tumor cells.

TUNEL assay Identifies apoptotic cells in situ by the characteristic fragmentation of their DNA. It uses TdT-dependent dUTP-biotin nick end labeling.

type I hypersensitivity Immediate hypersensitivity reactions involving IgE responses and the triggering of mast cells.

type II hypersensitivity Hypersensitivity reactions involving IgG antibodies against cell surface antigens that result in direct killing of the cell.

type III hypersensitivity Hypersensitivity reactions that involve antigen–antibody complexes depositing in filtering organs and triggering cytotoxic reactions.

type IV hypersensitivity T-cell-mediated, delayed hypersensitivity reactions involving T$_H$1 cells and monocytes.

tyrosine kinases A family of enzymes that phosphorylates proteins on tyrosine residues, a critical step in lymphocyte activation. The key tyrosine kinases in T-cell activation are Lck, Fyn, and ZAP-70; those in B-cell activation are Blk, Fyn, Lyn, and Syk.

unresponsiveness Inability to respond to antigenic stimulation. Unresponsiveness may be specific for a particular antigen (see tolerance) or broadly nonspecific as a result of damage to the entire immune system such as that occurring after whole-body irradiation.

urticaria Swelling and redness of the skin caused by localized and transient leakage of fluid and plasma proteins from small vessels into the dermis during an immediate hypersensitivity reaction.

vaccination Any protective immunization against a pathogen. Originally referred to immunization against smallpox with the less virulent cowpox (vaccinia) virus.

variable (V) region The N-terminal portion of an Ig or TCR which contains the antigen-binding region of the molecule; V regions are formed by the recombination of V(D) and J gene segments.

V(D)J recombination Mechanism for generating antigen-specific receptors of T and B cells. The process is mediated by the enzyme complex V(D)J recombinase and products of the *RAG-1* and *RAG-2* genes and involves the joining of V, D, and J gene segments.

virion A complete virus particle.

virus An organism comprising a protein coat and DNA or RNA genome; it requires a host cell for replication.

V region See variable region.

Western blotting A technique to identify a specific protein in a mixture; proteins separated by gel electrophoresis are blotted onto a nitrocellulose membrane, and the protein of interest is detected by adding radiolabeled antibody specific for the protein.

wheal and flare Itchy reaction at skin site where antigen has been injected into an allergic individual; characterized by erythema (redness due to dilation of blood vessels) and edema (swelling produced by release of serum into tissue).

white pulp The part of the spleen that is composed predominantly of lymphocytes, arranged in periarteriolar lymphoid sheaths and follicles, and other leukocytes. The remainder of the spleen (the red pulp) contains sinusoids lined with phagocytic cells and filled with blood.

Wiskott–Aldrich syndrome An X-linked immunodeficiency disease characterized by eczema and thrombocytopenia (reduced blood platelets). Individuals with this disease are highly susceptible to bacterial infections. The defective gene encodes a cytosolic protein involved in signaling cascades and regulation of the actin cytoskeleton.

xenoantigen An antigen expressed by a graft from another species.

xenogeneic Originating from a foreign species.

xenograft Tissue transplantation between individuals belonging to two different species.

X-linked agammaglobulinemia A disease in boys (also known as Bruton's agammaglobulinemia) in which B-cell differentiation does not progress beyond the pre-B-cell stage and so manifesting as absence of mature B cells; a tyrosine kinase btk is mutated in these individuals.

X-linked hyper-IgM syndrome Disease in boys manifesting as inability to synthesize Ig isotypes other than IgM; result of defect in either CD40 or CD154 (CD40 ligand).

ZAP-70 A T-cell specific tyrosine kinase involved in T-cell activation.

Partial List of CD Antigens

CD Antigen	Other Name(s)	Cellular Expression	Function/Comments	Ligand
CD1		Langerhans cells, dendritic cells, B cells, thymocytes	MHC class I–like molecule, presents lipids and glycolipids to T cells	Lipids, glycolipids
CD2	T11, LFA-2	T cells, NK cells	T-cell adhesion molecule	CD58
CD3	T3	T cells	TCR signal transduction	
CD4	T4	Thymocytes, major set of mature T cells (MHC class II restricted), monocytes, macrophages	T-cell coreceptor, signal transduction	MHC class II, HIV-1 and HIV-2, gp 120
CD5	T1, Tp67	B-cell subset, T cells	B-cell expression associated with polyreactive IgM production	
CD8	T8	Thymocytes, major set of mature T cells (MHC class I restricted) = cytotoxic T cells	T-cell coreceptor, signal transduction	MHC class I
CD11a	LFA-1 chain	Leukocytes	Subunit of adhesion molecule CD11a/CD18 (LFA-1)	ICAM-1, -2, -3
CD18		Leukocytes	Integrin chain that associates with CD11a, b, c, or d	

CD Antigen	Other Name(s)	Cellular Expression	Function/Comments	Ligand
CD19		B cells	B-cell signal transduction	
CD20		B cells	Ca^{2+} channel in B-cell activation	
CD21	CR2	B cells, follicular dendritic cells	Involved in B-cell activation	Complement component C3d and EBV
CD25	TAC	Activated T cells, B cells	IL-2 receptor α chain	IL-2
CD28	Tp44	T-cell subsets	T-cell costimulator molecule	B7 (CD80 and CD86)
CD32	FcγRII	Monocytes, granulocytes, B cells, eosinophils	Low-affinity receptor for IgG	Aggregated IgG and antigen–antibody complexes
CD34		Endothelial cells, hematopoietic precursors	Marker for early stem cells	L-Selectin (CD62L)
CD40		B cells, macrophages, dendritic cells	Involved in T-cell interactions with APC and class switching; receptor for costimulatory signals	CD154 (CD40L)
CD44	Pgp-1, H-CAM	Leukocytes, erythrocytes	Lymphocyte adhesion to HEV	Hyaluronic acid
CD50	ICAM-3	Broad (not on endothelial cells)	Adhesion molecule	LFA-1
CD54	ICAM-1	Broad	Adhesion molecule	CD11a/CD18, rhinovirus
CD55	DAF	Broad	Dissociates C3 convertases of complement cascades	C3b, C4b, CD97
CD58	LFA-3	Leukocytes, endothelial cells, epithelial cells, fibroblasts	Adhesion molecule	CD2
CD62L	L-Selectin, MEL-14	B cells, T cells, monocytes, NK cells	T-cell adhesion to HEV	CD34
CD74	Invariant chain	B cells, macrophages, monocytes, activated T cells	Associated with MHC class II in endoplasmic reticulum	
CD79a, CD79b	Igα, Igβ	B cells, pre-B cells	Signal transduction molecules associated with Ig in of BCR	
CD80	B7.1	B cells, macrophages, dendritic cells	Costimulatory molecule on APC	CD28, CD152 (CTLA-4)
CD81	Target of antipro-liferative antibody (TAPA-1)	Broad	Associates with CD19 and CD21 on B cells to form B-cell coreceptor	
CD86	B7.2	Activated B cells, macrophages, dendritic cells	Costimulatory molecule on APC	CD28, CD152 (CTLA-4)
CD95	Fas, Apo-1	Activated T and B cells, NK cells	Induces apoptosis following ligation with Fas ligand (CD178, CD95L)	CD178 (Fas ligand, CD95L)

CD Antigen	Other Name(s)	Cellular Expression	Function/Comments	Ligand
CD97	GR1	Granulocytes, macrophages, activated T and B cells	Counter-receptor for CD55	CD55
CD102	ICAM-2	Endothelial cells, resting lymphocytes, platelets	Adhesion molecule	CD11a (LFA-1)
CD152	CTLA-4	Activated T cells	Negative regulator for T-cell activation	CD80 (B7.1) and CD86 (B7.2)
CD154	CD40L	Activated T cells	Binding to CD40 on B cells induces B-cell proliferation and class switching	CD40
CD178	Fas ligand, CD95 ligand	T cells and NK cells	Induces apoptosis in cells expressing CD95; humans and KO mice with CD178 mutation show severe autoimmune disease	CD95 (Fas)
CD210	IL-10 receptor	T and B cells, NK cells, monocytes, macrophages	Receptor for IL-10; binding to IL-10 inhibits macrophage, monocyte, and dendritic cell cytokine production	IL-10
CD212	IL-12 receptor β chain	Majority of T cells, NK cells, some B cell lines	Dimerizes and associates with an unknown chain to form the IL-12 receptor; IL-12 directs immune responses preferentially toward T_H1-type responses.	IL-12
CD213	IL-13 receptor	Broadly expressed in hematopoetic tissue, nervous system, and other tissues	Binding to IL-13 mediates signals to suppress inflammatory cytokine production by monocytes and macrophages; IL-13 induces B-cell proliferation and Ig production	IL-13
CD217	IL-17 receptor	Broad tissue distribution; cord blood lymphocytes, peripheral blood lymphocytes, thymocytes	Binds IL-17 with low affinity; IL-17 induces proinflammatory cytokine secretion	IL-17
CD220	Insulin receptor	Ubiquitous, including erythrocytes, liver, muscle, adipose tissue	Cellular receptor for insulin; mutation in CD220 leads to insulin-resistant diabetes mellitus	Insulin

CD Antigen	Other Name(s)	Cellular Expression	Function/Comments	Ligand
CD247	T-cell receptor ζ chain, CD3 ζ	All T cells	Part of CD3 complex; couples antigen recognition to intracellular signal transduction pathways	Not applicable
CD281	Toll-like receptor 1, TLR1, TIL	Monocytes and neutrophils; detectable in breast milk	Plays role in innate immunity; induction of signal cascade leads to proinflammatory cytokine release	Recognizes outer surface protein A lipoprotein of *Borrelia burgdorferi*, mycobacterial lipoprotein, and triacylated lipopeptides
CD282	Toll-like receptor 2, TLR2, TIL4	Peripheral blood leukocytes; high expression in monocytes in bone marrow, lymph nodes, and spleen; detectable in other tissues	Plays role in innate immunity; induction of signal cascade leads to proinflammatory cytokine release	Recognizes molecular patterns of fungi, protozoan pathogens, and bacteria
CD283	Toll-like receptor 3, TLR3	Fibroblasts, myeloid dendritic cells, microglia, and astrocytes; mostly intracellular	Response to double-stranded viral RNA; activation leads to initiation of caspase-dependent apoptotic cascade	
CD284	Toll-like receptor 4, TLR4	Monocytes, macrophages, granulocytes, dendritic cells, and activated CD4$^+$ T cells	Activation of signaling pathways by binding to LPS ligand results in inflammatory cytokine production favoring a T_H1 response	LPS, taxol, RSV fusion protein, endogenous ligands include fibronectin, hyaluronic acid
CD288	Toll-like receptor 8, TLR8	Endosomal compartments of macrophages and subsets of dendritic cells	Part of innate defense against RNA viruses. Ligation triggers secretion of inflammatory and regulatory cytokines.	Single-stranded GU-rich viral RNA
CD289	Toll-like receptor 9, TLR9	High-level expression by plasmacytoid dendritic cells, by primary and secondary lymphoid organs, and at low levels by peripheral blood leukocytes	Receptor for DNA present in endosomes during bacterial and viral infection; triggers adaptive response towards T_H1	Unmethylated CpG DNA motifs

INDEX

Immunology: A Short Course, Sixth Edition, By Richard Coico and Geoffrey Sunshine
Copyright © 2009 John Wiley & Sons, Inc.